S0-CUF-283

COLLEGE MISERICORDIA LIBRARY
RECEIVED $13 75
DEC 5 1972
DALLAS, PENNSYLVANIA

Principles of
Public health
administration

Principles of

Public health administration

John J. Hanlon
M.S., M.D., M.P.H.

Assistant Surgeon General, Public Health Service, and
Deputy Administrator, Consumer Protection and Environmental
Health Service, U. S. Department of Health, Education, and
Welfare; formerly Commissioner of Health, City of
Detroit and County of Wayne, Michigan; Professor and
Chairman, Department of Community Medicine, Wayne State
University School of Medicine; Adjunct Professor of Public
Health Administration, University of Michigan School of
Public Health

With 45 illustrations

Fifth edition

NURSING DEPARTMENT
COLLEGE MISERICORDIA
DALLAS, PENNA. 18612

The C. V. Mosby Company

Saint Louis   1969

614
H19
1969
c

Fifth edition

Copyright © 1969 by

THE C. V. MOSBY COMPANY

All rights reserved. No part of this book may be
reproduced in any manner without written permission
of the publisher.

Previous editions copyrighted 1950, 1955, 1960, 1964

Printed in the United States of America

Standard Book Number 8016-2044-9

Library of Congress Catalog Card Number 69-11518

Distributed in Great Britain by Henry Kimpton, London

To
Florence, Frances,
Don, and Jon

75675

Foreword

The methods of providing our people and the communities in which they dwell with adequate health services are never static. They must ever be reconciled with the changing patterns produced by social, economic, educational, and professional characteristics. Man constantly adjusts to the environment in which he lives. He is affected by the health status of his family and neighbors. Changes in the way of life and the new aspects of an industrial age demand a continuous evaluation of methodology in the creation and functioning of agencies, both official and voluntary, personal and collective, which serve to prevent disease and accident and to promote positive health. The type of agency required will change with new problems. Trained manpower must be made available with which to staff such agencies, including private enterprise and industry. Costs must be considered in relation to goals and results; duplication of effort must be avoided. Public and family wants and needs must be studied in relation to the mores and attitudes of society. Economy demands maximum results compatible with the trend toward a longer and more wholesome life-span.

It is therefore most appropriate that our distinguished author, fortified with a vast and impressive service in the health sciences, should review and reconcile his text with the scientific, educational, and political aspects of a fast-moving world, seeded by an ever enlarging population, alert to the needs and fruits of an environment in which man can live best with himself and his fellowman.

Henry F. Vaughan, Dr.P.H.

Preface

It is now about 20 years since in a surge of dissatisfaction and as a personal challenge the decision was made to write this book. After several abortive efforts, it finally appeared in 1950. Much has happened to me, the nation, and the world during the years that have since transpired. I well remember doing the final writing of the last chapter on the first edition while waiting in an anteroom for the birth of my second son and some months later struggling through the drudgery of page proofing in the almost unreal environment of the Bolivian *altiplano,* $2\frac{1}{2}$ miles above sea level. Since then, my experiences have fortunately been many—in public health practice and teaching, in many countries and localities, and on many levels of government. Each has enriched my personal life and hopefully my perspective. Perhaps a few glimmers will show through in this fifth and latest edition.

Concurrently, much has changed in the nation and the world. In 1950, when the first edition appeared, our nation's population was 150 million. Now it has passed the 200 million mark. Similarly, the world's people have multiplied from 2.5 billion to approximately 3.5 billion. During the brief number of years that have passed, there has been a phenomenal agglutination of people in urban centers. In 1950 there were 48 states instead of 50, and only 18 cities in the nation had populations over .5 million; now the number is 30. In addition to the growth of existing communities, myriads of others, predominantly of a suburban nature, have appeared. Rural living has become the unusual in our scheme of things. In 1950

there were only 60 members of the United Nations; now there are 122.

Public health has also changed dramatically. When this book first appeared there was no Department of Health, Education, and Welfare, and the original Social Security Act had only recently been enacted and was undergoing implementation. Now the former has become an enormous organization with a budget just for medical and health-related programs of well over $4 billion annually. For its part, Social Security legislation has been significantly amended to provide not only greatly expanded retirement and related benefits but also to include medical care insurance benefits of far-reaching social consequence. Trust funds for these purposes now total about $3.3 billion.

The perimeters of public health have undergone considerable change. Gone is the long-standing dichotomy of disease prevention and health promotion in contrast to therapy and rehabilitation. Gone is the categoric approach. Disappearing is the distinction between official and voluntary action. Now the watchword is statewide and community-wide comprehensive planning for universal continuity of comprehensive neighborhood health services. The credit for these changes is shared by the Public Health Service, the Office of Economic Opportunity, and the Social Security Administration. Of paramount importance have been the interest and leadership of the President and Congress in health matters. During the week in which this preface was written, President Johnson signed the thirty-second major health bill placed before him in the course of his 4 years' incumbency. He was able to point out proudly that this is more health legislation than was passed in all of American history. Certainly this bodes well for the future of the health of our people. Certainly there will be no lack of challenges for public health workers of the future. The tools have been placed in our hands. Let us make the most of them.

In the preparation of this fifth edition, I have become greatly indebted to Mrs. Ethel Thurovat, my extremely able secretary, who has shepherded the preparation of the manuscript so efficiently. In addition, Miss Margaret Maki helped immeasurably in recasting material on government, and Miss Lynn Goossens assisted similarly with the material that deals with nutrition. Finally, much thanks is extended to John D. Pierson of Palo Alto, Calif., whose many suggestions and meticulous proofreading were particularly helpful. To each of you, a most sincere thanks.

John J. Hanlon

Preface
to
first edition

The policy which has developed in the United States and elsewhere is to place at the executive helm of organizations conducting public health programs individuals whose primary qualification is the possession of a medical education. Time was, in the formative days of the profession and in a less complex society, when that single qualification perhaps sufficed. But neither public health thought nor society has been static. Remarkable and intimately interrelated changes and progress have occurred at a rapid pace containing far-reaching implications for those who would successfully strive for the protection and promotion of the public health. No longer is it adequate merely that the health officer be a good diagnostician and therapist. If his ability and inclination are restricted to these, his most fruitful and satisfactory work will be performed in the private practice of medicine.

Should the physician, on the other hand, have a deep-seated wish to participate in the promotion of the well-being of the public en masse through the work of the increasing numbers of public health agencies, he soon finds himself involved in fields and problems whose importance, even existence, he was hardly aware of throughout the period of his medical education. In discussing the role of the governmental executive, Donald C. Stone, while Assistant Director of the Bureau of the Budget, pictured the problems in a manner worth repeating here:

The specialized conditions surrounding governmental programs put extraordinary demands on their directors in terms of knowing to weave the competing and disparate elements into a unified whole and producing an organization capable of accomplishing its mission. Public pressures, the need to adjust to the views of legislative bodies, the rigidities in procedures attendant upon management according to law and executive regulation are elements present in any public service enterprise. All of these are related to that central characteristic that distinguishes executive positions in the public service from those in private management—the fact that the government executive is the guardian of the public interest and is accountable to the electorate, directly or indirectly, for what he does. This is very different from the concern for the public which the private executive has in relation to the marketability of his product and the good name of his firm.*

In a more specific sense, the neophyte in public health administration, when he first opens the door providing entry to the organization for which he is to provide leadership, finds himself face to face with a series of problems of quite unexpected types and for which he usually has been unprepared. His record of clinical prowess and acumen may be excellent, but he will find it of little value in solving these particular problems. When he pulls on the knob and enters, his first problem is always one of personnel management. In rapid succession he finds himself concerned with problems implying an understanding

*Stone, D. C.: Notes on the government executive: his role and his methods; new horizons in public administration, a symposium, University, Ala. 1945, University of Alabama Press, pp. 47-48.

of the principles of organization, government, and law. Before much of his first day has passed, he is certain to have participated in a number of situations requiring personal relationships with the public, the press, the medical profession, and others. He then realizes that, while a satisfactory bedside manner is one thing, an acceptable public manner is another. Sooner or later he awakens to the fact that the program and the personnel he is directing involve the expenditure of money. Where does it come from? How to go about obtaining it? The probability is that his acquaintance with the word "budget" was in connection with his personal financial struggles at the end of each month. Now demands are made upon him to produce in some baffling manner what seems to him a complicated document depicting the financial working, past, present, and future, of the agency he directs.

These are but a few of the unforseen and unprepared-for headaches which are encountered by the man who decides to devote his professional life to the field of public health administration. What is expected of him appears to be the impossible. Physician, engineer, lawyer, political scientist, economist, sociologist—must he be all of these and more? In the literal sense this, of course, would not be possible. It is not too much to expect, however, that he have at least an understanding of the fundamental principles involved in the various fields related to his office. Experience will teach him much, but at least a modicum of information beforehand might be helpful. It is with this in mind and with the hope of stimulating an interest for further study that this book is presented.

•   •   •

He who writes a textbook is one of the most indebted of men. So many persons contribute and assist in so many direct and indirect ways that complete recognition and repayment becomes an impossibility. Who can ever adequately evaluate the influence of past friends, associates, and teachers? Yet their influence upon us and anything we undertake is deep and lasting. For most, all that can be done is humbly to acknowledge their value and influence.

There are always a few, however, who stand out—those without whose help and encouragement the immediate task would not have been possible. In the case at hand, the writer wishes to express particular thanks to a few such specific individuals: to Dr. Henry F. Vaughan for his many years of professional guidance and inspiration and for critical review of many of the following chapters; to Dr. Carl E. Buck, long-time Field Director of the American Public Health Association, for many valuable suggestions concerning the contents of this book; to Dr. Louis I. Dublin, Dr. Joseph W. Mountin, Professors F. Alexander Magoun and Leonard D. White for their kind permission to make generous use of much of their material. Much credit is due the writer's wife not merely for her many suggestions but for her constant prodding and encouragement.

John J. Hanlon
Ann Arbor, Michigan, 1950

Contents

Part V   The future of public health

List of figures

List of tables

Part I

Roots of
public health

Before embarking on the main purpose of this book it is perhaps worthwhile to consider certain fundamental and background aspects of public health. It has been interesting and enlightening to hear the replies of fellow workers and particularly those of students when they are asked why they are in or planning to enter the public health profession. It must be admitted that the occasional vague and indefinite replies have been most discouraging. It is desirable, therefore, to admonish students to question seriously the advisability of becoming public health workers, as, of course, they should question the pursuit of any calling. The disadvantages as well as the advantages which are honestly believed to exist should be considered. Each of us has but one life to live, and for practical if not selfish reasons we should each exercise jealous care of what we do with it. It is foolish indeed for an individual to cast away his one great experience in a field for which he is unsuited or unhappy or to work for a cause in which he does not sincerely believe. Every enterprise requires understanding and belief to be satisfying and fruitful. Part of the purpose of these introductory chapters is to indicate the high degree of satisfaction and fruitfulness to be found in public health work.

An acquaintance with the history of society, its health problems, and its attempts to solve them contributes to greater understanding and satisfaction. Similarly an awareness of man's state of illness or health is important. These are but a few of the phases of the subject which are presented in brief form. This is done in the hope of stimulating interest in more extensive reading, analysis, and thought.

Chapter 1

Philosophy of public health*

PUBLIC HEALTH AS A PROFESSION

It is significant that many outstanding persons who unquestionably could have gained greater material benefits in some other type of activity have devoted their lives to the public health movement. One of their predominant characteristics has been a dedicated enthusiasm for their work. It is appropriate to wonder what has made such ardent proponents of those who have given sincere thought and effort to the public health movement. Is there some unique challenge to be found? Perhaps here more than in any other field of human endeavor, be it of a professional, economic, or artistic nature, man for the first time has the opportunity successfully to adapt the creatures and environments of nature to himself and his welfare rather than to submit helplessly to them.

But, one might ask, what can a sincere and honest person hope to accomplish in the face of superstition and ignorance of a large part of the people, political interference, inadequate funds, and sometimes personnel of poor quality? Is not impatience justified? One is reminded of a statement by the Irish parliamentarian Edmund Burke (1729-1797) in the face of repeated criticism: "Those who carry on great public schemes must be proof against the most fatiguing delays, the most mortifying disappointments, the most shocking insults, and what is worst of all, the presumptuous judgments of the ignorant." Sir Henry Cole

once showed this statement to his close friend, the public health pioneer Edwin Chadwick, with the comment that he should have it pinned to his sleeve as an epigraph.

Perhaps the essential point is that, despite all handicaps, spectacular successes of far-reaching consequences have been achieved during a very brief period of man's history. At the time of Cole's comment to Chadwick in the midnineteenth century the average age at death in large English cities was only 36 years for the gentry, 22 years for tradesmen, and 16 years for the laboring class! More than one half of the children of the working class and one fifth of the children of the gentry died before their fifth birthday. During the century and a quarter since, the average life expectancy at birth has been increased in the United States and several other countries to over 70 years, and deaths before the fifth birthday have decreased about 95%.

A justification for patience was suggested to the author by the late Milton J. Rosenau. Briefly his reasoning was that relatively few generations have existed throughout the recorded history of Western civilization. Only 3,500 years have passed since the time of Moses; and if the average length of one generation were considered to have been approximately 35 years, there have been only about 100 successive generations or direct steps back to the time of Moses. To pursue this reasoning further, when one considers that the majority of those generations might be ignored on the basis of their failure to contribute significantly to the knowledge and social advancement of

---

*For a detailed discussion, see Hanlon, Rogers, and Rosen: Amer. J. Public Health.[1]

man, there remains perhaps a scant dozen, most of them in the immediate past, to whom we owe a real debt.

The practice of medicine is commonly referred to as one of the oldest professions. Yet modern medicine can hardly be considered more than a century old, and the present-day practice of medicine is quite different from that of only a decade ago. Still more recent in origin is the public health movement, which, though presaged by occasional sporadic earlier glimmerings, dates back but a brief half century. We are naturally led to a consideration of the significance and purpose of this public concern for health. Far from being a thing apart, it is intimately related in its conception and development to a broad philosophic and social revolution of many facets which has as its driving force a growing appreciation of the innate dignity of man. It has been an accompaniment of a spectrum of social reforms which include public education, public welfare, rights of labor, humane care of the mentally ill, and penal management, to mention but a few of the more outstanding developments.

DEFINITION

There have been many attempts to define public health. When the various definitions are arranged chronologically, it is interesting to observe that they present a word picture of the evolution and progress of the field. Early definitions limited public health essentially to sanitary measures invoked against nuisances and health hazards with which the individual was powerless to cope and which when present in one individual could adversely affect others. Insanitation and, later, communicability were the criteria followed in deciding whether a problem fell within the concern and jurisdiction of public health. Following the great bacteriologic and immunologic discoveries of the late nineteenth and early twentieth centuries and the subsequent development of techniques for their application, the concept of prevention of disease in the individual was added. Public health then came to be regarded as an integration of sanitary science and medical science.

As far back at 1847, Solomon Neumann

in Berlin propounded that "medical science is intrinsically and essentially a social science, and as long as this is not recognized in practice we shall not be able to enjoy its benefits and shall have to be satisfied with an empty shell and a sham." Despite this, it is only recently that medicine and, indeed, public health have become widely recognized as applied social science. Many writers still find it necessary to emphasize this relationship.[2,3] The enigma of the delay in acceptance of this relationship has been particularly well analyzed by Rosen[4]:

In Great Britain, as in the United States, interest in the development of a concept of social medicine is a recent phenomenon. The social relations of health and disease had been recognized by physicians and laymen, but owing to a number of causes no concerted effort had been made to organize such knowledge on a coherent basis and thus make it available for practical application. In part this was due to the dominant role that laboratory sciences and techniques had come to play in medicine, in part to the concurrent rise and expansion of medical specialism, and in part to the limited view of public health that had been current in both countries. Furthermore, the bias created by these factors was reinforced by powerful social ideologies still rooted in the nineteenth century version of natural law.

During the past few decades, however, influences within medicine itself and in society as a whole have acted to overcome these factors. The development of such branches of medicine as endocrinology, nutrition and psychiatry tended to break down the compartmental thinking of the physician, and to bring back into mental focus the sick person, the patient. Moreover, within society as a whole, the ideology of the complacent individualism was wearing thin, and the consciousness of social problems, including those involving health, became exceedingly acute.

One of the most forceful advocates of this broader point of view was Winslow,[5] who crystalized his thought into what has become perhaps the best-known and most widely accepted definition of public health and of its relationship to other fields. For analytic purposes it is presented in the following manner:

Public Health is the Science and Art of (1) preventing disease, (2) prolonging life, and (3) promoting health and efficiency through organized community effort for
(a) the sanitation of the environment,
(b) the control of communicable infections,

(c) the education of the individual in personal hygiene,

(d) the organization of medical and nursing services for the early diagnosis and preventive treatment of disease, and

(e) the development of the social machinery to insure everyone a standard of living adequate for the maintenance of health,

so organizing these benefits as to enable every citizen to realize his birthright of health and longevity.

Winslow's definition certainly cannot be criticized for lack of comprehensiveness; it provides for inclusion of almost everything in the fields of social service and reform. In addition, it provides a rather complete summary not only of public health and its administration but also of the sequence of its historic development as well as present-day and probable future trends.

From a somewhat different viewpoint the multifaceted relationships of health and public health may be considered in the following terms:

Health is a state of total effective physiologic and psychologic functioning; it has both a relative and an absolute meaning, varying through time and space, in both the individual and in the group; it is the result of the combination of many forces, intrinsic and extrinsic, inherited and contrived, individual and collective, private and public, medical, environmental, and social; and it is conditioned by culture and economy, and by law and government.

Accordingly,

Public health is dedicated to the common attainment of the highest level of physical, mental and social well-being and longevity consistent with available knowledge and resources at a given time and place. It holds this goal as its contribution to the most effective total development and life of the individual and his society.

There are two other definitions to which attention should be directed. The first is the official statement of the House of Delegates of the American Medical Association, formulated in 1948. This statement defined public health as:

The art and science of maintaining, protecting and improving the health of the people through organized community efforts. It includes those arrangements whereby the community provides medical services for special groups of persons and is concerned with prevention or control of disease, with persons requiring hospitalization to protect the community and with the medically indigent.

From its inception the protection and promotion of public health has been one of several stated concerns of the American Medical Association. This somewhat narrow definition of public health is of particular interest and significance in view of and in the context of recent social and legislative trends.

The second definition is that of the World Health Organization and is included in its constitution:

Health is a state of complete physical, mental and social well-being and not merely the absence of disease or infirmity.

In one sense this may be considered not so much a definition as a statement of aims and principles.

It is evident from the various definitions that there has occurred a gradual extension of the horizons of public health. In conformity with the advances of medical and scientific knowledge and keeping pace with social and political progress, public health work has expanded from its original concern with gross environmental insanitation to, in sequence of addition, sanitary engineering, preventive physical medical science, preventive mental medical science, positive or promotive as well as social and behavioral aspects of personal and community medicine, and, more recently, organization of comprehensive health services.

An appropriate note of caution has been voiced by Mountin[6] with regard to the question of definition. He points out:

The progressive nature of public health makes any restricted definition of the functions and responsibilities of health departments difficult. More than that—there is a real danger in attempting to narrow down a moving or growing thing. To tie public health to the concepts that answered our needs 50 years ago, or even a decade ago, can only hamstring our contribution to society in the future.

THERAPEUTIC MEDICINE, PREVENTIVE MEDICINE, AND PUBLIC HEALTH

The question sometimes arises with reference to the distinctions between therapeutic medicine, preventive medicine, and public health. Up to the present the private practive of medicine has been concerned essentially with diagnosis and therapy of damage already done—the realignment of a broken limb, the healing or removal of a diseased organ, or the readjustment of an unsettled mind. By virtue of the nature of the problems involved, its efforts necessarily have been highly personalized and individualized. Preventive medicine goes a step further, but its primary goal still represents a negative ideal: prevention of disease in the individual. In this sense preventive medicine can be said to consist of three areas of activity[7]:

1. The prevention by biologic means of certain preventable diseases such as acute communicable and deficiency diseases
2. The prevention of some of the consequences of preventable or curable chronic diseases, such as syphilis, tuberculosis, cancer, and diabetes
3. The prevention or retardation of some of the consequences of nonpreventable and noncurable diseases, such as many cardiac ailments

More recently it has become increasingly obvious that, as the number of possible applications of preventive care to the early diagnosis and treatment of incipient or established diseases are multiplied, preventive medicine becomes all but indistinguishable from good clinical medicine in general. Among the results have been the increased teaching of community medicine, comprehensive medicine, continuity of care, and the growing tendency of private physicians to incorporate preventive medicine in their practices.[8]

We must go still further and promote the development of constructive and promotive medicine in which the center of interest is still the individual, but now as a social or community integer, a member of a family and social group. We must not be content with the mere preservation of his health, but must strive for the development of its maximum potentialities. Referring again to Professor Winslow's definition, it is of interest to note that the emphasis in public health has changed from physical environment or sanitation to preventive medicine and, more recently, back to the individual and his environment, but now in terms of his relationship with his complex social environment. With this change in emphasis has come a more

mature realization on the part of both organized medicine and public health workers that each is an adjunct to and a true partner of the other. Murphy,[9] in attempting to answer whether health is a public or a private matter, indicates that "it is neither and it is both." In considering the many and complex health and medical problems that challenge us, he argues that "their effective resolution will be hastened as we blend public and private effort on the basis of logic and need." Appropriately, he concludes, "There may be times when we can afford the luxury of foolish, unproductive infighting, but this is not one of them." A quarter century ago, Vaughan,[10] while extolling the striking success of various types of public health programs, nevertheless cautioned:

Notwithstanding these reasonable and warranted activities, supported in the main by tax funds cheerfully and eagerly appropriated by our elected officials, public health will never rise higher than the level of health established for the individual. The health of the many is but a summation of personal health. A nation can never be healthier than its citizens, and it is upon the welfare of the latter that our effort must be concentrated.

In the final analysis it would be preferable if the private physician or medical practice group were to serve in the total sense—as personal or family health counselor, therapist, and provider of all preventive and health promotive services. One method of great potential by which this might be accomplished is through the application of what may be referred to as prospective medicine. The widespread acceptance and use of this developing approach will probably depend upon effective cooperative efforts of public health organizations, schools of medicine, and practitioners of medicine. Briefly the concept is based upon the fact that, while a given individual theoretically may be subject to a vast array of health risks that may lead to a large number of possible illnesses or injuries, i.e., causes of death, in actuality at any given point in life, for a particular type of individual, a very few conditions, perhaps five or six, constitute most of the risk for the succeeding 5 to 10 years. This is a period of time which the usual

Name *William Smith* Age *45* Sex *male* Race *white*

Rank	Cause of death	Average risk*	Pertinent observations	Present personal risk†	Prescription	Adjusted personal risk‡
1	Arteriosclerotic heart disease and chronic endocarditis	35.07	10 lbs. overweight, 2 packs cigarettes/day, coronary thrombosis in 35er	350	weight reducing exercise and coagulant regime, alcohol and tobacco	70
2	Malignant neoplasms, pulmonary	4.86	2 packs cigarette/day	50	stop smoking	25
3	Vascular lesions of central nervous system	4.28	see 1	14	same as 1	5
4	Cirrhosis of liver	3.70	heavy smoker, heavy drinker (8-12 oz./day)	15	reduce alcohol intake	4
5	Suicide	3.13	other release	2		2
6	Accidents, vehicular	3.13	overweight, heavy drinker, hypertension	9	same as 1, seat belts, periodic vision tests	3
7	Chronic rheumatic heart disease	2.20	no history	1		1
8	Pneumonia	1.85	no significant findings	2		2
9	Malignant neoplasms, intestinal, rectal	1.85	"	2		2
10	Other diseases of the heart	1.50	"	1		1
11	Malignant neoplasms, stomach, esophagus	1.50	"	1		1
12	Hypertensive heart disease	1.50	160/110 overweight, history of coronary	15	hypertensive treatment regime	7
13	Lymphosarcoma	.93	no significant findings	1		1
14	Tuberculosis	.93		1		1
15	Diabetes		family history	2	periodic blood sugar tests	1
16						
17	All other causes	25.24		25		
18	Total risk	91.67		490		124

* Chance in 1,000 of the individual dying from this cause during next ten years (based upon 1960 data)
† Present personalized risk—average risk modified by personal history, physical, laboratory and social findings
‡ Adjusted personalized risk—present personalized risk as it might be modified by certain specific preventive measures

Fig. 1-1. Probability of death in next decade from specific causes.

8   *Roots of public health*

person is able to comprehend and more willing to plan for. For the specific type of person, based upon age, sex, race, and perhaps occupation and location, the probability of illness or death from each of the predominant conditions during the next 5 or 10 years is presented. These probabilities are then adjusted in terms of the patient's history, habits, and physical examination. Indicated laboratory and clinical tests may refine them more. It is then possible to tell the individual that, while people of his age, race, sex, and occupation have, let us say, 780 chances out of 1,000 of surviving the next decade, his chances are only 590 out of 1,000. It is also possible then to pinpoint the specific changes that might be made in order to raise his chances to those of the average person of his type. For example, a certain amount of weight reduction would lower the chances of heart attack, a reduction in alcohol consumption would reduce the risk from accidents, and elimination of smoking would lower the chances of carcinoma of the larynx and lungs. An example of such a health hazard chart is shown in Fig. 1-1.

The various shifts in opportunity, attitude, and practice that have occurred over the years have led inevitably to a reevaluation of the meaning and purpose of health. Until recently, to the extent that it has been possible, many people, including not a few health workers, have tended to pursue health as an ultimate goal in itself. Increasingly, however, it is being realized that health has value only to the extent that it promotes efficiency and a satisfactory totality of living. After all, it is the quality of life that is meaningful, not the quantity. Health in and of itself is therefore of little if any use. Its true value lies in worthwhile activities made possible by virtue of it. One must also be cautious not to fall into the trap of regarding complete and lasting health as attainable. Dubos[11] has used this point as the theme of his provocative book, *Mirage of Health.* In it he points out that health and happiness, for so long regarded as absolute and permanent values supposedly achieved by some in the golden

ages of the past and still universally sought after as man masters the arts of living through power and knowledge, now in our time appear to be illusions. To be otherwise is unnatural because, as he indicates, complete freedom from disease, from stress, from frustration, and from struggle is incompatible with the process of living. He muses, "Life is an adventure in a world where nothing is static, where unpredictable and ill-understood events constitute dangers that must be overcome, often blindly and at great cost; where man himself, like the sorcerer's apprentice, has set in motion forces that are potentially destructive and may someday escape his control. Every manifestation of existence is a response to stimuli and challenges, each of which constitutes a threat if not adequately dealt with. The very process of living is a continual interplay between the individual and his environment, often taking the form of a struggle resulting in injury or disease." He adds wryly, "Complete and lasting freedom from disease is but a dream remembered from imaginings of a Garden of Eden designed for the welfare of man."

HEALTH AND GOVERNMENT

Occasionally one encounters objection to the concept that the protection and promotion of the public's health is an appropriate responsibility and activity of government. It must be realized that social and political philosophy was not always such as to lead to acceptance of this idea. The Roman Empire is notable for its wise concern for the protection and enhancement of the health and well-being of its people. During most of history, however, the prevailing attitude has been to regard any such proposition as constituting either unnecessary and dangerous pampering of the masses or, later on, as unwarranted and improper interference on the part of government in the private rights of the individual. Ann Beck-Storrs[12] describes the dilemma well in her discussion of the beginning of public health legislation in England as recently as the late nineteenth century, against a background of liberalism and individualism. She points to the conflict presented by the basic concept of public health and the prevailing idea of freedom of the individual:

It suddenly dawned upon Englishmen that the modern apostles of health challenged the tradition of local government. They thought that they were called upon to make a decision between two evils, namely, either to let disorder and disease continue as before, or to suffer the monster of a civilized state.

She points out that public health threatened the Englishman's "right to be dirty" if he were so inclined. The well-to-do and the legislators, in the face of widespread communicable disease, were willing to agree to certain changes in order to protect themselves, but they did not want to go too far. The recommendations of The Royal Sanitary Commission of 1869 required the services of inspectors—but how could their authority be limited? To control the spread of infectious diseases, a system of compulsory notification would be necessary. Rules would have to be enforced for slum clearance. Minimum specifications for low-cost housing for workers were apt to force landlords and landowners to spend more money than they had intended. "Here for the first time in the modern period, arose the problem of state supported welfare measures which threatened to interfere with the economic activities of private citizens. And this happened at a time when economic liberalism was believed to be the principle reason for the prosperity of the 19th century."[12]

To the extent possible, the government of England attempted to present the desired changes in a positive context—rights rather than restrictions, protections rather than prohibitions. Thus the state was empowered to ensure that a man was no more apt to have his well poisoned through the neglect of his neighbor than he was to be robbed with impunity. Health inspectors were given the responsibility of surveillance over drainage and sewerage systems, water supplies, bathhouses and washhouses as well as health conditions in workshops, mines, and bakeshops. Under the existing circumstances the inspectors were natural targets of a public very sensitive to its freedoms. Success depended upon their training

and tact and also upon whether the instinctive resentment against such invasions of a person's private affairs could be overcome. The Royal Sanitary Commission, anticipating this reaction, therefore recommended "employment of only well-trained men, capable of administering on a national level the measures instituted by the proposed central authority." It may be worth observing parenthetically that this recommendation is as valid now and in America as it was in England at the time it was made.

In the developing United States, attitudes were if anything more individualistic. As Roemer[13] has pointed out, the Western world's negative attitude toward government has deep roots, especially in America, where the colonists revolted against a domineering British monarchy. One result was the explicit limitations placed upon the central government in the Constitution and the absence of Constitutional reference to health, either as a personal right or a governmental responsibility. He also emphasizes that the medical profession, having much earlier achieved independence from feudal landlords and religious authority in Europe, was doubly suspicious of governmental interference. In this latter connection Shryock[14] reasons that medicine had little tangible impact upon society prior to 1875. Since then, however, medicine and related fields, either by their presence or absence, have had increasingly significant effects upon the problems and very nature and even survival of society. This no government can afford to ignore.

Mustard,[15] in *Government in Public Health*, analyzes the situation in more colorful but effective terms:

Public health service at any given time and place represents, in a way, the confluence of two streams in human progress. First there is the fairly clear and clean, but somewhat cold, trickle that filters down through the very fine sands of science; and second, there is the somewhat muddy flow of varying temperature that gushes intermittently from the rich but unpatrolled sociopolitical pastures. Taking their rise as they do in such entirely different sources, it is not astonishing that these tributaries do not completely or smoothly mix on their conjunction; nor need one be discouraged because there are eddies and backwashes, flotsam and froth.

It is a powerful stream and one that will continue to flow.

There is no longer any question concerning health as a human right and its protection as a governmental responsibility. Thus, commenting upon the National Hospital Act of 1940, Senator James E. Murray said, "It is the function of government to preserve the person as well as the property of man. . .and there can be no natural progress except through promoting the health and welfare of the citizens of the Nation." The same thought has been emphasized on a number of occasions by each of our recent Presidents and other leading governmental figures.[16]

In our society there are numerous reasons for governmental action in public health. Many public health activities can be carried out only by group or community action. This is particularly true in urban areas, which are so characteristic of our increasingly mechanized industralized societies. Sanitary water systems and sewage disposal facilities are obvious examples. Many necessary health activities must have an authoritative and legal base such as is available only to government. Isolation and quarantine regulations and many aspects of environmental health work offer examples in this category. Still other activities such as the collection, protection, and analysis of vital records can be carried out only through a well-organized, well-staffed, stable, and continuing governmental agency. The most important organizing force is government, which passes, enforces, and finances health legislation which in the final analysis determines the content and pattern of health services and protection for all of the people. It is the only mechanism that can do this in the total sense. However, as Kruse[17] indicates, "This concentration of political, economic, and social power, with its vast organization, is at the expense of the individual. . . . He surrenders liberty for opportunity and security."

SCOPE OF PUBLIC HEALTH

The perimeters of generally acceptable areas of public health concern have been moving outward during recent years at a rapid rate. One may now state with assurance that, whereas not long ago many would limit public health matters to general sanitation and the control of infectious disease, today all aspects of Winslow's famous definition are not only included but even surpassed. With reference to the environment of man we now think in the broadest possible terms—the total ecologic relationship between man and his environment. This forms one of the bases of a recent comprehensive study of environmental health.[18] Similarly, with reference to personal health services, health agencies are already deeply involved not only in problems of distribution of facilities and standards of their quality but also in providing medical care at an increasing rate. The latter has become possible primarily as a result of a number of very significant federal legislative acts, among them the Economic Opportunity Act (P.L. 89-794), the 1965 Amendments to the Social Security Act (P.L. 89-97), and the Regional Medical Programs or Heart, Cancer, and Stroke Amendments of 1965 (P.L. 89-239).

In general terms it has been stated that public health is concerned with two broad areas: (1) environmental problem sheds and (2) health service marketing. More specifically, public health activities appear to fall into the following seven categories:

I. Activities which must be conducted on a community basis
    A. Supervision of community food, water, and milk supplies
    B. Insect, rodent, and other vector control
    C. Environmental pollution control, including atmospheric, soil, and aquatic pollution control, prevention of radiation hazards, and noise abatement
II. Activities designed for prevention of illness, disability, or premature death from
    A. Communicable diseases, including parasitic infestations
    B. Dietary deficiencies or excesses
    C. Behavioral disorders, including alcoholism, drug habituation, narcotic addiction, certain aspects of delinquency, and suicide
    D. Mental illness, including mental retardation
    E. Allergic manifestations and their community sources

F. Acute and chronic noncommunicable respiratory diseases
G. Neoplastic diseases
H. Cardiac and cerebrovascular diseases
I. Metabolic diseases
J. Certain hereditary or genetic conditions
K. Occupational diseases
L. Home, vehicular, or industrial accidents
M. Dental disorders, including dental caries and periodontal disease
N. Certain risks of maternity, growth, and development
III. Activities related to provision of medical care
    A. Promotion of equitable distribution of personnel and facilities
    B. Assistance in development and maintenance of the quality and quantity of community resources and facilities, including establishment and application of standards for hospitals, nursing and convalescent homes, and day care centers
    C. Operation of screening programs for early detection of disease
    D. Operation of treatment centers, varying from disease-specialty clinics to comprehensive medical centers
    E. Facilitation of and participation in pregraduate and continuing professional education
IV. Activities concerned with collection, protection, and analysis of vital records
V. Public education in personal and community health
VI. Comprehensive health planning and evaluation
VII. Research—scientific, technical, and administrative

Obviously, many public health agencies do not find it possible or necessary to engage in all of these activities. In each case it is desirable to determine local needs, wishes, resources, and capabilities and to adapt the program of the community to them. Various administrative and planning tools exist to aid in accomplishing this; one is the *Guide to a Community Health Study*,[19] developed by the American Public Health Association. This and a number of others are considered in the chapter on planning and evaluation.

In addition, it must be realized that public health agencies cannot and should not attempt to carry out the foregoing activities by themselves. To be successful and acceptable requires that most if not all of them be done in cooperative partnership with many other agencies, organizations, professions, and community groups.

PUBLIC HEALTH VERSUS NATURAL SELECTION

A final consideration deals with the objection that public health is dangerous because it promotes the survival and propagation of the biologically or genetically unfit. Advocates of this viewpoint claim that public health activities interfere with or negate the forces of natural biologic selection, which in a coldly impersonal manner supposedly weeds out "the lame, the halt, and the blind" as well as protoplasm of poor quality. Thus referring to public health as unnatural, Aldous Huxley[20] called it the very essence of the myth of progress. In general, the argument he and others propound is that public health and preventive medical measures serve to protect and promote the unfit at the mental, moral, physical, and financial expense of the fit and that this jeopardizes future generations by interfering with the process of natural selection. One British writer[21] concludes that, while modern public health measures will continue to make life comfortable during the few remaining generations of our Western civilization, a few good old-fashioned epidemics such as the Black Death might be desirable because they tend to wipe out many mental and physical weaklings who at present are coddled through life. Other examples among many that can be cited are those of a sociologist,[22] on the one hand, and a physician,[23] on the other, who point to the public health efforts which protect the unfit while more desirable human specimens are sent off to war.*

On the other hand, one may ask how the "fit" (whoever they may be) can survive if disease is allowed to run rampant among the "unfit." It is true that uncontrolled disease tends to eliminate those who appear to be weak or inferior according to certain standards. Those who are chronically tired, hungry, and cold are indeed

---

*An interesting analysis of these various arguments may be found in Goldstein: J. Nat. Med. Ass.[24]

more apt to succumb. In the majority of instances, however, uncontrolled disease strikes blindly, producing malaria, tuberculosis, and other diseases that attack with limited selectivity among allegedly superior individuals if they are unprotected as well as among so-called inferior individuals. Disease and death have often entered palaces and mansions through the back door. A normal infant, or for that matter a gifted infant, may be disastrously affected by the presence of disease. Generally speaking, the use of the terms "unfit," "undesirable," or "inferior" represents psychologic, socially produced blind spots based upon subjective judgments.

The risk involved in uncontrolled disease is strikingly exemplified by the entries on the church register at Stratford-on-Avon. At that shrine of civilization, enclosed in a carefully guarded glass case, is a church register opened at the page on which is entered the statement of birth of William Shakespeare. Several lines above may be seen the entry "juli 11, 1564, Oliverus Gume—hic incipit pestis." Altogether, during the year 1564, that little village suffered 242 deaths from plague. This probably represented from one third to one half of the population at that time. During the upswing of the epidemic, there was born a helpless infant who easily could have been one of those affected but who, by chance alone, was spared to subsequently give us some of the greatest cultural treasures of our civilization. If he had become infected and died, would that infant have been considered unfit or inferior?

The question arises, therefore—just who are the fit and the unfit? Close observation indicates that the definition varies with time and place. Steinmetz was a congenital cripple, Toulouse Lautrec was afflicted with hereditary osteochondritis fragilitas, Mozart and Chopin died at early ages from tuberculosis,* and Schumann died from typhoid fever. Would anyone dare label these and thousands like them unfit? Americans can least afford to point the finger. A majority

of the citizens of this great nation are descendants of persons who by one standard or another would have been considered undesirable or unfit. The reasons have varied—religious, national, economic, social, political, and cultural—whatever reason has been most expedient at the moment. Recognition of this is given by the statement by Emma Lazarus which is enshrined in the Statue of Liberty:

> Give me your tired, your poor,
> Your huddled masses yearning to breathe free,
> The wretched refuse of your teeming shore.
> Send these the homeless, tempest-tossed to me.
> I lift my lamp beside the golden door.

While some individuals or even groups admittedly may suffer from physical or other handicaps, it is false reasoning to suppose that they are necessarily stigmatized for all time. No public health worker would deny that his profession now makes it possible for many to live who otherwise would have died. These beneficiaries have lived, and, while much yet needs to be done, they have prospered. Each new Olympic Tournament sees the establishment of new records of physical prowess. The descendants of immigrants are taller and of greater physical stamina than were their forebears or are their counterparts in the old country. This is not meant to deny the need to apply the increasing knowledge of genetics in personal and marital counseling, which will be considered subsequently in relation to maternal and child health. At this point, however, one cannot help pondering the potential magnitude of the benefits that would accrue to the human race from a truly vigorous application of the knowledge we have at the present time. Rosenau had this in mind when he wrote concerning preventive medicine and public health:

It dreams of a time when there shall be enough for all, and every man shall bear his share of labor in accordance with his ability, and every man shall possess sufficient for the needs of his body and the demands of health. These things he shall have as a matter of justice and not of charity. It dreams of a time when there shall be no unnecessary suffering and no premature deaths; when the welfare of the people shall be our highest concern; when humanity and mercy shall replace greed and selfishness; and it dreams that all these things will be accomplished through the wisdom of man. It dreams of these things,

---

*For a long list of notable persons who were tuberculous, see *Tuberculosis and Genius* by Moorman.[25]

not with the hope that we, individually, may participate in them, but with the joy that we may aid in their coming to those who shall live after us. When young men have vision the dreams of old men come true.

Some people may easily dismiss all this as starry-eyed, impractical idealism. But to achieve the greatest success and satisfaction in a social field such as that represented by public health demands a full share of idealism. This must, by elimination, be the answer, since it can be said fairly that public health officials through their efforts have rarely aimed at the improvement of personal fortunes or the creation of new positions in which they have a private personal interest. But, after all, idealism and practicality are not necessarily immiscible as are oil and water. In fact, their admixture is sorely needed now more than ever before in this newborn atomic age. The prefacing statement by A. Lawrence Lowell[26] in his book, *Conflicts of Principle,* is as timely and pertinent now and to our present public health purpose as when he wrote it:

People often call some men idealists and others practical folks as if mankind were by natural inclination so divided into these two groups that an idealist cannot be practical or a man of affairs have a lofty purpose whereas in fact no man approaches perfection who does not combine both qualities in a high degree. Without either he is defective in spirit and unscientific in method; the idealist because he does not strive to make his theory accurate, that is consonant with the facts; the so-called practical man if he acts upon the impulse of the occasion without the guidance of an enduring principle of conduct. Hence both lack true wisdom, the idealist more culpably for he should be diligent in thought and seek all the light he can obtain. It is useful to repeat that many men have *light* enough to be visionary, but only he who *clearly sees* can *behold* a vision.

REFERENCES

1. Hanlon, J. J., Rogers, F. B., and Rosen, G.: A bookshelf on the history and philosophy of public health, Amer. J. Public Health **50**:445, Apr. 1960.
2. Boek, W. E., and Boek, J. K.: Society and health, New York, 1956, G. P. Putnam's Sons.
3. Terris, M.: Social medicine as an academic discipline, J. Med. Educ. **33**:565, Aug. 1958.
4. Rosen, G.: Approaches to a concept of social medicine, Milbank Mem. Fund Quart. **26**:7, Jan. 1948.
5. Winslow, C.-E. A.: The untilled field of public health, Mod. Med. **2**:183, Mar. 1920.
6. Mountain, J. W.: The health department's dilemma, Public Health Rep. **67**:223, Mar. 1952.
7. Smith, G., and Evans, L. J.: Preventive medicine, attempt at definition, Science **100**:39, July 21, 1944.
8. National Commission on Community Health Services: Comprehensive health care, Washington, 1967, Public Affairs Press.
9. Murphy, F. D.: Health—public or private? Amer. J. Public Health **46**:15, Jan. 1956.
10. Vaughan, H. F.: The way of public health, Trans. Coll. Physicians Phila. **9**:86, June 1941.
11. Dubos, R. J.: Mirage of health, New York, 1959, Harper & Row, Publishers.
12. Beck-Storrs, A.: Public health and government control, Social Stud. **45**:211, Oct. 1954.
13. Roemer, M. I.: The influence of government on American medicine, Oslo, 1962, Gyldendal Norsk Forlag, p. 226.
14. Shryock, R. H.: The interplay of social and internal factors in the history of modern medicine, Sci. Month. **76**:221, Apr. 1953.
15. Mustard, H. S.: Government in public health, New York, 1945, Commonwealth Fund.
16. Government and public health, Bull. N. Y. Acad. Med. **43**:4, Apr. 1967.
17. Kruse, H. D.: The great bane, Bull. N. Y. Acad. Med. **42**:2, Feb. 1966.
18. Linton, R. M., et al.: A strategy for a livable environment, Washington, 1967, U. S. Government Printing Office.
19. American Public Health Association: Guide to a community health study, New York, 1961, The Association.
20. Huxley, A.: Brave new world, Life **25**:63, Sept. 20, 1948.
21. Bowes, G. K.: Epidemic disease; past, present, and future, J. Roy. San. Inst. **66**:174, July 1946.
22. Gillette, J. M.: Perspective of public health in the United States, Sci. Month. **53**:235, Sept. 1941.
23. Johnson, A. S.: Medicine's responsibility in the propagation of poor protoplasm, New Eng. J. Med. **238**:715, May 27, 1948.
24. Goldstein, M. S.: Theory of survival of the unfit, J. Nat. Med. Ass. **47**:233, July, 1955.
25. Moorman, L. J.: Tuberculosis and genius, Chicago, 1940, University of Chicago Press.
26. Lowell, A. L.: Conflicts of principle, Cambridge, 1932, Harvard University Press.

Chapter 2

Background and development of public health*

REASONS FOR REVIEW

While the primary purpose of this book is to consider the various administrative factors involved in the practice of public health, it is also important to consider the genesis of the present situation. This is done not merely to pay tribute to the great figures in public health but also for practical reasons. Osler[4] once claimed it to be a sign of a dry age when the great men of the past are held in light esteem. One practical reason for historic review is that we might thereby grasp the social significance of the public health movement.

Another reason is to achieve a better understanding of where we are and in which direction we should be going; we must occasionally glance backward to see whence and how we came. Many circumstances and events that have occurred in the past help to explain some of the present-day administrative problems and trends which otherwise might be puzzling. As with all other constructive social movements, numerous difficulties have been encountered in the field of public health; superstition, public apathy, political interference, inadequate funds and, too often, personnel of poor quality are but a few that have been mentioned. One sometimes hears shortsighted, impatient, and intolerant persons, even within the public health profession itself,

condemn past and present public health practices in terms of these factors or because progress appears to be slow. These persons should learn something of the background of our social structure and of the public health movement so that they may better understand the relative importance of these factors and the reasons why they may yet exert some influence. This is not meant to condone or encourage an attitude of complacency or comfortable self-satisfaction but merely to point out that sound planning for the future is best accomplished by honest evaluation and understanding of the past and present.

THE PRECHRISTIAN PERIOD

Little is known concerning the prehistoric origins of either personal or community hygiene. Some hints may be gleaned, however, from a study of the customs and tribal rules of contemporary groups that are low in the scale of civilization. With few exceptions, notably the Eskimos, primitive tribes have a certain amount of group and community hygienic sense. Rules against the fouling of family or tribal quarters are almost universal. Many tribes of American Indians, for example, have a long-standing custom of using the downstream side of the camp site for excretory purposes. Burial of excreta is not uncommon. However, this practice often is based more on superstition than on sanitary intent. Many groups have elaborate provisions for the burial or burning of the dead. Practically all primitive people recognize

*For two extensive and scholarly presentations of this subject, see *A History of Public Health* by Rosen[1] and *The History of American Epidemiology* by Top.[2] See also Hanlon, Rogers, and Rosen: Amer. J. Public Health.[3]

the existence of disease and engage in forms of voodoo, quarantine, tribal dancing, and the use of smoke and noise to drive away the evil spirits of disease. With this in mind, it is difficult to resist calling attention to the practice of burning pitch and firing cannons as a means of combating yellow fever in American communities as recently as the end of the nineteenth century.

Archeologic evidence and other historic records show that the Minoans, 3000 to 1500 B.C., and the Cretans, 3000 to 1000 B.C., had advanced to the point of constructing drainage systems, water closets, and water-flushing systems. The Egyptians of about 1000 B.C., as described by Herodotus, were the healthiest of all civilized nations. They had a marked sense of personal cleanliness, possessed numerous pharmaceutical preparations, and constructed earth closets and public drainage pipes. The Hebrews extended Egyptian hygienic thought and behavior by stating in Leviticus, written about 1500 B.C., what is probably the world's first written hygienic code. It dealt with a wide variety of personal and community responsibilities, including cleanliness of the body, protection against the spread of contagious diseases, isolation of lepers, disinfection of dwellings following illness, sanitation of campsites, disposal of excreta and refuse, protection of water and food supplies, and the hygiene of maternity.

The Grecian civilization is of particular interest for two reasons. It was here that personal hygiene was developed to a degree never previously or subsequently approached. Much concern was given to personal cleanliness, exercise, and dietetics rather than to matters of environmental sanitation. Another point of interest is that, in contrast with present-day public health thought, the weak, the ill, and the crippled were ignored and in some instances deliberately destroyed.

The Roman Empire is well known for its administrative and engineering achievements. At its zenith this civilization had laws providing for the registration of citizens and slaves, the taking of a periodic census, the prevention of nuisances, ruinous buildings, dangerous animals, and foul smells, the destruction of unsound goods, the supervision of weights and measures, the supervision of public bars, taverns, and houses of prostitution, and the regulation of building construction. Steps were taken by the government to ensure an uninterrupted supply of good and cheap grain to the population. Many public sanitary services were provided. Many streets were paved, some even had gutters and were drained by a network of drains. Provision was made for the cleaning and repair of streets and the removal of garbage and rubbish. Numerous public baths were constructed. An adequate and, for that time, a relatively safe public water supply was made available by the construction of magnificent aqueducts and tunnels to transport water. It is of interest to note that several of the aqueducts and subsurface drains (cloacae) constructed by the Romans are actually still in use, having been incorporated in the present-day water and sewerage systems of Rome.

THE MIDDLE AGES

With the dawn of the Christian era there developed a reaction against anything reminiscent of the Roman Empire and its attendant paganism. The early Christian Church, representing the consensus of the period, took the attitude that the Roman and Grecian ways of life pampered the body at the expense of the soul. Accordingly, belittlement of worldly and physical matters and "mortification of the flesh" became the preferred patterns of behavior. This philosophy expanded to such an extent that there resulted the prolonged intermission in the progress of civilization known as the Dark Ages, marked by superstition, mysticism, and the rigorous persecution of freethinkers.

So intense was the reaction that it even included a marked change in attitude toward sanitation and personal hygiene. It was considered immoral to see even one's own body; therefore people seldom bathed and wore notoriously dirty garments. This is said by some to have been partly responsible for the eventual widespread use of perfume in the latter part of this period. Diets in general were apparently poor and consisted of badly prepared or preserved foods. This contributed to the eventual great interest in the use of spices and in the development of trade routes for obtaining them. There was utter disregard for sanitation; refuse and body wastes were allowed to accumulate in and around dwellings. Slops were customarily emptied out of windows, giving rise eventually to the familiar password *gardez l'eau*. These and other customs lasted until relatively recent times, as evidenced by Hogarth's prints of life in eighteenth century England.

However, some important medical and hygienic developments did occur during this period. Generally speaking, they were forced upon the people by the untoward effects of an uncontrolled nature and as fruits of their self-made, ill-conceived habits and customs. Terrifying pandemics of disease occurred which were among the most commanding and intense experiences in the entire history of the human race. During the seventh century a new religion, Mohammedanism, had arisen. The philosophy of Islam spread and gathered many followers in Africa, the Near East, Asia, and to some extent the Balkans and the Iberian peninsula. Following the death of Mohammed, it became a religious custom to make a pilgrimage, usually in the company of a large number of people, to Mecca, the birthplace of the prophet. During each great pilgrimage, among the many thousands converging on the small city were some from far-off Asia, especially India, which was and still is the endemic center of cholera. Cholera naturally spread rapidly throughout the thousands of pilgrims, who on turning homeward disseminated it along their routes of travel and throughout their respective homelands. Thus each great pilgrimage was almost invariably followed by a pandemic of cholera. Added to this were the hordes of Christian crusaders from all parts of Europe whose wanderings inevitably resulted in periodic seeding of the European continent with the vibrio of cholera as well as other agents of disease. The vibrio prospered in a gradually

urbanizing Europe, whence centuries later it was transferred to America by the invading settlers. During the period from 1830 to about 1880 cholera repeatedly reentered America, spreading along the water routes and accompanying the prospectors to the gold fields of California. At one time or another most settlements were affected by cholera, often resulting in the death of one third to one half of the population.

During the early Dark Ages leprosy spread probably from Egypt to Asia Minor, whence it was broadcast throughout Europe, aided again by the Crusades and other great migrations. It apparently was a far more acute and disfiguring disease than those presently observed in the Western world and, because of the terror to which it gave rise, laws were passed all over the continent regulating the conduct and movement of those afflicted. In many places lepers were declared civilly dead and were banished from human communities. They were compelled to wear identifying clothes and to warn of their presence by means of a horn or bell. This had a twofold result in that it was a most effective isolation measure and usually brought about a relatively rapid death from hunger and exposure as well as from lack of treatment and care. These measures, inhuman as they were, practically eradicated leprosy in Europe, but by no means in the world, by the sixteenth century and may be regarded as the first great, although unplanned, victory in epidemiology.

The Black Death
No sooner had leprosy passed its zenith and begun to decline than an even deadlier menace appeared in the form of bubonic plague. Its spread was largely the result of the development of trade contacts between Europe and the Near East and Asia. It has been said with considerable justification that nothing before or since so nearly accomplished the extermination of the human race. To quote a few historic figures,[5] during the 1340's more than 13 million are said to have died from the disease in China. India was practically depopulated; Tartary, Mesopotamia, Syria, and Armenia were literally covered by dead bodies. When the

disease was raging in its greatest violence, Aleppo lost about 500 and the larger city of Cairo, from 10,000 to 15,000 daily. In Gaza, 22,000 people and most of the animals were carried off within 6 weeks; Cyprus lost all of its inhabitants, and ships without crews were often seen in the Mediterranean, as afterward in the North Sea, drifting about aimlessly, spreading the plague wherever they were driven ashore. When Pope Clement VI asked for the number of the dead, some said that half of the population of the known world had died. The figure he was finally given was about 43 million. The total mortality from the Black Death is thought to have been over 60 million.

Europe, particularly during 1348, was devastated. Florence lost 60,000, Venice 100,000, Marseilles 16,000 in 1 month, Sien 70,000, Paris 50,000, St. Denys 14,000, Strasbourg 9,000, and Vienna 1,200 daily. In many places in France not more than 2 out of 20 people were left alive.

In Avignon, where 60,000 people died, the Pope found it necessary to consecrate the Rhone river in order that bodies might be thrown into it without delay, the churchyard no longer being able to hold them. In Vienna, burial within churchyards or churches was prohibited; the dead were arranged in layers by thousands in six large pits outside of the city, as had already been done in Cairo, Paris, and other cities. Crossing the channel, it destroyed one half of the population of medieval England, at least 100,000 in London alone.

Altogether it is estimated that Europe's tribute in the pandemic of the midfourteenth century was about 25 million. Furthermore, this one horrifying visitation was just beginning; plague continued to ebb and flow like a tide, periodically sweeping over the dirty, miserable European continent. For example, in the city of London in 1603 over one sixth of the population succumbed to the disease, in 1625 another sixth, and in 1665 about one fifth. During 1790, Marseilles and Toulon lost 91,000; in 1743, Messina 70,000; and in 1759, about 70,000 died on the island of Cyprus.

Growing out of these terrifying experiences, and despite the then current view of divine or cosmic causation of disease, certain groping attempts were made to forestall the apparent inevitability of epidemic disaster. In 1348 the great trading port of Venice banned entry of infected or suspected ships and travelers. In 1377 at Rogusa it was ruled that travelers from plague areas should stop at designated places outside the port and remain there free of disease for 2 months before being allowed to enter. Historically this represents the first quarantine measure, although it involved a 2-month interval rather than the literal 40 days. This procedure is of particular interest in that it implied a vague realization of the existence of an incubation period for a communicable disease. Six years later, in 1383, Marseilles passed the first actual quarantine law and erected the first quarantine station. These are historic landmarks in public health administration and epidemiology, but unfortunately their effectiveness was impaired by the fact that great attention was paid to humans, but the role of the rat and the flea was not discerned.

Other diseases

Some mention, even if necessarily inadequate, should be made of the rapid dissemination of syphilis throughout Europe and the Near East following the discovery of America. Some measure of its incidence and devastation is obtained by considering the name, "the great pox," which was applied to it in order to distinguish it from smallpox, which we now consider serious enough in its present generally milder form. Incidentally, it is curious that little historical reference is made to many of the other diseases which are known to have existed with incidences far exceeding any now occurring, e.g., diphtheria, the streptococcal infections, the dysenteries, typhoid, typhus, and others. The most probable reasons for the paucity of mention of these diseases are that, in the first place, people undoubtedly became accustomed to their inevitable endemicity and accepted them as part of the routine risk of life, and, second, that they were so dramatically overshadowed by the tremendous impact of the great periodic pandemic killers as to merit relatively little mention in the historical writings of the times. In summary, therefore, the peoples of Europe emerged from the Middle Ages and, as a matter of fact, came all the way to very recent times with little or no comprehension of any principles of public health other than those of crude, inhuman, and inefficient isolation and quarantine.

THE RENAISSANCE

In a period of history marked by increasing tendencies toward social concentration, expanding trade, and population movement, the risks involved in pursuing these trends in the face of rampant disease were necessarily great. The great pandemics of the Middle Ages, therefore, must have caused considerable social and political frustrations which could lead only to attitudes of fatalism and general disregard for the welfare of individuals. Hecker,[5] philosophizing along these lines, commented:

The mind of nations is deeply affected by the destructive conflict of the powers of nature, and . . . great disasters lead to striking changes in general civilization. For all that exists in man, whether good or evil, is rendered conspicuous by the presences of great danger. His inmost feelings are aroused—the thought of self-preservation masters his spirit—self denial is put to severe proof, and wherever darkness and barbarism prevail, there the affrighted mortal flies to the idols of his superstition, and all laws, human and divine, are criminally molested.

The way of life of a people likewise has a marked effect on their state of health or illness. In this respect, it is of interest to learn from a letter of Erasmus to the personal physician of Cardinal Wolsey, as quoted by Winslow,[6] the manner of life in the average English household of the sixteenth century:

As to floors, they are usually made with clay, covered with rushes that grow in the fens and which are so seldom removed that the lower part remains sometimes for twenty years and has in it a collection of spittle, vomit, urine of dogs and humans, beer, scraps of fish and other filthiness not to be named.

Winslow, in his incomparable presentation of the development of the modern public health movement, points out how long it has taken the human race to improve such conditions, presenting examples even more disgusting than the above from

England of 1842 and New York City in 1865. As a matter of fact, even at the present time it is necessary to work but a short time in a sociologic field in either urban or rural areas in order to see conditions not much different from those to which reference is made.

There gradually developed in the minds of a few some doubt of the teleologic origin of disease as a punishment for sin. It might be noted in passing, however, that this stigma has only recently been removed from cancer and tuberculosis and that venereal infection is still considered by many as a punishment for immorality. By the end of the Middle Ages, differentiation of a number of diseases had been accomplished. Among the conditions recognized as distinct entities were leprosy, influenza, ophthalmia, trachoma, scabies, impetigo, erysipelas (St. Anthony's fire), anthrax, plague, consumption, syphilis (the great pox), smallpox, diphtheria and scarlet fever considered as one, and typhus and typhoid fever also considered together.

The people of Europe, coming out of this dreadful, depressing period of history, slowly and cautiously began to open their eyes and to think as free individuals. There began to appear a few outstanding thinkers, the number increasing with the passage of time. Among them are found the names of Descartes, Lyell, Lamarck, Cuvier, Boyle, Bentham, Smith, Voltaire, and Darwin, to mention but a few. Each in his own way hammered at the bars imprisoning the minds and bodies of men. Their combined efforts resulted in remarkable accomplishments, especially in the late eighteenth century and throughout the nineteenth century. The concept of the dignity of man began to be emphasized more and more. The search for scientific truth was at last advocated for its own sake.

THE EIGHTEENTH AND NINETEENTH CENTURIES

The plight of children

However, other changes were occurring at the same time. Among them was the development of nationalism, imperialism, and industrialization, with their tragic and degrading influences. The false gods of power and profit were placed on higher pedestals than they had ever before occupied, and individual liberties, labors, and lives were sacrificed on a scale probably unprecedented since the building of the pyramids. As an example, in one of the most shameful actions in the history of the human race, there came about in England a legally condoned practice of apprentice slavery, whereby pauper children were indentured to the owners of mines and factories. The socially accepted pattern was for parishes to assume responsibility for orphans and pauper children. This responsibility was met at first by paying private "nurses" for taking the infants and younger children into their homes for a few years and putting them out to work as apprentices when they became older. Partly because of the increasing numbers and partly as a remedy for frequent abuse of the young children, parish workhouses began to be established in the late seventeenth and early eighteenth centuries as a substitute for parish nurses.

Theoretically the workhouses were also intended to provide some training for the children, but this was kept at a minimum and was largely concerned with inculcating the ideals of labor and industry, virtue and religion. It was hoped that the workhouses would ". . . cure a very bad practice in parish officers, who to save expence, are apt to ruin children by putting them out as early as they can to any sorry master that will take them, without any concern for their education and welfare."[7]

In her authoritative review of life in England in the eighteenth century, Dorothy George[7] gives a picture of these methods and ideals in practice by describing the London Workhouse in Bishopsgate Street in 1708:

. . . thirty or forty children were put under the charge of one nurse in a ward, they lay two together in bunks arranged round the walls in two tiers,"boarded and set one above the other . . . a flock bed, a pair of sheets, two blankets and a rugg to each." Prayers and breakfast were from 6:30 to 7. At 7 the children were set to work, twenty under a mistress, "to spin wool and flax, knit stockings, to make new their linnen, cloathes, shooes, mark, etc." This work went on till 6 P.M. with an interval from 12 to 1 for "dinner and play." Twenty children were called away at a time for an hour a day to be taught reading, some also writing. Some children, we are told, "earn a halfpenny, some a penny, and some fourpence a day." At twelve, thirteen or fourteen, they were apprenticed, being given, at the master's choice, either a "good ordinary suit of cloaths or 20s, in money."

When children reached an age when they might be apprenticed, their lot became infinitely worse. "A most unhappy practice prevails in most places," said a writer on the Poor Laws in 1738, "to apprentice poor children, no matter to what master. Provided he lives out of the parish, if the child serves the first forty days we are rid of him for ever. The master may be a tiger in cruelty, he may beat, abuse, strip naked, starve or do what he will to the poor innocent lad, few people take much notice, and the officers who put him out the least of anybody. . . . The greatest part of those who now take poor apprentices are the most indigent and dishonest, in a word, the very dregs of the poor of England, by whom it is the fate of many a poor child, not only to be half-starved and sometimes bred up in no trade, but to be forced to thieve and steal for his master, and so is brought up for the gallows into the bargain. . . ." Children apprenticed to chimney sweepers fared among the worst. In 1767, Hanway, a leading reformer of the period, described the miseries of their neglect and ill-treatment, of their being forced up chimneys at the risk of being burnt or suffocated, and of their being forced to beg and steal by their masters. "Chimney-sweepers," he says, "ought to breed their own children to the business, then perhaps they will wash, clothe and feed them. As it is they do neither, and these poor black urchins have no protectors and are treated worse than a humane person would treat a dog." In apprenticing children in large groups the provision was not uncommon to require that for every 30 normal children 1 idiot would have to be taken. These unfortunates, forced to work from 15 to 18 hours a day, sometimes literally chained to their machines, fed a minimum of food scarcely fit for consumption, and housed under the most crowded and filthy conditions, usually were released from their sufferings and abuse by early death.

In 1842, Edwin Chadwick pointed out that more than one half of the children of the working classes died before their fifth birthday and that in cities such as Liverpool the average ages at death of the various social classes were 36 years for the gentry, 22 years for tradesmen, and 16 years for laborers![8] The breakdown for London, obtained by the Sanitary Commission for the Metropolis in 1843, is given in Table 2-1.

Sanitary conditions

During this period the condition of the streets became deplorable, due in part to nightmen and scavengers emptying their carts in the streets instead of in the places assigned for the purpose. The accumulated filth of the eighteenth century house was in many cases simply thrown from the doors or windows.

Although eighteenth-century London was incredibly dirtier, more dilapidated and more closely-built than it afterwards became, was there no compensation in its greater compactness, the absence of straggling suburbs, the ease with which people could take country walks? This is at least doubtful. The roads round London were neither very attractive nor very safe. The land adjoining them was watered with drains and thickly sprinkled with laystalls and refuse heaps. Hogs were kept in large numbers on the out-

skirts and fed on the garbage of the town. A chain of smoking brick-kilns surrounded a great part of London and in the brick-fields vagrants lived and slept, cooking their food at the kilns. It is true that there was an improvement as the century went on. In 1706 it was said of the highways, "tho" they are mended every summer, yet everybody knows that for a mile or two about this City, the same and the ditches hard by are commonly so full of nastiness and stinking dirt, that oftentimes many persons who have occasion to go in or come out of town, are forced to stop their noses to avoid the ill-smell occasioned by it.[7]

These conditions under which so many hundreds of thousands of people lived and worked had dire results indeed from a hygienic standpoint. Smallpox, cholera, typhoid, tuberculosis, and many other diseases reached exceedingly high endemic levels, and the contamination of sources of water became so extensive as to prompt that famous statement in Parliament on the condition of the empire in 1859: "India is in revolt and the Thames stinks." Southwood Smith pointed out at the time that the annual slaughter in England and Wales from typhus and typhoid fevers was double the number of lives lost by the allied armies in the battle of Waterloo.

ENGLISH SANITARY REFORMS

Concern with the economic consequences of existing social and sanitary conditions

Table 2-1. Deaths by social class, London, 1840*

Class	Proportion of deaths from epidemics to total deaths of each class (%)	Proportion of deaths of children under 1 year to births in that year	Proportion of deaths of children under 10 years to total deaths of each class (%)	Mean age of death of all who died— men, women and children	Mean age of all who died above age 21 years
Gentry, professional persons, and their families	6.5	1 to 10	24.7	44	61
Tradesmen, shopkeepers, and their families	20.5	1 to 6	52.4	23	50
Wage classes, artisans, laborers, and their families	22.2	1 to 4	54.5	22	49

*Adapted from Chadwick as quoted by Richardson, B. W.: The health of nations, a review of the works of Edwin Chadwick, London, 1887, Longmans, Green & Co., vol. II, p. 80.

began to appear, providing leaders in sanitary reform with forceful arguments. Thus Chadwick[8] reported:

This depressing effect of adverse sanitary circumstances on the labouring strength of the population, and on its duration, is to be viewed with the greatest concern, as it is a depressing effect on that which most distinguishes the British people, and which it were truism to say constitutes the chief strength of the nation—the bodily strength of the individuals of the labouring class. The greater portion of the wealth of the nation is derived from the labour obtained by the application of this strength, and it is only those who have had practically the means of comparing it with that of the population of other countries who are aware how far the labouring population of this country is naturally distinguished above others.... The more closely the subject of the evils affecting the sanitary condition of the labouring population is investigated, the more widely do their effects appear to be ramified. The pecuniary cost of noxious agencies is measured by data within the province of the actuary, by the charges attendant on the reduced duration of life, and the reduction of the periods of working ability or production by sickness. The cost would include also much of the public charge of attendant vice and crime, which come within the province of the police, as well as the destitution which comes within the province of the administrators of relief. Of the pecuniary effects, including the cost of maintenance during the preventible sickness, any estimate approximating to exactness could only be obtained by very great labour, which does not appear to be necessary.

Public health went unrecognized in a legal sense in England until 1837, when the first sanitary legislation was enacted. It established a National Vaccination Board and appropriated 2,000 pounds for its support. As a result a few vaccination stations were set up in the city of London. This modest beginning was followed shortly in 1842 by Edwin Chadwick's momentous *Report on an Inquiry into the Sanitary Condition of the Labouring Population of Great Britain,* one of the results of which was the establishment in 1848 of a General Board of Health for England. Significantly, the same year saw the appointment as first medical officer of health for London of John Simon, who 7 years later was to assume that office for the nation as a whole. Improvements rapidly followed one another. These advances in sanitation and hygiene did not go forward alone. Legislation was passed concerning factory management, child welfare, care of the aged, the mentally ill, and the infirm, education, and many other phases of social reform.

It was not long before the horrors of previous conditions were forgotten, and the standards of order, decency, and sanitation began to be taken for granted.

... pride was based on real achievements, which had an undoubted effect on the health of the town, and in which London was a pioneer among large cities. The foot-pavements, the lamps, the water-supply, the fire-plugs, the new sewers, defective enough by later standards, were admired by all.... Beneath the pavements are vast subterraneous sewers arched over to convey away the waste water which in other cities is so noisome above ground, and at a less depth are buried wooden pipes that supply every house plentifully with water, conducted by leaden pipes into kitchens or cellars, three times a week for the trifling expense of three shillings per quarter.... The intelligent foreigner cannot fail to take notice of these useful particulars which are almost peculiar to London.[8]

The seeds of sanitary and social reform spread rapidly to other large urban centers of England. However, participation in these benefits by the smaller towns and rural areas was understandably slower. As early as 1830, Chadwick had recommended the employment of a large number of local sanitary officers, including medical personnel, for the adequate coverage of the nation. As might be expected, his proposals originally met with considerable opposition, some of which continued, even when he subsequently was able to demonstrate the economic soundness of the costs incurred.

ENGLISH INFLUENCE ON AMERICA

It may appear to the more casual reader that conditions and developments in Great Britain have been unduly stressed. Considering the primary concern of this book, any discussion of backgrounds must necessarily emphasize those extraterritorial developments which have exerted the greatest influence upon America. It is quite true that many advances had been made elsewhere, notably in the Low Countries, in Germany, and on the Scandinavian peninsula. By midnineteenth century, France had long since embarked on significant studies and activities relating to public health and sanitation, and many scientific papers were being published. The very establishment of the *Annales d'Hygiene Publique* gives testimony to this. The work of the Belgian, Quételet, was already widely known, and Pettenkofer, in Munich, and Virchow, in Berlin, already had far-reaching influences.

Nevertheless, the early intimate ties, social, economic, and otherwise, between the North American continent and Great Britain made happenings in the latter of particular signficance to the former. The relationship was aptly described by Dr. Henry I. Bowditch,[9] first president of the Massachusetts State Board of Health:

> But by far the greatest influence has been exerted upon us in America by England, who, by her unbounded pecuniary sacrifices and steady improvement in her legislation, and her able writers, has far outstripped any country in the world in the direction of State Preventive Medicine. . . . The consumate skill in the discovery, removal, and prevention of whatever may be prejudicial to the public health, shown under the admirable direction of Mr. Simon, late Medical Officer of England's Privy Council, by his corps of trained inspectors is wholly unequalled at the present day, and unprecedented, I suspect, in all past time in any country on the globe.

While scientific researchers may have progressed further in some other countries, the application of the new knowledge, especially in terms of administrative organization and procedure, occurred more rapidly and more successfully in England than elsewhere. Since the administrative organization depends to a considerable degree upon legal procedure, it is of additional significance that America, from the beginning, followed the pattern set by English law. Thus, when the time came for American cities to pass sanitation ordinances, they did so in the tradition of the English common law.

COLONIAL AMERICA

Transferring attention to the newly developing North American continent, it appears that certain public health problems were soon recognized by the colonists. They had good reason for being conscious of the threat of disease. Many of the early settlements had been completely obliterated by epidemic diseases, particularly smallpox.

Among these were the colonies at Jamestown and undoubtedly the colony at Roanoke Island. On the other hand, it was probably due to disease that the colonies were able to establish their eventual footholds in the new continent. The settlers of the Massachusetts Bay Colony, for example, came to a territory the natives of which were by no means peaceful. Yet by the time the Pilgrims landed at Plymouth the hostile natives of the surrounding countryside had been all but eliminated, apparently by smallpox introduced by the Cabot and Gosnold expeditions. Smallpox also appears to have played a role to some degree in the weakening and eventual conquest of the Aztec Empire. In this instance it is known to have been introduced by a servant of Narvaez who joined Cortez in 1520.[10] It has been estimated that during the early periods of colonization of Central and North America, the Indian population was decimated by diseases introduced by the invaders, whether peaceful or otherwise.[11]

The registration of vital statistics is generally considered to be one of the essential cornerstones of sound, efficient public health awareness and practice. It is not without interest that the recording of these data was a very early concern of the New England colonists. As early as 1639 an act was passed by the Massachusetts colony ordering that each birth and death be recorded; subsequent acts outlined the necessary administrative responsibilities and procedures. Not only was the information made available locally but copies had to be made by the town clerks and transmitted to the clerks of the county courts. The law also provided for fees and penalties. Similar laws were enacted at about the same time by the Plymouth colony.[12]

Most of the early activities of a public health nature in America were concerned with gross insanitation and attempts to prevent the entrance of exotic diseases. For example, as early as 1647 the Massachusetts Bay Colony passed a regulation to prevent pollution of Boston Harbor. Between 1692 and 1708, Boston, Salem, and Charleston passed acts dealing with nuisances and trades offensive or dangerous to the public health. In 1701, Massachusetts passed laws providing for the isolation of smallpox patients and for ship quarantine, to be used whenever necessary. The difficulty with these and other early measures was that no continuing organization or even committee existed in order to assure ready recognition of undesirable situations or noncompliance with the requirements of the legislation enacted.

In the century during which the American colonies developed, drew together, and eventually formed a federation of states very little progress of a public health nature was made. Following the American Revolution, the threat of various diseases, particularly yellow fever, led to widespread interest in the development of legislation for the establishment of permanent boards of health. Permissive legislation of this type was passed in 1797 by both the states of New York and Massachusetts, followed in 1805 by Connecticut. There is some controversy over the establishment of the first permanent local board of health. Boston is commonly said to have organized the first in 1799, with Paul Revere as its chairman. However, this has been contested by the cities of Petersburg, Va. (1780), Philadelphia (1794), New York (1796), and Baltimore (1793). The latter claim has been supported more or less by the American Public Health Association.[13]

By the end of the eighteenth century, New York City, with a population of 75,000, had formed a public health committee concerned with the "quality of the water supplies, construction of common sewers, drainage of marshes, interment of the dead, planting of trees and healthy vegetables, habitation of damp cellars, and the construction of a masonry wall along the water front." In July 1798 the new American Congress created a Marine Hospital Service in order to provide for the care of sick and disabled merchant seaman. This service was later to become of interest and significance for three reasons; First, it was the origin of what eventually became the United States Public Health Service; second, it was to furnish the organization for effecting national quarantine; and, third, it represents

one of the earliest examples of prepaid medical insurance. For 20 cents per month each merchant seaman was provided with medical and hospital care. As early as 1800 the first marine hospital was constructed in Norfolk, Va.

THE NINETEENTH CENTURY IN AMERICA

Between 1800 and 1850 the United States underwent great expansion, but public health activities remained stationary. What did not remain stationary, however, was the development of threats to public health and welfare and the resulting incidence of disease. Many epidemics, especially of smallpox, yellow fever, cholera, typhoid, and typhus, repeatedly entered and swept over the land. Tuberculosis and malaria reached high levels of endemicity. In Massachusetts in 1850, for example, the tuberculosis death rate was over 300 per 100,000 population, the infant mortality was about 200 per 1,000 live births, and smallpox, scarlet fever and typhoid were leading causes of deaths. As a result, by 1850 the average life expectancy in Boston and most of the other older cities in America was less than that in London, which at that time was itself the object of wide criticism for its sickening scenes of misery and depravity. The American social scene was the subject of scathing comments by visitors from abroad who were impressed with the crudity and "barbarism" of life in the United States and the generally unkempt appearance of its communities. As so often has happened, improvements in sanitation and public health were delayed by lack of progress in other fields. Sir Arthur Newsholme,[14] the noted British hygienist, described this period of American social history in the following manner:

The rapid growth of cities tended to out run the forces of law and order and to smother under the weight of numbers any attempts at civic reform. Before public health measures could be adopted or enforced, other more pressing problems had to be solved. An effective police force, the first requisite of community life, did not make its appearance in the Atlantic seaboard cities until 1853, and satisfactory fire prevent came even later. Protection against the dirt and filth of human aggregation, which threatened the life of every man, woman, and child, had to wait upon the adequate enforcement of law and order.

The inadequacies of the times were reflected in the low quality of medical care available to the people. Professional teaching facilities were few and inadequate. Many "physicians" were self-designated and itinerant. The prestige of the medical profession was at its lowest ebb, and its ranks were disorganized and split by the development of numerous healing philosophies and cults. One writer[15] summarized the situation: "The doctors were victims of their own want of knowledge, of the absence of adequate medical standards and of a chaotic educational system." Healing agents used included not only empiric remedies left over from medieval Europe but, in addition, many newly discovered "remedies" often borrowed from the American aborigines. This state of therapeutic affairs led Oliver Wendell Holmes[16] to remark that "if the whole materia medica as now used, could be sunk to the bottom of the sea, it would be all the better for mankind—and all the worse for the fishes."

CITY HEALTH DEPARTMENTS

The first half of the nineteenth century saw a gradual trend toward the more or less full-time employment of persons to serve as the functional agents of local boards of health, which now were increasing in number. This represented the first step in the formation of full-time local health departments. Some of the earlier of these organizations were established in Baltimore (1798), Charleston, S. C. (1815), Philadelphia (1818), Providence (1832), Cambridge (1846), New York City (1866), Chicago (1867), Louisville (1870), Indianapolis (1872), and Boston (1873). The last is of interest in illustrating the lag, in this instance three quarters of a century, that occurred between the formation of many local boards of health and the establishment of functional health departments. As might be expected, the activities of these health departments were determined by the current epidemiologic theories that placed particular emphasis on the elimination of sanitary nuisances. For example, at the mid-point of the nineteenth century the population of New York City had reached 300,-000. Its board of health was concerned only with crowded living conditions, dirty streets, and the regulation of public baths, slaughterhouses, and pigsties.

THE SHATTUCK REPORT[17]

In terms of American public health history, the midnineteenth century is most notable for the extraordinary *Report of the Sanitary Commission of Massachusetts*. Its author, Lemuel Shattuck (1793-1859), a most unusual man, led the diversified life of teacher, historian, book dealer, sociologist, statistician, and, finally, legislator in the state assembly. Although in a medical sense a layman, he had a keen interest in sanitary reform, originating apparently with his work when gathering and tabulating the vital statistics of Boston. Because of his persistent complaints regarding the current lack of sanitary progress, he was appointed chairman of a legislative committee for the study of health and sanitary problems in the commonwealth. From this committee, and essentially from Shattuck's pen issued the report to which reference is made. With remarkable insight and foresight the report included a detailed consideration not only of the present and future public health needs of Massachusetts but also of its component parts and of the nation as a whole. This most remarkable of all American public health documents, if published today, in many respects would still be ahead of its time.

The content of the Sanitary Commission report may be appreciated in its true light when it is realized that at the time it was written there existed no national or state public health programs and such local health agencies as by that time had been organized were still in an embryonic stage of development. Medical practice in general was then far from scientific; facilities for medical training were few and in a most confused state; and provisions for nurses' training entirely lacking. Almost another half century was to pass before the spectacular era of Pasteur, Koch, and the other contributors to the golden age of bacteriology would begin. Among the many recommendations made by Shattuck a century ago were those for the establishment of state and local boards of health, a system of sanitary police or inspectors, the collection and analysis of vital statistics, a routine system for exchanging data and information, sanitation programs for towns and buildings, studies on the health of school children, studies of tuberculosis, the control of alcoholism, the supervision of mental disease, the sanitary supervision and study of problems of immigrants, the erection of model tenements, public bathhouses, and washhouses, the control of smoke nuisances, the control of food adulteration, the exposure of nostrums, the preaching of health from pulpits, the establishment of nurses' training schools, the teaching of sanitary science in medical schools, and the inclusion of preventive medicine in clinical practice, with routine physical examinations and family records of illness.

Unfortunately, while this document laid down the principal ideas and modes of action which would ultimately form the basis of much of today's public health practice, its importance was not appreciated at the time it was submitted, and it was destined to lie dormant for nearly a quarter of a century. One of the earliest appraisals of it was given in 1876 by Henry I. Bowditch, first president of the State Board of Health of Massachusetts, in an address before the International Medical Congress at Philadelphia[9]:

The report fell flat from the printer's hand. It remained almost unnoticed by the community or by the profession for many years, and its recommendations were ignored. Finally, in 1869, a State Board of Health of laymen and physicians, exactly as Mr. Shattuck recommended, was established by Massachusetts. Dr. Derby, its first secretary, looked to this admirable document as his inspiration and support. In giving this high honor to Mr. Shattuck, I do not wish to forget or to undervalue the many and persistent efforts made by a few physicians, among whom stands pre-eminent Dr. Edward Jarvis, and occasionally by the Massachusetts Medical Society, in urging the State authorities to inaugurate and to sustain the ideas avowed by Mr. Shattuck. But there is no doubt that he, as a laymen, quietly working, did more towards bringing Massachusetts to correct views on this subject than all other agencies whatsoever. Of

Mr. Edwin Chadwick, I need say nothing. You all know him. Fortunately for himself, he has lived to see rich fruits from his labors. That was not granted to Mr. Shattuck.

The comparison of Shattuck, the American, and Chadwick, the Englishman, is of more than passing interest. Some lessons may be learned by comparing the effects of the work of the two men. Shattuck's report consisted essentially of straightforward, unembellished, unillustrated statements of fact, followed by specific and detailed recommendations. This is in contrast with Chadwick's *Report on an Inquiry into the Sanitary Condition of the Labouring Population of Great Britain,* which included many vivid descriptions of the appalling conditions in existence. The latter caused an immediate emotional response on the part of all those who read or heard of the report. One is lead to wonder if Shattuck's report might have had a more immediate effect had it provided the reader with mental images of existing conditions for contrast with further mental images of desirable conditions attainable. Another point of contrast is that, although Chadwick's report brought about a prompt reaction resulting in the establishment of a General Board of Health in 1848, the response was not long lasting. Chadwick's overenthusiasm and impatience demanded immediate action, for which the British people were not yet ready[18]. Certain aspects of this were discussed in Chapter 1. Considerable antagonism and resistance was generated in many quarters, resulting in the early demise of the General Board of Health after only 4 years of existence. This reversal caused an unfortunate delay in the ultimate development of a sound national health program in Great Britain. The reports of Chadwick and Shattuck, therefore, remarkable as they were, provide us with examples of administrative failure, one because of underpromotion and the other because of overpromotion.

THE FIRST STATE HEALTH DEPARTMENT

The repeated outbreaks of yellow fever and other epidemic diseases caused the state of Louisiana in 1855 to set up a board or commission to deal with quarantine matters in the port of New Orleans. This has led some to claim priority for Louisiana in the establishment of a state board of health. However, in terms of the more usual concept of the general functions of a state board of health, it is generally considered that Massachusetts, despite its lack öf response to Shattuck's recommendations, merits recognition for establishing the first true state board of health in 1869. The act creating it directed:

The board shall take cognizance of the interests of health and life among the citizens of this Commonwealth. They shall make sanitary investigations and inquires in respect to the people, the causes of disease, and especially of epidemics, and the sources of mortality and the effects of localities, employments, conditions and circumstances on the public health; and they shall gather such information in respect to those matters as they may deem proper, for diffusion among the people.*

In determining policy at early meetings the board, under the leadership of Dr. Henry I. Bowditch, decided to concern itself with public and professional education in matters of hygiene, various aspects of housing, investigations of various well-known diseases and measures for their partial or entire prevention, prevailing methods of slaughtering, sale of poisons, and conditions of the poor. It was decided also to send a circular letter to local boards of health in order to inquire about their powers and duties and to collect for publication the number and prevailing causes of deaths in the most populous cities and towns in the state. The board requested that each community designate a physician to act as correspondent. Patterson and Baker,[19] in discussing the early history of this board, made the pertinent observation that "one by-product of this correspondence was the beginning of a productive cooperation between the state and local authorities." One reads with annoyance of the merger in 1878 of the Massachusetts Department of Health with the Department of Lunacy and Charity because of political pressure and a desire for "economy." As a result matters dealing with the public

*Act of 1869, General Court of Massachusetts.

health were effectively submerged by the weight of the other two interests. Eventually the light was seen, and a sound program was made possible by reestablishment of the health agency as an entity.

It is interesting to note the establishment of the second state health department the next year, on the opposite side of the continent in California. By the end of the nineteenth century 38 other states had followed suit. Eventually, with action by Texas in 1909 and by New Mexico in 1919, all of the states in the Union had boards of health and health departments.

THE QUARANTINE CONVENTIONS AND THE AMERICAN PUBLIC HEALTH ASSOCIATION

Other events of great public health potential were occurring in the midnineteenth century. Those concerned about the public health felt the need to maintain closer contact in order to solve problems of mutual concern. Due particularly to Wilson Jewell, the health officer of Philadelphia who had recently attended the Conference Sanitaire in Paris in 1851-1852, there was called a series of National Quarantine Conventions.[20] The first, a 3-day meeting, was held in Philadelphia in 1857. It organized itself formally, and the 54 members in attendance discussed many subjects of common interest, including prevention of the introduction of epidemic diseases such as typhus, cholera, and yellow fever, port quarantine, the importance of stagnant and putrid bilge water, putrescible matters, filthy bedding, baggage and clothing of immigrant passengers, and air that has been confined. It recommended that immigrants not previously protected against smallpox be vaccinated. The second convention, held in Baltimore in 1858, was noteworthy for proposals for a uniform system of quarantine laws and the organization of a Committee on Internal Hygiene or the Sanitary Arrangement of Cities. It is interesting that 42 of the 86 persons attending the second convention were not physicians. Two more conventions were held, New York in 1859 and Boston in 1860, before the outbreak of the American Civil War precluded further meetings.

The seed planted by the quarantine conventions by no means died. On April 18, 1872, following the termination of the war, 10 men, including Elisha Harris and Stephen Smith, met informally in New York City for the purpose of reactivating interest in national meetings for the consideration of public health matters. Meeting again at Long Branch, N. J., in September with several additional representatives, they chose a name, adopted a constitution, and elected Dr. Stephen Smith first president of the American Public Health Association. In a later discussion of the early days Dr. Smith[21] said, "The American Public Health Association had its origin in that natural desire which thinkers and workers in the same fields, whether of business or philanthropy, or the administration of civil trusts, have for mutual council, advice and cooperation."

Since the National Quarantine Conventions were necessarily concerned primarily with quarantine matters, the formation of the American Public Health Association represented a considerable advance in that the scope of interest was greatly broadened. This was reflected in its earliest meetings, wherein were presented papers on many aspects of sanitation, on the transmission and prevention of diseases, on longevity, on hospital hygiene, and on other diverse subjects. In addition, discussions on quarantine were held. Through the years of its continued existence the Association has served its members well, providing a common fount of knowledge, information, and encouragement and a means of presenting a united front for the improvement of the health of America.

THE NATIONAL BOARD OF HEALTH

One of the earliest concerns of both the Quarantine Conventions and the American Public Health Association was with the need for a national board of health. Smillie[22] described the circumstances which led to the ultimate formation of such a national board, its controversial 4 years' existence, and its painful, premature death from deliberate financial starvation. Meetings were held in Washington in 1875 attended by representatives of many state and city health departments for the purpose of considering plans for the formation of a federal health organization. The meeting degenerated into a jurisdictional dispute on the part of the Army, the Navy, and the Marine Hospital Service, the three existing governmental departments already providing certain services in this field. In 1878 a devastating epidemic of yellow fever swept over a large part of the country. Since the disease was known to have entered through the port of New Orleans, the Louisiana authorities were charged with laxity. Public sentiment was aroused; as a result not only the Army and the Marine Hospital Service but also the American Public Health Association sponsored national health department bills. It was the latter bill that was finally passed by Congress in 1879. This bill transferred from the Marine Hospital Service all health duties and powers, including maritime quarantine. The act created a board of presidential appointees consisting of seven physicians and representatives from the Army, the Navy, the Marine Hospital Service, and the Department of Justice. About 2½ months later another act was passed which gave the board extensive quarantine powers and authorized an appropriation of $500,000 for its work. This second act included an unfortunate clause which limited the powers to 4 years, necessitating a reenactment of the bill in order for the work to continue.

The membership of the first board was notable, including J. L. Cabell, J. S. Billings, J. T. Turner, P. H. Bailhoche, S. M. Bemiss, H. I. Bowditch, R. W. Mitchell, Stephen Smith, S. F. Phillips, and T. S. Verdi. The 4 years of life of the National Board of Health were marked by an ambitious and efficient program of studies and services marred by the persistent and vociferous opposition of Dr. Joseph Jones, secretary of the Louisiana Board of Health, who objected to the presence of "Federal agents and spies" and seized every opportunity to belittle and misrepresent the activities of the National Board. Intent as he was on destroying the new organization, he was saved the trouble by Dr. John Hamilton, the Surgeon General of the Marine Hospital Service. Dr. Hamilton, although professionally inept, possessed considerable political astuteness. Realizing that the National Board of Health would pass out of existence unless the law of 1879 was reenacted in 1883 and that in such an event its powers and functions would revert to the Marine Hospital Service, he worked quietly and effectively to prevent reenactment. Charging misuse of funds, extravagance, and incompetence, he succeeded in bringing the National Board of Health to an untimely death.

One of the members of the Board, Stephen Smith, from the first had favored conferring all national public health duties and powers on the National Board of Health but incorporating in it the officers, staff, and activities of the Marine Hospital Service and any other agencies concerned with public health matters. Smillie[22] analyzed the situation in the following terms:

He foresaw that Congress would lose interest in the National Board of Health, but would continue to support a service agency that had full-time career officers and was incorporated as an integral part of national government machinery.

In retrospect we realize that Stephen Smith was right. The unwieldy board of experts, each living in a different community and attempting to carry out administrative duties, with no cohesion, no real unity of opinion and no central authority, was an impossible administrative machine. A centrally guided service, such as actually developed, had unity and purpose, but unfortunately lacked intelligent leadership. The public health policies for a great nation for many years were determined solely by the opinions—sometimes the whims and personal prejudices—of a single individual. It would have been a much better plan if Dr. Stephen Smith's half formulated plan of 1883 could have been carried out, thus salvaging the really important features of the National Board of Health and incorporating in it a service agency with a full-time personnel, an esprit de corps, and a strong central administrative machine. The members of the Board of Health selected by the President of the United States because they were public health experts, should have been continued as a Board of Health and should have served as a permanent policy-forming body, advising and aiding their administrative officer. The Marine Hospital Service was the most logical existing national agency with which to vest this national public health function. The Surgeon General should have been made the executive officer of the Board, and all actual administrative responsibility should have been centered in him. It was a great opportunity to have organized a

close-knit, effective National Health Service, but there was no single man who had the vision or the power to solve this simple problem.

THE PUBLIC HEALTH SERVICE

To consider the history and development of the Public Health Service, the most important federal health agency, it is necessary to retrace our steps to the year 1798. The United States of America had just come into existence. Though still largely undeveloped, it was already vigorous and enterprising. One manifestation of this was its already expanding maritime trade. Sailing ships for world commerce were coming down the ways at an ever increasing rate, and the maritime service was becoming one of the nation's most important occupations.

The farmer of Virginia and the tradesman of Boston had roots which were firmly established in their respective communities, which they were helping to support in the form of taxation. The merchant seaman, on the other hand, led a precarious existence somewhat resembling that of the itinerant or vagabond. In a great many instances he had neither a permanent abode nor a permanent route. His ship was the closest approach to a home, and his ship might be in New York harbor one week, in Charleston the next, and in Liverpool within a month. Despite this, he too was an American citizen and deserving of what security and assistance his nation could find possible to provide its citizens. For a period, however, things did not work out that way. Like anyone, the sailor was subject to injury or illness. In fact, because of the hazards of his occupation he was subject to greater than average risk. Furthermore, he was not overpaid, and what payment he received at the end of a journey was more often than not quickly removed from him in the taverns and brothels which thrived in the vicinity of the wharves. As a result he usually found it difficult or impossible to pay for whatever medical or hospital care he needed. Because he paid no local or state taxes and usually was not a member in good standing of whatever port city he happened to be in when ill, responsibility for him was usually avoided by the local authorities.

The young American Congress, becoming conscious of this undesirable state of affairs, passed the Marine Hospital Service Act in June 1798, which authorized the President to appoint physicians in each port to furnish medical and hospital care for sick and disabled seamen. Twenty cents per month was deducted from the pay of each man, the money being collected from the paymasters by the customs officers of the Treasury Department. Since the money was placed in the custody of the Treasury Department, there came about the somewhat anomalous situation whereby until 1935 the majority of federal public health services were carried out under the egis of the Treasury Department. The small sum of 20 cents per month, subsequently increased to 40 cents per month, is of particular interest in that it actually represented a sickness insurance payment and provided the precedent for the first prepaid comprehensive medical and hospital insurance plan in the country, under the administrative supervision of what eventually became a public health agency. In 1884 the tax of 40 cents per month was discontinued and replaced by a tonnage tax. The tonnage tax is still collected but now goes into the general Treasury, from which the hospitals are supported through appropriations to the Public Health Service.

At first the physicians serving the plan were also engaged in the private practice of medicine, but before long the demands for service became so great that the full-time employment of physicians was indicated. Originally, sailors needing hospital care were placed in whatever public or private hospitals existed at the ports. However, as in the case of the physicians, the demand for hospital services soon became so great that within 2 years (1800) the first marine hospital was constructed at Norfolk, Va. This was followed by similar hospitals throughout the country, at first at certain seaports and later at a number of places along inland waterways. By September 1963 there were 11 hospitals officially referred to as Public Health Service Hospi-

tals. Ten are general hospitals located at Staten Island, Baltimore, New Orleans, Seattle, San Francisco, Norfolk, Boston, Detroit, Savannah, and Galveston. The remaining hospital is the National Leprosarium at Carville, La. The total capacity is approximately 3,179 beds. In addition, outpatient facilities are operated in 28 cities. The Service also maintains contract arrangements in about 120 cities, where the use of non-Service facilities is economically more feasible. In addition, 49 hospitals, 46 community health centers, and about 300 other health stations are operated exclusively for American Indians and Eskimos by the Division of Indian Health. Two clinical research centers for drug addicts and certain mental patients are in operation at Lexington, Ky., and Fort Worth, Tex., by the National Institute of Mental Health.

Through time, eligibility for admittance to Public Health Service Hospitals has been broadened, and now United States merchant seamen constitute less than 50% of all patients. Eligibility now includes:

1. Seamen employed on vessels of the United States, registered, enrolled, and licensed under the maritime laws thereof, other than canal boats engaged in coastal trade
2. Enrollees in the United States Maritime Service on active duty and members of the Merchant Marine Cadet Corps
3. Cadets at state maritime academies or on state training ships
4. Federal Civil Service employees injured or taken ill in line of duty and falling within purview of regulations governing the administration of Federal Employee's Compensation Act
5. Officers and enlisted men of the United States Coast Guard, active or retired, and their dependents
6. Officers of United States Public Health Service, active or retired, and their dependents
7. Ships' officers and crew members of vessels of the United States Environmental Science Services Administration (formerly, Coast and Geodetic

Survey), active and retired, and their dependents

8. Officers and enlisted men of the United States Army, Navy, Marine Corps, and Air Force, active or retired, and their dependents
9. Any person requiring immunization for yellow fever

Foreign seamen and nonbeneficiary emergency cases are charged for outpatient and/or inpatient medical care according to rates established by the Bureau of Budget.

It is interesting that a medical director or supervising surgeon for the Service was not appointed until 1870. Compensation at the time amounted to a salary of $2,000, plus travel expenses. This position was later to become that of Surgeon General.

The growing concern of the federal and state governments with the need for preventing the introduction of epidemic diseases led to the passage in 1878 of the first port quarantine act. Entry into the country was limited to its ports, and as a consequence it was readily realized that the ports were the nation's first line of defense against epidemic diseases. Since the incidence of these diseases was invariably greater at ports, the physicians of the Marine Hospital Service had more opportunity to see and become acquainted with them. In addition, since epidemics usually began at the ports and frequently got out of hand, the states had developed the custom of asking or authorizing the federally employed Marine Hospital Service physicians to aid in the control of local situations. It was logical, therefore, that the responsibility for carrying out the new port quarantine activities should have been placed in the Marine Hospital Service. Quarantine stations presently operate in 23 ports.

The law of 1878 embodied another most important new departure, since it gave authority for investigating the origin and causes of epidemic diseases, especially yellow fever and cholera, and the best methods of preventing their introduction and spread. With but little delay, attempts were begun to prevent the entry of communicable disease by control measures carried out at the ports of origin of those who might potentially be carriers of disease. Marine Hospital Service physicians were attached to the offices of the consular service in major foreign ports, and a system of reporting communicable disease through the consular service was put into effect. In 1890 domestic quarantine was added, providing for interstate control of communicable disease. This was an immediate outgrowth of a particularly devastating epidemic of yellow fever that began at New Orleans and spread throughout the Mississippi Valley. Between the time of the Louisiana Purchase, in 1803, and the beginning of the twentieth century, New Orleans experienced no fewer than 37 severe epidemics of yellow fever, to say nothing of constantly recurring outbreaks of cholera, plague, and smallpox.

In 1890, Congress gave the Marine Hospital Service authority to carry out medical inspections of all immigrants. This was intended first to bar lunatics and others unable to care for themselves, but the following year "persons suffering from loathsome and contagious diseases" were added. In that year Congress also saw fit to provide quasi-military status for the personnel of the Marine Hospital Service, so the men were given commissions and uniforms. The year 1901 saw the establishment of the Hygienic Laboratory. Fortunately, from the start it was developed with such skill, imagination, and foresight that it soon became one of the world's leading centers of public health and medical research. Originally organized in three divisions of chemistry, zoology, and pharmacology, its functions were expanded in 1912 by an act authorizing the laboratory to "study and investigate the diseases of man and conditions influencing the origin and spread thereof including sanitation and sewage, and the pollution directly or indirectly of navigable streams and lakes of the United States and may from time to time issue information in the form of publications for the use of the public." Under consistently able direction the Hygienic Laboratory, which was later to become the National Institutes of

Health, attracted and developed a steady stream of outstanding investigators, including Carter, Sternberg, Rosenau, Goldberger, Frost, Leake, Armstrong, Stiles, Lumsden, Francis, Spencer, Maxcy, and Dyer, to name but a few. The contributions of these men and their co-workers caused Dr. William H. Welch to state publicly that there was no research institute in the world which was making such distinguished contributions to basic research in public health. The subsequent development of the National Institutes of Health will be discussed later.

In 1902, recognizing that the Marine Hospital Service had come of age, Congress renamed it the Public Health and Marine Hospital Service and gave it a definite form of organization under the direction of a surgeon general. The reorganization act was of further significance in that for the first time the Surgeon General was authorized and directed to call an annual conference of all state and territorial health officers. In 1912 the Service experienced another change in title, this time to the United States Public Health Service.

From this point on the Public Health Service grew rapidly under the impetus of an increasingly complex society, two great wars, and an economic depression. In 1917 the National Leprosarium at Carville, La., was established. In the same year the Service became responsible for the physical and mental examination of all arriving aliens. The year 1917 is also noteworthy for congressional appropriation of $25,000 for the Public Health Service to spend in cooperating with the states on studies and demonstrations in rural health work. This modest appropriation represented the beginning of a new administrative approach in federal-state public health relationships. In 1918, because of problems brought to public awareness by our entry into World War I, a Division of Venereal Diseases was created, with power to cooperate with state departments of health for the control and prevention of these diseases. In 1929 a Narcotics Division, later renamed the Division of Mental Hygiene, was created with hospital facilities at Lexington, Ky., and Fort

Worth, Tex., for the confinement and treatment of narcotic addicts.

Developments of far-reaching consequence occurred in 1935 with the passage of the Federal Social Security Act. Title VI of the act, which relates to the Public Health Service, was written "for the purpose of assisting states, counties, health districts, and other political subdivisions of the states in establishing and maintaining adequate public health service, including the training of personnel for state and local health work. . . ." Associated with the act was an appropriation which made possible grants-in-aid to the states and territories according to budgets submitted to the Surgeon General and approved by him. This brought with it a most difficult administrative problem for the Service, which has constantly attempted to determine an equitable basis on which the funds may be distributed. While subject to frequent adaptation, an attempt has been made to allocate these funds on the basis of four factors: (1) population, (2) public health problems, (3) economic need, and (4) training of public health personnel. The method of allocation has carried with it an educational value for state legislators since considerable proportions of the grants-in-aid must be matched by existing state and local appropriations. Results were rapidly forthcoming. More than a year after the funds were first made available, not only was there a marked increase in the number of new local health departments but, in addition, 19 states which did not already have such service set up central facilities for the promotion and supervision of local health administration; 33 state health departments strengthened their public health engineering forces; 11 states added new units for the investigation and promotion of industrial hygiene; preventable disease control groups were materially strengthened in 24 states; laboratory facilities were augmented in 27 states; 19 states made needed improvements in the personnel and equipment for vital statistics; public health nursing was strengthened either directly or indirectly in practically all states; 11 states provided special measures for syphilis control; and 13 states provided measures for the control of tuberculosis.[23] In 1938 a second Federal Venereal Disease Control Act was passed, designed to promote the investigation and control of the venereal diseases and to provide funds for assistance to state and local health agencies in establishing and maintaining adequate measures to that end.

In 1939, as part of President Roosevelt's program for the reorganization and consolidation of federal services, a Federal Security Agency was created for the purpose of bringing together a large part of the health, welfare, and educational services of the federal government. After 141 years, only 9 years less than the life of the nation itself, the Public Health Service left the now anachronistic administrative jurisdiction of the Treasury Department. At that time the Service had the following eight divisions, each under an assistant surgeon general:

    I. Division of Scientific Research (including the National Institute of Health and the National Cancer Institute)
    II. Division of Domestic Quarantine (including State Relations)
    III. Division of Foreign and Insular Quarantine
    IV. Division of Sanitary Reports and Statistics
    V. Division of Marine Hospitals and Relief
    VI. Division of Mental Hygiene
    VII. Division of Venereal Disease Control
    VIII. Division of Personnel and Accounts

Since that time, in order to achieve greater organizational efficiency and to bring the benefits of research and federal health legislation more quickly and effectively to the people of the nation, the Public Health Service underwent a number of reorganizations in 1944, in 1954, and again in 1963. Recently its goals, programs, and organization have been the subject of several intensive studies and reviews.[24,25] As a result it has again been reorganized in 1968. The present structure is shown in Fig. 11-4.

During the interval many further developments of consequence have occurred. In 1946, Congress passed the Hospital Survey and Construction (Hill-Burton) Act, which placed upon the Public Health Service administrative responsibility for a na-

tionwide program of hospital and health center construction. Each year since 1947, Congress has appropriated from $75 million to $150 million for this purpose; the federal contributions must be matched by from one third to two thirds state and local funds. In 1954, Congress enlarged the program to permit federal assistance in the construction of other types of health facilities as well as hospitals and health centers. Now eligible are general hospitals, mental hospitals, tuberculosis hospitals, chronic disease hospitals, public health centers, diagnostic and treatment centers, rehabilitation facilities, nursing homes, state health laboratories, and nurse training facilities.

The research activities of the Public Health Service date back about three quarters of a century to a one-room Laboratory of Hygiene in the Marine Hospital on Staten Island which was devoted to bacteriologic studies of returning seamen. This grew slowly to become the National Hygienic Laboratory, later renamed the National Institute of Health, which was located on a farm in Bethesda, Md., about 10 miles from Washington. From these humble beginnings has grown the greatest medical research center in the world. In 1937, Congress indicated its concern over a rapidly growing health problem by passing the National Cancer Act, which provided for the establishment of a National Cancer Institute for research into the cause, diagnosis, and treatment of cancer, for assistance to public and private agencies involved with the problem, and for the promotion of the most effective methods of prevention and treatment of the disease. In 1946 the National Mental Health Act was passed. This measure authorized $7.5 million for the construction and equipment of hospital and laboratory facilities to be operated by the Public Health Service as a stimulating center for research and training in the field of mental health; $10 million for grants to states; and an additional $1 million for demonstrations and personnel to assist the states.

In 1948 the National Heart Institute was authorized by Congress, and three other institutes—the Microbiological Institute, the Experimental Biology and Medicine Institute (these two joined in 1955 to form the National Institute of Allergy and Infectious Diseases), and the National Institute of Dental Research—were established by regrouping existing units; the National Institute of Health became the National *Institutes* of Health. In 1949 the activities of the Mental Hygiene Division were transferred from the Bureau of Medical Services to the National Institutes of Health to form the National Institute of Mental Health. In 1950 the National Institute of Neurological Diseases and Blindness was founded, and in 1959 the National Institute of Arthritis and Metabolic Diseases came into being. In 1962, legislation raised the Division of General Medical Sciences to institute status and also established an Institute of Child Health and Human Development.

As time passed, an increasing amount of the NIH's function came to be fulfilled by grants to universities and other extramural research centers. By now about 80% of its budget goes to finance research in such centers throughout the United States and abroad. At this time the federal government supports more than 16,000 separate research projects and the advanced training of about 25,000 scientists in the health field. Because of the evergrowing grant programs, the NIH found it necessary to establish certain organizations to handle them. In 1947 it formed a Division of Research Grants, in 1955 a Division of Research Services, and in 1962 a Division of Research Facilities and Resources. With the burgeoning of the pharmaceutical industry and market it also became necessary to establish in 1955 a Division of Biological Standards.

In order to accelerate research and its confirmation and final application, the Public Health Service in 1952 completed and opened the National Clinical Center on the grounds of the National Institutes of Health in Bethesda, Md. This is a research hospital of 516 beds, with twice as much space for laboratories (about 1,000 of them) as for patient care. Each institute of the National Institutes of Health has space for patients and laboratories in close proxim-

ity. Patients are admitted only when they meet the requirements of a particular study being conducted by one or more institutes. A patient chosen by a particular institute, for example, may be one of a group of patients having the same type of condition at the same stage and site. Often factors such as the patient's sex, age, and weight must also be taken into consideration. Patients may be accepted from any part of the country.

The planning and conduct of research in the Clinical Center is the responsibility of each institute. When a problem is selected, the methods of approach are determined by a research team, which may include scientists from more than one institute and from other research organizations. Special provisions are made so that outstanding laboratory scientists and research physicians from other institutions may work in the Clinical Center for periods ranging from a few months to a year or more on problems of their own choosing. As a result investigations involve numerous scientific fields and widely varying viewpoints, bringing laboratory and clinical workers into close daily association in a search for answers to both basic scientific and practical problems.

The staff of the Clinical Center immediately responsible for the care of a patient maintains intimate morking relationships with the physicians and institutions who send patients to the Center. This professional liaison is so close that for all practical purposes the referring physician is a member of the research team and the Clinical Center becomes a major addition to the resources available to the physician for the study and benefit of his patient. Through the years Congress has shown an intense and growing interest in health research. Necessarily appropriations have had to be constantly increased to the point where in 1966 the total budget of the National Institutes of Health reached $1.2 billion. It is also noteworthy that in 1965, Congress authorized an additional $280 million for the construction of other laboratories throughout the nation during the next 3 years.

To return for a moment to 1956, another significant event was the transfer of the Army Medical Library to the Public Health Service, which has since established it as an expanded National Library of Medicine in an excellent structure on the grounds of the National Institutes of Health. A very important activity at the Library has been the development and implementation of the computer-based MEDLARS (Medical Literature Analysis and Retrieval System). This is an automated bibliographic service to assist users in selecting material pertinent to their area of interest. It has become necessary because of the inability of conventional methods to keep current with the tremendous growth of medical literature. This development probably leads the way for the National Library of Medicine to become, among other things, a center for research in biomedical communications. In this regard a Division of Computer Research and Technology is developing as a component of the National Institutes of Health. Another recent unit in the Public Health Service is the Division of Regional Medical Programs, established in 1967 in relation to the Heart, Cancer, and Stroke Amendments.

Mention should be made of a number of other important post-World War II additions to the resources of the Public Health Service. One was the development of the National Office of Vital Statistics, later renamed the National Center for Health Statistics. This valuable staff unit provides a vast amount of detailed data concerning health, illness, injuries, and death. Of very great significance was the establishment at the end of World War II of the Communicable Disease Center in Atlanta, Ga. This outstanding organization has grown to become not only one of the world's great epidemiologic centers but also an outstanding training center for various types of health personnel as well as a leading center for health communications and educational methods. Another important postwar development was the establishment in 1954 of the Robert A. Taft Sanitary Engineering Center in Cincinnati as a center for research and training in vari-

ous aspects of environmental health. In 1966 this institution and the responsibility for water-pollution control were transferred to a new Federal Water Pollution Administration in the Department of Interior. Meanwhile, plans are underway for the construction in Cincinnati by the Public Health Service of a National Environmental Health Research Center that will be particularly concerned with research in the engineering aspects of solid waste disposal and occupational health. Also, there is under construction in North Carolina a large Environmental Health Science Center which is to be concerned especially with the biomedical aspects of environmental hazards.

Mention has been made of the growing interest of Congress in health affairs. This has by no means been limited to research. In fact the past several Congresses have raised repeated question about the application of the growing fund of knowledge in the health and medical field—how to close the gap between the acquisition of knowledge and its application for the welfare of the people. The Eighty-ninth Congress was especially notable in this regard. It had the distinction of being known as the most "health minded" Congress in our history.[26] An astounding number of legislative acts were passed which, if wisely used by public health workers, will completely recast the nature, structure, and effectiveness of public health in the United States. There appear to have been three great turning points in public health history in the United States, and it is interesting that they have been about 50 years, or two generations, apart: the 1860's, when the Shattuck Report began to exert an influence; the 1910's, when the groundwork was laid for so much of public health development since; and the 1960's, when public health really began to broaden its horizons and abandon the barrier between it and medical care and when Congress decided to make undreamed of resources available for undreamed of accomplishments. It would appear that public health has now come of age.

Included in the legislation with pertinence to health that was passed by the Eighty-ninth Congress were:

The Drug Abuse Control Amendments (P.L. 89-74)

The Federal Cigarette Labeling and Advertising Act (P.L. 89-92)

The Mental Retardation Facilities and Community Mental Health Centers Construction Act Amendments (P.L. 89-105)

The Community Health Services Extension Amendments (P.L. 89-109)

The Health Research Facilities Amendments (P.L. 89-115)

The Public Works and Economic Development Act (P.L. 89-136)

The Water Quality Act (P.L. 89-234)

The Heart Disease, Cancer, and Stroke Amendments (Regional Medical Programs) (P.L. 89-239)

The Clean Air Act Amendments and the Solid Waste Disposal Act (P.L. 89-272)

The Health Professions Educational Assistance Amendments (P.L. 89-290)

The Medical Library Assistance Act (P.L. 89-291)

The Appalachian Regional Development Act (P.L. 89-4)

The Older Americans Act (P.L. 89-73)

The Social Security Amendments (Medicare, Medicaid, Comprehensive Child Health Care) (P.L. 89-97)

The Vocational Rehabilitation Amendments (P.L. 89-333)

The Housing and Urban Development Act (P.L. 89-117)

The Extended Comprehensive Health Planning and Public Health Services Amendments (P.L. 89-749)

The Allied Health Professions Personnel Training Act (P.L. 89-751)

The Demonstration Cities and Metropolitan Development Act (P.L. 89-754)

The Traffic Safety Act (P.L. 89-563)

This partial list represents a formidable health legislative record indeed! Its significance is well summarized by Forgotson[27]:

The deep and long-term significance of the 1965 federal health legislation ... lies in the changing role of government in the direction of widening the responsibility of the public sector (as exemplified by the Medicare amendments) and in developing new patterns of medical service and continuing education (as exemplified by the Regional Medical Programs). The introduction of systems engineering and operations analysis into the total health endeavor (see Chapter 14) will permit the development of sound priorities, effective controls, and improved administration. Comprehensive legislation covering every facet of resources and services makes 1965 the turning point in health legislation.

The cumulative effect of all of the foregoing developments has been a remarkable growth in the size and usefulness of the Public Health Service. This growth may be illustrated in one way in terms of expenditures. In 1900 the budget of the Marine Hospital Service was about $1.4 million; by 1950, almost $120 million; by 1960, it had reached about $300 million. Seven years later, in 1967, federal expenditures for health totaled well over $3 billion, of which about two thirds or $2.03 million was budgeted for the Public Health Service. Through the years since 1798, great responsibilities have been placed upon the Public Health Service. It is fortunately appropriate to state that the Service has met its responsibilities and opportunities as a governmental agency remarkably well, as is readily evident from its admirable record. It is probable that no one in the nation passes a day without being affected by its efforts in some way.

THE CHILDREN'S BUREAU

Next in importance to the Public Health Service in federal health activities is the Children's Bureau. The conception, establishment, and development of this specialized agency is worthy of considerable study by students of public administration. While appearing on the surface to be concerned with matters of a noncontroversial nature, the Bureau from its inception has been a principal in many disputes and the target of not a few administrative and ideologic struggles.

The idea of a separate Children's Bureau was first suggested to President Theodore Roosevelt in New York City.[28] As pointed out later by Julia C. Lathrop,[29] who served as the first chief of the Bureau from 1912 to 1921, it was no coincidence that "this bureau was first urged by women who have lived long in settlements and who by that experience have learned to know as well as any person in this country certain aspects of dumb misery which they desired through some governmental agency to make articulate and intelligible."

The support of numerous protagonists was obtained, with little delay, among them the National Consumers League, the National Child Labor Committee, and many national women's organizations and church groups. Arguing for a center of research and information concerning the welfare of mothers and children, they maintained an active lobby and pressure group in Washington until their goal was ultimately obtained. One of their most effective arguments was that the federal government had already set a precedent by establishing centers of research and information in other fields relating to national resources and that it might well become similarly concerned with its most important resource, the mothers and children of the nation. Between 1906 and 1912 many bills concerned with the establishment of a Children's Bureau were introduced and extensive hearings held on each. Both President Theodore Roosevelt and, later, President Taft gave support to the movement, which incurred but little opposition. Eventually Congress was spurred to final action and passed a measure sponsored by Senator Borah on April 9, 1912.

One of the reasons for delay was controversy over the placement of the bureau in the federal governmental structure. The three possibilities suggested were the Bureau of Labor and the Bureau of the Census, both in the Department of Commerce and Labor, and the Bureau of Education, in the Department of the Interior. It should be noted that the United States Public Health Service, then a part of the Treasury Department, was not considered. This may have been due to the submergence of the health aspects by the broader social service aspects of the proposed Bureau. The failure on the part of the Public Health Service to concern itself with the problem at the time was to lay the groundwork for subsequent controversies over administrative jurisdiction and organization.

The Act of 1912, which established the Children's Bureau,[30] placed it as an agency in the Department of Commerce and Labor. When this Department was divided the following year, the Bureau was retained by the Department of Labor. The act directed that the "said Bureau shall investigate and report . . . upon all matters pertaining to the welfare of children and child life, among all classes of people, and shall especially investigate the questions of infant mortality, the birth rate, orphanages, juvenile courts, desertions, dangerous occupations, accidents, and diseases of children, employment, legislation affecting children in the several states and territories." While originally given authority merely to *investigate* and *report,* the Bureau trained a highly technical staff of experts who rapidly gained in experience. The Bureau thus became the natural agency to be entrusted with new programs dealing with problems of maternal and child welfare. During the early years of its existence the Bureau, in accordance with Congressional direction, followed a path of extensive and fruitful scientific research and dissemination of information. Many studies were made of the effect of income, housing, employment, and other factors on the infant and maternal mortality rates. These studies led to the White House Conferences on child health, the first of which was held in 1919. Evidence gathered in some of the investigations was used by the National Child Labor Committee in obtaining the passage of the Federal Child-Labor Law in 1915. This law, with the Children's Bureau designated as the administering agency, was effective from 1917 to 1918, when it was declared unconstitutional by the Supreme Court.

Study of maternal and infant care problems in rural areas led to the introduction of bills intended to encourage the establishment of maternal and child welfare programs by means of grants-in-aid to the states. The Children's Bureau, designated in the bills as the administering and supervising agency, quickly found itself the subject of attacks from a number of quarters. It was argued that the adoption of the Sheppard-Towner Bill would provide an entering wedge for socialized medicine, that it would centralize power in the hands of federal bureaucrats, and that personal, family, and states' rights would be violated. The American Medical Association, the Anti-Suffragists, the Sentinels of the Republic, and a number of other organizations arrayed themselves in opposition.

During the hearings a controversy that had begun to smolder between the Public Health Service and the Children's Bureau broke through. Some of the opponents of the bill were willing to compromise by favoring administration by the Public Health Service. The decision depended on whether the chief concern of the bill was with health or with general child welfare. Congress, deciding upon the broader viewpoint, retained the Children's Bureau as the administering agency when final approval was given in 1921. One authority[31] has pointed out that unquestionably the Bureau was able to maintain its position "by right of discovery and occupation and that the Public Health Service had been derelict in not promoting this type of work with sufficient vigor to maintain its belated claim to jurisdiction." In their analysis of the Emergency Maternity and Infant Care Program, Sinai and Anderson,[32] in referring to this conclusion, observe that it merits reading and rereading by public health officers today. They point out that, when the suggestion of a governmental health plan arises, one of the first concerns is with the agency of administration and that control by right of occupation has occurred more often than not in government.

The Sheppard-Towner Act established in a very real sense a pattern for maternal and child health programs throughout the country. It provided for federal assistance to states in the form of grants-in-aid for use in attacking problems of maternal and infant welfare and mortality. The states were given authority to initiate and to administer their own plans subject to approval by a Federal Board of Maternity and Infant Hygiene, consisting of the Chief of the Children's Bureau, the Surgeon General of the Public Health Service, and the Commissioner of Education. Prior to the passage of the act, 32 states had established divisions or bureaus of child hygiene. During the following 2 years an additional 15 states developed programs of this nature. While it is difficult to conclusively prove a causative relationship, the Children's Bureau is generally given major credit for the increased interest and action.

The original act provided for a 5-year program. In 1926 a bill was introduced for the extension of the act to 7 years. This provided opponents with another opportunity for attack. The 2-year extension, although granted, signaled the end of the program, further efforts to continue it being fruitless. The importance of the federal aid was well illustrated by the fact that following expiration of the program 35 states decreased appropriations, 9 eliminated appropriations, and only 5 reported increases for the maternal and child health program.

With the adoption of the Social Security Act in 1935 the Children's Bureau not only regained its lost functions but added to them. Under Title V of the Social Security Act the Children's Bureau was given responsibility for the administration of programs dealing with maternal and child health, crippled children, and child welfare services. To implement these ends, the Bureau was allotted an annual budget of $8.17 million for grants-in-aid exclusive of administrative costs. In 1939 this sum was increased to $11 million and in 1946 to $22 million. Within 10 months after the grants-in-aid became available all of the 48 states, the District of Columbia, Alaska, and Hawaii submitted requests and plans for approval. In this way, state maternal and child health programs received a much needed transfusion.

Through time there has been ample evidence of the success of the pioneering and stimulating efforts of the Children's Bureau. Thus in 1940, federal contributions accounted for 48% of the total sum spent for maternal and child health activities; since then, state and local governments have assumed increasing proportions of the costs.

With the entrance of the United States into World War II and the subsequent draft of a large proportion of the male population many wives, expectant mothers, and infants found themselves in somewhat precarious economic positions, reflected in their inability to pay for private obstetric and medical care. Congress, becoming aware of the problem in 1943, decided to take action, and established the Emergency Maternity and Infant Care Program, which functioned throughout the war years.[32] It considered the Children's Bureau to be the logical federal agency for the administration and supervision of the program of aid which it decided upon. Once again the factor of prior interest and occupation decided the issue of administrative jurisdiction. The Children's Bureau had attempted, to the best of its ability and using some of its grants-in-aid funds, to do what it could to alleviate the situation. Congress decided to take action by means of supplementing the grants-in-aid funds of the Bureau. As a result a series of appropriation acts were passed involving a total of more than $130 million. The use of these sums made possible the provision of much needed obstetric care for about 1.2 million expectant mothers and pediatric care for about 200,000 infants. An incidental but significant result was that the staffs of the Children's Bureau and of many State Health Departments obtained an invaluable experience in medical care administration.

The Children's Bureau has continued to expand its leadership in many fields, including audiology, perinatal mortality, prematurity, rheumatic fever, epilepsy, cerebral palsy, mental retardation, juvenile delinquency, nutrition of growth and development, problems of children of migratory workers, and children's dentistry.[33]

The Children's Bureau shared in the momentous legislative advances of the mid-1960's. Because of increased awareness of and concern about the relatively high rate of perinatal mortality as well as premature births, handicapping conditions, and mental retardation, Congress passed the Maternal and Child Health and Mental Retardation Planning Amendments of 1963. This law authorized project grants to meet up to 75% of the costs of projects to provide comprehensive maternity care for high risk mothers in low income families and care for their children. Two years later, in 1965, when Section 532 of Title V, Part 4, of the Social Security Act was amended, provision was made for the development of high quality comprehensive health services for children and youth.

The combined objective of these two pieces of legislation is the reduction of maternal, infant, and child morbidity and mortality by assisting communities to organize and use their services and resources to maximum efficiency. For improved maternal and infant care, funds are used for the establishment of prenatal and postpartum clinics, hospitalization, medical salaries or fees, salaries of public health nurses, health education, and various other services. The Social Security Amendments of 1965 make possible some major departures from traditional public health services. Comprehensiveness and continuity of care are stressed. There is no separation of preventive and promotive health services from treatment and rehabilitation, nor are services limited to particular illness categories. All health problems of the children involved are to be taken care of by the program, either by direct services or by referral to appropriate resources in the area concerned. Medical, dental, and emotional health problems are all included and, since particular emphasis is placed upon children of families often unaccustomed to seeking care, outreach casefinding is provided. These two programs are especially needed in areas where there are many people of low incomes and where there are apt to be few practitioners of medicine and dentistry, a situation common to city slums. These efforts are bringing convenient, well-organized, high quality comprehensive health services to those who need them the most and have obtained them the least.

In the process the public health agencies of some cities have developed some new, very interesting, and effective working relationships with medical schools and other organizations in their jurisdictions. Also, wherever programs exist through the egis of the Economic Opportunity Act to assist the socioeconomically disadvantaged, the new maternal and child health programs have been intimately coordinated with them.

From the standpoint of organization, early in 1963, soon after its fiftieth anniversary, the Children's Bureau became part of a new Welfare Administration in the Department of Health, Education, and Welfare. Subsequently, in August 1967 it became part of a new major unit in the Department. This unit, named the Social and Rehabilitation Service, also includes the functions of the former Welfare Administration, the Vocational Rehabilitation Administration, the Administration on Aging, and the Mental Retardation Division of the Public Health Service. The new agency is designed to join under single leadership both the income-support programs for those in need and the social service and rehabilitation programs that many individuals and families require.

THE DEPARTMENT OF HEALTH, EDUCATION, AND WELFARE

In 1946 the Federal Security Agency underwent further accretion and the various federal health services were further consolidated by the transfers of the Children's Bureau from the Department of Labor and the Food and Drug Administration from the Department of Agriculture. At about the same time the National Office of Vital Statistics was transferred from the Bureau of the Census of the Department of Commerce to the Public Health Service. In this way the activities of the agencies concerned with various aspects of health and sanitation were brought into closer working relationship. Then in 1953 the first move taken by President Eisenhower to reorganize the Executive Branch of the Government was to propose that the Federal Security Agency be granted Cabinet status.

The proposal became fact on April 11, 1953, when Congress established the Department of Health, Education, and Welfare. On the same day the first Secretary of the newly created Executive Department of Health, Education, and Welfare was sworn into office.

The purpose of this plan was to bring together and improve the administration of the important health, education, and social security functions then being carried on by the federal government. Up to the present this plan has succeeded only partially; the functions, relations, and organization of the basic components have not yet changed in a fundamental sense. This has led some to refer to the Department as an enormous social welfare "holding company," a "bureaucratic maze" for which no effective guide exists.

The Department of Health, Education, and Welfare, therefore, is not an administrative or functional unity designed to accomplish a specific mission. It consists of units of differing organization, expertise, and interests. Most units have strong traditions and histories which antedate the Department considerably. Many have separate, strong, and effective Congressional ties and do not hesitate to use them unilaterally. Yet the tide of recent events has made quite clear the need to bring about a more effective operational relationship among those working in the fields of health services, education, and social security. This, as indicated earlier, has led to increased attention to the exceedingly difficult problem of bringing about a truly effective reorganization of the Department.[24,25] The most recent organization, effective in early 1968, is shown in Fig. 11-4.

VOLUNTARY HEALTH AGENCIES

While the official, governmental, or public health agencies were still in the process of development, a complementary and supplementary force appeared in the form of voluntary or nonofficial health agencies. This is considered in detail in Chapter 12. Beginning with the establishment of a local antituberculosis society in 1892, the voluntary health movement soon developed considerable force and magnitude. Spurred by public interest, by desire for private philanthropy, and sometimes by impatience or dissatisfaction with governmental programs, over 20,000 such agencies were established during the ensuing half century. They draw voluntary support from literally millions of persons and serve millions of others.

Not infrequently the development of these agencies has been intimately bound to certain strong and appealing personalities such as Beers, Trudeau, Wald, and Franklin Roosevelt. One interesting aspect of their development is that, while some agencies, such as the antituberculosis associations, began locally and spread upward to state and national levels, others, such as the National Foundation for Infantile Paralysis, began on the national level and spread downward. Still others, notably the mental hygiene associations, began on the state level and spread both upward and downward.

One phase of the voluntary health movement, visiting nursing, deserves particular mention. Dr. William Welch once singled out public health nursing as perhaps America's greatest contribution to the public health movement. It had its origin in 1877 in the Women's Branch of the New York City Mission and was organized for the purpose of teaching hygiene in the homes of the underprivileged. In 1902, Lillian Wald organized the first school nursing program in New York City, setting up a pattern which was rapidly followed throughout the nation. Largely from these modest beginnings developed the adoption of public health nursing as a most important part of any public health program. Among the important recent developments, as discussed in Chapter 33, is the move toward merger of official and voluntary visiting nursing programs and the development of and experimentation with new types of auxiliary personnel, such as Home Health Aids.

COUNTY HEALTH DEPARTMENTS

In the year 1910-1911 there occurred in Yakima County, Wash., one of a series of

severe typhoid fever epidemics. Because it was uncontrolled by local authorities, Dr. Lumsden of the United States Public Health Service was loaned to bring it under control. In his own colorful manner, Dr. Lumsden not only solved the particular epidemiologic problem but went on to suggest ways of preventing its recurrence. One of his strongest recommendations dealt with the desirability of establishing a full-time resident staff to deal with all public health matters. Meanwhile the Rockefeller Sanitary Commission, which had been working in the southeastern United States as well as in Central and South America, came to the conclusion that no single disease, sanitary problem, or public health problem could be successfully attacked without concurrent efforts aimed at all phases of public health. As a result they also strongly recommended the establishment of local full-time resident public health staffs. There resulted the interesting situation whereby at almost the same moment at two different places for two different although related reasons, the first full-time county health departments were established: Guilford County, N. C., June 1911 and Yakima County, Wash., July 1911.* The fundamental soundness of the approach is given testimony by the continual adoption of the principle so that at the present time the majority of the population has local health services. The pursuit of the principle to its ultimate, complete coverage of the nation now represents one of the chief aims of all who are interested in public health, sociology, and medicine. With the increased trend toward core city-suburbia complexes as well as metropolitanization, there is underway a growing movement toward merger of city and county health departments in many situations. This trend, while fraught with difficulties of a political and fiscal nature due to an outdated intergovernmental system, to the extent that it succeeds can only bring about greater efficiency and improved public service. In discussing county health or-

---

*Some difference of opinion exists with regard to priority, many contending that Jefferson County, Ky., was the first in 1908.

ganization one should mention the Association of County Health Officers, which is related to the National Association of County Officials, an organization of ever growing significance and national influence.

DEVELOPMENT OF PROFESSIONAL TRAINING

The appointment of health officers for many towns and districts in midnineteenth century England led to the establishment of a course of lectures on public health at St. Thomas' Hospital, in London. This was the first training of its kind in England and led to the development of a number of excellent curricula and schools devoted specifically to the subject. Despite the many parallel interests and activities, no facilities existed in the United States for specialized training or education in public health until 1910. Since sanitary science and engineering were perhaps of predominant interest at the time, it is not illogical that the first teaching of public health was carried out particularly in relation with engineering. The first specific public health degree was awarded in 1910 at the University of Michigan. Beginning in 1912, a program of study was organized at the Massachusetts Institute of Technology by William T. Sedgwick, whose strong personality sent forth a large number of outstanding disciples in the new profession. After a few years, realizing that the environmental phases represented only a part of the total public health picture, there was formed a joint Massachusetts Institute of Technology-Harvard School of Public Health, which later divided when Harvard established its own separate School of Public Health. Meanwhile the first school of public health (now defunct) was organized at the University of Pennsylvania.

In considering these early attempts to establish public health training on a high professional level we again encounter the name of Rosenau, who served as codirector of the joint M.I.T.-Harvard school, whence he left to assume chairmanship of the division of preventive medicine in the Harvard School of Medicine. It was about this time (1913) that Rosenau brought out the first edition of his world-famous volume,

Preventive Medicine and Hygiene. One public health authority, Wilson G. Smillie, has commented that there can be little doubt that this one book has done as much to advance public health as any other single factor. It is of interest in passing that Dr. Rosenau in his perennial youthfulness of mind, on reaching the age of retirement at Harvard in 1936, went on to establish and direct another school of public health at the University of North Carolina before his death in 1946.

In connection with professional education and training in public health, recent years have seen many worthwhile developments. In the process the Committee on Professional Education of the American Public Health Association has played a most significant role in stimulation of thought and discussion, crystalization of ideas, and development and implementation of programs for the improvement of the quality of public health personnel. This is exemplified in its current activities, which include the accreditation of schools of public health, the development of statements on educational qualifications of personnel in the various public health disciplines, the development of field-training methods and standards, the conduct of a professional examination service, the development of recruitment programs, and the study of public health salaries. Mention should also be made of the great professional development value of the scientific sessions at its annual meetings.

Returning for the moment to academic training, as more and more demand developed for public health services, many schools and universities began to offer a wide variety of degrees in public health, often on a questionable basis. In 1941, the leading schools formed the Association of Schools of Public Health. This stimulated a study by the Committee on Professional Education of the American Public Health Association which led to the development and application by the Committee in 1946 of a system of accreditation for the granting of recognized degrees in public health. At the present time (1968) there are 17 schools so accredited—University of California at

Berkeley, University of California at Los Angeles, Columbia University, Harvard University, University of Hawaii, Johns Hopkins University, Loma Linda (Cal.) University, University of Michigan, University of Minnesota, University of Montreal, University of North Carolina, University of Oklahoma, University of Pittsburgh, University of Puerto Rico, University of Toronto, Tulane University, and Yale University. The Association maintains contact with other centers of public health education elsewhere in the world, especially those in Latin America, Great Britain, France, and the American University at Beirut in Lebanon. In recognition of the fact that the accredited schools in the United States serve regional, national, and, indeed, international needs a number of bills calling for the provision of federal subsidization have been introduced into Congress during the past few years. The first definitive result occurred in 1958 when the sum of $1 million was appropriated for strengthening the accredited schools by providing grants for construction and improvement of teaching facilities. The present law also provides funds for scholarships and loans to students who otherwise would be unable to pursue professional education.

In early 1949, recognizing that the full-time practice of preventive medicine and public health had long since become a specialty in the medical profession, the American Board of Preventive Medicine and Public Health was organized under the joint sponsorship of the American Medical Association, the American Public Health Association, the Association of Schools of Public Health, The Canadian Public Health Association, and the Southern Medical Association. Rigid standards and requirements with regard to training and experience were developed, and an examination system was established, upon the satisfactory completion of which candidates become certified as specialists in this field of medical practice. Soon after, in 1950, steps were taken for the development of approved field residency programs in acceptable public health organizations. Supervision and accreditation of these are under the joint egis of the American Board of Preventive Medicine and Public Health and the Council on Medical Education and Hospitals of the American Medical Association.

Since these last developments apply only to physicians, several of the other professional disciplines involved in public health work have developed or are now in the process of developing similar procedures for the accreditation of field training in their respective specialties.

As a result of these many activities the past decade has seen extensive improvements in all aspects of training, education, experience, and status of those who are devoting the energies of their professional lives to the improvement of the health of the public. Some aspects of these training and accreditation subjects are discussed further in the chapter on personnel.

REFERENCES

1. Rosen, G.: A history of public health, New York, 1958, MD Publications, Inc.
2. Top, F. H.: The history of American epidemiology, St. Louis, 1952, The C. V. Mosby Co.
3. Hanlon, J., Rogers, F., and Rosen, G.: A bookshelf on the history and philosophy of public health, Amer. J. Public Health 50:445, Apr. 1960.
4. Osler, W.: The functions of a state faculty, Maryland Med. J. 37:73, May 1897.
5. Hecker, I. F.: The epidemics of the Middle Ages, Philadelphia, 1837, Haswell, Barrington and Haswell.
6. Winslow, C.-E. A.: The evolution and significance of the modern public health campaign, New Haven, 1923, Yale University Press.
7. George, M. D.: London life in the XVIIIth century, New York, 1925, Alfred A. Knopf.
8. Richardson, B. W.: The health of nations, a review of the works of Edwin Chadwick, London, 1887, Longmans, Green & Co., vol. II.
9. Bowditch, H. I.: Address on hygiene and preventive medicine, Transactions of the International Medical Congress, Philadelphia, 1876.
10. Prescott, W. H.: History of the conquest of Mexico, New York, 1936, Random House, Inc.
11. Woodward, S. B.: The story of smallpox in Massachusetts, New Eng. J. Med. 206:1181, June 9, 1932.
12. Chadwick, H. D.: The diseases of the inhabitants of the commonwealth, New Eng. J. Med. 216:8, June 10, 1937.
13. Editorial: Has Baltimore the oldest health department? Amer. J. Public Health 35:49, Jan. 1945.
14. Newsholme, A., Sir: The ministry of health, London, 1925, G. P. Putnam's Sons, Ltd.

15. Kramer, H. D.: The beginnings of the public health movement in the United States, Bull. Hist. Med. **21**:369, 1947.

16. Holmes, O. W.: Writings, IX, medical essays, Boston, 1891, Houghton, Mifflin & Co.

17. Shattuck, L., et al.: Report of the Sanitary Commission of Massachusetts: 1850 (Dutton and Wentworth, State Printers, Boston, 1850), Cambridge, 1948, Harvard University Press.

18. Beck-Storrs, A.: Public health and government control, Social Studies **45**:211, Oct. 1954.

19. Patterson, R. S., and Baker, M. C.: Seventy-five years of public health in Massachusetts, Amer. J. Public Health **34**:1271, Dec. 1944.

20. Cavins, H. M.: The National Quarantine and Sanitary Conventions of 1857 to 1860 and the beginnings of the American Public Health Association, Bull. Hist. Med. **13**:404, Apr. 1943.

21. Smith, S.: Historical sketch of the American Public Health Association, Public Health **5**:7, 1889.

22. Smillie, W. G.: The National Board of Health, 1879-1883, Amer. J. Public Health **33**:925, Aug. 1943.

23. Annual Report of the Surgeon General of the Public Health Serivce, 1936.

24. Investigation of Health, Education, and Welfare, Report of the Special Subcommittee on Investigation of the Department of Health, Education, and Welfare of the Commission on Interstate and Foreign Commerce, House of Representatives, Eighty-Ninth Congress, second session, Oct. 13, 1966, House Report No. 2266.

25. Advisory Committee on Health, Education, and Welfare Relationships with State Health Agencies, Report to the Secretary of Health, Education, and Welfare, Dec. 30, 1966.

26. Rusk, H.: Congress and medicine, The New York Times, Nov. 20, 1965.

27. Forgotson, E.: 1965, The turning point in public health law—1966 reflections, Amer. J. Public Health **57**:934, June 1967.

28. The Children's Bureau, yesterday, today and tomorrow, Washington, 1937, U. S. Government Printing Office.

29. Lathrop, J. C.: Children's Bureau, Amer. J. Sociol. **18**:318, Nov. 1912.

30. 37 Stat., 79, 737, 1912.

31. Key, V. O.: The administration of federal grants to states, Chicago, 1937, Public Administration Service.

32. Sinai, N., and Anderson, O. W.: E.M.I.C., a study of administrative experience, 1948, University of Michigan.

33. Eliot, M. M.: The Children's Bureau, fifty years of public responsibility for action in behalf of children, Amer. J. Public Health **52**:576, Apr. 1962.

Chapter 3

World health problems*

INTRODUCTION

The ultimate strength of a nation is to be found in the quantity and quality of its people. Everything else, including agricultural, mineral, and industrial potential, is of value only to the extent and manner in which it may be related to people. The quantitative measure of a people is, of course, the population, especially the number of persons who are able to produce goods or children. The qualitative measure of a people is largely determined by the degree of illness or health and the rates by which it dies or survives. Four factors influence the growth or decline of a nation's population: the numbers of births, deaths, immigrants, and emigrants. At the moment we are not concerned with the last two. The first two, numbers of births and deaths, are of major social, economic, political, public health, and medical importance to every nation. Beyond this, their relationship to similar factors in other countries, especially those nearby, is frequently of utmost importance. It is therefore fundamental to any consideration of international problems or relationships that there be readily available an adequate fund of accurate statistical data relating to the number of persons in each nation as well as the rates and manner in which they are born, live, and die. Unfortunately, this is not the case. The student of international health problems is confronted at the outset by gross inadequacies in this respect and is forced to work to a considerable degree on the basis of impressions, estimates, and generalizations.

*The reader is referred to the final pages of Chapter 11 for a brief discussion of international health organization and programs.

It is not the purpose here to evaluate the completeness, accuracy, or comprehensiveness of various national or international vital statistics. However, it may be worth pointing out that, generally speaking, the most complex, industrialized, and highly developed countries have the most exact and adequate vital data whereas the least developed and youngest nations, and unfortunately many of those with the most outstanding health problems, tend to have the least satisfactory information about their people. One might generalize that population enumeration and birth and death registration are relatively good in the countries of Northern and Western Europe, parts of Central and Southern Europe, the British Isles, North America, Australia, New Zealand, and Japan. Conversely, they are less accurate, to varying degrees of course, in most countries of Central and South America, parts of Eastern and Southern Europe, and practically all of Africa, the Middle East, and Asia.

GENERAL OBSERVATIONS

Despite these limitations, there is sufficient knowledge and information to indicate considerable variation among countries with regard to the fertility, health, and longevity of their populations. For detailed information the reader is referred to the various statistical and epidemiologic reports of the World Health Organization. In evaluating these variations it is important to realize that many biologic, environmental, and social factors are involved. Thus climate, the nature of the soil, food consumption and habits, physical inheritance, and habits of work or exercise may affect the fertility, health, and mortality experiences of populations. Beyond these there are, of course, the influences of public health facilities, medical and nursing services, housing standards, and occupational conditions.

The key factor in determining the size of a population is the extent to which it can reproduce and maintain or increase itself. Various methods have been devised in order to measure this, the most common of which is the birthrate. In general, there appears to exist an inverse relationship between the birthrate and the degree of development of complexity of a nation. Thus the greater the degree of industrial and scientific progress, urbanization, and elevation of the standard of living, the more the birthrate tends to be depressed. There are, of course, a number of exceptions to this generalization. Nevertheless, birthrates have declined rather consistently in the European countries, the British Isles, North America, and Japan. By contrast, birthrates have tended to fall more slowly or to increase in the countries of Asia, Africa, and Central and South America.

The birthrate in itself is neither a true measure of human fertility nor indicative of the extent to which the number of births is sufficient to maintain or to increase the population of a nation. Because of this, additional indices such as the rate of natural increase and fertility rates have been devised. The rate of natural increase is simply the annual excess of births over deaths per thousand population. In general this rate is highest in the countries of Africa, the Middle East, Asia, Southeastern Europe, and parts of Central and South America and is lowest in Northern and Western Europe and North America. Even this rate of numerical excess of births over deaths, however, is not a conclusive indication of the ability of a country's population to reproduce itself. A particular country at a given time may have a very large excess of births over deaths, yet its birthrate, especially when determined in relation to the number of persons of childbearing age, may not be high enough to eventually maintain the present population. This can occur when a country has a temporarily high pro-

portion of young adults due to immigration or as a result of a mass delayed genetic action such as occurs during a period of warfare followed by the return home of large numbers of young men. As a result of such circumstances the birthrate temporarily may be much higher than the death rate, but the gross number of births may not be large enough to permanently maintain such a favorable age distribution. There results eventually a population with a relatively high proportion of older persons and a concomitant fall of the birthrate, even below the level of the death rate.

In view of the foregoing, one might conclude that, if the variations presently observed continue, the trends of population growth in various countries will differ in the future as compared to the past and present. North America, the British Isles, and many of the nations of Europe will probably experience stabilized or even decreasing populations unless net reproductive rates increase, mortality rates decrease even more than they have, or major immigrations occur. The countries of Asia, Africa, the Middle East, and Central and South America, on the other hand, will have increasing populations if present fertility rates continue. In addition, barring the influence of other factors, these increases will tend to be greatly magnified if mortality rates are subjected to any considerable extent to even present-day scientific knowledge. It must be remembered, however, that there are many factors which might change or even reverse these trends. Among the most important of these, it is believed, is the apparently inevitable result of a lower birthrate in the face of a continuous and sustained elevation of the standard of living.

The crude death rate is one of the most common and convenient indices of the state of health of a community or nation. In viewing the world scene, despite inadequate information, it is readily observed that in general the highest death rates occur in the countries of Africa, the Middle East, Asia, and parts of Central and South America as well as in a few Southern and Eastern European nations. Significantly lower death rates are experienced by Western Europe, the

British Isles, Australia, New Zealand, North America, Japan, and a few countries in South America. It is immediately apparent that the difference observed in the case of birthrates between more highly developed industrialized countries and less developed and primarily agricultural countries exists also in the case of death rates but in a reciprocal sense. Progress in combatting preventable disease and reducing mortality has been closely related to the widespread application of advances in medical, physical, and chemical sciences. This has occurred to the greatest extent in the Western European countries and in North America, the most highly industrialized and urbanized areas in the world. One may generalize, therefore, that death rates are lower in the more highly developed countries and higher in the more underdeveloped countries. Similarly, death rates tend to be lower in the more urbanized and industrial countries and higher in the more rural and predominantly agricultural countries.

While this relationship appears to apply to many specific death rates, it is by no means universally true. Certainly the relationship applies to the infant death rate and the maternal mortality rate, as it also applies to the specific rates of death from almost all of the communicable diseases which can be controlled by public health, sanitation, and immunization methods. One outstanding group of exceptions, however, does exist. Death rates for the degenerative diseases of middle and later life, such as cancer, hypertension, and the like, are generally much higher in the economically more priviledged and industrially and scientifically advanced countries of Western Europe, the British Isles, North America, Australia, New Zealand, and Japan. This apparent difference is undoubtedly due to the higher proportion of persons who reach later life as a result of public health measures and also to more accurate cause-of-death reporting in the more advanced countries.

In addition to birthrates and death rates, but as a function of the latter, average expectation of life should be considered briefly. The average life expectancy varies considerably among the different nations of the world, from a low of perhaps about 30 to 35 years to a high of about 70 years. As would be expected from the preceding consideration of death rates, the average life expectancy is much greater in Western Europe, the British Isles, North America, Australia, New Zealand, and Japan than it is in most of the rest of the world. The differences between countries in this respect are significant at all age levels, but appear to diminish consistently as one approaches the older ages. The logical conclusion, upheld by a consideration of age-specific death rates, is that the greatest risks to life in the underdeveloped and less priviledged countries are experienced most by infants and young children and that once an individual has reached a certain age he stands a reasonable chance in most places of attaining advanced age.

One final interesting aspect of the variation in death rates and life expectancies relates to the differences that are observed between races. That such differences generally exist is not subject to question. It is not known, however, whether the differences are related to inherent racial characteristics or to social and economic environment. In general, one is inclined to feel that the difference is circumstantial rather than inherent. This appears to be borne out by the fact that the Negro in the New World, although he still has a somewhat lower life expectancy and higher death rate than his white compatriot, nevertheless is in a decidedly more advantageous situation than the members of his race who are still living in Africa. Furthermore, the discrepancy between the rates for whites and Negroes in the Western Hemisphere has consistently become less. That the problem is not simple, however, is indicated by the situation in Hawaii, where the life expectancy of native Hawaiians is significantly less than for other races at every specified age except under 1 year. In fact, Caucasian-Hawaiians also have a shorter life expectancy than Caucasians, Japanese, and Chinese who live on the islands. The explanation for this and similar phenomena remains to be determined.

EXTENT OF WORLD HEALTH PROBLEMS

When one attempts to reduce a study and analysis of world health problems to the lowest common denominators, the conclusion is inevitable that a sound knowledge and consideration of two important but related fields is a prerequisite. These are the sciences of biology and climatology in their broadest senses. Man is a biologic being whose behavior, cultural development, physical development, feeding habits, clothing, housing, and, it would appear at least to some degree, methods of political organization are determined largely by biologic factors, particularly his reaction to his environment. By like token, the majority of the preventable illnesses to which man is subject involve other biologic beings: bacteria, viruses, protozoa, helminths, insects, and the like. Intimately influencing the extent of favorable development of man on the one hand and those factors which may act to his detriment on the other is the climate of the environment in which man and these agents are cast. A few examples serve to illustrate these obvious points. Since man is a satisfactory host for the plasmodium of malaria and since he shares this unfortunate role with the mosquito, it is obvious that, in the absence of scientific interference, human beings affected by malaria are most frequently found in areas where the climate is most conducive to the propagation of the mosquito. Such conditions are found especially in the warm and moist tropical and subtropical zones of the world. In contrast, it is to be expected that the serious pulmonary infections are found most frequently in the less temperate climates that have wider and more frequent variations in temperature. These climatic conditions are conducive to frequent upper respiratory illnesses which so often are the precursors of more serious diseases of the pulmonary system. Between these two situations one might point to typhus fever, which requires environmental and climatic conditions that are not so cold as to discourage the propagation of the louse vector yet are cold enough to cause the human host to wear considerable clothing, usually in a continuous and unwashed manner. If climatic conditions are such as to combine a certain degree of coldness with continued inadequacy of water, thereby precluding bathing and the washing of clothing, that is better yet for the rickettsiae and lice which carry them.

In view of the foregoing one would rightly expect to find that the greatest incidence of preventable disease at the present time is in the warmer areas of the earth. If the factors of biology and climatology were correlated with the degree of economic development and applied scientific knowledge (and, indeed, the latter would appear to be a function of the former), it would be possible to sketch a broad zone on a globe, with necessarily indefinite borders and certain variations, which in general would overlap the equator about 20 to 25 degrees in both directions. This band or zone would include the areas in which the bulk of preventable infectious diseases and premature deaths are now found.

To most of those who reside permanently outside of this zone the extent of preventable disease seems incomprehensible. Nevertheless, as Paul Russell has said, "Nothing on earth is more international than disease."

Consider first malaria, which is still the leading cause of death in the world. In India, "no less than 75 million persons suffer from it every year, and during epidemic years the incidence may reach up to twice as much or even more. It has been calculated that approximately half of the 5.5 million annual deaths in India are accounted for by fevers. Nearly one seventh of these fever deaths are directly attributable to malaria. Apart from this high annual mortality, malaria is also responsible for untold sickness and suffering. Untreated or partially treated malaria leads to general debility and anaemia, and reduces the resistance of the individual to other diseases. This results in an unduly high rate of morbidity. Thus, by sapping the vitality of whole groups of population, malaria has been largely responsible for impeding the development of the country's agricultural and other natural resources. The economic loss to the nation is therefore incalculable."[1]

In Liberia, 90% of the children under 5 years of age have positive blood smears and 70% of the adults are continuously infected. It is a constant scourge of a large part of the lowlands of South and Central America, large parts of Africa, and practically all of South and Southeast Asia. For the world as a whole, it has been estimated that malaria claims about 300 million people and causes from 4 to 6 million deaths each year.

Schistosomiasis affects the populations of large parts of Africa, northeastern South America, Japan, and southeastern China. In Egypt about three fourths of the population is affected. In the Middle East it has been estimated that from 20 to 30 million people, or 90% of the rural population, suffer from this debilitating disease, which in general reduces the productivity of the population by at least one third.[2] Wright[3] estimates its cost to Egypt to be about 20 million pounds per year. Lower Egypt is affected more than Upper Egypt. It is significant that 22% of army recruits from the former must be rejected because of physical defects, as compared with only 3% from the latter.

Helminthic or worm infestation represents one of the greatest drains on human energy and health. Some careful estimates have been made of their extent, and the resulting figures are staggering. To give a few examples, hookworm, the aptly termed assassin worm, one of the worst scourges to suck the lifeblood and strength of a population, affects about 460 million persons throughout the world, over 200 million in India alone. For the roundworm, *Ascaris,* an interesting and dramatic picture has been painted by Stoll.[4] The total case load approaches 650 million persons. China's load alone has been computed to be about 335 million cases, with an estimated 6 billion adult ascarides. This number of worms is equivalent to the combined weight of almost a half million adult men, and they consume enough food annually from the bellies of the already hungry Chinese to feed the entire populations of Guatemala and Costa Rica. It has been further calculated that this many worms produce about 18,000 tons of microscopic eggs, which are broadcast continuously over the landscape.

In 1947, Stoll estimated that while there were just under 2.2 billion people on earth there were, considering multiple infestations, just over 2.2 billion cases of helminthic infestation. The largest amounts of infestations were in the so-called underdeveloped areas of the world. He describes their significance dramatically by saying, "Helminthiases do not have the journalistic value of great pandemics like flu or plague . . . but to make up for their lack of drama, they are unremittingly corrosive."

In India there are more than 2 million blind persons, mostly from trachoma, gonorrhea, and syphilis. Many millions more are affected by trachoma to a degree less than total blindness. An idea of the economic burden involved may be obtained from figures from a much smaller country. Tunisia, with only 3.5 million inhabitants, loses an estimated 25 million workdays per year because of trachoma. Leprosy claims a world total of from 5 to 7 million people. It is estimated that 1 million persons in India and 2 to 4 million persons in China suffer from this disease. In Africa there are probably about 1.5 million affected persons. Some estimates for Latin America include Brazil, 40,000; Bolivia, 12,000 to 15,000; Paraguay, 10,000 to 12,000; Argentina, 12,000; Mexico and Colombia, 9,000 each; and Peru, Venezuela, and Cuba, about 3,000 each. Yaws is one of the most important economic disease handicaps. Throughout the world it is estimated that there are 30 million cases, approximately half of them in the Republic of Indonesia.

With regard to tuberculosis, which may rightfully be considered a disease of poor economy, there are probably about 50 million cases and about 5 million deaths each year throughout the world. Studies have indicated the existence of about 1.3 million cases and 35,000 deaths each year from this disease in the Philippines; India has an estimated 2.5 million cases and about 500,000 deaths annually. China, with 50% more people than India, has a tuberculosis rate about twice as high as India. Recognizing the fact that in most of the world there is no, or at best only poor, reporting and statistics, several interesting attempts have been made to analyze the world prevalence of tuberculosis. One such study, although somewhat out of date, is particularly illustrative. It divides the countries of the world into the following four groups:

Group		
I	Very low prevalence	Rates under 49 per 100,000
II	Low prevalence	Rates from 50 to 99 per 100,000
III	Medium prevalence	Rates from 100 to 149 per 100,000
IV	High prevalence	Rates over 150 per 100,000

At the time of the analysis in 1946 the rates ranged from a low of 34 for Denmark to 550 for Greenland. Only four countries, Denmark, Australia, Netherlands, and the United States, were in group I. Thirty-two countries were in group II, 26 were in group III, and 34 were in group IV. Even this does not tell the whole story. The picture became more skocking when populations affected, rather than numbers of countries, were considered. When this was done, there appeared the following:

Group	TB death rates	Number of countries	% of world population
I	Very low	4	8
II	Low	32	14
III	Medium	26	8
IV	High	34	70

This, it should be realized, was correlated on the basis of considering death rates of from 100 to 149 per 100,000 as medium!

It is impossible even to estimate the number of cases and deaths attributable to typhoid and paratyphoid fevers, the diarrheas and dysenteries, and other related illnesses acquired through the gastrointestinal tract. That their incidence is tremendous is common knowledge. An indication of this is shown by the statement of the Director General of the World Health Organization,[5] who said, "One-fifth of all deaths throughout the world are due to faulty environmental conditions." He pointed out that "probably three-fourths of the world's populations drink unsafe water, dispose of human excreta recklessly, prepare milk and food dangerously, are constantly exposed to insect and rodent enemies, and live in primitive condition of insanitation." By virtue of the circumstances which tend to bring about such undesirable environment it is again obvious that these diseases are most widespread in the predominantly rural agricultural nations of the world.

Filarial infestations are another widespread cause of physical incapacitation and economic loss. *Wuchereria bancrofti* is found in most tropical countries, particularly in the Republic of Indonesia, northern Australia, parts of South Asia, Japan, Africa, the West Indies, the northern coast of South America, and the eastern coast of Brazil. In addition, *Wuchereria malayi* occurs frequently in the Malay peninsula, Sumatra, Borneo, New Guinea, India, Indochina, Ceylon, and southern China. Onchocerciasis is the best-known filarial disease of the western hemisphere, occurring in Mexico, Guatemala, and Venezuela, It is also found on the west coast of Africa from Sierra Leone to the Congo Basin, then eastward across Africa through the Congo and the Sudan to Uganda, Nyasaland, and Kenya. The number of persons affected by filariasis is difficult to determine but is known to be large. Some idea of the magnitude is indicated by the incidence of infestation by one other filarial worm, *Dracunculus medinensis,* or the guinea worm; approximately 50 million people act as hosts to it.

Another geographically very widespread disease is leishmaniasis. While its victims are unnumbered, it is known to occur in various forms across South and Southeast Asia, the Middle East, North and Central Africa, and in a number of South and Central American countries. A somewhat related disease, trypanosomiasis, is of particular significance since along with malaria it bars effective use of the tremendous area of Central Africa, which many consider to contain some of the best agricultural and grazing land in the world, equal to or surpassing in quality that of Argentina or the central United States. The total area involed is about 4.5 million square miles, 50% again as large as the continental United States. The potential importance of the effective use of this tremendous area to the future world food supply is obvious.

The venereal diseases are truly worldwide in occurrence, but again their true extent is unknown. Guthe and Hume[6] have pointed out that if the discovered incidence of syphilis in Denmark and Finland in 1946, i.e., 100 to 200 new cases of syphilis per 100,000 persons per year, were applied to the then world population of 2 billion, the result would be from 2 to 4 million newly acquired cases of syphilis annually. There is of course good reason to consider this incidence rate as low for the world as a whole. Beyond this, if the conservative ratio of 1 case of syphilis to 3 of gonorrhea is applied, the result is an estimated minimum of from 6 to 12 million new cases of gonorrhea per year. In terms of prevalence, if the probably low rate of 2% is applied, an estimated total of 40 million cases of syphilis results.

ECONOMIC, SOCIAL, AND POLITICAL RELATIONSHIPS OF WORLD HEALTH PROBLEMS

From what has gone before, it is obvious that the major portion of the vast mass of preventable disease in the world is concentrated in what is commonly referred to as underdeveloped areas or countries. At this point it should be recognized that the term "underdeveloped" is unsatisfactory and that citizens of countries so described naturally object to it. Perhaps such understandable objection based upon commendable national pride may be somewhat assuaged by pointing out that the term implies that there is something worth developing—a situation not without its desirable aspect. It would seem equally obvious that one cannot speak, think, or act about the health problems of these countries or areas within an isolated substantive framework. Large proportions of the human beings who live in these areas, and they constitute a majority of the population of the earth, eke out a miserable existence under circumstances which are undesirable from many different standpoints, of which ill health is only one. Their housing is inadequate, their economy unbalanced, their food supply pre-

carious, their methods of performing daily tasks primitive, their educational horizons limited, and their daily work relatively inefficient and unproductive. What is cause and what is effect? Widespread preventable disease unquestionably serves as a barrier to progress in any direction, be it economic, social, or political. A population that is chronically ill understandably has a decreased productivity. Thus, in planning a program in the mid-1950's to provide safe water in rural Venezuela, it was found that about 2 million man-days of work were lost annually because of typhoid, paratyphoid, the dysenteries, and enteritis. This was estimated to represent a total productive loss of 2,321,000 bolivars. It was further estimated that the cost of medical treatment and care of persons stricken with these preventable diseases amounted to 1,643,000 bolivars per year, approximately $5.5 million. The loss of manpower in Southern Rhodesia due to malaria has been reported to be from 5% to 10% of the total labor force, with the greatest incidence of the disease occurring at the peak period of agricultural production. Similarly in Indonesia a program for the mass treatment of yaws returned large numbers of incapacitated persons to work and increased the national production significantly.

It has been estimated by Paul Russell[7] that any nation which imports the products of a highly malarious country pays the equivalent of a 5% malaria tax. For what the United States imports from such areas each year this would amount to an additional hidden cost of about $175 million per year. Widespread disease also serves as an effective barrier to the development of agricultural lands and natural resources. The effective settlement of such areas as Sumatra, Borneo, Central Africa, large areas of South America, and, until recently, the Terai of India, Pakistan, Nepal, and large parts of Sardinia, to mention but a few examples, has been prevented by disease, primarily malaria and other insect-borne diseases. The accomplishments in the last two locations give some indication of the potential elsewhere. The control of malaria in Sardinia during the past decade has paved the way for the resettlement of about 1 million Italians from the overcrowded mainland. Similar measures in the Terai have made it possible to begin the opening of this great fertile area so badly needed to feed the people of India. From 1949 to 1954, 35,000 acres were cleared and put into production and 11 new industrial undertakings, such as flour and rice mills and food preservation plants, were initiated. By 1951 the population had already grown to about 300,000 persons.

For the individual, educational and intellectual development is difficult, if at all possible, when the body is chronically drained of its energy by illness and parasites. This was illustrated in the Philippines, where it was found that malaria control reduced school absenteeism from about 50% daily to 3%. At the same time industrial absenteeism was reduced from 35% to under 4%. Uncontrolled disease in the environment and the continuance of conditions that breed unproductivity and

illiteracy also effectively discourage investment from within or without as well as industrial development. Finally, a low economy and standard of living attributable directly or indirectly to widespread ill health is a constant encouragement to political instability. Under such circumstances people have many reasons for discontent and have very little to lose in resorting to violence.

We are dealing here, of course, with a vicious circle. Disease breeds poverty, and poverty in turn breeds more disease. A similar relationship exists between disease and illiteracy, political instability, and many other factors. It is difficult or impossible to state which factor is primary, which is cause, and which is effect. Once the cycle is established, however, it is clear that each factor contributes to the continuance of all other undesirable factors. This has been referred to as cumulative causation. The relationships are illustrated in Table 3-1, which presents data for countries of the Free World, distributed by regions—more

Table 3-1. Comparison of economic, health, and educational conditions in the more developed and less developed regions of the Free World

Condition	More developed regions	Less developed regions
Population in millions, 1950	534.0	1061.0
National income ($ per capita), 1949	690.0	70.0
Nonhuman energy (metric tons of coal per capita or equivalent), 1950	3.8	0.2
Males in nonagricultural employment (%)	73.0	33.0
Births per 1,000 population, 1950	21.7	43.5
Deaths per 1,000 population, 1950	10.5	25.9
Infant mortality per 1,000 births, 1950	45.0	183.0
Expectation of life (years)	63.0	34.0
Crop yields (bushels per acre)		
Wheat, 1949-51	26.0	13.0
Rice, 1949-50–1951-52	69.0	30.0
Calories person per day	2,800	2,000
Animal protein per day (oz.)	1.4	0.4
Persons per physician, 1945-50	1,000	14,000
Daily newspapers per 100 persons, 1948-51	31	2
Radio sets per 100 persons, 1948-51	28	1
Illiterates per 100 persons		
Males	5	64
Females	7	83
Elementary school teachers per 1,000 persons	3.6	1.3
Motor vehicles per 100 persons, 1950	12	0.4
External trade ($ per capita), 1949	140	32
Consumption of textiles (pounds per capita), 1948	21	5

developed regions and less developed regions. While based upon data collected about 1950 and while some changes and improvements have unquestionably occurred, the relative picture remains essentially unchanged. For the sake of depicting broad geographic areas of relative development and for the sake of convenient general statistical handling, certain individual countries that are obvious exceptions to the region in which they are located are nevertheless included in that region. The more developed regions include North America, Western Europe, the British Isles, Southern Europe, Australia, New Zealand, and Japan. The less developed regions include Latin America, Southeastern Europe, the Near East, Africa, and South and Southeast Asia. It will be observed, first of all, that twice as many people live in the less developed regions than in those that are more developed. Beyond this, it will be noted that in the case of every index (and they measure health, agricultural development, industrial development, education, trade, and food consumption), the less developed regions are significantly disadvantaged as compared with the more developed regions.

The solution to the problem is not easy. Certainly it cannot be accomplished by an attack upon health problems alone. In fact, such an approach would carry with it certain very real dangers, if indeed it were to really succeed at all. Advancement must be made in many fields simultaneously. In this regard the statement of Gunnar Myrdal[8] at the Fifth World Health Assembly is worthy of note in summarizing the complexity of the situation and outlining a guide for effective, lasting action:

The task of social engineering is to proportion and direct the induced changes in the whole social field so as to maximize the beneficial effects of a given initial financial sacrifice. One important corollary to the theory of cumulative causation is that a rational policy should never work by inducing change in only one factor; least of all should such a change of only one factor be attempted suddenly and with great force. This would in most cases prove to be a wasteful expenditure of efforts which could reach much further by being spread strategically over the various factors in the social system and over a period of time. What we are facing is a whole set of interrelated adverse living conditions for a population. An effort to reach permanent improvement of health standards aimed to have a maximum beneficial effect on the well-being of the people will, in other words, have to be integrated in a broad economic and social reform policy. Such a policy will have to be founded upon studies of how in the concrete situation of a particular country the different factors in the plane of living are interrelated and how we can move them all upwards in such a fashion that the changes will support each other to the highest possible degree.

REFERENCES

1. Summary Proceedings of the First Meeting of the Central Council of Health, Hyderabad, Jan. 29-31, 1953, Government of India, Ministry of Health.
2. United Nations Document E/1327/Add. 1.
3. Wright, W. H.: Medical parasitology in a changing world, J. Parasit. 37:2, Feb. 1951.
4. Stoll, N. R.: This wormy world, J. Parasit. 33:1, Feb. 1947.
5. Hyde, H. V.: Sanitation in the international health field, Amer. J. Public Health 41:1, Jan. 1951.
6. Guthe, T., and Hume, J. C.: International aspects of the venereal disease problem, New York, 1948, American Social Hygiene Association, Inc.
7. Russell, P.: A lively corpse, Trop. Med. News 5:25, June 1948.
8. Myrdal, G.: Economic aspects of health, Chronicle of World Health Organization 6:207, Aug. 1952.

Part II

Sociology of public health

The manner in which those engaged in public health view themselves and the field of activity in which they are engaged has undergone an interesting evolution through the years. Originally they regarded their work as a part of medicine. As specialized knowledge and techniques were developed and applied, it came to be considered as a separate science—sanitary science. With the involvement of increasing numbers of individuals other than physicians, public health became known as a distinct discipline, then a profession in itself. More recently, as the effects or end results of public health programs upon other aspects of life and society manifest themselves, those in the field have begun to recognize themselves for what they truly are—agents of social change. This places the public health worker squarely in the arena of applied sociology, sharing kinship with a broad array of other social scientists. It is some of the more pertinent of these fields with which the following section is concerned.

Chapter 4

Social science and public health

INTRODUCTION

Although the term "public health" has been used for several generations, the significance of the *two* words seems often to be overlooked. It should be realized that we are dealing both with a product—health— and a recipient—the public—and that the most complete knowledge and understanding of the one is pointless without corresponding knowledge and understanding of the other. This is what Leavell[1] had in mind when he wrote:

Two major types of changes with which public health must deal are going on in the modern world: "public" changes and "health" changes. Our professional training helps us most with the health changes. Our knowledge of biology, chemistry, and physics and their medical sub-specialties helps us find and use the proper immunizing agents to prevent disease, the right kinds of food to eat, the best sprays to kill mosquitoes, and so on. We can usually adjust rather readily to rapid changes demanded as a result of research which provides better tools with which to combat health problems.

The public changes that are so important in public health work are in many respects more difficult for us to appreciate. Most of us have limited backgrounds in the basic social sciences—sociology, anthropology, psychology, economics, and political science— that might help us understand better the people with whom we must work. Yet public changes are often of even greater importance than health changes.

. . . we need a great deal more research to be able to translate the findings of biological investigation into social application. When we meet a health problem, we must recognize that two kinds of diagnosis and treatment are necessary. We must understand and deal with the health problem. We must also understand and treat the social or public part of the situation. Our pharmacopeia in both fields must be

strong. It is no longer sufficient to prescribe drugs and neglect the social factors in a given case.

THE MEANING OF HEALTH TO SOCIETY

It is only natural that each of us tends to view his particular interests and activities as being of paramount significance. Because of this, there is some danger that public health workers may consider public health goals as ends in themselves and the activities required for their achievement as necessarily of primary interest to society. Few attitudes are more conducive to disappointment and disillusionment. This is particularly true if, as is sometimes the case, goals have been arbitrarily determined and activities planned and carried out by "experts" who themselves are necessarily prejudiced, without concern for the needs, ideas, and wishes of the group. The group or public may look upon the goals and activities quite differently. Furthermore, for reasons of group pride, cohesion, or self-assertion, the group may be forced into the psychologic position of objecting or resisting.

The fact is that although health is a common need and the effort to attain it represents a common drive it is actually of secondary rather than of primary importance. Even in the primitive state man is concerned with the achievement of a total or integrated way of life. Because of its complexity, this is not easy to define. Some distinctions are possible, however, especially through study of certain situations such as primitive societies and societies under stress. In such circumstances one cannot avoid the conclusion that, while man and his societies are subject to many needs, urges, or drives, only a few of them are primary or basic, i.e., the need for food, shelter, and sexual expression or propagation. As for many other goals, of which health is only one, most individuals and society in general are interested in them to the extent that they make possible the achievement of related goals, especially those which are primary in nature. It may be argued that the desire for comfort, the absence of pain, and the achievement of physical well-being are very relative terms. In societies where the majority of individuals acquire malaria or trachoma, these conditions come to be looked upon as part of the normal pattern of life and are adapted to as well as possible. Under such circumstances ill health tends to be considered as the presence of any condition which is unusual or beyond these. It might perhaps be said that man will strive for food, shelter, and sexual expression in the absence of complete health, but he will not strive for complete health in the absence of the others.

A few examples may help to place the desire for health in its proper perspective. A man and woman stranded on an island will ordinarily seek to assure themselves of food, shelter, and sexual satisfaction before giving attention to other needs. In most instances they will seek to satisfy these three needs or urges in the order given because of the differing critical intervals involved. Furthermore, they will do so in the face of potential threats to their health or safety. Thus, if the only source of food or of materials for shelter are in or near an insalubrious spot, they will still seek them out. Later, perhaps, they may seek out a more desirable alternative. Undoubtedly syphilis could be completely eradicated by abstinence from sexual intercourse on the part of all members of society. The chances of this procedure's being followed are obviously nil because, when faced with a choice between

the two, the risk of infection will be readily accepted by the majority. The example is more than theoretical, as the suggestion has been made on more than one occasion to individuals or special groups to no avail.

Another example of health's being relegated to a secondary position is observed in relation to technical assistance activities in malaria control in North Africa. In that area the date is the basic element in the food supply. Despite the recognized relief from malaria, the activities eventually were somewhat opposed in several communities because the DDT killed not only the malaria-transmitting *Anopheles* but also the species of fly which normally carried the pollen from the male to the female date palm. In order to assure both desirable ends, modifications in control techniques had to be developed.

There are some situations in which health measures as deterrents to ultimate death are actually regarded as somewhat undesirable. The realization of this comes as a shock to those accustomed to regarding health and the preservation of life as universally desired goals. Where conditions for life and survival are difficult and especially where disease and premature death are common, the social attitude toward death may be quite different from ours. Not uncommonly, especially in the case of infants and very young children, death is not necessarily too sad an event. The young child, as a child, does not yet have a fully developed personality and may be regarded as an added economic burden to the family. The child's timely removal may mean more food and other things for the rest of the family and less suffering and misery for itself in the long run. An impression of this may be obtained by observing funeral ceremonies in less developed societies with high death rates. The difference between the funeral of a productive adult and that of a very young child or an elderly person is quite striking. In the former instance there usually is genuine regret shown by the mourners. The adult has been around long enough for people to know him as a personality; beyond this, his death is recognized as the economic loss of a producer for his family and the community. In the case of funerals of elderly persons there is again genuine regret, but not as much as in the former case. True, the elderly individual's personality is well known and familiar in the local scene. However, he has served his economic purpose in life, as he has also served his social purpose in producing offspring and in transmitting through his life the mores of the group. He now has become an economic or even a social burden that has to be supported, and anyhow he is now entitled to his well-earned release to the rewards and security of the hereafter. In the case of infants and young children the difference may be even more marked. Often there appears to be surprisingly little mourning; the physical appearance of the funeral procession, if anything, tends to be much brighter and, among some peoples, even rather cheerful. Songs may be sung, bands may play, and, when the small body is finally removed, there may be a somewhat enthusiastic social event, with dining, drinking, dancing, and indulgence in all other pleasures of the flesh. Even in our more sophisticated societies gradations of these differences in attitudes may be observed. Suffice to point to the oft-expressed ameliorating thought that a deceased child was "pure of heart" hence much more apt to achieve everlasting happiness.

Finally, recognition may be given to certain societies in which to be ill and suffering is considered saintly or godlike. Similarly, in these and other societies in which it is common to undertake religious pilgrimages to holy places, to become ill and die during a pilgrimage is regarded as a good omen for the hereafter.

The foregoing discussion is not intended to belittle or discourage efforts toward the improvement of public health; rather, the purpose is to point out that health is a relative concept, that its definition and value vary from one place to another, and, even in a given society through time, that it is only one facet of the total interest and welfare of the individual and his society and as such is in constant competition with all other factors of greater or lesser importance to that individual and that society. It is

necessary that we realize these things, for as Koos[2] has pointed out: "What we can expect a community to provide, and its members to accept, in the way of health activities must therefore be viewed in a framework which is peculiar to that community. This in no way prevents the establishing of uniform goals or standards for health, but it does mean that community efforts directed toward better health are necessarily custom-built."

SOCIAL ANALYSIS AND COMMUNITY ORGANIZATION FOR HEALTH

Each of us is many things. First of all, we may consider ourselves individuals, a composite or compromise of various strengths and weaknesses, interests and prejudices, abilities and failings. But, as some philosophers have claimed, perhaps there is no such thing as a true individual; each of us is the product and a part of a series of environments beginning with the womb. Beyond being individuals we are members of families and beyond that, members of varying numbers and types of social groups with shared and common needs and interests—complexes of interrelated families, the guild, the village, the clan, eventually agglutinating to form various types of cultural and national entities.

Human beings everywhere are members of groups. As such they may be dependent upon one another within the groups for sustenance, education, inspiration, economic welfare, and entertainment as well as for many other needs. The individual needs the group, but not necessarily only a particular group, or always the same group, or the same group for all needs. The same conditions also apply to the group's need for the individual. While the bonds which link the individual to the group must be strong if they are to be of value, they are not necessarily fixed. They may be and in fact often are broken or transferred. It is in line with this that individuals are seldom found to be members of only one group. Different groups are needed for different purposes. Although this is not so apparent in primitive societies, even there individuals have multigroup attachments—to the family, to a larger kinship group, to a totem group, and to a maturation cult or secret society as well as to the tribe. In more highly developed societies the plurality of group membership is more evident. In addition to the family there is the school, the church, the social club, the athletic club, the business and professional associations, and many, many others.

The question inevitably arises whether all of these many groups are necessary and important or whether, for our purposes or those of others, it is possible successfully to approach and influence all individuals through one group. This is another way of asking if it is possible to focus all of man's interests toward one group. Is it possible to have one group which would satisfy all needs? Clearly the answer is found in reality. Innumerable groups exist because people develop them to meet their various and varying needs. An individual requires a social complex of many differing groups in order to obtain sufficient significant or fruitful relationships which will satisfy the various facets of his personality and interests. Repeated attempts have been and are still being made to relate the complete allegiance and interest of people to one single supergroup, e.g., the state.

All previous attempts along these lines have failed, and one might safely guess that all future attempts will experience the same fate. Life devoted exclusively to one group is necessarily very narrow and self-limiting. "The man who can live without society," said Aristotle, "is either a beast or a god. But the man who can live exclusively for the state, if indeed such a being exists, is either a tyrant or a slave."

Granted that it is the nature of man to belong to various groups, how does this affect his behavior and his receptivity? It should be recognized at the onset that man's behavior as an individual is usually quite different from his behavior as a member of a group or of society and that his social or group behavior varies from group to group. Furthermore, when a point of common concern or mutual interest exists and can be adequately indentified, widely differing groups may join forces and with

regard to this particular interest jointly behave differently from the way each behaves alone. This does not mean that any one group forfeits its identity. As Skinner[3] points out, "Social behavior arises because one organism is important to another as part of its environment. A first step, therefore, is an analysis of the social environment and of any special features it may possess." Since our intention here is social analysis for the purpose of community or social organization for public health improvement, it is important to distinguish and identify groups which may be of significance toward that end. There are three general categories of identifiable groups the existence of which the specialist in community organization should be constantly aware and which are important "because community organization for health cannot be carried on in an icy apartness from the social worlds in which people live for whom it is designed, and because community organization cannot ignore the strength of the factors which create distinctive values regarding health and which place these values high or low in the whole hierarchy of values that are a part of . . . life."

The first of these groups provides for ethnic identification. This identification is represented by religious, racial, or nationality groups, each with its own prescriptions, prohibitions, and ideals, any one of which may be of significance in matters of health and sickness.

A second category is related to ethos identification, i.e., bonds which identify individuals as belonging to the same ethical, economic, or social group (sometimes coincident with a neighborhood). The economic, educational, or moral nature of the group may determine the extent or manner of participation in activities designed for the improvement of the public health.

Finally, there is the family, which usually represents the most powerful example of social cohesion. To ignore the position of predominant influence of the family in the development or conduct of a public health program usually guarantees failure. The pertinence of Koos'[2] remarks in this regard justifies their repetition here:

NURSING DEPARTMENT
COLLEGE MISERICORDIA
DALLAS, PENNA. 18612

We may well question the logic of industry- or school-centered programs that ignore the importance of the family as a "conditioner of attitudes," and which may send the individual back into his family to face conflicting ideologies about health and its value. This is not a plea to abandon school- or industry-centered programs; it is to point out that such programs can work effectively only if they send the individual back to his family prepared to adjust differences that may have been engendered; to make him, in effect, a health organizer in his own small family world. If the individual is not so prepared . . . the cost in tensions and frustrations can outweigh any small good the program may have accomplished.

SOCIETY AND CULTURE

Since up to this point reference has been made to several closely related fields, it is important that distinction be made between society, the subject matter of sociology, and culture, the subject matter of social or cultural anthropology. The society is any community of individuals drawn together by a common bond of nearness and interaction, i.e., a group of people who act together in general for the achievement of certain common goals. A society has both quantitative and qualitative characteristics. Thus it is possible to count and measure the number of individuals who constitute a society. One of the qualitative characteristics is its culture or the manner in which the group as a unit tends to think, feel, react to stimuli, believe, in other words, its basis for behavior. As Kluckhohn[4] describes it, "a culture refers to the distinctive ways of life of such a group of people . . . a culture constitutes a storehouse of the pooled learning of the group." Every society has its own distinctive culture, and, since there are innumerable societies in each community, in each country, and on each continent of the world, there are therefore innumerable cultures, each differing to a greater or lesser degree from all of the others. The study of these cultures, their components, and their relationships with each other is the subject matter of cultural anthropology, the purpose of which is to aid man in understanding himself. Kluckhohn graphically states, "Anthropology holds up a great mirror to man, and lets him look at himself in his infinite variety."

Throughout the entire course of history every member of the human race was born into some sort of culture. Some cultures were primitive, simple, and crude, whereas others were complex and highly developed. Some dwindled and died while others flourished and grew. All of them, however, regardless of their degree of complexity or simplicity, developed some form of techniques, religious beliefs, social systems, and art forms. Every child born into his particular group culture is certain to be influenced more by it than by anything else in his entire life. "As a matter of fact," says White,[5] "his culture will determine how he will think, feel and act. It will determine what language he will speak, what clothes if any he will wear, what gods he will believe in, and how he will marry, select and prepare his foods, treat the sick, and dispose of the dead. What else could one do but react to the culture that surrounds him from birth to death?"

This behavioral determining effect of culture on the individual and the importance of understanding it is further stressed by Benedict[6]:

. . . The life history of the individual is first and foremost an accommodation to the patterns and standards traditionally handed down in his community. From the moment of his birth the customs into which he is born shape his experience and behaviour. By the time he can talk, he is the little creature of his culture, and by the time he is grown and able to take part in its activities, its habits are his habits, its beliefs his beliefs, its impossibilities his impossibilities. Every child that is born into his group will share them with him, and no child born into one on the opposite side of the globe can ever achieve the thousandth part. There is no social problem it is more incumbent upon us to understand than this of the role of custom. Until we are intelligent as to its laws and varieties, the main complicating facts of human life must remain unintelligible.

Beyond this she says:

The study of different cultures has another important bearing upon present-day thought and behaviour. Modern existence has thrown many civilizations into close contact, and at the moment, the overwhelming response to this situation is nationalism and racial snobbery. There has never been a time when civilization stood more in need of individuals who are genuinely culture-conscious, who can see objectively the socially conditioned behaviour of other peoples, without fear and recrimination.

The importance of culture and the con-

tribution which cultural anthropology may make to action programs in the field of public health have perhaps become somewhat more evident to those public health workers who have been working in lands and countries other than their own and in the field of international health. They have come to realize, with Carothers,[7] that "the visitor to foreign lands is always most impressed by the general peculiarities of peoples, whereas in his homeland . . . he notices only the individual divergencies." It should be pointed out that the choice of words in this statement is rife with significance. It is important to call attention, however, to the oft-overlooked fact that it is not necessary to visit foreign or exotic lands to encounter cultures. It is fundamental that the domestic health worker realize that he too has been born into and grown up in a culture, received his training in possibly still another culture, and in the conduct of his work must deal with a great many cultures in his own community. It is well for each of us to realize that, as Oliver Wendell Holmes so aptly remarked, "The people in every town feel that the axis of the earth passes through its main street." That is why so many tribal and national names, when traced to their origins, are found to mean "the human beings," "real or principal people," and similar accolades. Thus, as Gittler[8] has discovered, "The Greenland Eskimo believes that Europeans have been sent to Greenland to learn virtue and good manners from him. Their highest form of praise of an outsider is that he is or soon will be as good as a Greenlander." This is also why our language contains such often-used phrases as "beyond the pale" or "the other side of the tracks." It is most certainly unnecessary to go to the ends of the earth to find other cultures; we can find them, must understand them, and must live and work with them in our own communities.

In this connection, sound action in a field like public health presupposes sound evaluation of circumstances and situations, and it is important to recognize that our evaluations are determined by our own cultural background. In discussing the relationship between science and culture, Bernard[9] says,

"We have come to use the term 'definition of the situation' to describe the process which people go through in perceiving, evaluating, and interpreting what goes on about them. Even within a given culture, among people using the same language, the student and the teacher, the husband and the wife, the parent and the child, the employer and the employee, define an identical situation quite differently. They all see, hear, and perceive different things, and what they see, hear, and perceive, has different meanings for each." According to Benedict,[6] "The truth of the matter is that the possible human institutions and motives are legion, on every plane of cultural simplicity or complexity, and that wisdom consists in a greatly increased tolerance toward their divergencies. No man can thoroughly participate in any culture unless he has been brought up and has lived according to its forms, but he can grant to other cultures the same significance to their participants which he recognizes in his own."

What is the purpose of culture? All cultural traits, habits, prejudices, and the like are based essentially on a mixture of conscious and subconscious urges for individual and group survival and perpetuation. As Kluckhohn[4] indicates: "Any cultural practice must be functional, or it will disappear before long; that is, it must somehow contribute to the survival of the society or to the adjustment of the individual." Every society has developed institutions and methods of behavior to safeguard and perpetuate the practices and beliefs which its members consider the most important and valuable. In every society social arrangements or organizations have been developed over long periods of time on the basis of proved group experience to meet life's basic needs. Programs such as public health necessarily involve the introduction of new practices and changes in these arrangements into the culture of the society. If such programs are to be constructive rather than disruptive forces, the social structure and the traditional cultural way of life of the community must be taken into account and utilized.

Not only are the accepted value systems of a culture deeply ingrained, but disadvantaged people adhere particularly strongly to their attitudes and beliefs. This is to be expected since people who for a long time have been accustomed to crowded living conditions, low economic status, discrimination, and philosophic systems that serve to make life under these conditions bearable look upon change or suggested change with misgivings and suspicion. Their greatest fear is that things might get worse, and to them, on the basis of their experience, change often implies that very possibility. Advantageous incentives to change and demonstrations of the value of new ideas, techniques, or actions are necessary to overcome the natural reluctance of people to change their ways and their fear of the possible risks involved in following new practices. They need to have proved to them in one way or another that the suggestions will make possible real improvements in their standard of living, and they need to be assisted in their attempts to implement the suggestions made and to integrate them with the rest of their cultural pattern. A public health program must demonstrate to people that the continued improvement in their welfare and level of living is its main purpose. It is insufficient merely to enunciate general principles or objectives of health as if they were the end and to think of the people involved merely as a means to that end. Instead, people must be able to see clearly and unequivocally that the public health activity or program is one which attacks the problem not just in terms of increasing community health in the abstract but in terms of all the needs of people with much the same aspirations the world over for their families and for their neighbors.

It is true, therefore, as Paul[10] says:

The cultural system does limit the range of individual behavior and in this sense customs exert a restraining influence. Culture defines the values men hold, the goals they seek, the means they use. By thus organizing their outlook, culture is also a guide to action, a positive force that channels motivation and imparts meaning to existence. We are too inclined to perceive the negative and overlook the positive when we behold the customs of others. . . . Now a health program strikes at the uncertainties of death and disease, and it may seem ironical

that the dissemination of improved medical practices should be impeded precisely by those superstitions that owe their vitality to the hazards of life deriving from inadequacies of medical knowledge. But faith is strong where risks are great, and people act slowly when it comes to shifting their faith from a familiar system of security to an unfamiliar one, however efficacious the new system may prove to be in the long run. It should not be overlooked that faith gives psychological security, whether faith is placed in magic, religion or science.

One aspect of culture which is easily overlooked is the fact that it is more than a collection of customs; it is a system of customs, each one more or less related to the others in a meaningful fashion. A culture has structure as well as content; it is not just like a haphazard pile of bricks. This gives a clue to the reason for the tenacity with which societies hold on to their customs. Each one is like a gear in a transmission system, important and necessary for the total function and directly or indirectly related to all of the other gears. As it is impossible to remove a gear from a transmission system and still have the system function without an adequate substitute, so it is impossible to remove a custom from a culture without providing for an equally satisfactory or better substitute custom. To carry the analogy further, the end result of a transmission system is the product of its component gears, not merely their sum. Similarly a total culture is the product of its component parts or customs—not merely the sum—and if any one basic part is destroyed or reaches zero, the entire culture collapses. Former President Eisenhower had this in mind when, speaking at Supreme Headquarters Allied Powers Europe, he said: "The strength that a nation, or a group of nations, can develop is the product obtained by multiplying its spiritual or moral strength, by its economic strength, by its military strength . . . . There can be no army unless there is a productive strength with a productive power to support it. There can be neither a strong economy nor an army if the people are spiritless, if they don't prize what they are defending."

Benedict[6] narrates a significant and touching anecdote in this regard. She tells of her conversations with a chief of the Californian Digger Indians who had been "civilized" and integrated to a greater or lesser degree with our Western civilization. He told her of life in the olden days, of the ceremonies, the agriculture, the tribal economy, and of how each of these and other customs were so meaningful to the tribe: "In those days," he said, "his people had eaten 'the health of the desert' and knew nothing of the insides of tin cans and the things for sale at butchershops." It was such innovations that had degraded his people in the latter days. Then he added one day: "In the beginning God gave to every people a cup, a cup of clay, and from this cup they drank their life. They all dipped in the water, but their cups were different. Our cup is broken now. It has passed away."

In discussing the social disorganization which developed in the little Guatemalan town of Tiquisate, site of an experiment in agricultural productive efficiency, Hoyt[11] warns:

The potential economic effects of increasing production cannot be abstracted from the actual psycho-social effects; and it is possible, if we are not careful, that the disorganization accompanying the latter may be greater than the constructive services of the former.

She continues:

If Tiquisate is an outstanding example of productive efficiency, it is also an outstanding example of social disorganization, even to the extent that the latter threatens the former. This is evidenced by a great deal of drunkenness and prostitution—which the people themselves deplore—by lax family relations, and by strong social antagonisms . . . . Although new values appeared, they did not take the place of the old; neither did they furnish a framework within which the psychic aspects of the people's old life could find their place and get the necessary response.

I encountered a somewhat similar phenomenon on the lovely island of Bali. The government of the new nation of which Bali is a part, wanting to take its rightful place in the modern society of nations, apparently deplored any custom which might cause other nations to consider it backward or primitive. It therefore passed a law requiring the women of Bali to cover their breasts. According to observers who had lived there for some time, there has come about a noticeable change in the Balinese males' attitude toward female breasts and toward women, and it is significant that in the short time since that law was passed prostitution has appeared on the island for the first time. That a causal relationship actually exists in this case, of course, is not possible to determine. The circumstances and timing, however, give some cause to wonder.

In summary to this point, therefore, all human beings are members of societies, each with its own culture consisting of a complex mosaic of interrelated customs. These customs have developed through the ages as a result of group experience in its struggle for survival and for a reasonably satisfactory life. Accordingly people relinquish customs reluctantly, and it is well that they do, because each custom or a truly adequate substitute is fundamental to the continued existence of the society. The great contribution of cultural anthropology to the conduct of programs such as public health is constantly to identify and point out the importance of cultural patterns of the groups or societies which constitute a community or a nation. Social evolution inevitably disturbs cultural patterns, but that is one price of progress. However, cultural patterns need not be disturbed more deeply or more rapidly than the people are able to tolerate. This principle should underlie all of our actions.

EFFECT OF CULTURAL PATTERNS ON HEALTH

With the previous considerations in mind it is obvious that many if not all cultural patterns bear some relationships to the degree of health of a people and the extent to which they will accommodate themselves or be receptive to efforts that might be made to improve their state of health. It does not seem necessary to discuss here the positive or scientifically desirable contributions of certain cultural patterns to health or the even more obvious contributions of sound public health measures in general to cultural development. Let us therefore concern ourselves with some examples of cultural patterns that may have a disadvantageous effect on the health of a people.

There are many reasons for ill health, only a few of which will be discussed at this time. One easily recognized reason is ignorance or lack of knowledge about the factors involved in the causation of illness and death. It is recalled that during a period when the infant mortality rate for the city of Detroit in general was undergoing a consistent and significant decline there were several areas of the city which did not appear to be sharing in the improvement. Analysis of those areas and comparison with other sections of the city indicated that they were populated to a major degree by foreign-born individuals of a particular European nationality. A study of their cultural habits indicated that there was considerable family attachment to the infant and that the environmental circumstances were relatively clean. However, further inquiry brought out that the infants traditionally were taken off the breast at a very early age, following which they were fed essentially adult foods, often directly from the family table. Concurrent analyses of the causes of infant mortality in these areas indicated a high incidence of death due to severe digestive disturbances and intestinal infections. It was necessary over a period of several years to bring to bear the efforts of a reoriented and rather specialized public health nursing program, assisted by appropriate nutritional and pediatric consultation. In addition to this instance there are many groups in which it is the custom for mothers to prechew solid foods for their babies and young children, not realizing the bacteriologic risk in their attempt to carry out what appears on the surface to be a logical procedure.

Very often economic factors are cultural reasons for ill health. Until recently in the United States, and even now in a number of other countries, certain methods of earning a living have resulted in high incidences of tuberculosis and other diseases. This has been particularly true of certain industrial and manufacturing activities and in areas where trading, with its increased contacts,

forms the economic basis of a group. Difficult as it may be for some to believe, there are many societies in which excrement, both human and animal, represents the most valuable if not the only valuable commodity. The reason may be that it is used either as a fertilizer or as fuel. The extent of the use of human feces for fertilizer and the inherent dangers involved are rather well known and need not be dwelt upon.

With regard to the use of excrement as fuel, the following example may be pertinent. Recently an attempt was made to improve health conditions in several villages in Egypt by installing latrines, constructing wells, and killing flies with insecticides.[12,13] The project was regarded as less than successful, not just because the fly population repeatedly developed resistance to the insecticides used, but particularly because of various cultural features of the situation which could not be changed within the scope of the project. One factor was that the dung of the *gamous* or cow was exceedingly valuable as the only form of fuel for heating and cooking. Accordingly, all members of each household were constantly on the lookout for dung and would collect it, pat it into cakes, and store it within the confines of the household where it would be safe from thieves. There it constituted a continuous and most effective breeding ground for flies, which for centuries have multiplied at a tremendous rate. An additional factor was that each house served as the home of both the family and its livestock. A significant and permanent improvement in the health of the people of these villages, of which there are many thousands, must depend upon effective separation of the family and their livestock, especially the gamous. But, aside from extremely difficult problems of finding adequate space and building materials for stables in a land where every inch of arable soil is at a premium and trees are extremely rare, it was found that not inconsiderable social problems would arise from such a contemplated change. One of these was the safety and security of the animals. In addition, however, it was brought out by careful interviews that many women in the villages found the gamous their only source of companionship within the home during the day while the men and boys worked in the fields and that they might resist attempts to end this sociable relationship. It was concluded therefore that an attack on health conditions in the villages by methods of sanitary engineering and fly control was not enough. The abominable conditions could not be materially improved without an attack on a very broad front involving economic and social measures as well as those which had been carried out.

Bogue and Habashy[14] have also described the attitude of the Egyptian villager toward his animals and its effect on attempts to improve health conditions by quoting a villager involved: "The fellah has his own habits and traditions which have come down with his long heritage. Many of these habits are good but many contribute to bad health because of lack of experience or ignorance of their effect. The poorest farmers keep their cattle and other animals in the same house they live in themselves . . . In attempting to get at the basis of such a peculiar habit in this modern time, many approaches were made by the social workers. One old man explained it to a health educator simply that: 'We like our animals and want them where we can see them at night . . . They are our wealth. They are our most prized possessions on which we depend for our very food and livelihood.' Such a realistic answer causes social maneuverers to stop and think before making a casual suggestion to move them to a shed." While these examples may seem somewhat bizarre, recognition should be given to the presence in innumerable homes in our own societies of all sorts of animal pets, some of which are none too clean, others transmitters of specific diseases such as psittacosis, and to many of which humans may become allergic. Despite all of this, they are maintained on a sentimental or a companionship basis similar to the Egyptian village woman and her gamous.

An example of misguided effort and of the effect of economic limitation deals with the attempts by some outsiders to change

what they felt were unhygienic traditional menstrual habits of the Chamorro women, as observed by David M. Schneider while making a cultural study of the island of Yap. The attempts to make them give up their practical, time-proved although strange custom were successful, and they were persuaded to use sanitary napkins. However, these are not made locally, the supply is limited, and the native economy provides little cash for the purchase of manufactured goods. As a result each individual pad is worn throughout the entire menstrual period, during which time the Chamorro women, following the example of their American sisters, continue to be active in their society where previously they were separated from it. This is cited by Paul[15] as an example of unforeseen, undesirable consequences of supposedly progressive social action. I am reminded of a rather impressive phenomenon of this nature which I observed in several communities in Java. Apparently at sometime in the recent past a very effective selling job on the merits of the brushing of teeth must have been carried out. Imported toothpaste, however, is well beyond the economic capacity of many of the people. Nevertheless, it is extremely common to see individuals with toothbrushes in their pockets stopping to brush their teeth at the edges of the many canals which run through the streets. Since these are actually open sewers used for bathing, laundering—and for brushing the teeth—one could not help wondering if the dental hygienic gains might not better be forfeited in the interests of other sanitary considerations.

Conflict of desirable health practices with other cultural values that are considered more important forms another basis for the development or perpetuation of health problems. Few things are as important to people as their religious beliefs. As a result, if it is a custom not to eat a certain type of food such as animal protein, individuals will tend to avoid them even if an adequate nonanimal substitute is unavailable. Similarly, although it is well known that certain of the great traditional pilgrimages mean sickness and death for many people, nothing can deter them from the tremendous cultural drive to participate in the event. Modesty or moral values are factors of considerable import to most people. There have been periods in history and there are still societies in the Western world where to see the naked body, even one's own or that of one's child, is considered immodest and immoral. In such instances personal cleanliness and hygiene tend understandably to reach a low ebb. The type of clothing customarily worn is part of the culture of a people and often has been developed in conformance with the environment. Sometimes, however, clothing acts as a deterrent to health and a spreader of disease. The barracan, worn by many people in North Africa, is a very practical garment from the standpoint of protection from the environment. However, coupled with the dearth of water and soap, the exceedingly common use of the long loose sleeves to wipe one's eyes, nose, and mouth and those of one's children most certainly is a factor in the spread of disease, particularly trachoma, which is so widely prevalent in the area.

Hyde[16] gives an example of a cultural value, this time the wish for fertility, that supersedes not only health but even convenience*:

> I recall being told in Egypt of a wealthy land-owner who had dug good wells, out of which his fellaheens could obtain clear and pure drinking water. After some three days' use of this safe water, the fellaheens returned to drinking the polluted water of the Nile. On inquiring into their reasons, the landowner was told that the people preferred the Nile water, that it was obviously better because the Nile made the fields fertile and would therefore make the people fertile.

One might speculate on the possible value of an explanation of the relationship between the river water and the ground water through subterranean diffusion as well as evaporation and precipitation. In addition, it might have been possible to point to families of desirable size who used water from a well rather than from the river.

---

*See also *Health Education Pilot Project in Three Villages in Egypt* by Bogue and Habashy.[14]

EFFECT OF CULTURAL PATTERNS ON PUBLIC HEALTH ACTIVITIES AND PROGRAMS

From the examples that have been given it should be evident that public health programs are frequently hampered by failure to inquire into or attempt to understand customs which the members of the group involved hold very important. The public health worker is rare indeed who can truthfully claim unqualified success of every program or activity he has undertaken. Every one of us has had the experience at some time of planning a program with meticulous care, bringing together every possible bit of technical knowledge available, only to be thwarted or disillusioned by an apathetic or resistant public. Very often the explanation of failure may be found in the field of cultural anthropology.

There are many barriers to public health success. One of the simplest is the matter of communication. It is a common trap to feel that just because we understand what we are thinking and saying that everyone else interprets it the same. Whorf[17] analyzes this in the following way: "Western culture has made, through language, a provisional analysis of reality and, without correctives, holds resolutely to that analysis as final. The only correctives lie in all those other tongues which by eons of independent evolution have arrived at different but equally logical, provisional analyses . . . An important field for the working out of new order systems . . . lies in more penetrating investigation than has yet been made of languages remote in type from our own." Even within the confines of our own communities language differences may serve as a communication barrier. Particularly in our larger communities there are sizable groups whose ability to speak and understand our traditional tongue is limited. Certainly more than one patient has received inappropriate treatment in a hospital, clinic, or health center because he could not understand his examiner and his examiner could not understand him. Perhaps the tragedy of such situations is that the more educated of the two is the least apt to admit to his handicap or failing.

Even where the same language is ostensibly spoken, there may easily be differences in interpretations of what is said. There are also such factors as regionalism and provincialism; many words and phrases in our language have quite different meanings in different sections of the country, not to mention the varying accents which those who speak them may use.

I received an interesting and valuable lesson on communication as a barrier in connection with a health education program in Bolivia. Very few of the rural people could read, so the use of educational films along with other techniques was indicated. At first, for lack of others, films on health which had been produced for use in the United States were shown. As would be expected, they meant little if anything to those who saw them. The people, their clothes, houses, foods, behavior, in fact, everything in the pictures was strange and foreign to the viewers. The medical and hospital environments presented conditions much too advanced to be of any practical use or applicability to the local situations. Then several health agencies in the United States had cartoon-type health education films made. These were better in that the characters shown had a more or less universal appeal. However, they were first used with English sound tracks, followed sometimes, it is true, by verbal explanations in the native language. But the crucial moment of maximum impact had passed, and their chief function had still been that of entertainment. Following this, the films were made with Spanish sound tracks, since that was the official language of the country. Now they became useful as health education films in some areas, notably in a few of the larger cities. However, they still did not apply to the majority of the people who needed them the most, because they were Indians and a great many spoke little or no Spanish. Therefore we undertook to translate and dub in the sound tracks in the two chief native languages of the Andes. Now the films really meant something to the people for whom they were intended, and they began to respond well. Inciden-

tally, to my knowledge these were the first films with speech in the Quechua language of the Incas and the much more ancient and rarely heard language of the Aymara.

A slightly different type of communication barrier results from the communicator's being held in awe, with the other person ill at ease and nervous. Foster[18] relates that, in the Cerro Baron Health Center in Valparaiso, Chile, one of the finest in Latin America, 13 women were asked as they emerged from the physician's room to repeat his instructions. The remarks of 10 indicated that they had failed to profit from the visit. This prompted similar investigations in other countries, and the results were similar. A variety of reasons were responsible for the failure to comprehend the physician's instructions. Often a woman patient would be nervous and uneasy in the presence of a man, particularly since she usually was in a lower social class than he. She would therefore be unable to concentrate or to grasp what was being said. The problem was partially resolved by having the physician write the instructions on the patient's record card, following which a more "sympatico" nurse would explain the instructions in greater detail and more in terms that the patient would understand.

Differences in behavioral patterns may negate carefully planned and well-intentioned public health endeavors. More than one American public health worker has learned by bitter experience that the manner in which people relieve themselves may be subject to a good deal of variation. A great many American-type privies have gone unused for failure to realize that some people by tradition are "sitters" while others are "squatters." Actually, as Leavell[1] points out, it is unimportant for its public health purpose whether the privy has a seat or whether the squatting method is used in defecation. Even where they are adopted and used, surprising cultural handicaps may appear. I recall seeing privies designed by Westerners using local materials in rural Burma that were used by the people. The use of handy, inexpensive local materials is always praiseworthy. However, the fact that paper in Burma as in many other places is a luxury was overlooked. But of even more consequence was the failure to learn that, by custom, pieces of bamboo were used for the same purpose that paper is in the Western toilet. As a result, before long the privy superstructure tended to assume a rather moth-eaten appearance, and the privy hole became clogged with pieces of bamboo. I recall also talking one day, through an interpreter, with a rural Thai who really made me think. He said, in effect, "You Americans are strange. Before you came here, if I felt like relieving myself, I found a quiet spot in the open with gentle breezes and often a pleasant vista. Then you came along and convinced me that this material that comes from me is one of the most dangerous things with which people can have contact. In other words, I should stay away from it as far as possible. Then the next thing you told me was that I should dig a hole, and not only I, but many other people should concentrate this dangerous material in that hole. So now I have even closer contact not only with my own but everyone else's, and in a dark, smelly place with no view at that." Frankly, I wondered, and I still wonder, which of us was the more logical.

People will seek to attain and maintain health provided that there are no other conflicting cultural forces. Even in our more sophisticated societies, people may react in what they know are illogical or ill-advised ways because of deep-seated folkways or cultural traits of which they are sometimes not even aware, much less understand. Here, too, cultural anthropology may be of great assistance to the public health worker, either through analysis of the situations at hand or by explanation of the same or similar problems in purer cultures, i.e., in more simple or primitive societies. For example, why do some people resist hospitalization? It may be that their group customarily looks upon a hospital as a place to go to die. Beyond that, cultural anthropologists have found that a very common if not universal cultural trait is a strong feeling of continuity with the land

or, in a nonrural situation, at least with the home. Remote in our history, but in many places even yet, is the feeling that when one dies one should die at home, that the spirit will reside in the place where one dies, and that the spirit's place is with the family. To some people death away from home means that the spirit must wander homeless and that it is in an unfavorable position from which to intercede with the gods on behalf of the family which remains behind.

Another common reason for resistance to hospitalization is reaction against tendencies to break down the cultural feeling of responsibility for a member of the family in distress. In addition to pride this may be on the basis that the individual is continuous with his family unit. Too, another reason may be a customary shame in admitting that one is sick, weak, or inadequate. This last is closely related to a common cultural reason for resistance to surgery, i.e., shame or a feeling of incompleteness. This is emphasized particularly if by custom much importance is placed upon the part removed, notably a breast, the uterus, or the testes. Again one does not have to leave the domestic scene to observe this. Closely related to the concept of continuity of the individual with the land is the fear that the excised part or, in the case of obstetrics, the placenta or the dead fetus will not be destroyed or will be separated in space from the environment of the rest of the body or from the family. In more primitive societies, of course, the thought enters into the picture that the excised part, if not destroyed, may be used against oneself as a fetish.

In relation to obstetrics and gynecology there are innumerable taboos or cultural barriers. A hint as to one of the reasons for this is obtained from a study of Yap culture by Schneider.[19] The Yap woman feels that her genitals are the locus of power over her husband. Since her sex organs have enabled her to secure and keep a husband and to raise a family, they constitute her personal "trade secrets" which must not be revealed to women rivals. Yap women never allow other women to view their genitals; therefore, attempts to use native female attendants in the delivery rooms have met with resistance. The substitution of nonindigenous female attendants has proved somewhat more acceptable. They are women, to be sure, but they are alien to the native system of power and sex competition. A husband may see his wife's secrets, but she knows that no self-respecting Yap husband would tolerate any man, including an American obstetrician, seeing and manipulating his wife's private parts. The wife herself does not feel that exposure before any man is as undesirable as exposure before another woman, but she is constrained by the knowledge that she would be violating her husband's personal rights if she allowed the former. A solution has been found in this situation by means of a compromise on both sides. It involves the use of nonnative female attendants and postponement of the mechanics of antisepsis and delivery by the physician until after the patient has been anesthetized.

This leads logically to a consideration of the difficulties encountered with regard to nursing in many parts of the world. Among many peoples the position of women is not only subservient or submerged but they are not even allowed to be seen or move as freely in public as the male. To develop much-needed training programs for nurses under such circumstances is difficult, to say the least. In some other cultures a woman who would touch, cleanse, or come in contact with the discharges or internal parts of other people is customarily held in very low regard. In such circumstances it is again most difficult to elevate nursing to the status of a useful, esteemed profession since, among other things, only the poorest, least educated, and least dependable women are free to engage in the activities necessary. As one other example of a cultural reason for resistance to nursing care there might be mentioned the fear which exists in some societies that to be touched by or given food by a female nurse might, should she be menstruating, bring impotence, illness, or death.

Spectacular curative measures are more readily accepted than are preventive measures which in the long run might be more beneficial. This has been found true in the development of public health programs in this country as well as elsewhere. In most parts of the world, therefore, it is quite impractical to completely disassociate promotive and preventive measures from those which are curative. Erasmus[20] points to the difference in reception and support of the campaigns against yaws carried on by the Institute of Inter-American Affairs in collaboration with the governments of Colombia and Ecuador in contrast with measures to prevent intestinal infections. The results of the yaws treatment were rapid and dramatic, and even the native healers readily admitted that the modern medicine was much more effective than their own herbal and magical treatments. In the case of preventive measures against intestinal infections, however, the story was quite different. Many looked upon the symptoms in a young child as a manifestation of the "evil eye," outside the realm of scientific medicine. Since the conditions under which they lived and their failure to understand the rationale of the suggested measures made obvious rapid improvement impossible, the latter measures were not successfully adopted.

Summarizing his findings, Erasmus[20] concludes:

. . . Needs created by the process of specialization and the desire for increased production and profit actually seem the easiest for technicians from another culture or subculture to meet. The solution is often largely technical, fewer cultural barriers to a common understanding are presented, and the perception and feeling of needs are more easily shared by the innovators and the people.

However, when change is being attempted in a field not directly related to increased production in a cash economy, in other words not directly in terms of profits, the difficulties increase. In the field of public health, for example, the innovator may consider it highly desirable to introduce basic disease prevention measures into an underdeveloped area. But the folk still subscribed to an age-old system of beliefs about the cause, prevention, and treatment of disease, a system so different that the preventive measures of the innovator were meaningless. Lacking an understanding of the modern concepts of the etiology of disease and consequently the reasons for modern methods of prevention, they may feel no need to adopt the prescribed changes. Thus, despite the fact that they feel a general need for assistance in combatting the ailments common among them, they may fail to perceive the need for the specific measures proposed and may actively resist them.

An important fact which should always be remembered by public health workers, particularly the medical component thereof, is that they are constantly in competition with very ancient folklore, superstitions, and well-accepted ideas, even in the most modern societies. The practice of the healing arts is the oldest specialized activity known and one of the very few, along with the priesthood (with which it is closely allied), that appears to be a universal characteristic of all cultures. In spite of this fact, the phrase "world's oldest profession" is commonly applied to a rather different type of human activity. Yet, as Murdock[21] points out, "Prostitution, historically, is a relatively recent phenomenon. I have personally read accounts of many hundreds of primitive societies, and in not a single one of them is genuine prostitution reported. Many of them exhibit forms of such behavior that we would regard as exceedingly lax, but such laxity does not take the specific form of prostitution except in the so-called 'higher' civilizations... Specialized occupations are exceedingly few in the simpler societies, and with a single exception, none occurs more than sporadically. This exception is the medical profession. Specialized practitioners of the healing art are found, to the best of my knowledge, in every known society, however primitive. The 'medicine man,' in one form or another, is universal and hence must be regarded as the oldest professional specialist."

If this is true, it would appear that medical and public health programs have an edge over other types of social programs, provided that they are designed so that there is a ready possibility for adequate transference from the old way to the new. The purpose here is to stress the need to recognize the existence and acceptance of the old ways. If medical and public health measures have an edge over the other social measures, it is also true that the medi-

cine man, the *curandero,* and the medical superstitions and folkways have an edge over the new and strange ideas of modern medicine and public health.

In all instances, from primitive societies in the most underdeveloped areas to the most sophisticated groups in our most modern Western cities, there would appear to exist an interesting dichotomous attitude toward illnesses and what might be done about them. If the reader will bear in mind the continued extensive use of patent medicines and the enormous amount of self-medication as well as the extent to which various types of quacks, faith healers, and pseudophysicians are used by our sophisticated modern societies, it may be of value to explore the background of these tendencies in less complex circumstances. In connection with a 10-year evaluation of the cooperative health programs of the Institute of Inter-American Affairs, Foster[18] has brought out the significance of this pronounced distinction between folk illnesses and those recognized by medical science. As he says, people know that certain types of disease which do not respond to treatment methods of *curanderos* can be cured or prevented by the scientific physician. On the other hand, they feel that there are other illnesses that are best treated by home remedies or with the aid of curanderos, i.e., illnesses which are not understood by modern physicians and the very existence of which they deny. These illnesses, which may be referred to as "folk diseases," are particularly those considered to be of magical or psychic origin. "If an illness is diagnosed, for example, as 'evil eye,' obviously it is poor judgment to take the patient for treatment to a person who denies the very existence of the disease." (See Table 4-1). Now it may be that the illness is actually admitted and recognized by a modern physician. Even in this case, if individuals of the society involved, on the basis of past experience and social custom, regard the condition as due to magical or psychologic etiology, they will tend to rule out the potential usefulness of the modern physician—and it must be remembered that it is they who are in the position to make the primary decision as to what they will do about it.

In connection with the Latin American studies several attempts have been made to measure the extent of the practical effect of the distinction between "folk diseases" and "doctors' diseases." In Ecuador, under Erasmus' direction, a list of the most common complaints was given to 48 schoolchildren of both sexes, ages 11 and 12 years. On the assumption that the opinions expressed would correspond reasonably well with those which they had heard from their parents and other adults, the children were asked to indicate which illnesses they would take to a doctor and which they would treat with home remedies or take to a curandero. The results are shown in Table 4-1. They indicate quite clearly that even some distinctly physical ailments as well as certain psychologic conditions may

tend to be cared for by other than an orthodox physician.

Similar surveys were carried out in Chile and Colombia, and the results were similar. If conditions were customarily thought to be due to the evil eye, bad air, fright, shock, or other magical or psychic causes of which most people felt modern physicians were ignorant, they were almost universally treated at home with folk remedies or by a curandero. This, of course, often prejudiced their chances of ultimate recovery since many times the symptoms were those of serious illnesses. On the other hand, certain clear-cut conditions such as anemia, appendicitis, hernia, meningitis, pneumonia, smallpox, typhoid, and the like generally, but not invariably, were considered to be within the province of a modern physician.

It is all too easy for those of us who

Table 4-1. Percentage of 48 schoolchildren in Quito, Ecuador, who would consult a doctor or a curandero for specified illnesses*

Illness	*Would consult a curandero or treat with home remedies* (%)	*Would consult a doctor* (%)
Fright†	98	2
Air†	93	7
Witchcraft†	86	14
Colic	79	21
Evil eye†	75	25
Stomatitis	72	28
Pasmo†	66	34
Open infections	66	34
Urinary complaints	64	36
Skin disorders	61	39
Diarrhea and vomiting	58	42
Emaciation	49	51
Smallpox	31	69
Dysentery with blood	25	75
Pneumonia	25	75
Whooping cough	20	80
Liver complaints	16	84
Paralysis	9	91
Typhoid	7	93
Bronchitis	6	94
Malaria	5	95
Tuberculosis	4	96

*Adapted from Foster, G. M.: Use of anthropological methods and data in planning and operation, Public Health Rep. **68:**853, Sept. 1953.
†Diseases with magical or psychologic etiologies.

have been exposed in our culture to modern scientific thought glibly and arbitrarily to belittle, toss aside, or ignore the practitioners of folk medicine as if they were completely unworthy of consideration. The illogic of so doing is expressed by Elkins[22]:

Aboriginal medicine men are far from being rogues, charlatans or ignoramuses. They are men of high degrees . . . men who have undergone tests and have taken degrees in the secrets of life much beyond that which ordinary men have a chance to learn. This training involves steps which imply a discipline, mental effort, courage and perseverance. In addition, they are men of respected, and often of outstanding personality. Thus, they are of immense social significance, with the health of the group depending largely on faith in their powers. Furthermore, the various psychic powers attributed to them must not be readily dismissed as mere "make-believe," for many of them have specialized in the workings of the human mind and in the influence of mind on mind and mind on body. And, what is more, they are deeply convinced of their powers, so much so, that as long as they observe the customary discipline of their "order," their professional status and practice continues to be a source of faith and healing power to both themselves and their fellows.

Returning to the Latin American scene, which is much closer to ours in the United States, Foster's[18] analysis of the relationship between the modern physician and the curandero is of particular pertinence and may be applied to our domestic scene with adequate provision made, of course, for differences in degree and type of social camouflage.

The conflict between folk medicine and scientific medicine is summed up in the persons of the physician and *curandero*. Each represents the highest achievement in his field. The attitudes of the people of Latin America towards each, therefore, are pertinent to this study. Unfortunately, the physician frequently comes off second best. This is due in part to the inherent nature of the situation, and in part to native suspicion of individuals in other social classes, particularly those above them. The *curandero* operates under conditions that are relatively more favorable than those of the physician, from the point of view of impressing the patient with concrete results and apparent success. He treats folk illnesses, the symptoms of which often are so ill-defined that he cannot help but succeed in alleviating them. If the vague physiological symptoms identified with the illness persist or reappear after the cure, the *curandero* can always say that the case has become complicated and requires another series of cures or a different

cure, or that a new and different illness has attacked the patient. Also, most *curanderos* do not claim to cure all illnesses, and in many cases can even recommend that a patient consult a physician. These factors establish the *curanderos* in the minds of the folk as fair, open-minded individuals willing to admit their limitations. Finally, the *curandero's* diagnostic techniques do not require elaborate and exhaustive questioning of the patient as to symptoms, case history, and the like. He has certain magical or automatic devices which he applies to specific situations, and the answers follow almost like clockwork. Moreover, there are many cases reported by field observers in which a physician failed to cure an individual and a *curandero* had apparently genuine success.

The physician enjoys few of these advantages. His diagnosis is seldom cut and dried, he cannot guarantee quick results, and he seldom enjoys the faith and confidence accorded the *curandero* because he is from a social class instinctively distrusted by the majority of his patients. Moreover, the physician seldom admits that a *curandero* can cure things which he is incapable of treating, and this is interpreted as meaning that he conceitedly and selfishly believes himself to be the sole repository of medical knowledge—a point of view which the villager is loath to accept.

Criticisms of physicians and their professional methods are rife among the patients of the lower class, and such criticisms are usually based on a complete lack of comprehension of medicine, its methods, and its limitations. Several patients pointed out that physicians asked them questions about their symptoms, which showed that the physicians were not as smart as they thought they were. A good *curandero* doesn't have to ask questions, so why should a man who pretends to know a great deal more have to do so? Another patient scornfully pointed out that a President of Colombia died "even though he had 50 physicians at his bedside." The implication was that if 50 physicians could not keep a man from dying, a single doctor in a short interview was almost worse than worthless.

A final handicap of the physician is the general tendency of the people to exhaust home remedies and the arts of the *curandero* before appealing to the physician. The physician, therefore, gets many cases too late to effect a cure and many others which are simply incurable. Hence, the failures of folk medicine as well as those of his own profession are heaped upon his shoulders.

In fairness it must be admitted that there are many points of value to be found in folk medicine. In fact, one might consider our modern scientific medicine as a natural extension and elaboration of folk medicine on a scientific basis, thereby representing our "scientific folk medicine." The number of effective drugs which have originated in folk medicine is rather impressive: quinine, rauwolfia, mescaline, chaulmoogra, opium, coca, curare, and many laxatives, to mention but a few. As to physical techniques one might mention massage, baths, sweating treatments, surgery, and even inoculation. In the field of mental health and psychotherapy, a great deal can be learned from the practitioner of simple folk medicine.

It is interesting that, although knowledge of the causative agents was lacking, certain illnesses traditionally have been considered as communicable, and it was believed that those who suffered therefrom should be kept apart from the other members of society. Beyond this it is commonly felt that individuals subject to certain debilitating illnesses are in a weakened condition and that visitors may unintentionally harm the patient as a result of strong "humors" which they may carry. Therefore, even without regard to the possible communicability of the patient's illness, isolation is carried out for the patient's own good. It is worthy of note that our own attitude toward the value of isolation in a great many instances has shifted to exactly this point of view. Where concern exists with regard to the evil effects of *aire,* strong humors, or similar folk influences, it may be possible to take advantage of this; for, whatever the reasoning, an essentially hygienic practice is followed, one that can with value be made use of by physicians and nurses in the treatment and prevention of spread of communicable diseases. Physicians need not express an opinion on the potential danger of *aire;* they can simply say that visitors are undesirable for the patient's sake, and the family will probably follow the recommendation, even though the physicians are thinking in terms of contagion and the family in terms of magic.

In most if not all instances it is probably ill advised merely to ignore the patient's ideas about his illness and the relationship of established folkways to it. Foster[23] warns, "The common tendency on the part of doctors and nurses to ignore, if not to ridicule, folk concepts of illness, probably reduces their effectiveness . . . ." He illustrates this with a number of instances

in which modern physicians and especially nurses wisely listen to patients' complaints and to their ideas of magical and metaphysical relationships thereto, then follow up by relating their suggestions for modern scientific treatment to those familiar, accepted ideas. This accomplishes several things. It puts the modern physician and nurse a notch higher in the patient's estimation since not only did they not belittle the patient's valued ideas and the folk traditions, but they actually exhibited some interest and understanding of them. From this starting point there develops a greater understanding and receptivity by the patient of scientific medicine and its practitioners. This is one of the most important ways that erroneous folk practices may eventually be dropped and more effective and suitable scientific practices substituted for them.

It would sometimes appear that we, as well as others, tend to make a fetish of terminology. After all, words and titles are of little consequence—the fundamental concept and what is done about it is truly important. I had the experience of working at one time as the health officer of a county in a southeastern state, the county seat of which was the international headquarters of a very fundamentalist religious group. It not only refused to recognize the germ causation of some diseases but actually refused to admit the very existence of illness of any kind. If there was something the matter with an individual, he was not sick —rather, God was displeased with him or with something in his environment, and when God became happy again, the individual would recover. Meanwhile, of course, he might die from an otherwise preventable disease. These ideas were deeply ingrained in the religious beliefs of these people. It was obviously futile to try to convince them otherwise. In terms of their religious tenets, in which they had absolute faith, they knew they were right, and, after all, they were entitled to whatever religious beliefs they wished. Nevertheless, this posed a very serious problem with regard to not only their welfare but also the welfare of everyone with whom they had contact.

Actually it worked out reasonably well. I went out of my way to become a good friend of the elderly bishop who was head of the church. He was obviously a good and sincere man. He believed that he and his people were doing the right thing. Who was I to say no? One day as we sat chatting I said to him, in effect, "Look here, Bishop, you and I may disagree on a philosophic basis about certain things. We do however have one very important common interest —we are both honestly interested in the well-being of your people and of all people. Furthermore, we also have a very important point of common agreement, we each recognize that at certain times something undesirable happens to people. Let us not argue about what causes that something to happen. After all, the cause is incidental to the effect. If you want to say that it is displeasure on the part of God, that is all right with me. On the other hand, if it makes me happy to think that it is a bacterium, it can do no harm for me to think so. But, let us, you and I, work together in doing something about the result." After that I had no more difficulty. If I wished to impose isolation on a person with a communicable disease, it was on the basis of preventing contact of the general public with influences that had displeased God. If I wanted to use immunizing agents, it was on the basis of injecting God-inspired material to help keep away unknown, displeasing factors which might harm people. If I wished to prescribe drugs and medicines, it was on the basis of giving materials to assist in driving out or removing from the body the things that had displeased the Lord. In fact, we got along so famously that I finally found myself being consulted on various church matters.

How does all of the foregoing tie together? We may gain a clue if we accept the idea that our goal as public health workers must be to make good personal and community health practices an accepted part of the way of life and culture of people. This cannot occur spontaneously, and it cannot be done merely by destroying what to us may seem to be erroneous customs. It must be carefully planned and worked at over a long period of time. We have long since learned the inadequacy of doing things to or even for people. We realize now that the best way is to do things with people, and in order to do so we must understand as thoroughly as possible the cultural factors which make them act the way they do and tailor our suggestions and programs to the accepted general cultural pattern of the group. We should constantly relate our efforts to something familiar, something most people already know, do, and accept. In addition, we must recognize that our own communities, sophisticated as they may appear to be on the surface, consist of numerous societies and numerous cultures. We must recognize that so-called sophistication may merely substitute city ways for folkways and that many of our customs are fundamentally the same as those found elsewhere, having merely been transferred, transformed, or adapted to a new environment or set of social conditions.

EFFECT OF PUBLIC HEALTH ACTIVITIES ON CULTURAL PATTERNS

Discussion up to this point has centered on the effect which cultural patterns may have on the public health and on public health activities. A brief consideration of inverse relationship would seem to be in order. If public health programs are successful in their attempts to improve the state of physical and mental health of a people, it should be obvious that there are complex far-reaching effects on many if not all other phases of the culture of the people. Thus, if workers are made healthier and more alert mentally, their ingenuity and inventiveness tend to increase. To the extent that they may produce more and better mechanical aids to their labors, they then find it not only possible to produce more, but they do it more easily and in less time. This makes possible a shorter workday for the average person and, concomitantly, more time for leisure. With more time of their own on their hands people tend to engage more in the pursuit of some of the less tangible cultural activities, i.e., recreation, study, reading, and the fine arts, and gradually, because of an increased standard of living, they have more and more money for such activities.

A measurable effect of public health activities is a decrease in the number of deaths and an increase in the average life expectancy. Thus in the United States since the beginning of the twentieth century, infant death rates have been lowered from about 200 per 1,000 live births to about 25 per 1,000 at the present time. This means that instead of every fifth baby's dying, only every fortieth baby now dies. In the same period of time the average life expectancy has been raised from about 49 years to over 70 years. The social consequences of such a rapid effect of public health activities are many and far reaching. There are more mouths for the family and the nation to feed, greater housing needs, more schools to be built and more school buses to be supplied, and more recreation facilities and other civic and social activities are needed. On the other hand, it also means that less money is needed for the care of preventable illnesses, much less family worry and sadness, and it means a changed attitude toward illness and death and healthier children who in a short time become more alert, better informed, and capable citizens and workers. One might generalize by saying that in many or all such situations rapidly improved health conditions tend to result first in increased social pressures and problems and a little later in greatly multiplied social benefits.

The provision of more and healthier people, then, sets off a whole chain of events, all aimed at improvement of our national culture and all resulting eventually in an improved standard of living for everyone. There are more people available to work in our offices, businesses, farmlands, and factories, and, because they are on the average healthier than their parents and grandparents, they can produce more, which means an increase in the individual share of the material things of life. At the same time attitudes toward marriage and family life are strongly affected by the results of public health measures. To approach this negatively, if death rates are high in general and if maternal mortality rates are high in particular, family structure must be adapted accordingly. The husband and children must accept the possibility of having several wives and mothers, and, for the woman, childbirth is surrounded by real fear and many superstitions. Because of the frequency of deaths of the mothers, the position of the older surviving female relatives is much more important in the total family picture than in our present typical American situation. Also, because of high infant and child mortality, husbands, public opinion, and nature conspire to keep the woman pregnant most of the time. One might say further that the generally pregnant wife results in the most marked accentuation of the double standard. The male tends toward more widespread promiscuous relationships, which tend to be accepted more readily by society, and this, of course, invites a greater prevalence of venereal diseases.

Lowered infant mortality and maternal mortality rates, on the other hand, tend eventually to bring about a pattern of smaller families which, in some respects at least, have stronger immediate family bonds. In our current American society this has had a marked effect on the size of houses and even their architecture as well as on the use which is made of the home. A social complication has resulted, however, by virtue of the concurrent lengthening of life and a growing number of elderly individuals. This fact, related to a change in social attitude or interpretation of family constituency and responsibility as well as to the change which has occurred in the size and layout of the modern small home, leaves a sizable proportion of the population, the grandparents and other elderly persons, with little or no home base. The development of a social problem of this unfortunate type results inevitably in a social reaction. Some symptoms of this are evident in the increasing literature and social legislation dealing with the elderly or senior citizens' needs for medical care, housing, and other things.

Successful public health programs may bring about a marked change in attitude toward previously deep-seated customs. The wearing of charms of all sorts is a remarkably common practice in this as well as many other countries. Usually they are not readily relinquished. Because of the success of certain phases of the health technical assistance programs in Haiti, it was found necessary to place boxes at the treatment and health centers as receptacles for the charms and fetishes which some of the now convinced patients discarded in large numbers.

One final example of an effect which public health activities may have upon a society illustrates that the results may be not only quite unexpected but even undesirable. A truly effective venereal disease control program, like any other special health program, should take into consideration the social and behavioral problems and attitudes of the people and the social and cultural consequences of the activity. The many ramifications of a program of this nature were brought out dramatically in a joint international attempt to eradicate venereal diseases. Many United States soldiers were located in training camps close to communities in another nation. Large numbers of these young soldiers, when off duty, had no place else to go except those communities. Because of this, prostitution in its worst form flourished, and large numbers of these soldiers were reported infected with venereal diseases. United States public health officials got together with their counterparts in the other nation's government to solve the problem. From a strictly scientific and public health standpoint their jointly devised program provided a solution. However, some other things happened upon which they had not counted. In line with recently developed antibiotic therapy and prophylaxis the basis of their approach was to require all of the regular prostitutes to receive large injections of residual penicillin each week, whether or not they appeared to be infected. Failure to be able to present evidence of the weekly injection meant a loss of permit to work in the carefully regulated and registered houses of prostitution. The first result was a dramatic drop in

the incidence of new infection among the United States soldiers, the local population, and the prostitutes. Next, apparently as word of the situation got around, it was realized that these were desirable places in which to practice prostitution and relatively safe places to visit for such purposes. Understandably, nonpublic health officials of the other nation thereupon complained that the program was actually promoting and increasing their prostitution problem. Finally, a totally unexpected result began to appear: many of the prostitutes had been suffering from gonorrheal inflammations which had prevented their becoming pregnant; now, with the repeated routine injections of penicillin, those inflammations were cleared up and some of them became pregnant by totally unknown fathers. The social welfare aspects of this problem are obviously enormous.

We should always be conscious of the very delicate balance in which society operates. This applies particularly to activities in a field that may have as prompt and far-reaching influences as does public health. While it is axiomatic that progress in one cultural direction inevitably results in progress in other aspects of a culture, it is equally true that the artificial stimulation of great sudden advancements in one phase of a culture alone may bring about at least a temporary social difficulty, if not even chaos. Thus we may actually be wielding a two-edged sword if we suddenly, rapidly, and exclusively apply all of our present public health knowledge to a situation. If we do so without considering the other basic social needs of the additional people, there is real danger of causing irreparable distortion and harm to a culture or a society. There may develop increased food problems, social and economic imbalance, and political unrest, to mention but a few potential results. We need not be pessimistic about this, however. The important thing is to realize the potentialities and implications and to emphasize the absolute necessity for public health workers to move consciously ahead, hand in hand with workers in other fields, i.e., agriculturists, educators, political scientists, social service workers, and many others, including the cultural anthropologist, who can contribute greatly to this by indicating needs, ways, and means.

CONTRIBUTIONS OF SOCIAL SCIENTISTS TO PUBLIC HEALTH

In *The Epic of America,* James Truslow Adams claims that America's greatest contribution to the total human culture is the "vision of a society in which the lot of the common man will be made easier and his life enriched and ennobled." Most certainly a well-chosen and successfully pursued public health program is one of the significant handmaidens to this goal of social order. But, as Kluckhohn[4] warns:

Order is bought too dearly if it is bought at the price of the tyranny of any single set of inflexible principles, however noble these may appear to be from the perspective of any single culture. Individuals are biologically different, and there are various types of temperament which reappear at different times and places in the world's history. So long as the satisfaction of temperamental needs is not needlessly thwarting to the life activities of others, so long as the diversities are not socially destructive, individuals must not only be permitted but indeed encouraged to fulfill themselves in diverse ways. The necessity for diversity is founded upon the facts of biological differences, differences in situation, varying backgrounds in individual and cultural history.

It is part of the function of the social scientist to study these differences, to serve as pilot when in the planning and operation of our activities we attempt to sail through the complex seas of societies and their cultures. Further, they can send out storm warnings when we appear to be in danger of serious error because of misunderstanding the motivations of individuals and groups. Finally, if we do find ourselves in inexplicable difficulty, the social scientist, by virtue of his somewhat different way of looking at things, may be able to find out why and to point to a way out of our dilemma. For example, the health educator, as Paul[10] describes, may approach his assignment with the preconception that his job is merely to convey information to people who are "uninformed." If he does so, he is not too apt to succeed, whereupon he may conclude that the slow acceptance of his ideas is attributable to intellectual deficiency or willful stubborn resistance on the part of those he seeks to benefit. In most if not all instances, his job is really to help people reorganize their existing conceptual system. As Paul states, "Knowledge of the local belief system enables the imaginative educator to present his data in such order and in such a way as to be most readily grasped by the recipients. It also enables him to anticipate the directions that 'misunderstanding' will take."

Meltzer[24] has provided an excellent example or illustration of the manner in which the approach to activity or program analysis previously suggested may be of value. The study relates to topical fluoride demonstration programs in six communities; three were successful and three were failures. The purpose was to determine if possible the reasons for the failures as well as for the successes. By way of introduction, she complains that, "We in public health work have an unfortunate habit of talking and writing only about our successes, ignoring our failures, and seldom examining the principles we were trying to use when we failed. It does little good to study the methods that led to program success in one community, if we forget that the identical methods have failed miserably in other similar communities. When that happens, it is a case of using methods based on untested assumptions, rather than on sound principles." In the analysis of the dental programs, as might be expected, it was found that there was neither one reason for success nor one reason for failure since each of the six communities was a case into itself with its own cultural pattern. The failures were ultimately attributed to a variety of reasons, including inadequate communication between the public health workers and the public, the impression that the program was a self-contained short-term experiment, that it needlessly disrupted the school routine without real purpose, and that some significant groups in the community were not brought into the planning. The example illustrates that action teams such as groups of public health workers often define the reaction or the anticipated reaction of a community in their own way and according to their own standards. They see the community and interpret the situations they encounter according to their own preconceptions, which of course are rooted in the subculture of there own professional as well as social class. As Paul[10] emphasizes, this need to understand and overcome cultural differences "applies not only in the case of a health mission operating in a foreign country, but also in the case of a team working in a community within its own country. The difference in the two cases is one of degree."

The relevancy of the subject to public health has been formally recognized by the American Public Health Association in a resolution unanimously adopted at its Eighty-first Annual Meeting in New York on November 11, 1953:

WHEREAS, the field of health education is concerned basically with human behavior, its nature and how it may be altered for the improvement and promotion of individual and community health, and

WHEREAS, the social sciences contribute to knowledge of human nature and behavior, therefore be it

RESOLVED, that the American Public Health Association encourage collaboration between public health workers and social scientists to better promote the utilization of social science findings toward the solution of public health problems.

In discussing the ways in which social science may be of significance to the field of public health, Foster[23] has presented a list of factors to be considered, which, he warns, are intended to be merely suggestive and illustrative and not a definitive catalog. The list is sufficiently thought provoking, however, to merit repetition here:

Although it is desirable to know as much about a culture as possible, there are obviously strict limitations as to what can be known. Social scientists have barely made a beginning in the formidable task of describing the elements of the cultures of the world and interpreting their significance. It must be assumed that for any given program there are certain categories of information about the culture in which the work is to be carried out which are of primary importance, and others that are of lesser importance. A "trial run" in compiling a list of primary classes of data for public health programs gives the following picture.

Folk medicine and native curing practices. The

importance of this has been discussed at some length above and need not be commented on further at this point.

Economics, particularly incomes and costs of living. Since in the final analysis the success of public health programs rests upon major changes in the habits of people with respect to diet, housing, clothing, agriculture, and the like, knowledge of the economic potential of an area is paramount.

Social organization of families. A bride often lives in her husband's home, under the domination of her mother-in-law. There are cases in which pregnant women failed to follow, or had difficulty in following, health center recommendations because these conflicted with what the mother-in-law thought was best.

Men and women who live together are frequently not legally married. Under such circumstances, a man is less likely to recognize obligations to his companion and their children, and it is therefore more difficult to persuade him to come to the health center for venereal or other treatment. Recognition of these and similar problems makes the responses of patients more intelligible.

Education and literacy and comprehension. Ability to comprehend the real nature of health and disease, to profit by health education, and to understand and follow the physician's instructions depends on the education and literacy of the people.

Political organization. Local conditions under which physicians and other staff members are appointed, the local attitude toward nepotism, bureaucratic rules which govern operations, and the like, are factors which will affect public health programs. In one country, for example, a large health center, not yet placed in operation, was seriously threatened by the conflicting interests of the state governor, the local nurses' union, and other bureaucratic factors.

Religion. A basic analysis of religious tenets is not essential, but some parts of the religious philosophy of the people should be known. Are there any beliefs which hinder or directly conflict with proposed programs? Is death, for example, at any age considered a welcome relief from a world of suffering? Are there food taboos based on religious sanction which should be taken into consideration in planning diets?

Basic value system. What are the goals, aspirations, fundamental values, and major cultural premises, consciously or unconsciously accepted, which give validity to the lives of the people in question? What is the practical significance, for example, of a fatalistic approach to life and death? What part does prestige play in determining customary behavior patterns of the people? Is male vanity and ego a factor to consider? What are the ideas of bodily modesty? What are the types of stimuli and appeal to which people respond most readily?

Other types of data. Planners and administrators of public health programs should also have at hand such information as credit facilities and money usages, labor division within the family, time utilization, working and eating schedules, cooking and dietary practices, and the importance of alcoholism.

Categories of culture in which precise knowledge would appear to be of lesser importance include agriculture, fishing, and other primary productive occupations, industrial techniques (except as working conditions may affect health), trade and commerce, religious fiestas and church observances, wedding ceremonies, burial customs, and music and folk tales.

In bringing to a close this brief consideration of social science in relation to public health, it is appropriate to call attention to one final value which it has for public health workers. It has been stated by Murdock[21] in the following manner: "One of the greatest potential contributions of anthropology is to make those who are professionally concerned with health problems aware of the broad sweep of culture history and of their position in it."

REFERENCES

1. Leavell, H. R.: New occasions teach new duties, Public Health Rep. **68**:687, July 1953.
2. Koos, E. L.: New concepts in community organization for health, Amer. J. Public Health **43**:466, Apr. 1953.
3. Skinner, B. F.: Science and human behavior, New York, 1953, The Macmillan Co.
4. Kluckhohn, C.: Mirror for man: the relation of anthropology to modern life, New York, 1949, Whittlesey House.
5. White, L. A.: Man's control over civilization, an anthropocentric illusion, Sci. Month. **66**:238, Mar. 1948.
6. Benedict, R.: Patterns of culture, New York, 1934, The New American Library of World Literature, Inc.
7. Carothers, J. C.: The African mind in health and disease, World Health Organization Monograph Series, No. 17, 1953, Geneva.
8. Gittler, J. B.: Man and his prejudices, Sci. Month. **69**:44, July 1949.
9. Bernard, J.: Can science transcend culture? Sci. Month. **71**:270, Oct. 1950.
10. Paul, B. D.: Respect for cultural differences, Community Development Bull., University of London Institute of Education **4**:42, June 1953.
11. Hoyt, E. E.: Tiquisate: a call for a science of human affairs, Sci. Month. **72**:114, Feb. 1951.
12. Miller, W. S.: Some observations on enteric infection in a delta village, J. Egypt. Public Health Ass. **25**:45, 1950.
13. Wier, J. M., et al.: An evaluation of health and sanitation in Egyptian villages, J. Egypt. Public Health Ass. **27**:55, 1952.
14. Bogue, R., and Habashy, A.: Health education pilot project in three villages in Egypt, 1955, Unnumbered Publication of World Health Organization Regional Office, Alexandria.
15. Paul, B. D.: American medicine on the island of Yap, Harvard School of Public Health, 1951 (published paper).
16. Hyde, H. V.: Education and world health, Progressive Education Mar. 1949.
17. Whorf, B. L.: Languages and logic, Techn. Rev. **43**:250, Apr. 1941.
18. Foster, G. M.: Use of anthropological methods and data in planning and operation, Public Health Rep. **68**:853, Sept. 1953.
19. Schneider, D. M.: In Paul, B. D.: Health, culture, and community, New York, 1955, Russell Sage Foundation.
20. Erasmus, C. J.: An anthropologist views technical assistance, Sci. Month. **78**:148, Mar. 1954.
21. Murdock, G. P.: Anthropology and its contribution to public health, Amer. J. Public Health **42**:8, Apr. 1952.
22. Elkins, A.: Aboriginal men of high degree, Sydney, 1944, Australasian Publishing Co., Ltd.
23. Foster, G. M.: A cross-cultural anthropological analysis of a technical aid program, Washington, 1951, Smithsonian Institution.
24. Meltzer, N. S.: A psychological approach to developing principles of community organization, Amer. J. Public Health **43**:198, Feb. 1953.

Chapter 5

Social pathology
and
public health

INTRODUCTION

Now that we have viewed public health in relation to cultural behavior and the development of society, it is important to consider some of the social factors which play significant causal, effectual, or companionship roles with regard to the state of health or illness of the group or society. Simmons and Wolff[1] neatly state that "culture sets the stage, ascribes the parts, and defines the terms whereby society's drama is enacted." On the other hand, society is the instrument, the mechanism, the organization that provides the environment for a culture to develop, grow, and manifest itself. This is an area to which insufficient attention has been given not only by public health workers but also by those in other disciplines who think, plan, and strive for the protection and promotion of the total well-being of society.

Paradoxically, as far as public health is concerned, the appearance of the great era of bacteriology actually resulted in delaying broad effective progress. The discovery that very specific living organisms are related to plague, anthrax, and many other disease conditions and that these clinical syndromes could not occur in the absence of their respective causative organisms brought about a great flush of enthusiasm and hope. An unfortunate result, however, was the development of an attitude on the part of some that effective bacterial exposure was the alpha and omega of disease causation.

Indeed, this had much to do with the broad acceptance and support of certain sanitary measures in the late nineteenth and early twentieth centuries since it became recognized that bacteria could invade the town house and the palace through the servants' quarters and that *Corynebacterium diphtheriae* could strike the children of the wealthy and privileged as well as the children of the poor.

As long as etiology was still indeterminate or uncertain, men tended of necessity to cast about widely in their search for causal relationships. Once a scientific or, better yet, a laboratory answer was forthcoming, there was a tendency to close the issue with a Q.E.D. This comparative attitude was well put by Stern[2] in a discussion of living conditions and health:

In contrast with the narrower focus of public health work after the modern science of bacteriology had developed, the objective of the pioneers of public health included demands for better housing conditions, nutritious food, unpolluted water, cleaner streets and improved working conditions. These men anticipated the fundamental truth of modern preventive medicine, that the health of the individual is intimately and indivisibly tied up with the social as well as the physical environment in which he resides.

The reader is asked to refer back to Chapter 2 on background and development and to note that it was no coincidence that the midnineteenth century reports and recommendations of men like Southwood Smith, Chadwick, and Shattuck were so extensive and far reaching. Similarly it was no coincidence that they "fell flat from the printers' hands," and were underrated or cast aside, appearing when they did on the eve of the era of great bacteriologic discoveries. They simply had to wait until the more palatable and more easily dealt with vogue had run its course. It is equally interesting to note that those diseases for which etiologic agents were difficult to determine or were matters of controversy continued to be related, to some extent, to social conditions and to environmental factors. This was true, for example, of tuberculosis, pneumonia, and influenza. One might state as an axiom that the easier it was to determine a specific relationship between a microorganism and a disease, the more social and environmental factors were ignored.

In recent years it has been increasingly realized that man in his entirety is a combination of physical, psychologic, social, and cultural factors. If the recognition and acceptance of this is to be at all meaningful, practitioners of public health and medicine must cease to evaluate and treat man by the first of these factors alone. Sir Farquhar Buzzard,[3] Regius Professor of Medicine at Oxford, has stressed that our aim should be as follows:

> . . . to expose the sources and bases whence arise ill health and disability, by investigating the influence of social, genetic, environmental, and domestic factors on the incidence of human disease . . . [taking into consideration] . . . such varying agents as heredity, nutrition, climate, and occupation . . . [as well as] . . . the part played by the individual and mass psychology.

A similar conclusion was reached by Ryle,[4] who after 30 years as a student and teacher of clinical medicine accepted the chairmanship of the first Department of Social Medicine (Oxford, 1942). He contemplated that during those 30 years he saw disease studied ever more thoroughly but not more thoughtfully, as if through the high power of the microscope, and more and more mechanically. He commented:

> Man, as a person and a member of a family and of much larger social groups, with his health and sickness intimately bound up with the conditions of his life and work—in the home, the mine, the factory, the shop, at sea, or on the land—and with his economic opportunity, has been inadequately considered in this period by the clinical teacher and hospital research worker. [And may I add—by a large number of public health workers!]

In his prefacing statement Ryle avers:

> We no longer believe that medical truths are only or chiefly to be discovered under the microscope, by means of the test tube, and the animal experiment, or by clinical examination and increasingly elaborate pathological studies at the bedside. Psychological and sociological studies have as important a part to play. Even so, it is not yet appreciated how intimately disease and social circumstance are interrelated. The whole natural history of disease in human communities, as well as in individuals, is ripe for a fuller and more exhaustive study.

Reference has now been made to social medicine and social pathology. These terms are much better known and understood in Europe than in America as a result of the outstanding writings of Pettenkofer, Neumann, and Grotjahn of Germany, Sand of Belgium, and Southwood Smith, Chadwick, Simon, Buzzard, and Ryle of Great Britain. Nevertheless, the relationships between factors in the social environment and disease have long been a matter of concern in the United States, although it is only relatively recently that they have been considered under the term "social medicine." Unfortunately, in this country the term is often confused with socialized medicine and its content similarly confused with concerns about the organization and economics of the provision of medical care. Some have tried to solve this dilemma partially and indirectly by use of the term "comprehensive medicine." In its present form this tends to limit itself essentially to the relationship between an individual's physical illness and his psychosociologic stresses. It is done essentially toward the end of diagnosis, treatment, and prevention of recurrence of the particular malady.[5,6] The United States does have its share of individuals who have contributed notably to the philosophy of social medicine and social pathology, albeit not always by their European designations. Among those who may be mentioned are Shattuck, Smith, Sydenstricker, Mountin, and Winslow. More recent contributions of significance have come from Galdston, Dunham, Rosen, and Wolff.*

The need to recognize the reality of the fields of social medicine and social pathology becomes more imperative in view of the twin revolutions now being witnessed in medicine and society. As an example, attention is directed to the dramatic changes in the types and extents of illnesses and deaths and in the resources with which to combat them. Thus the rate of major medical discovery has accelerated from one per century before 1900, to one per decade between 1900 and 1940, and to one or more per year since 1940. In the United States at the time of this writing 90% of the prescriptions written are for substances which did not even exist 10 years ago.[11] The nature and extent of the social revolution is discussed in Chapter 32, "The Past as Prologue." Suffice to point out here the tremendous increase in the population, its significant aging, the dramatic extent of urbanization and mechanization, and the marked increase and equalization of the standard of living.

DEFINITION

There have been numerous attempts to definite social medicine and social pathology. One of the earliest and still one of the best definitions is that of Grotjahn,[12] who approached the problem of definition by enunciating several principles which, as he saw it, were necessary considerations in the proper study of a disease. These principles may be summarized as follows:

1. The social significance of a disease is determined primarily by its frequency. This emphasizes the importance of accurate medical statistics.
2. The most common form of a disease, its sociopathologic prototype, is also of social significance—more significant

than its unusual or complicated rarer forms.
3. The etiology of every disease includes both biologic and social factors. The latter may affect a disease in several ways—they may be causative, predisposing, or they may influence the transmission or the course of illness.
4. The prevalence and outcome of disease may be influenced by attention to social and economic factors as they relate to the individual and the group.
5. It is important to determine the influence of successful treatment of a disease upon the subsequent prevalence and upon other social factors.
6. Diseases may themselves affect social conditions for the individual or for the group through recovery, predisposition to other illnesses, chronic infirmity, degeneration, or death.

The British Journal of Social Medicine attempted to clarify the issue editorially in January 1947 by the following statement:

Social medicine is that branch of science which is concerned with: (a) biological needs, inter-actions, disabilities, and potentialities of human beings living in social aggregates; (b) numerical, structural and functional changes of human populations in their biological and medical aspects. . . . Social medicine takes within its province the study of all environmental agencies, living and non-living, relevant to health and efficiency, also fertility and population genetics, norms and ranges of variation with respect to individual differences and finally, investigation directed to the assessment of a regimen of positive health.

The importance of statistics of mass phenomena and relationships has again been stressed by Wolff[13] in his definition of social pathology:

The relation between disease and social conditions is the content of social pathology; its method is necessarily a sociological description of this relationship which, for simplicity's sake is mostly based on a statistical analysis of the quantitative findings.

It is obvious that in the discussion so far the terms "social medicine" and "social pathology" have been used almost interchangeably. Although similar and related, they are different. The following definitions are suggested, therefore, in an attempt to synthesize and simplify the several state-

---

*For historical review the reader is referred to *The Concept of Social Medicine as Presented by Physicians and Other Writers in Germany, 1779-1932* by Kroeger,[7] *Social Pathology and the New Era in Medicine* by Ryle,[8] *The Meaning of Social Medicine* by Galdston,[9] and *Approaches to a Concept of Social Medicine* by Rosen.[10]

ments to which reference has been made and to indicate the relationship and the difference between the two terms:

1. *Social pathology* is a state of community imbalance evidenced by significant prevalence of disease and its related social disorders.
2. *Social medicine* is the study of the manner in which disease may result from, cause, or accentuate social problems and of the ways in which medical and public health efforts may contribute to their solution.

MAN AND ENVIRONMENT

Even the most cursory consideration results in the empiric conclusion that there is some direct interrelationship between undesirable living circumstances and various types of problems. This is especially true and especially evident in urban situations, where sheer numbers and crowding accentuate all such problems. The numerous social difficulties of cities are commonly observed to be concentrated particularly in the slum or substandard sections. Here houses tend to be small and crowded together, with a maximum amount of the area devoted to profitable subsistence living space. Little or no consideration is given to recreational needs. Often, and through no accident, industry is located nearby—close to a supply of labor eager for employment. The crowding of buildings, the generally narrow streets, the absence of open recreational areas, and the smoke of factories limit considerably the amount of sunshine and fresh air. Cleanliness and sanitation are difficult to maintain. Death or injury is invited by the narrow traffic-laden streets, the rickety abandoned structures, and the poorly planned flammable dwellings. Both education and nutrition also tend to be substandard and combine with insanitation and overcrowding to maintain a high incidence of illness. Lack of privacy encourages immorality and is conducive to a lowering of self-respect. This and other psychologic maladjustments in the developing child and adolescent breed attitudes of hopelessness, constant frustration, cynicism, resentment, and explosive pent-up hostility. Responsi-

bility and initiative appear pointless, and what seem to be the only roads to self-expression and escape are socially undesirable. There tend to occur undesirable positive reactions of rebellion such as destructiveness or crime or negative reactions of defeat such as addictions or prostitution. It is perhaps not coincidental that the word for town dweller *(pagani)* has the etymologic root that it does.

These relationships have been repeatedly and conclusively shown to exist. Much of the writings of Southwood Smith and Chadwick dealt with this subject. Earlier, in 1828, Villermé, one of the originators of social statistics, presented to the French Academy of Medicine a memoir comparing the death rates of the rich and the poor. Studies during the early 1930's in the United States showed about 20% of the land area of a number of metropolitan areas to be of a substandard, blighted, or slum quality. These areas, aside from factories, included the living quarters of a third of the populations of those cities. However, they accounted for 35% of the fires, 50% of the disease in general, 65% of the tuberculosis cases, 55% of the juvenile delinquents, and 50% of the arrests. Although they contributed only 6% of the tax revenue of the cities, they required 45% of the cities' expenditures.[14]

In the study of a specific community, Cleveland, O., in 1934, the relationships shown in Table 5-1 were found to exist in connection with a slum section.

As in other studies, while the area contributed only $225,000 per year in taxes, it required eight times that amount or $1.97 million per year to sustain it.

With specific reference to the relationship of general environment to disease and death a considerable body of data has now accumulated. Several examples may be worth while for purposes of illustration. One is a study in Liverpool, England (1923-1929), which showed the comparisons presented in Table 5-2 with regard to the effect of the social environment upon health.

At about the same time the National Health Survey in the United States brought to light many correlations between environment and health. Thus for urban white persons the relationships of crowding to amount of illness were found to be very significant (Table 5-3).

The incidence of tuberculosis was found to be almost twice as high in group C as in group A, pneumonia was about one and a half times as frequent, and diphtheria occurred almost three times as often.

In a search for "the causes behind the causes of death" in the city of Cincinnati, O., in 1949-1951 it was found that, while significant declines in illness and death had taken place throughout the community during the previous quarter century, the death rates still varied considerably from section to section. This was emphasized by the Basin area, the oldest section, which comprised about one seventeenth of the city's area but contained one fourth of the popu-

lation. Most of the dwellings were substandard. In the Basin area, infant mortality was twice as high, home accident fatalities were three times as high, the pneumonia death rate was eight times as high, and the tuberculosis death rate was thirty times as high as the corresponding rates for the remainder of the city. Interestingly there were no appreciable differences in the rates inside and outside the Basin for the noncommunicable diseases of the older ages.[15]

Admittedly it is difficult to determine direct cause and effect relationships between poor housing and ill health. Nevertheless, the consistency of their occurrence together cannot be ignored. As Pond[16] has reasoned:

A cautious and critical analysis of available data relating to the effects of housing on health leads to but one conclusion: one cannot state that substandard housing alone begets ill health. However, no

Table 5-1. Slum section of Cleveland, O., 1934, compared with entire city

Slum section	Percent of total in Cleveland
Population	2.5
Homicides	21.0
Prostitution	26.0
Tuberculosis deaths	12.0
Illegitimate births	10.0
Police protection expenditure	4.5
Fire protection expenditure	14.5
Health department expenditure	8.1

Table 5-2. Deaths by social area, Liverpool, England, 1923-1929

City of Liverpool	Crude death rate	Tuberculosis death rate	Infant mortality
Entire city	13.9	123	98
Corporate tenement area	18.2	164	131
Slum area	28.4	299	171

Table 5-3. Illness and crowding, United States, 1934

Group	Degree of crowding (persons per room)	Percent of persons with illness 1 week or longer
A	1 or less	14.8
B	1 to 1½	15.7
C	More than 1½	17.8

reasonable student of the subject has yet stated that bad housing is compatible with good health. In the absence of irrefutable proof that housing has no ill effect on health, it may reasonably be hypothesized that good housing promotes the attainment of good health.

The quality of housing is, of course, only one reflection of socioeconomic status, and there are a number of other indicators of the latter which may be and have been used for comparative purposes. Thus Lawrence[17] followed a significant number of persons and families over a period of 20 years. He divided them into five socioeconomic groups and determined the prevalance of chronic illness as shown in Table 5-4.

A similar relationship has been found to hold true with regard to maternal and in-

fant mortality. For example, Yerby[18] points to the very significant differences between the mortality rates of Negro and Puerto Rican infants and mothers in the slum areas of New York City and the rates of the white population in that city (Table 5-5).

Even more striking are the results of a more recent study in Aberdeen, Scotland, by Baird.[19] His method of distinction was to compare women who could afford delivery in private nursing homes with those who could not and were therefore delivered as charity patients in the Aberdeen Maternity Hospital. He found the results shown in Table 5-6.

Especially interesting is Baird's comparison of the characteristics of the two groups

Table 5-4. Prevalence of chronic illness in families by socioeconomic status*

Socioeconomic status	Adjusted† percent ill	
	1923	1943
Well-to-do	27.7	29.3
Comfortable	47.3	39.8
Moderate	55.0	41.1
Poor	57.7	50.6
Very poor	61.3	44.0

*Modified from Lawrence, P. S.: Chronic illness and socio-economic status, Public Health Rep. 63:1507, Nov. 19, 1948.
†Rates adjusted for age and family size.

Table 5-5. Infant and maternal mortality by race, New York City, 1963*

Ethnic group	Infant mortality	Neonatal mortality	Puerperal mortality
Nonwhite	39.2	28.1	11.8
Puerto Rican	28.2	20.7	10.2
White	19.9	15.0	4.1

*From Yerby, A. S.: The problems of medical care for the indigent populations, Amer. J. Public Health **55:**1212, Aug. 1965.

Table 5-6. Infant deaths by place of delivery, Aberdeen, Scotland, 1950

Place delivered	Stillbirth rate	Neonatal death rate	Combined death rate
Charity hospital	2.23	1.78	4.01
Private nursing home	0.99	0.50	1.49

of mothers. He points out that all the women received the same standard of prenatal and postnatal care so that the differences in results were due to differences in health, physique, and intelligence. His epitomization is summarized in Table 5-7.

If one looks for them, relationships with factors in the social environment may be found with regard to almost all diseases. Their significance varies with regard both to the particular group of individuals and their social environment and to the particular disease. In the case of diseases such as tuberculosis, silicosis, or gastric ulcer the relationship may be readily evident, whereas in others it may be somewhat obscure. The number of social factors potentially related to disease is undoubtedly legion. Furthermore, they are of several different types and affect health in a number of different ways—some directly, some indirectly. Certain factors such as tendencies to develop certain mental conditions, physical malformations, or blood dyscrasias are inherent in the members of the group; other such as exposure to silicious dust or to fumes are related to occupation. Factors such as overcrowding or proximity to brothels are dangerous because they are conducive to exposure. Still others such as certain dietary habits or infant feeding customs are related to cultural factors.

In their stimulating discussion of social science in medicine Simmons and Wolff[1] present the interplay of the several aspects of man and his social and physical environment in an unusually descriptive manner well worth repeating:

. . . as an organism man is borne along by his physical environment, but he is also buffeted about by some of its elements. As a member of society, he is supported and reinforced by some fellow agents, while he may be frustrated, handicapped, or even vanquished by others. Similarly, as a personality, he is both a product of his culture and a potential victim of its compelling or conflicting norms and codes. Anyone may be carried along comfortably in his milieu for awhile, only to be torn down miserably after a time as these various environmental components of his life converge and impinge upon him. During long stretches of time, harmful and helpful forces may blend and balance, permitting him a workable and safe equilibrium amid many minor fluctuations. What is most important for us to realize, however, is the possibility that the scales may be *tipped* critically at a particular time by a clustering of forces from any one area, or from a combination of the triad of environmental pressures, and that, for the individual, a landslide of ill effects is started.

The following represents one possible classification of a few of the many group and social factors that may be related to disease. It is admittedly general and is presented merely to illustrate the variety and to provoke consideration of others:

    I. Factors in the members of the group
        A. Inherent characteristics
           1. Group susceptibility
           2. Tendency to inherent defects
        B. Cultural characteristics
           1. Racial, national, or religious customs
           2. Agricultural customs and methods

Table 5-7. Comparison by income group of women at delivery, Aberdeen, Scotland, 1950

Characteristic	Low-income group	High-income group
Stature	Small	Tall
Physical grading	Poor	Good
Pelvis	Flat	Round or long
Functional grading	Poor	Good
Hygiene	Poor	Good
Knowledge	Limited	Adequate
Prenuptial conception	Frequent	Seldom
Housing	Poor	Good
Premature labor	Frequent	Infrequent
Fetal deaths	High	Low
Repeated pregnancies	Frequent; unplanned even when contraindicated	Limited; planned
Premature aging	Common	Seldom

3. Dietary habits or customs
4. Educational limitations
5. Linguistic barriers
6. Traditional family size
7. Relative status of sexes
8. Relative status of age groups
9. Relative importance of family in total social life

II. Factors in the activities of the group
   A. Political
      1. Stability
      2. Quality
      3. Honesty
      4. Foresight of leadership
   B. Occupation and income
   C. Economy
      1. Basis
      2. Stability
      3. Trade
   D. Leisure behavioral pattern
   E. Mobility
      1. Travel
      2. Migration
   F. Traditional household habits
   G. Traditional purposes of household

III. Factors in the environment of the group*
   A. Geologic and climatic
      1. Severity of winters and summers
      2. Amount of rainfall and available water
      3. Mineral content of soil
      4. Degree of geographic isolation
   B. General environment
      1. Atmospheric pollution
      2. Soil and water pollution
      3. Amount of arable land available
      4. Proximity to detrimental factors (railroads, highways, industries, brothels, bars, fire hazards)
      5. Availability of recreation areas and facilities
   C. Home environment
      1. Size (persons per room)
      2. State of repair

3. Type of structure
4. Sanitary facilities
5. Natural and artificial light
6. Ventilation

It is well to give constant consideration to these social and environmental influences in order to emphasize the importance of regarding public health work for what it really is, i.e., an applied social science, through which is brought to bear appropriate medical, engineering, nursing, educational, and many other disciplines. It is only by considering the social and environmental conditions under which people live, sleep, work, recreate, procreate, and rear their young that we can hope to understand and control disease in the most complete sense. It is only in this way that we can eventually grasp the meaning of total health.

MODERN DEVELOPMENT

Over a long period social action to combat or remedy the various types of social problems was fractionated into separate, more or less insulated, activities. This was natural since the recognition of each specific problem and its espousements for public action usually originated with one or several visionary individuals. Sometimes these persons were dedicated to the amelioration of a particular problem because of some personal or familial experience. This was the cause above all causes which motivated them and those they gathered about them. The result was a parochialism of interest and action evidenced by separate health reforms, housing reforms, penal reforms, and so on. Gradually a relationship among all of these apparently unrelated social problems became recognized on more or less theoretical and empiric grounds, but attempts to correlate remedial action lagged essentially up to the present generation.

Perhaps the single most significant contribution to this recent development has been the recognition of an emphasis on the family, in contrast to the individual, as the basic social integer. Thus it is now accepted that the individual cannot be considered apart from his family or from the various and many forces in the physical and social environment which may influence his fam-

---

*For a much more complete list, see *Basic Principles of Healthful Housing*.[20]

ily. Further, it is increasingly recognized as usually futile to attempt to treat an individual problem without taking into consideration the family situation and all the forces which may affect it. This is even recognized to apply to the single individual on the basis of his having come from a family, living in a family substitute, and subsequently entering or establishing a family. In this regard Richardson[21] has written the following:

> The individual is a part of the family, in illness as well as in health . . . the idea of a disease as an entity which is limited to one person . . . fades into the background, and disease becomes an integral part of the continuous process of living. The family is the unit of illness, because it is the unit of living.

It is interesting to consider momentarily the multifaceted functions of the family, which provides, of course, the sole means of continuity and growth of the human species. As Ackerman[22] explains, it accomplishes this by providing a socially supported group pattern for the sexual union of man and woman and a stable situation that encourages a quality of parental partnership essential to the care of the resulting offspring. As he describes it, "The family is literally the cradle for the infant's tender mind as well as his body." The family, when properly established and conducted, presents a circumstance for the provision of food, clothing, shelter, and other materials necessary to life, for the proper emotional development of children and of their parents, for the guided evaluation of personal identities, for the development of normal and acceptable sexual patterns, for the establishment of social and ethical standards and the ability to accept social responsibility, and for the acquisition of knowledge and creative ability.

Children who grow up in a family setting acquire not only the general patterns of the culture of their particular society but also their parents' unique interpretation of it. Thus, although children of the same generation of a society develop in a more or less similar manner, the children in each family are somewhat different from those in other families. Part of the role of the family, therefore, is not only to nurture a new generation that fits into society but also to provide the great variety of personalities necessary for the society and its biologic and cultural evolution.

Many psychiatrists and sociologists have emphasized that one of the greatest values of the family is as a stabilizing force for the individual member, on the one hand, and for society, on the other. It accomplishes this by means of two apparently conflicting mechanisms. For purposes of long-term security the family tends to resist change. However, in times of trouble or emergency it provides a psychic and social cushion, a means for sharing difficulty, and a basis for accommodation to change. Unfortunately, all family structures are not such as to ensure this. As Ackerman[22] states, "In the meeting of new problems and crises, some families are weakened and others grow in solidity and emotional strength. Some families grow and learn from experience; others seem unable to do so because they are too inflexible and tend to disintegrate."

A subject for particular concern is the tendency toward small, urban families. As Bossard[23] says, "The very size of the family unit is important to the child . . . for the same reason that the size of the ledge from which we view the precipice below affects our sense of security." In families with one or few children and no grandparents, uncles, or aunts the child has few upon whom he may depend, and a single or, at most, a few difficulties may spell disaster.

In addition, as Schottstaedt[5] has emphasized, decreasing the number of people in the home tends to increase the frequency and intensity of emotional reactions because there are fewer people to absorb impacts and frictions. Furthermore, support tends to be concentrated in one wage earner since there are fewer people to contribute to the common family needs. Similarly the household duties and responsibilities of the housewife are increased in a relative sense, since such work must be done whether there is one or a number in the house, and are increased in an absolute sense, since there are fewer or none to share the work with her. Compounding this are the numerous extrafamilial distractions and demands upon the parents in the urban situation. Schottstaedt also points out how the burden and the risk are greatly increased in the small family when illness strikes one of its members. There are fewer people to perform nursing functions and fewer to assume the customary responsibilities of the one who is ill. As he states, "Available home resources for nursing chronically ill members of the family are therefore decreased and the percentage of people who require hospitalization, nursing home care, or institutional care is increased." With regard to the latter point Parsons and Fox[24] have suggested that the growth and increasing use of hospitals is not merely due to advances in medical knowledge and its application in an increasingly exacting technology but is also a response to a shift in family structure which is itself linked to the occupational structure.

Such considerations go far in explaining some of the difficulties encountered in the handling of certain types of illnesses and certain types of individuals. They provide, for example, one reason why in a substantial number of cases medical treatment alone of chronic diseases is ineffective because of tangential relationships to the family economy and other aspects of family and social life.[25] As a result of differences in the amount and type of stress on the male in our society, they explain, in part, the excess of gastric and duodenal ulcers in males. They further provide a logical reason for the recent increase of these conditions among women since their social and occupational emancipation. Also, as has been shown by several investigators, the diabetic individual fares less well in the competitive industrialized urban situation because of frequent and often intense stress. Thus stress threatens security, and the emotional response results in an increase in ketone bodies in the venous blood and fluctuations in blood sugar level.[26,27] Anyone who has worked with elderly persons is familiar with the frequent difficulty of maintaining their health or, indeed, their interest in it. Left to their own devices because they have passed their biologically and economically productive years, older

people tend to feel useless and unwanted. One result is a tendency to neglect themselves. Matters of personal hygiene may not be observed. Nutrition may suffer because of defective teeth, vicarious food preparation, poor eating habits, and lack of appetite caused by feelings of depression. As Schottstaedt[5] summarizes the situation, "Many of the diseases of older age are related to three things: nutritional deficiencies, circulatory disturbances, and general disuse."

INTERRELATIONSHIP OF SOCIAL PROBLEMS

From what has gone before it would appear evident that neither man nor his problems exist in vacuums. By virtue of being a product of a family and a participant in a society, innumerable external factors, both good and evil, impinge upon him as an individual. Some act to cause difficulty and problems; others serve to provide support and solution of problems. Thus it is now recognized that the state of personal or familial health or disease is the result of many interacting biologic, physical, and social factors. Depending upon the nature of the disease and circumstances, any one of these may be primary and the others contributory. Furthermore, given a state of disease, these same factors are involved in the chances for and mechanism of recovery and rehabilitation. This has led to the consideration of disease in the individual as more and more a social phenomenon involving a number of people and especially those immediately related to and around the patient. As Richardson[21] has put it, "Illness is one form of family maladjustment." An attempt to illustrate these relationships insofar as disease is concerned has been made in the previous discussion of man and his environment.

This leads to a still more significant aspect of the subject which requires consideration—the intimate interrelationships among a number of seemingly diverse types of social problems which may affect an individual, a family, and a society. One way to approach the subject is to consider the example of a man suffering from pneumonia who is brought into a hospital. Physical and radiographic examinations may conclusively determine the clinical diagnosis. Sputum examination may clearly implicate *Diplococcus pneumoniae* as the causative organism. However, is it as simple as this? Several questions remain unanswered. It is known, for example, that many more people are exposed to this organism than become clinically ill. Why did this particular individual become ill with pneumonia? True, he could not develop this particular disease in the absence of the organism. Nevertheless, a valid question may still be raised as to what actually caused the illness. Investigation may elicit circumstances such as the following: The patient suffered from overexposure because on the preceding night he slept on a park bench in the rain. He slept on a park bench because he did not know what he was doing. He did not know what he was doing because he was under the influence of alcohol. He indulged in an excess of alcohol because of discouragement and despondency over a bitter argument with a complaining wife. His wife complained because her husband was unemployed and had no income. He may have been unemployed because of inadequate training, intrinsic inability, or some complex interplay of business economics. Which of these factors caused his pneumonia? Obviously they all did.

Similarly, consider the case of an adolescent apprehended by the police as a juvenile delinquent. The immediate circumstance may have involved being caught while breaking into a store. Was the child intrinsically antisocial, and was the fault exclusively his? Investigation may bring out that he is only one of a group of similar adolescents who have formed an antisocial club or gang. It may be discovered that the group is sexually promiscuous, that venereal infections and abortions are common, and that alcoholism and narcotic addictions are present or incipient. In fact, the crystalizing store-breaking incident may have occurred to obtain money for alcohol or drugs. Why did this boy or, for that matter, any of the others belong to the gang and engage in such antisocial behavior? More often than not, discussion with a parent will result in

the statement: "I just can't do anything with him." Deeper inquiry and study, however, are certain to bring out a number of other causative factors, most of them relating to the family and the social environment. Often the family bonds are discovered to be frayed or parted. The home may have only a single parent because of illegitimacy, divorce, separation, illness, or absence of one or both parents due to their employment. In such instances, the gang is often a substitute family situation, i.e., something to belong to in which to socialize and exercise self-expression. On the other hand, both the parents and the children may live together. However, the home, because of economic stringencies due to ignorance, misfortune, or other reasons, may consist of just a few crowded rooms of a substandard quality with little or no privacy, ample opportunities for bickering and quarreling, and few facilities for cleanliness. Such a situation offers little incentive for the development of a sense of dignity, pride, or responsibility. The most intimate personal and sexual acts may be commonly observed, which encourages a cynical attitude toward them; there is little opportunity or reason to develop respect for the property of others even within the family; education, virtue, frugality, and social responsibility may be derided; dependence upon public welfare and public assistance may be the cornerstone of the family finances; parental bouts of alcoholism and physical as well as verbal abuse may be so common as to establish themselves as the standard of behavior. Under such circumstances one may properly ask: Why did this boy attempt to steal? Why was he sexually promiscuous? Why did he have gonorrhea? Why, perhaps, was he on his way to being an alcoholic or a drug addict? Why had he no respect or use for the concepts of family and society? Obviously none of the answers to these questions can stand alone; they are all interlinked. And they all devolve into the three fundamental questions: Where and how did it all begin? How can this chain be broken? How can similar complex situations be prevented from occurring in others?

One of the conclusions which such cases bring out forcefully is that the primary diagnosis of a situation is not always in the same field as that under immediate or initial consideration. Social problems tend to exist together like different vegetables in a stew, as it were, and occasionally a particular problem erupts on the surface of the simmering stew. Regarded singly and momentarily it gives a very limited and quite fallacious impression. To appreciate the total situation fully, one has to stir the stew, sample it, and observe it over a period of time. In terms of such an analogy it is important to realize that although each vegetable when dredged up and examined in the ladle appears to be discrete it is meaningful only in relation to the total stew and, if spoiled, can affect all other parts of the stew. Caudill[28] has stated this in more formal terms as the basic conclusion of a presentation in *Effects of Social and Cultural Systems in Reactions to Stress:*

. . . stress can manifest itself in one or more of a number of linked open systems, and . . . the strain on one system can be transmitted to others so that several become involved in the process of adaptation and defense. These linked open systems may be thought of as: physiology; personality; relatively permanent meaningful small groups, e.g., the family; and wider social structure, e.g., community and the nation or, variously, economic and political structures . . . .

Following this he points out:

. . . in very few studies [and it might be added parenthetically, in very few action programs] has the research design taken account of more than two of the possible systems as variables. Physicians have found relations between physiological phenomena and conditions that have been conceived as psychological (fear, rage), psychodynamic (unresolved dependency, anxiety), and environmental (cold, imprisonment). Social scientists have shown relations between the structure of the family and its position in the economic or social class system, and have attempted to work with a concept of basic or modal personality in relation to the patterns of child rearing found in a culture. But only a few studies have examined three such variables as more than static background phenomena . . . .

Simmons and Wolff[1] have attempted to present the concept of some of these interrelationships in tabular form. The essential point made by them is that physical, social, or cultural events or forces may constitute either or both sources and consequences of strength or weakness, good or evil. Thus a particular physical source, event, or force may have physical consequences, social consequences, or cultural consequences. This is similarly true of social and cultural sources, events, or forces. It is also important to recognize that the resulting consequences may in turn become sources or forces themselves. This method of presentation is adapted here to illustrate many of the issues raised in the preceding paragraphs.

With regard to the interrelationships among negative or undesirable sources, events, or forces and consequences we may consider as *sources* the following examples:

1. Physical: Disease, congenital defect, or injury to face
2. Social: Sudden industrialization with an influx of young adult workers
3. Cultural: Development of an urbanized living pattern

Each of these may have undesirable physical, social, and cultural *consequences*. (See Table 5-8.)

In a similar manner sources, events, or forces may be of a positive nature and result in desirable consequences. To illustrate this, the following *sources* may be used:

1. Physical: Improved nutrition, public health, and medical care
2. Social: Development of social security and medical care plans
3. Cultural: Provision of improved education

Each of these may have desirable physical, social, and cultural *consequences*. (See Table 5-9.)

MULTIPROBLEM FAMILIES

Everything that has been said thus far on the subject of social pathology points to the veracity of the common saying, "misery loves company." This is true in the sense that people and families in difficulty tend to be concentrated geographically, especially in urban situations. It is also true in the sense that difficulties seldom occur singly. In recent years this phenomenon has been described in several ways, one of them by the use of the phrase, disease-delinquency-dependency syndrome. This gives recogn

Table 5-8. Interrelationships of undesirable physical, social, and cultural factors*

Undesirable sources or events	Consequences		
	Physical	Social	Cultural
Physical			
Disease or injury	Facial deformity	Inability to obtain employment	Misanthropy Condemnation of parenthood
Social			
Industrialization	Increased venereal disease	Free sexual relationships and promiscuity	Changes in attitudes toward marriage and family
Cultural			
Urbanization	More accidents and insanitation	Overcrowding Development of gangs Alcoholism	Breakdown of kinship and family bonds

*Modified from Simmons, I. W., and Wolff, H. C.: Social science in medicine, New York, 1954, Russell Sage Foundation, p. 111.

Table 5-9. Interrelationships of desirable physical, social, and cultural factors*

Desirable sources or events	Consequences		
	Physical	Social	Cultural
Physical			
Improved nutrition, public health, and medical care	Less illness and longer life	Greater productivity	Stronger family and social responsibility
Social			
Social security plans	Fewer complications	Less pauperization of sick and aged	Changed attitude toward aged
Cultural			
Improved education	Earlier diagnosis, prevention, and treatment	Demand for better public health and medical care	Rational understanding of sickness and health

*Modified from Simmons, I. W., and Wolff, H. C.: Social science in medicine, New York, 1954, Russell Sage Foundation, p. 111.

tion to the fact that at any time in a society there are a certain number of individuals and, more significantly, families who get caught in a vortex of contributory social problems, each of which complicates the others in turn, making it more and more difficult to escape. For some the situation becomes so extreme and hopeless that there results an eventual condition which has been referred to as *cumulative degradation.*

There would appear to exist at least three types of families or situations which differ from each other essentially in the degree of ability to respond to assistance successfully.

One type of multiproblem family is self-sufficient under ordinary circumstances and goes along reasonably well until some catastrophe or crisis (medical, economic, or otherwise) sufficient in magnitude to throw the family off balance occurs. This crisis, if unsolved, eventually gives rise to problems in other areas. Unless some assistance is forthcoming, this type of family is in danger of irreparable damage and may become a permanent multiproblem family. If, on the other hand, significant assistance is rendered with regard to the original or to each of the several accumulated and related problems, this type of family is able to rehabilitate itself and assume and maintain its proper and desired role of self-sufficiency.

A second type of family is somewhat similar to the first. It has good intentions and wants to be self-sustaining but lacks good management and staying power. As a result every once in a while it slips below the surface. If appropriately aided, it is able to climb back and operate on a relatively even keel until some new crisis occurs. Then it slips again and must be helped back again.

The third type of family is the most discouraging to deal with. Either because of overwhelming crisis and catastrophies for which it has received no help, insufficient help, or, important to this discussion, unilateral help, or because it is an intrinsically defective family, no extent or type of assistance seems to enable it to achieve recovery. Often the desire for recovery, i.e., for a different way of life, is lacking, unacceptable, or incomprehensible. The roots of the difficulties of these so-called hard-core problem families go very deep. They are almost irretrievably caught in an exceedingly difficult situation which might be referred to as the syndrome of the seven D's:

> Disease
> Deficiency (often both
>   nutritional and mental)
> Destitution
> Dependency
> Despondency
> Delinquency
> Degeneracy

Williams[29] summarizes the same situation with regard to England in the following terms:

. . . after the Industrial Revolution with its child labor, cheap alcohol, poor wages, and bad landlords, there must have been a much higher proportion of our working-class families living under conditions far worse than anything we see today.

As social amenities became more readily available to the people so the great majority took advantage of the benefits and improved their conditions of life . . . Yet one finds a small minority, either through a temperamental instability or a mental defect, who fail to keep pace with the advancing times.

He cites five surveys conducted by the Eugenic Society of Great Britain which found an average incidence of such hard-core families to be 3 per 1,000 families. He adds, "We find that a large number of these people are in early middle life, able-bodied and capable of regular manual work, who have difficulty in adjusting themselves to the recognized standards of life."

In the United States a number of significant investigations of this problem have been carried out in recent years. They too have clearly indicated the importance of the family as the basic unit of social significance, the simultaneous or successive occurrence of social problems, and the existence of a small hard core of multiproblem families.

The most comprehensive and illuminating of these investigations was the study of St. Paul, Minn., a more or less typical American city.[25] The study was carried out by a group of consultants from the fields of health, maladjustment, dependency, and recreation, with the cooperation of 108 public and private community agencies. About 41,000 families, representing 40% of the total in the city, had contact with one or more agencies during the study month of November 1948. The types of problems for which services were rendered are summarized in Table 5-10.

It should be noted that health problems were among the most common encountered. In fact, during the month studied about 16,000 families, a rate of 147 per 1,000 families, received some services from the 12 pub-

Table 5-10. Incidence of social problems, St. Paul, Minn., November 1948

Type of problem for which assistance was rendered	*Percent of families studied*	*Percent of families in city*
Financial	17	7
Maladjustment	26	10
Health	38	15
Recreation	46	18

lic and 18 private health agencies in the community. About one half of these services were in relation to a chronic disease or handicap. With regard to age distribution of those receiving services for ill health, 32% were reported to be under 20 years, 41% were between 20 and 64 years, and 22% were over 65 years. Between one half and two thirds of those who suffered from chronic handicaps or diseases were heads of families; thus their ailments inevitably affected the family income, prospectives, and behavior.

A simple totaling of the figures in the table indicates that a number of families must have required and received aid for more than one type of problem. Upon investigation the facts substantiated this beyond expectation. Of the financially dependent families, 77% had problems of ill health and/or maladjustment; 56% of the families with problems of maladjustment had problems of ill health and/or dependency; and 38% of the families with health problems had problems of dependency and/or maladjustment.

The most striking finding of the St. Paul study was that there was a group of about 6,500 families, only 6% of the total in the city, who suffered from such an essentially continuing complex of problems that they absorbed 46% of the health services, 55% of the adjustment services, and 68% of the dependency services. This finding was further refined by the discovery that only 4% of these hard-core multiproblem families were financially dependent because of unemployment. Of the 6,500 families, 58% were dependent because of ill health and/or maladjustment which rendered them unable to be self-sustaining.

The question naturally arises as to reason for the development of multiproblem families, especially those that form the hard core in a community. Analysis of the reasons is even more difficult than analysis of the problem. Practically all observers agree on one thing; i.e., that the qualities of family stability and cohesiveness are usually weak in such situations. In connection with concern over the effects of mobility on the family, Foster[30] has itemized four factors which

make for family solidarity: (1) stability of location, with the development of an empathy with and a stake in the surroundings; (2) frequent contacts among the members of the family; (3) homogeneity resulting from common or shared experiences; and (4) an intangible dynamic element or life principle within the fabric of the family itself. Foster makes the very important point that this appears first as an ideal or common purpose shared by the two people who marry and establish the family. He also expresses the opinion that all four of these basic factors have been subjected to weakening influences during recent years.

It has been observed that multiplicity of problems tends to occur most frequently among recent immigrants to nations or communities. That this would be so is not surprising and is quite in line with the foregoing. Simmons and Wolff[1] make this observation as follows:

. . . when peoples migrate, many elements of the new homeland's culture are rapidly adopted while large parts of the original culture survive in the family or small mobile group. Striking examples are found in first and second-generation immigrants . . . who because of contemporary patterns of prejudice may be barred from full participation . . . and become, in a sense, "marginal men" trapped between two cultures and subject to the conflicts arising from both.

Their statement continues in a sense which gives some hint regarding the development of multiple social problems in another group, i.e., the residual aging group:

Furthermore, a person in the same physical surroundings . . . may continue to cling to attitudes, habits, and goals acquired in his youth, while the cultural norms are changing rapidly, with the result that he is not in harmony with the newly evolved patterns within his own society. He may be left as one stranded with his own personal and outmoded cultural values and attachments. The sweeping tides of cultural change frequently produce new areas of stress in personalities and not seldom leave their marks on the organism.

All human beings engage to varying extents in a search for status and goals. In recognition of this Simmons and Wolff[1] present a graphic picture describing the genesis of a third type of individual who tends to become enmeshed in a tangle of multiple problem situations. Approaching the subject from the standpoint of medicine they describe this person in the following manner:

Clinicians will often find, at the other type-extreme from the creature of culture, the socially deviant individual who also strives, although perhaps unconsciously, for "wayward" goals and who follows his own atypical and partly false clues in response to his life situation. His adaptations are out of harmony with socially approved behavior, as well as inappropriate on a physical basis. Under such circumstances social penalties are added to the physical injuries, and stress may be compounded in a kind of "vicious cycle," for the more the subject reacts the worse becomes his plight. Following his false clues, he simultaneously impairs his body and his social relationships, perhaps even alienating the very persons best qualified to help and support him and whose rejection leads to further deviation.

The last sentence of this statement might well be reread occasionally by persons engaged in social improvement, including those in the field of public health. Too often, it is feared, the natural or emotional reaction to confusion and despondency is hastily grasped as an excuse for taking the easy way out by condemning individuals as intrinsically bad or worthless.

Another interesting possibility that is worthy of consideration, especially in view of recent developments in psychosomatic medicine, is the use of illness as a response to social difficulty or dissatisfaction. It is known that some individuals who cannot achieve satisfaction and fulfillment in positive or socially acceptable channels, turn in their search to negative or antisocial channels. These may take the form of alcoholism, sexual deviation, dependency, or crime. It is entirely possible that for some individuals still another solution is illness, alone or in company with one or more of the other negative forms of behavior. In fact, of these various solutions, sickness used in this sense has the advantage of being the most acceptable and of eliciting the most sympathy and ready assistance. Furthermore, it provides other individuals and groups in society an opportunity for the achievement of their sense of fulfillment and self-satisfaction.

One final aspect of the subject must be mentioned. It is entirely possible that on occasion the exercise of unilateral zeal on the part of public health workers may actually give rise to social problems in families and may contribute to the establishment and continuation of a vicious social cycle. For example, the public health worker knows that tuberculosis is communicable and may insist on prompt hospitalization of a wife and mother if she has this disease. Without question this is scientifically the correct thing to do. It is best for the patient, for her family, and for society. Best, that is, from the public health viewpoint. If, however, at the same time that hospitalization of the wife and mother is arranged the public health worker neglects to work intimately with the total family and with other sources of assistance in the community, good intentions may lead to ultimate greater evil. Public health workers must recognize that hospitalization of a parent interferes with family structure and relationships. Removal of maternal care and guidance may result in decreased family cohesiveness and supervision, which may lead to delinquency on the part of the children. Prolonged absence of wifely companionship compounded by concern over increased expenditures for medical care and housekeeping may lead to alcoholism and philandery on the part of the husband. This in turn may lead to lowered income. Eventual dissolution of the family with firm establishment of a disease-delinquency-dependency syndrome is by no means an impossibility. If the woman's tuberculosis is successfully arrested or cured, the pleased staffs of the institution and the health agency may discharge her to quite a grim future with an excellent chance of relapse. And, worst of all, the undesirable set of circumstances which has been set in motion may very well carry over into a number of future generations. Therefore, at the risk of redundancy, it must be emphasized that public health workers should be most circumspect when considering any measure that may interfere with the integrity of the family, its economic base, or its social relationships. Public health workers should always ask themselves if a program or an action might in any way contribute to the disintegration of the family, even though it might aid the family or society in other ways. All such situations call for careful consideration of all possible alternatives, exhaustive attempts to educate those who may be guilty of infractions of sanitary and health regulations, and the use of a multidisciplinary approach to the existing and potential needs and problems of the total family unit.

POINTS FOR ACTION

Fortunately there exist in most communities a wide variety of resources which may be called upon for assistance. For some time, attempts have been made to provide for some degree of joint planning and action. Usually these take the form of a council of social agencies or a community health and welfare council in which there is membership by many of the agencies active in these fields. However, on the one hand, any joint activity which occurs is often general and on a high level, quite distant from the family in need; on the other hand, most health and welfare councils are too limited, agencywise and substantivewise. Not all of the health and welfare organizations in a community are members of the council, and they do not all participate in the joint planning. Furthermore, a number of other types of agencies should be involved. Among those often absent are agencies for recreation, rehabilitation, public assistance, law enforcement, and the courts.

Another source of partial solution has been the Social Service Referral Center, to which representatives of member agencies (and sometimes others) may refer cases for certain specific investigations or for certain specific services. One common difficulty is that individuals and families sometimes get lost in the referral system. Sometimes they are never referred back to the initiating agency for follow-up or for resumption and completion of care that may have been instituted but interrupted in order to provide time or opportunity for solution of a secondary or contributory problem. Mention must be made also of an unfortunate practice occasionally indulged in, consciously or subconsciously, by a few agencies. This is to avoid referral of cases for additional or auxiliary services because of fear that a sort of right of proprietorship over the case might be lost and this would reflect poorly on the agency when the time came to publish an annual report or to engage in a fund-raising activity based upon case load. Obviously such an attitude, however rare, is totally unwarranted and inexcusable if it detracts in any way from the earliest possible and most satisfactory solution of a family's problems.

In England several different approaches have been attempted.* In Southampton a rehabilitation committee consisting of heads of pertinent municipal departments has been established. This committee in turn established a subcommittee of principal officers concerned with the operation of various social welfare and relief programs and of representatives of various voluntary agencies. Weekly meetings are held under the chairmanship of the medical officer of health, who acts as coordinator. Any member may bring up specific cases on the basis of their complexity or because inadequate action has been taken. Responsibility for action is clearly placed and followed up. It is felt that this procedure results in consideration of all aspects of the family problem, places responsibility, results in efficient use of home-visiting personnel, and results in action. It is interesting that a committee of experts on delinquency, called together by the World Health Organization and consisting of forensic, general, and child psychiatrists, psychologists, prison directors, criminologists, social workers, and a judge, suggested that jurists, psychiatrists, psychologists, and sociologists collaborate as a sort of "treatment tribunal" to decide the nature of the diagnosis and course of treatment.[31] In many cases a public health worker might also be of assistance. In Bristol, Liverpool, and Manchester, family service units were established after the war. The work is done from hostels by recently graduated social science workers. In addition to using the hostels for clubs, meetings, cleansing, and feeding, the workers help in the homes and

---

*See pp. 992 and 995 in *Rehabilitation of Problem Families* by Williams.[29]

gain the confidence of the families so that more effective service and referral is possible. These methods have resulted in about a 10% rate of rehabilitation of problem families. Williams[29] concludes, "Although the methods of dealing with problem families appear at first sight to be fairly costly, it is far cheaper than leaving the problem untackled."

In reviewing the findings of the St. Paul and similar surveys, Kandle[32] concludes that two things are necessary: first, application of the principles and methods of epidemiology to chronic diseases, disabilities, dependency, and maladjustment; second, development by specialists in health, family services, mental hygiene, social casework, and other related fields of more effective means of working together in order to achieve a sound and complete collective diagnosis and a coordinated form of treatment.

Essentially what is called for is a synthesis of philosophy, interest, resources, and effort to be applied to total social problems of the community through its families. Certain specific suggestions may be made. Professional parochialism must be broken down. This might be accomplished in part by the provision of more intimate working relationships among the various disciplines and agencies involved. Health departments and health centers should at least provide office space for liaison personnel from certain other public and private agencies and in turn should assign public health personnel to other agencies for the same purpose. Multidisciplinary and multiagency committees or councils for *case* planning and review should be established as well as committees concerned with *program* planning and review. Some of the community agencies and services that might be included or at least consulted are health, welfare, public assistance, hospitals, police, courts, fire protection, voluntary health agencies, and the social service agencies. Beyond this any honest recognition of professional parochialism should lead to the development of some organized means of bringing those who are to be served and who know their problems only too well into the planning of

programs. Family reporting and filing systems instead of individual reporting and filing systems should be used whenever possible. All health and other social agencies should participate in a central social service referral center established on a family basis as well as on a case basis. Every problem should be studied and handled with the family considered as the unit, and every proposed solution must be regarded in terms of possible undesirable effects.

Since social problems, including health problems, are inevitably family problems and since it is the concensus that most multiproblem situations have their roots in the early period of married life, health and other social agencies should make more use of marriage reports as a means of contact with certain types of individuals and groups before trouble has an opportunity to occur. Undoubtedly some relatively limited assistance in the establishment of a household, alerting a newly married couple as to sources of assistance and counseling, would prevent the unimpeded progression of numerous problem situations. From the overall community standpoint, concentration of multiproblem families in one area, whether the problems are incipient or fully developed, should be avoided if at all possible. Crowded together, they tend to maintain each other as problem families and groups. Separated, they tend to learn and improve by contact with more stable families.

If by now the reader feels that he has been led somewhat afield from the basic issue of public health, he might do well to recognize with Koos[34]:

. . . community organization for health is in no sense an activity divorced from other forms of activity for community welfare . . . all community organization is interwoven in a common effort. Health, says modern research, is not to be found apart from a general welfare of the individual and the community. It consists not only of an absence of disease but also of a sense of general well-being, of adjustment to all of the forces that make up the intricacies of the society in which we live.

ECONOMIC OPPORTUNITY PROGRAMS

The philosophy that the general well-being of society is related to its level of health coincides with that which led to the recent "poverty" acts of Congress: The Economic Opportunity Act of 1964 (P.L. 88-452) and The Appalachian Regional Development Act of 1965 (P.L. 89-794). These significant pieces of legislation virtually threw down the gauntlet to the field of public health as well as others. In effect they said, "For years you have been talking about the relationship between poverty and ill health. Yet for years you have been merely treating the signs and symptoms, the diseases, the consequences rather than the root or source of the problem. Now with these new weapons against poverty itself, let us see what can be accomplished!"

The weapons, while obviously insufficient for a truly all-out attack upon poverty or the ill health consequences of it, are nonetheless formidable. On the basis of multiple causation of social problems the legislation and accompanying appropriations provide significant sums for a multipronged attack upon the roots of poverty; the areas of assistance include education and training, health services, housing, employment, small business loans, and many others. Several parts of the program are of particular importance to public health workers in that they provide opportunities for health services and accomplishments heretofore not possible.[35] One is Operation Headstart, the chief purpose of which is to provide preschool learning experiences to disadvantaged children who are destined to enter kindergarten or first grade the following September. In the process, provision is made for a health program so that the children will not begin school with health handicaps.[36] A similar opportunity for extensive health examinations and correction of defects is provided by the Neighborhood Youth Corps program, which is designed to assist young people who have dropped out of school and who are unprepared for employment. The Community Action Programs allow, if a community wishes, the inclusion of a variety of disease preventive, therapeutic, and rehabilitative activities within the operation of the multipurpose Neighborhood Community Action Centers. It is of more than passing interest to note that in several cities where large programs of this type have

been conducted practically no effect was noted on the demand for outpatient services at municipal hospitals, which traditionally serve as the family physician to the poor. In other words, the health service needs met at the Neighborhood Community Action Centers appear to be over and above those customarily met by hospital outpatient departments. Perhaps in the long run the Economic Opportunity program that will have the greatest effect upon public health practice is that which will provide for the establishment of truly comprehensive neighborhood medical centers of high quality. Already a number of these have been established in economically depressed areas of various cities. The concept is to provide under one roof all of the outpatient services needed by the poor of a circumscribed area —promotive, preventive, screening, diagnostic, outpatient therapeutic, inpatient therapeutic (in a back-stopping hospital), and rehabilitative—medical, dental, and emotional. Some of those already established are conducted by health departments, others by university medical centers. For many reasons the most desirable is an operating partnership which involves the health department, the university medical center, and a representation from the neighborhood itself. Where a comprehensive child health program is being conducted with Social Security funds through the Children's Bureau, it should, of course, be correlated with the activities of the Comprehensive Neighborhood Medical Center by providing all the services for those under 20 years of age.

Mention should also be made of the potential for developing extended public health and comprehensive medical and dental services through the channels of the Demonstration Cities and Metropolitan Development Act of 1966 (P.L. 89-754). This is one of the most significant pieces of urban legislation ever passed by Congress. It provides under the administration of the Department of Housing and Urban Development an opportunity for cities to attack all the problems of their slums and blighted areas, concentrating and coordinating all available federal aid with local public and private resources. The program will operate in two stages: first, funds and technical assistance to plan and develop comprehensive improvement and development programs for specific parts of a city; second, grants equal to 80% of the local share of any federally assisted activity included as part of the demonstration city program. Since the program will focus upon conservation and rehabilitation, much emphasis will be placed upon housing code enforcement, solid waste disposal, rodent control, and other environmental problems. The establishment of neighborhood health centers in conjunction with the efforts of local health departments and federal programs such as those of the Office of Economic Opportunity, The Public Health Service, and the Children's Bureau are contemplated.

Truly the opportunity for great advancement in health services appears to be here. The choice before us has been very well stated by James[37]:

There are really just two basic strategies for attacking the health problems of poverty:

We can act against poverty itself and raise the standard of living of the poor. We all know that much of the advance of medicine has been due to a general improvement in the basic standard of living.

We can act against disease without doing anything about poverty. We can more or less accept poverty as something that exists and try to do what is medically possible within this framework.

It is to be hoped that we have the imagination and courage to choose the former. We have tried the latter approach for a long time with limited results and no light at the end of the tunnel. If we do not choose the former, there are many individuals in other fields of endeavor who would then properly push us aside and get on with the task themselves.

REFERENCES

1. Simmons, L. W., and Wolff, H. G.: Social science in medicine, New York, 1954, Russell Sage Foundation.
2. Stern, B. J.: The health of towns and the early public health movement, Ciba Symposium 9:871, May-June 1948.
3. Buzzard, Sir F.: The place of social medicine in the reorganization of health services, Brit. Med. J. 1:703, June 6, 1942.
4. Ryle, J. A.: Changing disciplines, London, 1948, Oxford University Press.
5. Schottstaedt, W. W.: Comprehensive medicine in relation to public health, Amer. J. Public Health 44:1340, Oct. 1954.
6. Steiger, W. A.: Causality and the comprehensive approach, J. Med. Educ. 33:538, July 1958.
7. Kroeger, G.: The concept of social medicine as presented by physicians and other writers in Germany, 1779-1932, Chicago, 1937, Julius Rosenwald Fund.
8. Ryle, J. A.: Social pathology and the new era in medicine, Bull. N. Y. Acad. Med. 23:312, June 1947.
9. Galdston, I.: The meaning of social medicine, Cambridge, 1954, Harvard University Press.
10. Rosen, G.: Approaches to a concept of social medicine, Milbank Mem. Fund Quart. 26:7, Jan. 1948.
11. Item, Amer. Med. Ass. News, Dec. 29, 1958.
12. Grotjahn, A.: Soziale Pathologie, Berlin, 1915, August Hirschwald Verlag.
13. Wolff, G.: Social pathology as a medical science, Amer. J. Public Health 42:1576, Dec. 1952.
14. Sydenstricker, E.: Health and environment, New York, 1933, McGraw-Hill Book Co.
15. Allen, F. P.: People of the shadows, Cincinnati, 1954, Public Health Federation.
16. Pond, M. A.: How does housing affect health? Amer. J. Public Health 61:667, May 1946.
17. Lawrence, P. S.: Chronic illness and socio-economic status, Public Health Rep. 63:1507, Nov. 19, 1948.
18. Yerby, A. S.: The problems of medical care for indigent populations, Amer. J. Public Health 55:1212, Aug. 1965.
19. Baird, D.: Social and economic factors affecting the mother and child, Amer. J. Public Health 42:516, May 1952.
20. American Public Health Association: Basic principles of healthful housing, ed. 2, New York, 1939, The Association.
21. Richardson, H. B.: Patients have families, New York, 1945, Commonwealth Fund.
22. Ackerman, N. W.: Psychological dynamics of the family organism, Public Health Rep. 71:1017, Oct. 1956.
23. Bossard, J. H. S.: The sociology of child development, New York, 1954, Harper & Row, Publishers.
24. Parsons, T., and Fox, R.: Illness, therapy, and the modern urban American family, J. Soc. Issues 8:31, Apr. 1952.
25. Buell, B., et al.: Community planning for human services, New York, 1952, Columbia University Press.
26. Hinkle, L. E., Jr., and Wolf, S.: Studies in diabetes mellitus: changes in glucose, ketone, and water metabolism during stress, Res. Publ. Ass. Res. Nerv. Ment. Dis. (1949) 29:338, 1950.
27. Rosen, H., and Lidz, T.: Emotional factors in precipitation of recurrent diabetic acidosis, Psychosom. Med. 11:211, July-Aug. 1949.
28. Caudill, W.: Effects of social and cultural sys-

tems in reactions to stress, New York, 1958, Social Science Research Council.

29. Williams, H. C. M.: Rehabilitation of problem families, Amer. J. Public Health **45**:990, Aug. 1955.

30. Foster, R. G.: Effect of mobility on the family, Amer. J. Public Health **46**:812, July 1956.

31. Psychiatry and the treatment of delinquency, WHO Chron. **12**:330, Oct. 1958.

32. Kandle, R. P.: In modern philanthropy and human welfare, New York, 1952, Grant Foundation.

33. Eller, C. H., Hatcher, G. H., and Buell, B.: Health and family issues in community plan-

ning for the problem of indigent disability, Amer. J. Public Health **48**:(supp.) Nov. 1958.

34. Koos, E. L.: New concepts in community organization for health, Amer. J. Public Health **43**:466, Apr. 1953.

35. Kravitz, S. L.: Health aspects of the antipoverty crusade, N. J. Dept. of Health, Public Health News, Jan. 1965.

36. Editorial: Project head start and public health, Amer. J. Public Health **55**:1122, Aug. 1965.

37. James, G.: Poverty as an obstacle to health progress in our cities, Amer. J. Public Health **55**:1757, Nov. 1965.

Chapter 6

Population and public health

INTRODUCTION

It would now appear to be without question that the single most significant phenomenon in man's history is his tremendous and rapid increase in number during the past few generations. The potential consequences of this biologic surge are so great and far reaching in terms of local and world politics, economics, morals, and even ultimate existence as to justify a full measure of concern and even pessimism. Increasingly the criticism leveled at public health workers is that they compound the problems of the world by causing widespread overpopulation through their dramatic saving and extension of lives. Public health workers, sociologists, political scientists, and others have long been aware of a relationship between public health activities and increases in the populations of nations and of the world.[1] Awareness has been sharpened more and more by recent world events, especially the sustained postwar rise in birthrates in many areas and the growth and success of international technical assistance programs in health and sanitation. This awareness has reached the point of acute concern, which is voiced in part by more and more vocal questioning, indeed, even condemnation, of the activities of the "dangerous doctor," the "heedless hygienist," and the "cynical sanitarian."[2-8] On the other hand, there are those[9-11] who are optimistic concerning the ability of this planet to sustain us. In view of these divergent opinions it may be useful to consider some of the facts, problems, and interrela-tionships as well as some of the pros and cons of this important question.

HISTORY OF POPULATION CHANGE

On the basis of recent anthropologic research by Leakey and others[12] it would appear that man has existed as a distinct species for at least a half million years. It is logical to assume that throughout this long period, and in fact during any particular interval of it, man multiplied to the extent that his way of life and environment allowed. The best available evidence indicates that the increase was gradual and often precarious. It is estimated that by 6000 B.C. the total world population was probably only about 5 million, an amount which is now added to the present world population every month. At the time of Christ it had reached about 250 million. Over 16 centuries were to pass before it doubled to about 500 million in 1650. Then an acceleration began; the population suddenly doubled during the next two and a half centuries, then doubled again in less than another century. It took all of man's long history to reach the current figure of about 3.5 billion, but it will require only about 35 more years to double that figure to an anticipated 7 billion. If the current rate of increase—1.75% compounded annually—continues, by the year 2050 the world's population will reach an almost incomprehensible 20 billion, and this is only about 80 years in the future! This should be viewed in the context of calculations that the earth can support 15 billion people if the level of its land cultivation is brought up to that of the Netherlands. It should be pointed out, however, that calculations such as this are subjects of disagreement.

Overall the world's population is currently increasing at the rate of about 200,000 per day, or about 70 million per year. This is equivalent to adding a city the size of Sacramento, Calif., each day or the total combined populations of the United Kingdom and the Scandanavian countries each year. The annual increase is also equivalent to about one tenth the population of China. Indeed, the increase of the past decade is equal to the population of all of Europe, exclusive of the U.S.S.R. The rate of increase is not the same, however, in all parts of the world. In the well-developed nations it varies from only 0.5 to 1.7% per year. This is in contrast with rates of 2.0 to 3.5% per year in the lesser developed nations. This is illustrated in Table 6-1.

DYNAMICS OF POPULATION GROWTH

When population growth data are studied, it soon becomes apparent that forces in addition to public health have been at work. Thus the onset of the upswing in world population actually antedates the modern public health movement. As has been indicated, a significant quickening in the rate of population increase began about 1650. It is difficult to determine the relative importance of the various factors that must have been involved in the reduction of mortality and in the resulting increase in population. It is evident, however, that the changes during the first part of this period were not due to public health

measures because few if any existed. Rather, it would appear that the determining roles during that period were played by changing social organization, a rising standard of living, gradually improved nutrition and work conditions, and the appearance of certain social reforms.

In Europe a significant excess of births over deaths was already well established by the eighteenth century, producing a steady population increase despite fluctuations due to frequent epidemics and occasional famine. Then in the midnineteenth century there began a marked decrease in mortality with a consequent upsurge in the rate of population increase. This reached a peak in the early twentieth century, despite the large number of emigrations. This upsurge may be attributed to the development of new means of transportation which facilitated a wider distribution of goods and people; to the technologic progress manifested by the Industrial Revolution which ensured improved conditions of living for greater numbers of people; and, particularly more recently, to the widespread application of newer knowledge concerning the causation and prevention of disease. Subsequently, despite continued decrease in death rates, the rate of population growth in Europe slowed down because birthrates began to fall rapidly.

The picture of population growth in the United States differs from that of Europe in three respects. First, during the early nineteenth century the rate of natural increase was much higher than in Europe, probably because of the young average age of those who came to America. Second, throughout the rest of the century the rate of natural

Table 6-1. Rate of population increase by region*

Region	Annual increase (%)	Doubles in
Latin America	Over 2.5	25 years or less
Africa, Middle East, South and Southeast Asia	2.0 to 2.5	30 to 35 years
Eastern Europe and Asia	1.5 to 2.0	35 to 45 years
North America	1.0 to 1.5	45 to 70 years
Western Europe	Less than 1.0	80 years or more

*From United Nations provisional report on world population prospects, 1963, ST/SOA/SER. R/7, p. 41.

increase underwent a rapid decline due to rapidly dropping birthrates. Thus in the United States births per 1,000 women aged 15 to 44 years dropped from 276 at the beginning of the nineteenth century to 208 at the midpoint and to 130 at the end. Finally, despite this marked slowing in natural increase, the flood of immigrants prevented a drop in the rate of total population growth.

The relationship between population changes and economic and social conditions is reviewed in *The Determinants and Consequences of Population Trends*,[13] issued in 1953 by the Population Division of the United Nations Department of Social Affairs. This extensive review indicates not only that many basic aspects of the problem have been scarcely considered but also that much disagreement exists over the interpretation of a large part of what has been studied. One thing appears obvious: in relation to population change no single factor, e.g., public health activity, can be considered alone as if it existed in a social and historical vacuum. Indeed, an exceedingly complex series of interrelationships is involved in the dynamics of population growth, stability, or retrogression. An elementary list of factors to consider includes areal limitations; climate; present size, spatial distribution, and age structure of the population; present and potential resources for food; availability and use of efficient agricultural implements, machinery, and techniques; quality of housing; policies and practices with regard to public health and education; existence, availability, and utilization of natural resources and sources of energy; means of verbal and physical communication, with special emphasis on farm-to-market roads; trends toward urbanization and industrialization; tax and financial structure, especially the availability of short-term and long-term loans at reasonable rates of interest; policies relating to the composition, full employment, and adequate compensation of the labor force; and a multitude of cultural factors.

Space does not permit adequate consideration of these factors. A few examples, however, illustrate the manner and extent

to which some of them may increase a population. It is well known that the addition of new sources or types of nutrient will result in increased bacterial growth or increased size of a herd. That this applies also to human beings is not surprising. Thus in the eighteenth century the sweet potato was introduced into China as a cheap, easily grown, rich source of carbohydrate in place of or to supplement grain. As far as is known, no other significant factor was changed. Certainly no public health or sanitary activities were pursued. Within 50 years the population increased from an estimated 60 million to 160 million. It is interesting to note that the inception of the population spurt in Europe dates from about the time of the introduction of the white potato from the Andean region of South America.

It is also accepted that the larger the areas effectively available to a species the more the species tends to move and increase. Thus an inoculum multiplies and spreads throughout a container of broth. This has also been the experience of man, most noticeably when new lands were discovered or developed. It was obviously more than chance that caused the beginning population upswing in the world to coincide with the great period of discovery, colonization, and exploitation and with more widely available and more rapid means of transportation.

Life, in the final analysis, depends upon energy. Some members of the determinant school of sociology have analyzed the history of man from this viewpoint and have found that each time a new source of power or energy has been discovered there has occurred a period of unrest and strife resulting in a smaller number of units of people—clans, tribes, nations, or alliances. There then has followed an increase in production and a marked upsurge in population.[14]

However, as Sears[15] has observed, "No form of life can continue to multiply indefinitely without eventually coming to terms with the limitations of its environment. . . . Every wise gardener knows better than to crowd his luck by crowding his plants too closely. Even the most aggressive organisms, such as weeds, rodents, and noxious insects, do not increase and spread indefinitely."

Unquestionably, public health measures have contributed to the population increase of the past century. It has done so in four ways: (1) by improving the chances of fruitful conception, (2) by greatly increasing the chances of survival among infants and young children, (3) by preventing the premature deaths of many young adults who represent the most fertile component of our population and the group with the longest period of future fecundity, and (4) by greatly reducing the number of marriages dissolved by the death of one partner. This too has allowed a longer period of effective married life.

Among the social and economic factors related to the dynamics of population, consideration must be given to the degree of urbanization and industrialization. These are two of the most striking phenomena of our time, and, of course, they are closely linked. They have a curious two-phased effect upon population growth—initial encouragement followed by secondary retardation. The sequence of events is complex but basically appears to be about as follows: Industry, concentrated in centers of population and offering a means to obtain cash income, attracts especially the more vigorous and adventurous young adults. At first they tend to follow the old established essentially rural customs of their kind—marry young and aspire to large families. Sexual union among them is more fruitful because of their youth and because of the long average remaining period of fecundity. To this extent industrialization and urbanization result in a substantial initial increase in the rate of population growth.

However, with improved education, growing sophistication, stabilization of the labor force, the wish for an improved standard of living, social rivalries, and competition for time, energy, and income there occurs an emphasis on rationality of and independence from tradition, with a breaking away from the old conservative cultural ties. Marriages are delayed and families are kept small for the sake of more educa-tion, increased income, or improved social position. Children come to be considered less an economic asset and more an economic burden. Family life becomes less cohesive because individuals have many contacts outside the home. Since life becomes increasingly complex, sexual intercourse becomes less frequent and chances of fertilization decrease. Added to this is the more ready availability of methods of contraception and the knowledge to obtain and use them. Hence industrialization and urbanization result eventually in a decreased rate of reproduction and population growth. This has been found to hold true in Eastern as well as in Western civilizations.[16]

Reference has been made to the lesser developed areas of the world. Understandably there is concern over the rapidly declining death rates occurring in these areas in the face of high birthrates. Certain considerations should be borne in mind, however. There are a number of reasons for such rapid mortality decreases at this time. These areas are enjoying promptly the benefits of technical knowledge which required long periods of investigation and experimentation by the presently advanced areas to attain. The practical and immediate application of this lifesaving knowledge in the lesser developed areas is now possible at low per capita cost because of the development of relatively simple and inexpensive techniques and because of the present provision of international cooperation and assistance. It is unfortunate that during the early and critical phase of these assistance programs there were lacking both the technical knowledge and the inclination to plan for and maintain a proper balance between lifesaving measures and birthrates. Somewhat belatedly, family planning activities are now often encouraged and included in technical assistance programs to developing countries. One hopes that the ecologic balance has not been already so upset as to make these efforts too little and too late.

Another important reason is the great historical striving for independence and national identity throughout the world, with stress being placed on catching up as quickly as possible in education, in health, and in technical, industrial, and economic progress. Because so much is needed to be done, achievements have been rapid and dramatic. It would be unrealistic, however, to expect improvements in health or other fields to continue indefinitely at the present rate. In the field of health, preventable communicable diseases have accounted for a large part of the illness and death, and it is in this area that practically all the gains have occurred. Other gains will take longer and will be more difficult to achieve. This is borne out by the slowing in the rate of mortality decline in some countries such as Ceylon, British Guiana, Japan, and others.[17]

After studying many aspects of this question, Woytinsky and Woytinsky[18] have concluded:

> The growth of world population in the past three hundred years obviously does not express the secular trend and cannot be projected indefinitely into the future. Rather, it has been a unique, unprecedented and unrepeatable phenomenon of limited duration. It had a beginning in the not too distant past, and it will have an end, perhaps, in the not too remote future. The slowing down and levelling off of growth in world population seems unavoidable. The question is only when will growth stop and at what level.

The possibility of a reversal must always be kept in mind. Overwhelming uncontrolled population increase itself would eventually produce a stifling effect. Furthermore, despite the marked improvements that have occurred in the mortality picture, if concurrent progress in fields other than health does not occur, a slump in the curve of health progress may be anticipated. Thus Stolnitz,[19] who refers to social and economic factors more as elements which permit than as factors which precipitate, states, "It is obvious that the impact of medical skills on today's underdeveloped areas can be enormous. Whether the permissive elements will also be adequate is perhaps the foremost problem confronting half the world's population." It should not be overlooked that some of the same social and economic factors that affect mortality also affect fertility. Their relationship to mortality is not necessarily the same as their relationship to other factors that con-

tribute to population change. Thus factors which contribute to the decline in mortality may not necessarily raise the rate of population growth since they may also contribute to a decline in the birthrate. In this regard we have seen public health activities contribute to improved school attendance and cerebration, to industrial development and urbanization, to higher general income levels and improvement in the standard of living, and to an understanding of man's physiologic and reproductive functioning as well as a better appreciation of his place in society. Beyond this it is reasonable to expect that some of the same forces which have been speeding the decline in mortality will also effect the speeding of a lowered birthrate hence the deceleration of population growth. In other words, it is possible that the so-called dangerous time lag between lowered mortality and lowered fertility may be telescoped.

Of necessity, much has been left unsaid. No mention has been made of the great possibilities of more efficient land use, development of new agricultural techniques, improvement of plant and animal strains, application of nuclear energy to power development, irrigation, water distillation, food preservation, more adequate utilization of solar energy, reduction of food wastage by insects and vermin, chemical soil treatment, and hydroponics; nor has there been mention of the release of land for food use as a result of inexpensive artificial fibers and plastics, the food value of algae, the possibilities of sea farming and sea breeding, the possibility of more artificially manufactured foods, and the need for less energy food as a result of increasing mechanization on farms as well as in industry. The technologic possibilities of the future seem vast indeed and give some cause for reasonable optimism and hope.

POPULATION AND ECONOMIC PROGRESS

One of the most fundamental facets of a culture or society is the productivity of the individual and his group—the degree of success to which he can feed, clothe, and house himself and those dependent upon him. In the simplest sense this constitutes the economy of the individual or the group. The concept of both society and its economy implies people, and the plurality of the word people implies relationships, one type of which is interdependence and mutual support. But there is always the potential converse relationship of competitiveness and mutual destruction. Either relationship appears to be the result of the degree of balance or imbalance between the two dependent variables mentioned— the nature of a population, on the one hand, and of its economy, on the other. A population necessarily depends upon its economy, whereas economic development in turn requires a population and is pursued to serve that population's purposes. Theoretically at least the greater the population is, the more fruitful its productivity will be; however, the greater the population is, the more it must produce. And the more a population grows, the broader and deeper must be its economic base. The breadth and depth of the economic base are dependent in turn upon the resources which nature has made immediately and potentially available. These have tangible limits, and the avoidance of their depletion depends upon careful husbandry and conservation in order to allow for whatever natural regeneration and replenishment may be possible.

To this point the word population has been used in a loose and general sense. It is important to consider certain of its components. Each population contains a proportion of socially dependent nonproducers —the young, the elderly, the infirm, and the unemployed. It must be recognized also that these groups are constant consumers. Indeed, at least two of the groups, the young and the infirm, in many societies such as our own tend to consume proportionately more of the products and services of society than does the average individual. Obviously, therefore, the more dependents there are in a society, the larger must be the corps of producers. Any circumstance that alters the number and proportion of the various types of dependents and producers affects the economy. Similarly, any change in the extent or nature of the economy tends to affect the number and proportion of dependent nonproducers. The most obvious effect is an increase in unemployed persons. Usually close on the heels of unemployment, however, comes a decrease in the number of conceptions and births. Excellent recent examples of this sequence are provided by the economic recession and a major steel strike which occurred in the United States in the late 1950's.[20] If a lowered economy should persist, financial inability to obtain adequate nutrition and preventive and therapeutic medical care as well as other necessities and amenities results inevitably in an increase in the number and proportion of individuals who become acutely and chronically ill. Finally, because of the interplay between these last two effects, there eventually occurs at least a temporary increase in the proportion of dependent adults and elderly persons.

Much of the problem with which we are confronted results from the different rates and timings of these and other changes. To consider this in another dimension, certain highly and rapidly effective disease preventive measures have made it possible within a relatively brief period of history for large numbers of otherwise doomed infants and children not only to survive but also in turn to become parents. Not so prompt has been the effect upon the number and proportion of persons of advanced age. Not so prompt either have been changes in cultural attitudes with respect to family size, role of children in society, attitudes toward fertility, and control of conception in order to compensate in time for the population changes noted. As Sears[15] has pointed out, this delay, uncertainty, and confusion is understandable in view of the overwhelming force of the reproductive urge, "whose consequences are far less immediate and far more complex than those that may result from mixing a solution or throwing a switch." The individual beset by this natural urge is equally beset by inertia, custom, tradition, and the voices of his time, which, "despite their common belief in the dignity and worth of human life, do not always see eye to eye."

Brock Chisholm,[21] former Director General of the World Health Organization, has expressed a similar opinion in relation to underdeveloped areas. He considers it impossible under current circumstances for foreign development assistance to be increased sufficiently to make possible the necessary rapid economic development in the face of high birth and survival rates:

> There are limits to the amounts of capital that can be absorbed usefully in an underdeveloped country at a given time. There are limits to the speed with which the people can be educated or trained. There are limits to the rate at which public administration can be improved, and to the rate at which public service can be expanded. And clearly, all these limits are narrowed by rapid population growth.

Many insist, however, that we should be seriously concerned and pessimistic about the distribution of the world's food products and especially about the possibility of improving to any significant degree the standard of living of the average inhabitant of the earth during the remainder of this century.[22] Chisholm[21] illustrates this by pointing out that, while a per capita income of $100 annually in a situation with a 1% population growth per year would increase to $135 annually over a 10-year period it would increase to $106 annually in the face of a 3.5% population growth per year. As he indicates, there are already a number of places in the world that have approached or reached the latter high rate of population increase.

It has become commonplace to compare the economically advanced countries with those that are economically retarded. Fifty-four percent of the world's inhabitants exist in 12 countries with 9% of the world's income, whereas the 7% who live in the United States and Canada produce and consume 43% of the world's income. Similarly one can compile a long list of variables that measure different aspects of social and economic development as well as political stability and sophistication and find, as one would expect, a remarkable consistency of relationship. Then one can examine the densities of population and

their respective rates of increase and income; here the relationships are not so clear cut and evident. The populations of Japan and the Netherlands are as dense as those of Egypt and Ceylon; those of Great Britain and the eastern United States as dense as the populations of the Balkans and Indonesia. To pursue this further into another dimension, one might compare the natural resources of the eastern United States with those of Indonesia and still be left with some unanswered questions.

It would appear, therefore, that no simple direct relationship exists between socioeconomic status and population status. One is forced to conclude that the relationship is affected by or dependent upon a third set of variables, and evidence appears to be mounting to point to the importance of the degree to which the combination of mobility, urbanization, mechanization, and industrialization has become a fundamental part of the way of life. This even appears to hold true in areas devoted essentially to mineral extraction and agriculture. Thus the populations of those areas which pursue such ends in a large-scale, mechanized, or industrialized manner fare better than do those which still resort to more simple, primitive, and individualized approaches.

The implications of this for the future of population growth is illustrated by the comparison in Table 6-2 of three groupings of nations. The comparison indicates that the greater the degree of industrialization, hence presumably urbanization, mechanization, and mobility, the greater will be the degree of balance between birthrates and death rates.

The fact that there is a worldwide trend toward urbanization and industrial development as well as toward more efficient agriculture provides some basis for optimism. These twin changes not only will produce more food and goods for more people at less unit cost, and indirectly force facilities for greater mobility but will also tend to increase the ratio of those for whom a smaller family is recognized as an advantage. This will contrast sharply with outdated traditional beliefs, practices, and

Table 6-2. Vital balance in three world areas by degree of industrialization*

Nature of group	World population (%)	Death rate	Birthrate
Industrialized Relatively balanced and stationary populations with relatively low birth and death rates and incipient population decline (U.S.A., United Kingdom, Scandinavia, France)	20	10	15
Transitional Somewhat imbalanced and expanding populations with significant control of deaths and beginning control of births (Eastern and Southeastern Europe, U.S.S.R., Japan, Brazil, Argentina)	20	15 to 20	25
Preindustrial Relatively balanced populations with high birth and death rates but with high population expansion potential (Asia except Russia and Japan, Africa except South Africa)	60	30+	35+

*Adapted from Gordon, J. E., Wyon, J. E., and Ingalls, T. H.: Public health as a demographic influence, Amer. J. Med. Sci. **227**:326, Mar. 1954.

customs regarding family size, purposes, and relationships in general and roles of children and women in particular.

In this regard it may be worth emphasizing the conviction that some social scientists have done a disservice to the concept of economic development and to the recipients of its benefits by trying to minimize its effect upon local mores and social organization. To the contrary, one should frankly recognize that it is critically necessary to bring about changes in family and group attitudes and practices in order to reduce birthrates as well as illness and death rates and to improve individual, group, and national living standards. To do otherwise is most unrealistic. Some individuals have even gone so far as to advocate almost exclusive emphasis upon agricultural extension programs to the exclusion of efforts in other areas of economic development. Such an approach is especially apt to be disadvantageous in the long run because the life of the typical farmer is highly traditional and merely to make it tolerable would remove the necessity or incentive for him to alter or adapt his attitudes and behavior toward many things, especially his family's size and purpose.

To carry this line of reasoning into the area of health programs in relation to economic development and population con-

trol, it might be considered best during a transitional period to emphasize activities in certain selective fields or areas such as the following:

1. Activities that tend to emphasize urban industrial areas more than rural agricultural areas
2. Activities that tend to favor actual producing components of the population more than dependents
3. Activities that tend to aid potential producers more than postproducers
4. Maternal and child health activities that convince women of the advantages of having fewer but healthier children
5. Activities that tend to improve the social and political position of women
6. Activities that tend to develop new sources of security for the individual in place of traditional social institutions which tend to encourage large families

In the process of considering the foregoing, however, it must be realized that the circumstances which led to industrial and economic development in the West and those that confront efforts toward industrial and economic development in much of the remainder of the world, including Asia, Africa, and much of Latin America, are quite different in certain important respects.[23] In the West, as has already been indicated, urbanization and the introduction of successful attacks upon the resulting rising mortality have accompanied industrialization. In fact, for a significant period of time economic and industrial development in western Europe and the United States has depended upon a lowered mortality in company with a sustained high birthrate and immigration rate for its continuance. During that period of human history, industry could be considered to have consumed human life at a rate faster than it could be produced locally. By contrast, the present situation elsewhere in the world is quite different. By virtue of the sudden application of certain products and techniques of our industrial culture, mortality rates are declining rapidly in the face of sustained or increased birthrates. As a result populations are soaring. The significant point is that these changes are precedents rather than necessary concomitants of the hoped-for economic, social, and industrial development. Many authors have commented on the dangerous time lag between lowered death rates and lowered birthrates. Another dangerous time lag to which perhaps not enough attention has been given is summarized by Van den Haag[24] in the following way:

> The endogenous industrialization of the West was prepared for by a cumulative historical development starting at least in the Renaissance, and including the rise of individualism, rationalism, empiricism and science, the fall of feudalism, and numerous other changes which led to the attitudes associated with successful industrialization. The sudden introduction of an alien economic system without historical preparation is a far more difficult and dangerous operation. It is unavoidable by now, but we must be prepared for undesirable side effects.

This phenomenon is further compounded by the agglutination of large numbers of persons in urban centers, not because growing industries can absorb them but because of the magnetism of the hoped-for amenities of a culture which is not yet there to enjoy.

The foregoing general comments are but a few of the many complex aspects of the relationship of population to socioeconomic development. While concern over these problems is rapidly increasing, it is by no means new. The lack of reference to Malthus may have been noted. Instead, attention is called to a statement made in 1908 by the Reverend T. N. Carver[25]:

> Fundamentally there are only two practical problems imposed upon us. The one is industrial and the other moral; the one has to do with the improvement of the relations between man and nature, and the other with the improvement of the relations between man and man. But these two primary problems are so inextricably intermingled, and they deal with such infinitely ranging factors, that the secondary and tertiary problems are more than we can count.
> But whence arises that phase of the conflict with nature out of which grows the conflict between man and man? Is man in any way responsible for it, or is it due wholly to the harshness or the niggardliness of nature? The fruitfulness of nature varies, of course, in different environments. But in any environment there are two conditions, for both of which man is in a measure responsible, and either of which will result in economic scarcity. One is the indefinite expansion of human wants, and the other is the multiplication of his numbers.

Members of the human race, especially those responsible for education, industry, politics, theology, medicine, and public health, who play such determinant roles in the life and future of society, have now reached a point when a critical decision must be made, a decision which no degree of euphoria or optimism can allow to be delayed any longer. Something has to give. We must either face reality and take rapid and forthright steps toward the deceleration of the increase in man's numbers or accept the inevitable take-over by nature that would involve the loss of all of our hard-won gains through the mechanism of widespread political unrest, pestilence, and famine.

What may be concluded so far? First, public health effort has saved lives and has contributed to population increase; second, public health is only one of many factors involved in both social improvement and population increase; third, public health measures tend to be more rapidly successful than do activities in other fields; fourth, interrelationships of these fields and ours in terms of the effects are relatively little understood; fifth, technical assistance to underdeveloped communities or areas should be multidisciplinary and never limited exclusively to public health or any other single field of endeavor and should always be associated with family planning programs; and sixth, in carrying out public health programs anywhere, rather than attempt the impossible of bringing about public health changes entirely within existing cultural patterns, as if they were static, we should encourage changes that are consistent with the realities of desirable dynamic, social, and public health improvement.

FAMILY PLANNING PROGRAMS

In view of the foregoing discussions it is obvious that in company with any efforts toward agricultural or industrial development or individual family or community self-sufficiency, there is a need for population or fertility control. With specific reference to the individual or the family, there are many valid indications. There are data to indicate that the incidence of infant mortality, maternal mortality, prematurity, mental retardation, congenital malformations, and brain damage is significantly higher than average among fourth and subsequent births, among births to older women, and among first births to girls in their early teens. These results are more prone to occur when pregnancies follow each other rapidly in economically underprivileged women whose health is below normal due to poor living conditions, undernutrition, and inadequate medical care. It has been estimated that about 2,200 infants' deaths would be prevented annually among each 500,000 low income patients if they were provided with voluntary family planning services.[26] With respect to maternal risks it has been long known that puerperal death rates increase strikingly with increased age and multiparity of the woman. In addition, it has been noted in a study by the World Health Organization that 10% of maternal deaths are due to abortions, many of which are induced because of large families. The removal of the mother by premature death or by invalidism in such instances is a

family catastrophe. Practical availability of family planning services would go far to eliminate these needless causes of suffering and death. Parents with large families necessarily tend to be inextricably caught in the dependency vortex, and their children are born into it and escape only with great difficulty. All aspects of living tend to be inadequately attainable—housing, food, recreation, education, and medical care. Such families tend to be more frequently broken.

For these and many other reasons fertility control or family planning, as it is now commonly designated, has been promoted for many years in the United States. Until recently, however, the promotion has been largely by some private physicians and several voluntary agencies. Without question, the greatest credit must go to the Planned Parenthood Federation of America, founded by the courageous and dauntless Margaret Sanger, who persisted over long difficult years for the fulfillment of an idea she considered humane, honorable, and important. Progress was discouragingly slow due to a variety of cultural blocks, political opposition, and technologic inadequacies. Gradually more and more professional organizations took a stand. At present the list includes the American Public Health Association, The American Public Welfare Association, the American Medical Association, the National Academy of Science, and the United Nations and its various specialized agencies such as WHO, UNESCO, and UNICEF. These actions have coincided with several significant scientific and technologic advances, particularly the development of relatively inexpensive, easily used, and increasingly effective methods of contraception. At the same time and for a complex set of reasons a remarkable change in public attitude toward the subject has occurred. Greatly improved and extended public education, the rigors of economic depression and wars followed by great national affluence, the rather complete emancipation of women, the development of mass communications—these and many other factors have led to a considerable liberalization of public, religious, and political attitude. Of great impact have been the forthright favorable statements of the late President John F. Kennedy and of former President Lyndon B. Johnson. Another significant milestone was the invalidation by the Supreme Court of the United States on June 7, 1965, of the 1879 Connecticut antibirth control law. The Court ruled that such legislation violated the constitutional right of married couples to privacy. Justice Goldberg, however, pointed out that the interpretation was a two-way street and must be considered similarly to protect welfare clients against coercive promotional techniques.

Federal, state, and local health, welfare, and other types of agencies have adopted enlightened policies at an increasing rate. The first state-supported family planning services in local health departments were established in 1937 in North Carolina. Six other southern states followed (Alabama, Florida, Georgia, Mississippi, South Carolina, and Virginia). Services were incorporated into maternal health clinics and home nursing programs and served primarily rural rather than urban areas. Mention should also be made of the development and operation during the 1930's of a large number of birth control clinics in Puerto Rico using funds from the Children's Bureau. It is interesting that, while the federal government still does not have a firm overall policy on family planning, many of its present component agencies are actively involved in a wide variety of services, research, and training programs in this field.[27] By now the majority of the states and many cities are included. Unfortunately policies vary considerably, as does the effectiveness with which they are carried out.[28] With reference to this a study of 56 metropolitan counties with the largest number of infant deaths, accounting for 26% of the national need, has indicated that only about one fourth of the women who needed subsidized family planning services were actually obtaining them from some source. Only about one half of the services obtained were provided by health departments. By the mid-1960's schools of public health had begun to present special

seminars and curricula designed for the training of various types of professionals to work in family planning programs.[29]

Methodology

While it is not the intent of this book to be a technical manual in any sense, the nature and importance of the subject at hand are such as to justify a few words about methods of contraception. The origins of attempts to prevent conception are lost in primitive history. Some indications of the wide variety of materials used may be obtained from an interesting study by de Laszlo and Henshaw.[30] The Ebers Papyrus, 1550 B.C., includes an interesting recipe for a medicated tampon to control fertility. The compound consisted of a mixture of acacia and honey which was to be inserted into the vagina as a suppository. Interestingly, on fermentation acacia breaks down into lactic acid, a rather effective spermicidal agent.[31] At the present time there exists a wide variety of behavioral, physiologic, chemical, and physical methods of contraception. They vary widely as to effectiveness, acceptability, cost, and other factors, The use of many of them requires or indicates the assistance, advice, or supervision of a physician or other properly trained person. To a considerable extent the ultimate choice depends upon individual preference.[32] The amount of research that is being carried out in this field is such as to anticipate further radical discoveries, hence changes in methodology, at any time.

REFERENCES

1. Hanlon, J. J.: The public health worker and the population question, Amer. J. Public Health **46:**1397, Nov. 1956.
2. Vogt, W.: Road to survival, New York, 1948, William Sloane Associates.
3. Osborn, F.: The limits of the earth, Boston, 1953, Little, Brown and Co.
4. Cook, R. C. In Russell, P. F.: Public health practice and population pressure in the tropics, Amer. J. Trop. Med. **1:**177, Mar. 1952.
5. Cook, R. C.: Human fertility: the modern dilemma, New York, 1951, William Sloane Associates.
6. Rolph, C. H.: The human sum, New York, 1957, The Macmillan Co.
7. Brown, H.: The challenge of man's future, New York, 1954, The Viking Press, Inc.

8. Hill, A. V.: Nature **170:**388, 1952.
9. Boyd-Orr, J.: Proceeding International Congress of Population, Cheltenham, England, 1948.
10. deCastro, J.: The geography of hunger, Boston, 1952, Little, Brown & Co.
11. Coale, A. J.: The economic effects of fertility control in underdeveloped areas. In Hauser, P. M., editor: The population dilemma, Prentice-Hall, Englewood Cliffs, N. J., 1963.
12. Man's origin: mystery deepens, M.D. **9:**99, July 1965.
13. Population Division of the United Nations Department of Social Affairs: The determinants and consequences of population trends, New York, 1953, United Nations.
14. White, L.: Man's control over civilization, Sci. Month. **66:**235, Mar. 1948.
15. Sears, P. B.: Pressures of population, an ecologist's point of view, What's New **212:**12, 1959.
16. Tauber, I. B.: Population and labor force in the industrialization of Japan, 1850-1950; economic growth in Brazil, India, and Japan, Princeton, 1955, Princeton University Press.
17. Bourgeois-Pichat, J., and Pan, C.: Trends and determinants of mortality in underdeveloped areas, New York, 1956, Milbank Memorial Fund.
18. Woytinsky, W. S., and Woytinsky, E. S.: World population and production; trends and outlook, New York, 1953, The Twentieth Century Fund.
19. Stolnitz, J.: Comparison between some recent mortality trends in underdeveloped areas and historical trends in the west. In Bourgeois-Pichat, J., and Pan, C., editors: Trends and differentials of mortality in underdeveloped areas. New York, 1956, Milbank Memorial Fund.
20. Westoff, C. F., Potter, R. G., and Sagi, P. C.: Some selected findings of the Princeton fertility study, 1963, Demography **1:**1, 1964.
21. Chisholm, B. In Jones, J. M., editor: Does overpopulation mean poverty? Washington, 1962, Center for International Economic Growth.
22. Hauser, P. M.: Demographic dimensions of world politics, Science **131:**3414, June 3, 1960.
23. Coale, A. J., and Hoover, E. M.: Population growth and economic development in low-income countries, Princeton, 1958, Princeton University Press.
24. Van den Haag, E.: Population and economic development, What's New **214:**4, 1959.
25. Carver, T. N.: The economic basis of the problem of evil, Harvard Theological Review, **1:**1, Jan. 1908.
26. Family planning and infant mortality, an analysis of priorities (mimeographed report), New York, 1967, Planned Parenthood-World Population. p. 8 ff.
27. Report on family planning: activities of the U. S. Department of Health, Education, and Welfare in family planning, fertility, sterility, and population dynamics, Washington, 1966, U. S. Government Printing Office.
28. Eliot, J. W.: The development of family planning services by state and local health departments in the United States, suppl. on family planning, Amer. J. Public Health **56:**6, Jan. 1966.
29. Corsa, L.: Introduction, supplement on family planning, Amer. J. Public Health **56:**3, Jan. 1966.
30. deLaszlo, H., and Henshaw, P. S.: Plant materials used by primitive peoples to affect fertility, Science **119:**626, May 7, 1954.
31. The first prescription for control of fertility, M.D. **9:**58, July 1963.
32. Calderone, M. S.: Manual of contraceptive practice, Baltimore, 1964, The Williams & Wilkins Co.

Chapter 7

Economics
of
public health

INEVITABILITY OF HEALTH COSTS

There are two related objections that are occasionally heard with regard to public health activities. One is that the establishment and growth of public health agencies and programs have resulted in increasing costs to the public. The other is that public health workers are at a disadvantage in that they cannot point to their successes. This latter statement is made in contrast to the position of the private physician who with justification can point to the saving of many specific lives by judicious medical and surgical management. Granted that the public health worker cannot point to particular individuals who have been spared illness and premature death by public health programs, this is more than compensated for by the possibility of measurement in a larger and ultimately more dramatic sense. It must be realized that the fruits of our labors are in essence quite different from those of therapeutic medicine and that accordingly the bases of measurement cannot be expected to be the same. Public health work is not fundamentally concerned with the repair of damage already done. Rather, we deal with the prevention of damage in the first place and the promotion of positive health. Furthermore, by virtue of the fact that, although healthy living is expensive, illness is even more so, it should be possible to demonstrate that preventive and promotive health activities offer a sound financial investment to the individual and to the community.

Most intelligent people appreciate the reduction in human suffering that has resulted from the public health movement. It must be realized, however, that the further removed one is by time and space from the threat of personal suffering the less consideration is apt to be given to it. In other words, our very success in public health work tends to mask our value. It is appropriate, therefore, that the public and its elected representatives be given cause to appreciate the wisdom of expenditures for health from an altogether different viewpoint.

As will be pointed out elsewhere, the costs of all governmental services have persistently increased. Proportionately speaking, the expenditure for public health services represents an area of considerable expansion. This has caused some to point to public health programs as an added economic burden to the taxpayer. It is important to point out and to demonstrate that an increased sum of money spent wisely for health services represents not an increase but actually a decrease in the net bill for personal and community welfare and protection. The construction and maintenance costs of public water purification and sewage disposal plants are admittedly great. The costs, however, do not represent an addition to our economic burden. Their absence would cost us a similar if not greater sum for individual facilities, for increased medical care, and for lost earnings resulting from the illnesses that would not be prevented. Single or repeated outbreaks of typhoid fever, for example, would cost a community much more in the long run than would installation of engineering and other measures designed for their prevention. A sound financial policy for public health services, therefore, must take into consideration not only the humanitarian and social gains but also the economic advantages to be derived therefrom. The problem then is to make the public conscious and to organize costs which in any case are destined to occur either as hidden individual expenditures or as socially beneficial public appropriations. Public health is the best form of social and economic insurance.

WHY LIFE AND HEALTH ARE MEASURED

Beyond the inevitability of these expenditures is the added factor of the economic value of the lives made possible or continued by public health endeavors. To many the thought of placing a monetary value on human life appears to be improper, immoral, or inhuman. Essentially, our reactions to life and death are based upon emotion and sentiment, and ordinarily we deliberately avoid any thought of placing an economic or cost-value label on a human being. Yet, to be realistic, it must be admitted that life does have a monetary value. The death of a parent brings to society as a whole as well as to the particular family involved an economic as well as a sentimental loss which is quite real and irreparable. This may manifest itself in a lowered standard of living for the family, the necessity of public financial aid, or the loss of a trained worker. Furthermore, governmental recognition is given to the value of a life, and one seldom hears objections to the concept of income tax exemptions.

In addressing himself to this question, Fuchs[1] makes several telling observations:

What, then, is the justification for such an inquiry? The principle one is the fact that the question of the contribution of health services is being asked and answered every day. It is being asked and answered implicitly every time consumers, hospitals, universities, business firms, foundations, government agencies and legislative bodies make decisions concerning the volume and composition of health services, present and future. If economists can help to rationalize and make more explicit the decision making process, can provide useful definitions, concepts and analytic tools, and can develop appropriate bodies of data and summary measures, they will be making their own contribution to health and to the economy.

In the same vein it must be recognized that, while members of appropriating bodies may be very humane and sympathetic, collectively they are becoming increasingly coldly analytic and practical. As a result it is becoming more difficult to sell our programs, especially on the basis of sentimentality or intangibles. It is unfortunate, in a sense, that so many of our results, although of tremendous intrinsic value, are largely of an intangible nature, e.g., diseases and deaths prevented, problems avoided, and the like. This makes it all the more imperative that health program planning and evaluative procedures have incorporated in them from the beginning a consideration not only of economic costs but also the anticipated economic return. Such data, if successfully obtained, can be of inestimable value both in obtaining public understanding and support and in budgetary presentations.[2]

In attempting to do so, however, one is immediately confronted with two fundamental problems: (1) problems of definition—What is health? What is incapacitation? etc.; and (2) problems of measurement—How does one measure something that isn't there? What base line can one use? The seriousness of these problems varies with time, place, and circumstance, as indicated by Linnenberg.[3] He points out that, if a community or nation has a high incidence of a disease which existing knowledge and methods systematically applied can quickly bring under control, it is possible to make an advance estimate not only of the cost of the methods but also of the likely benefits in terms of worker time not lost and treatment costs avoided. But, he adds, drama of this sort stems only from a sudden breakthrough, as in the case of a new effective vaccine, or from an area's being widely afflicted with a serious and especially an economically detrimental disease, such as malaria or yaws, which is anachronistic from the standpoint of modern medicine and which can be brought under control quickly, even though little or nothing is done about other health problems. Our difficulty, he concludes, is that such classic simplicity is absent from most of our public health work in this country, where public health achievement has progressed so far that our health problems are not so much the yes or no kind as the more or less kind.

ECONOMIC VALUE OF LIFE

Many have tried to evaluate man or to put a price on his economic worth. One of the earliest attempts was that of Sir William Petty (1623-1687), who originated many ideas later used by the political economist Adam Smith in *Wealth of Nations* and other works. Petty[4] derived his estimate as follows:

Suppose the People of England be Six Millions in number, that their Expense at £7 per head be 42 Millions: Suppose also that the Rent of the Lands be 8 Millions, and the yearly profit of all the Personal Estate be 8 Millions more; it must needs follow that the Labour of the People must have supplied the remaining 26 Millions the which multiplied by 20 (the Mass of Mankind being worth 20 years purchase as well as land) makes 520 Millions as the value of the whole people; which number divided by 6 Millions makes about £80 the value of each Head of Man, Woman and Child and of adult Persons Twice as much; from whence we may learn to compute the loss we have sustained by the Plague, by the Slaughter of Men in War and by sending them abroad into the Service of Foreign Princes.

Later, Sir William Farr and Irving Fisher made more scientific computations, using the life table technique, which by their time had been developed. Subsequently this approach was explored more extensively and effectively by Dublin and Lotka.[5,6] Several of their publications have considerable social significance and have been drawn upon freely in the following discussion. More recently Weisbrod[7] has combined this approach with a number of

other approaches to place health and expenditures for it in the proper context.

The human body may be considered as being similar to a machine. Like machines, its proper function depends on the movement and interaction of various physical and chemical parts, complicated and augmented, however, by a third and much more complex factor—biologic reaction. To resort to a crude analogy, the body might be likened to an internal combustion engine with limbs in place of pistons and the organs of internal secretion acting as the carburetor. Superimposed upon these is the supervisory function of the human mind, which might be compared with the governor on an internal combustion engine. In a like manner the human body may be regarded as an economic unit brought into existence for measurable, potential, productive purposes.

A machine designed for the production of ball bearings, for example, is of no intrinsic value in itself, its true value being measurable only in terms of its capacity to produce ball bearings, thereby justifying its existence. Similarly, except in a completely paganistic and hedonistic society, the mere existence of life is of little if any value. It should be realized that life and health in themselves have real value only as they promote efficiency and happiness and that in the final analysis it is the quality of life that counts, not the quantity. Of themselves, life and health are valueless, their true value depending upon the activities engaged in by virtue of them.

To return to the example of the machine, it must pass through several phases or steps before it is even ready to be of productive value. First, it must be built, which presupposes the existence of a factory in which it may be constructed. Its construction, therefore, involves from the start a considerable capital outlay for factory site, labor, and tools. On completion the machine is not yet of true value. It must be prepared for use or function. This involves a series of installation expenditures for inspection and checking, for transfer to the site where it is intended to function, and for oiling, tuning up, and other preparations. Following this, the machine is ready to become productive, and the extent and efficiency of its usefulness depend on its original quality or lack of structural defects, the correctness of its installation, and the manner in which it is routinely cared for while in use. It must be carefully and repeatedly lubricated, fed the proper fuel, inspected, overhauled, repaired, and given proper rest intervals rather than constant grinding use which would lead to metal fatigue. During this period of use, therefore, a certain amount of expenditure and effort is constantly required to maintain the machine, and its ultimate value can be determined only after the value of that expenditure and effort is deducted from the gross value of its productivity.

With man as with machines, there are always debit as well as credit items during the period of productivity. It is the hope and goal of the manufacturer that his machine will continue to function with relative efficiency at least long enough to produce sufficient items for sale to offset all of the debits incurred by the capital investment and the installation and maintenance costs. In other words, from the moment the machine is purchased, the curve of the cumulative investment in it continues to rise, the curve of cumulative productive value lagging for a considerable period. It is not until these two curves cross that the manufacturer can breathe easily and begin to reap a net benefit from the use of the machine. If any untoward circumstances develop before the two curves cross, the manufacturer stands to lose a considerable investment.

Many things may go wrong after purchase. The machine may have been unsuspectedly defective, it may have been damaged during transportation and installation, or it may have worn out prematurely due to improper use or care. These are but a few of the undesirable potentialities the manufacturer must constantly guard against. Even after the two curves cross, all is not necessarily clear sailing because the longer the machine is used, the greater is the tendency for parts to wear out and for maintenance and repair costs to increase.

Sooner or later a time is reached when these costs become greater than the value of the items produced and the two curves cross again. Continued use is no longer profitable. The machine has now passed into the phase of obsolescence or, in the case of human beings, senility. More idealistically it may be considered the period of retirement or senior citizenship.

It is of interest to attempt to analyze the items that contribute to the debit and credit columns of human life. One such analysis, based upon data and crude calculations for the year 1955 as a convenient example, is presented on the following pages. Insofar as possible, an attempt has been made to calculate or estimate monetary values for the many factors considered. It must be stressed, however, that *this is done simply to illustrate a general principle,* and the reader should realize that *the values assigned are at best no more than very crude calculations and estimates* which are subject to innumerable influences such as changes in monetary values, wage levels, cost of living trends, and the extent of unemployment, to mention only a few. In other words, *the figures given are not intended to represent true dollar values to be quoted as such but are presented simply to illustrate a concept.* The entire picture is summarized in Table 7-1.

FACTORS ENTERING INTO THE VALUE OF A HUMAN LIFE
Period of initial capital investment
1. *Value of economic incapacitation of the expectant mother* —$500

All adult females as well as males have an economic productive potential. For the majority of women this potential is effected in either or both of two ways: employment for wages or occupation as a housewife. Ordinarily the latter is not thought of in an economic sense since it rarely involves the transfer of an agreed upon sum of money for services rendered. Nonetheless, the housewife and mother fulfills a function of real economic value. In fact, her absence would necessitate the employment of a paid substitute. The average period of incapacitation for childbearing might be estimated roughly at 3 months, the actual degree of incapacitation varying throughout the period of pregnancy and with individuals. In 1955 the average age of the pregnant woman was 24 years and the annual value of her real or potential earnings might be estimated at an average of $2,000. This considers her to be in

Table 7-1. Factors in the socioeconomic value of human life—summary

Capital cost*		
1. Economic incapacitation of mother	$	500
2. Risk of death to mother (prorated)		12
3. Risk of injury to mother with immediate or subsequent effect on her economic value (prorated)		?
4. Immediate costs of childbearing		488
5. Risk of infant death (prorated)		40
6. Risk of infant illness or injury		?
7. Interest on capital investment		30
	$	1,070
Installation cost†		
1. Shelter, clothing, and food	$	11,900
2. Value of time mother devotes to child care		15,750
3. Education—family and community contribution		4,500
4. Medical and dental care and health protection		600
5. Recreation and transportation		3,000
6. Insurance		100
7. Sundries and incidentals		900
8. Risk of death during first 18 years (prorated)		250
9. Risk of disability during first 18 years		?
10. Interest on installation costs		23,000
	$	60,000
Period of productivity‡		
Credit		
1. Earning potential	$	60,000
2. Interest on earnings		50,000
3. Noneconomic potential		?
	$110,000	
Debit		
1. Risk of disability during productive period	$	4,000
2. Medical costs		6,500
3. Risk of premature death		200
4. Risk of becoming substandard		5,500
5. Interest on debit items		15,000
	$	31,200

*The investment that society has in each infant by the time it is born.
†The investment that society has in each individual by the time he reaches 18 years of age.
‡The return that society can expect from its investment, with the risks involved during this period.

the most typical economic class for her sex, which in 1955 reported a maximum potential annual income of approximately $2,500. Incapacitation for about one fourth of her twenty-fourth year, therefore, represents about $500 as part of the capital investment in the anticipated child.

2. *Prorated value of the risk of maternal death* —$12

If the efforts of a housewife and mother have an economic value and if, as will be developed, she herself represents a considerable investment, her death as a result of childbearing will constitute a monetary loss to her family and to society. In 1955 there were about 1,950 maternal deaths related to the 4.04 million births which occurred in the United States. The average age of the women who died was 29 years. The average net value of the potential

future activity of each of them might be estimated at about $26,000. Therefore, the monetary loss as a result of maternal deaths was the product of $26,000 times 1,950 deaths, or about $50.7 million per year, which, if prorated among all of the births, amounts to $12 as the value of the risk of maternal death, which should be added to the cost of each child born alive.

3. *Value of the risk of injury short of death to the mother* —?

As a result of childbearing, many women suffer disabilities or illnesses which, although they do not cause death, have a subsequent effect on their well-being, economic productivity, and length of life. As in the case of maternal deaths, the total economic effect of this should be prorated among all infants born. Though extremely difficult if not im-

Table 7-2. Estimates of average cost of births for women in the $4,500 family income class

Type of service	Total cost	Hospital cost	Physician's fee	Housekeeper	Minimum layette	Incidentals
At home	$300	$...	$ 70	$150	$60	$ 20
Ward	325	95	...	150	60	20
Semiprivate	535	150	150	150	60	50
Private	735	200	225	150	60	100

possible to estimate or calculate, its effect appears elsewhere in terms of medical expenditures and shortened lives.

4. Immediate costs of childbearing   —$488

Here are found a number of readily recognizable items. Included are the costs of prenatal and postnatal care, hospitalization, delivery, and expenditures for special maternity clothes, layettes, and the equipment for the care of the newborn infant. There also should be included an item for housekeeping assistance. While some objection might be raised to this, it may be pointed out that in some households a housekeeper is actually employed for a period preceding and following delivery. Furthermore, since this is not possible for the majority of families, some housekeeping assistance is required and furnished by a relative, friend, or neighbor. Their time and effort has value, and calling upon them to assist in the home of the expectant mother ultimately involves their temporary removal from productive enterprise elsewhere. Estimates of these costs for the most typical economic class have been adapted from studies by the Metropolitan Life Insurance Company and the Maternity Center Association, New York City, and are presented in Table 7-2. The average figure may be considered to be about $488.

*5. Prorated value of the risk of
    neonatal death   —$40*

Like their mothers, infants may be subject to injury or death as a consequence of abnormal development or of the birth process. This is analogous to the machine that might be defective in construction or damaged shortly thereafter. During 1955 in the United States there occurred a total of 167,700 known nonproductive deliveries, consisting of 90,000 stillbirths and 77,000 neonatal deaths. Up to this point, there had been invested in each of them an average of $1,000, which, if multiplied by the number of known nonproductive deliveries, gives $167.7 million as the annual monetary loss they represent. If this figure is prorated among the year's 4.04 million live births, each infant bears as his share of the risk of not being born alive or surviving 1 month a sum of about $40.

*6. Value of the risk of injury short of death
    to the infant   —?*

As in the case of mothers, infants may suffer nonfatal damage before, during, or shortly after birth.

Again the economic significance of this is difficult or impossible to determine. However, it shows up subsequently in the form of medical expenditures and shortened life.

7. Interest on capital investment   —$30

If a man and woman originally considered the pros and cons of prospective parenthood and, deciding against it, invested the total of the sums listed above for a period corresponding to that of pregnancy, there would accrue at 3.5% compound interest about $30. While this may sound venal, the fact remains that a considerable number of people do just this.

The total capital value of a child at birth is therefore about $1,070, which represents the economic interest that the parents and society have in it by the time it leaves the human factory.

Period of human installation costs

While the mechanical contrivance upon purchase may be installed and made ready for productive performance in a relatively short time, a rather lengthy period and a considerable cash outlay are required in order to bring the newly born human mechanism to the point of social and economic productivity. Among the costs involved may be listed the following, the figures for which are in many instances extremely conservative in view of current prices.

*1. Shelter, clothing, and food for first
    18 years   —$11,900*

For 1955 a breakdown of this crude estimate was $4,240 for shelter, $1,690 for clothing, and $5,970 for food. Since exception may be taken to the inclusion of an item for shelter, it might be pointed out that, from an overall social standpoint, if the addition of a new family member did not result in overcrowding, necessitating an enlargement of living quarters, the family was previously occupying more living space than was fundamentally required.

*2. Value of the mother's time devoted to
    the care of the child   —$15,750*

Based on the average value of the potential earnings of a 24-year-old woman at home or at work as $2,500, the value of her time given to the care of the child is estimated to decrease arithmetically from $1,250 for the first year to $400 for the eighteenth year. The cumulative total is about $15,750.

3. Education   —$4,500

It is estimated that the average expenditure for education of a child is $4,500, of which the community bears the major share.

4. Medical and dental care and
health protection   —$600

This small item of expense if increased substantially would undoubtedly result in considerably enhanced personal value, productivity, and length of life. It is unfortunate that this is considered to be of the same magnitude as "sundries and incidentals."

5. Recreation and transportation   —$3,000

6. Insurance   —$100

Very few children's lives are insured. The average is found to be about the figure shown.

7. Sundries and incidentals   —$900

8. Prorated value of risk of death before
eighteenth year   —$250

Deaths that occur during the first 18 years of life are analogous to irreparable damage of a machine following its purchase and during the process of its installation. During 1955 in the United States there were about 42,000 deaths among persons between the ages of 1 month and 18 years. The average age at death in this group was 9 years. The monetary loss attributable to these deaths might be approximated roughly from the cost items previously listed as 9/18 ($1,070 + $36,750) of the costs of birth and of the installation period, times an annual loss of 42,000 persons, times 18 separate years, during any one of which the death might occur. The product of these figures is about $14 billion, which, if prorated throughout the 55.02 million persons in the age group under 18 years, gives about $250 as each individual's share of the risk of preproductive death.

9. Nonfatal disabilities during first 18 years   —?

As before, it is impossible to determine or estimate the value of this effect, but it shows up subsequently in costs of medical care and premature death.

10. Interest on installation costs   —$23,000

Again, if a decision had been made against conceiving the child in the first place and if all of the installation expenses had been invested instead, at the end of 18 years there would accrue at 3.5% compound interest an additional sum of about $23,000.

Total installation value, therefore, amounts to about $60,000 for each child who successfully reaches the age of 18 years.

Period of human productivity

Up to this point the new human mechanism not only has been constructed but has passed through all of the phases that constitute an installation or get-ready period. Instead of being bolted to a floor, oiled, checked, and tuned as in the case of a ma-

chine, the human being has been fed, clothed, educated, and otherwise prepared until he is ready to assume his place as a productive adult member of society. He is now in a position to begin to repay the considerable investment that his parents and society have made in him. From this point on the picture becomes complicated by the necessity of considering both credit and debit items. In order to make possible an ultimate balancing of the books, the individual's cumulative gross earnings must accomplish three things: full repayment of all that has been invested in him, provision of current maintenance costs both personal and community, and provision for future retirement in the postproductive period of life. Added to this is the hope of providing if possible some net surplus to pass on to the succeeding generation. It is upon this surplus that all familial and social progress, in contrast to stagnation, depend.

Credit items. Three items appear on the credit side of the human ledger. They may be considered as follows:

1. Net earning potential   +$60,000

In 1955 the most typical wage class into which working adult males fell was that which could look forward to a maximum annual earned income of $5,000. This maximum is approached gradually, beginning with a much lower income at the age of about 18 years when individuals begin productive work. The maximum is reached as the individual approaches his fortieth birthday, following which the annual net income begins to decline slowly to the time of death or retirement, when a marked or complete drop results. On the basis of his life expectancy the average 18-year-old male in the $5,000 maximum annual income class can look forward to gross future earnings totaling about $100,000. His total future cost of living based on 1955 figures would amount to about $40,000, leaving $60,000 as the net value of the future earnings of persons reaching 18 years of age. Taxes must, of course, be deducted from this.

2. Interest on earnings   +$50,000

Since interest has been considered in relation to the sums invested in the individual, to be consistent it should be applied also to his net future earnings. While the individual wage earner does not necessarily receive the interest himself, society as a whole may be considered to benefit since the mere fact that money is spent means that it has been put to use for gain. Therefore the $60,000 net future earnings will produce for the working individual or for other members of society to whom it may be transferred through purchases a certain amount of interest. If the interest is compound and the basis of it is scaled from ages 18 to 70 years, it will accumulate to the approximate amount of $50,000.

3. Noneconomic productive potential   +?

The human mechanism differs from the mechanical contrivance in that it has abilities or potentials to produce value in forms other than material. Thus a human being has a reproductive potential which in light of the foregoing is obviously worth something. One is reminded of the fact that the totalitarian dictators of recent European history actually placed a value upon the reproductive potential of women and paid the individual cash awards for producing children. Despite this, any attempt to evaluate correctly the reproductive potential of human beings in a monetary sense is pointless. Human beings also have social and intellectual potentials of incalculable value. Who would dare appraise da Vinci, Beethoven, Shakespeare? Yet the world is infinitely richer because of their existence.

• • •

Debit items. Attainment of the age of productive capacity does not necessarily imply that the individual will actually be able to or will even choose to contribute his share to society's material advancement. A number of things may act as deterrents, among which are the forces of disability and premature death and the possibility that the individual, although by now an adult, may be physically or mentally substandard or antisocial.

1. *Value of risk of disability after eighteenth birthday*   —$4,000

Various surveys have indicated that in the United States about 2.5% of working time is lost due to absenteeism or inefficiency attributable to illness or injury. Incidentally, a considerable amount of this is preventable. Since the national income in 1955 was about $324 billion, the average economic loss due to disability per potential wage earner, of whom there were about 102.4 million, may be computed as $\frac{\$324,000,000,000 \times 0.25}{102,400,000} = \$80$ per worker per year. With an average working life expectancy of 50 years, this would amount to a total of $80 × 50 years = $4,000, which represents each wage earner's prorated share of the nation's economic loss due to disability that must be deducted from his average net productive potential.

2. *Medical costs*   —$6,500

The cost of disability in a worker does not merely involve loss of productive power. Since the individual's actual take-home pay is usually affected, there results a loss of family income often necessitating cutting into the future income of the family or into the wealth of society at large. The extent to which this occurs during the average wage earner's life has been estimated by various groups who have studied the problem as about $3,500. In addition, disabilities require expenditures for medical and nursing care and sometimes for hospitalization, drugs, and appliances. The results of studies of these miscellaneous costs place them at an average of about $3,000 during an individual's lifetime. It is significant that one of the chief reasons for borrowing is inability to meet the costs of illness. If the illness happens to be of a communicable nature, there is the added risk of spread of the disease, upon which some value might be placed. The amount is difficult to estimate, but its effect shows up elsewhere in the form of society's total medical bill and as premature retirement and death. Another factor, the value of which cannot be calculated but which shows up later, is the risk of lowering the level of health of an entire family when disability of the breadwinner lowers the standard of living.

3. *Value of risk of premature death of wage earner*   —$200

The possibility of premature death of wage earners has been referred to. When this occurs, the worker in most instances has not been allowed to live long enough to neutralize the investment that has been made in him. By prorating the lost potential future earnings of those who prematurely die, each worker's share of this risk of not fulfilling his life expectancy may be very crudely estimated as follows at about $200 (Table 7-3).

4. *Risk of becoming substandard or antisocial*   —$5,500

A large number of individuals are brought to maturity only to be found defective in one way or

Table 7-3. Potential future earnings of persons prematurely dead, United States

Age group (years)	Median age (years)	Deaths (1955)	Individual net future earnings	Total lost future earnings
19 to 24	21	13,350	$61,000	$ 814,350,000
25 to 44	35	106,360	60,000	6,381,600,000
45 to 64	55	392,800	27,500	10,802,000,000
65 and over	72	819,000	750	614,250,000
				$18,612,200,000

Population over 18 years of age in United States, 1955 = 102,400,000.

$$\frac{\$18,612,200,000}{102,400,000} = \text{abcut } \$200$$

another. Many of them require the full-time attention of an additional large group of potential producers in the form of police, mental hospital attendants, and the like.

It is difficult or impossible to determine the total number of such individuals. Estimates vary considerably. For the United States in 1955 some of the estimates were as follows: blind, 330,000; mentally ill or defective, receiving some type of intramural or extramural institutional care, 840,000; attendants of mental institutions, 100,000; physically handicapped, 2,230,000; chronic nonproductive alcoholics, 750,000; narcotic addicts, 60,000; criminals, 400,000 detained and 600,000 at large; police, wardens, etc., 750,000; paupers, 80,000; and prostitutes, 250,000. Some of these figures undoubtedly are overstatements and some of them are duplicative. Nevertheless, they have a double significance for the average wage earner. First, he himself shares the risk of becoming substandard. Avoiding that, he finds he must assist in the support of these defectives. The cost is enormous. The annual bill for the care of the mentally ill alone has been estimated at well over $1 billion, and criminals and those who apprehend and guard them must cost about the same. The partially or totally blind, deaf-mutes, the physically handicapped, and some others contribute varying amounts to their own support, and more adequate programs for their training and rehabilitation would increase the degree to which they might be self-sufficient. The cost of support of the handicapped, the substandard, and the antisocial may be put very conservatively at $4 billion annually. Prorated among the wage earners over 18 years of age, this amounts to about $1,000 per wage earner.

In addition, society suffers a loss due to their lack of production. Estimates of this loss prorated among the wage earners over 18 years of age amounts to about $4,500 per wage earner. In toto, the prorated share of the cost of the risk of becoming substandard or antisocial might be considered about $5,500.

5. Interest on Debit Items   —$15,000

The total of each individual's share of all the debits that occur during the productive period of life amounts to about $16,000. If this sum were invested instead of being lost, there would accrue at 3.5% compound interest about $15,000 at the end of his productive life, bringing the total loss to about $31,000.

SUMMARY

If from the total net productive credit of $110,000 in the rough example presented previously, the $1,070 in capital cost, the $60,000 in installation costs, and the $31,200 in debits during the productive period are substracted, there remains a net balance of about $18,000 per person for the individual's and society's provision for the period of obsolescence, retirement, or senility.

ECONOMIC RETURN ON PUBLIC HEALTH INVESTMENT

A previous chapter on world health problems presented a number of examples of the contribution of public health measures to regional or national economic development and productivity. The economic soundness of expenditures for public health may also be demonstrated by still a different approach. This considers only expenditures saved on hospital bills, medical care, laboratory work, and similar facilities. One example that has been well worked out relates to the control of diphtheria in New York City some years ago, where an attempt was made to prove, among other things, that it is cheaper to prevent than to treat illness. In 1920 there occurred in New York City about 14,000 reported cases of diphtheria. Three thousand were hospitalized at an average cost of $112, totaling $336,000 for hospitalization. The remaining 11,000 patients were cared for at home at a cost to the city for various medical services of an average of $35 per patient, or a total of $385,000. On the average, public health nurses visited hospitalized patients two times and home patients six times. At 50 cents a visit this cost $36,000. The laboratory work, on the basis of 10 nose and throat cultures examined for each reported case at 5 cents per examination, cost $70,000. Of the patients, 1,045 died from the infection; at an average of $200 each their funerals cost over $200,000. The total cost up to this point, therefore, was $1,027,000. In other words, the city of New York in 1920 spent over $1 million for the support of the diphtheria organism.

From 1929 through 1931 the City's health department, aided partly by private funds, carried on an intensive, well-organized campaign to secure the immunization of infants and children against diphtheria. The cost of this campaign during those 3 years was $375,000. At the end of the 3 years the program was continued at a cost of less than $10,000 per year. Unquestionably, many persons considered these sums an added economic burden. However, let us see what was purchased with that money. During 1939, instead of over 14,000 cases, there were only 543 cases, despite known improved reporting. One half of these were hospitalized at $112 each. The total hospital bill, therefore, was $31,000. The medical bills for those remaining at home at an average of $35 per case totaled $9,625. Nurses' visits to the patients cost $1,100, and the laboratory work was reduced to only $2,750. Instead of over 1,000 deaths, there were only 22 for whom the funeral cost was $4,400. Even if we add to this the cost of $375,000 for the 3-year program plus seven times $10,000 to continue it between 1932 and 1939, the total bill for diphtheria was only $493,875 or one half of the 1920 bill.

Private enterprise has long recognized the soundness of expenditures for health and safety. Between 1911 and 1925 the Metropolitan Life Insurance Company spent over $20 million for health education, early diagnosis, and nursing service among its policyholders. During those 17 years the death rate for policyholders declined more than 30%, which was fully twice the reduction that occurred in the general population. In monetary terms the $20 million spent resulted in a saving to the company and its policyholders during that period of $43 million. This is good business. While the length of life for the general public increased 5 years during the period under consideration, policyholders enjoyed an increased life expectancy of 9 years.

Even more spectacular savings become evident when the economic value of life is considered with regard to such situations. Charles Bolduan,[8] for example, pointed out that in 1935 lobar pneumonia caused the death of 2,039 males in New York City, 809 of them between the ages of 20 and 50. He computed that these 809 deaths occurring among working males represented an economic loss of about $20 million. This fact was used in requesting $500,000 to provide adequate pneumonia control work. It was estimated that the expenditure of this amount would result in a saving of $5 million.

Further examples may be found in relation to other diseases. Parran has pointed out that, whereas the $2 million of state and federal funds used in 1937 for the prevention and control of syphilis seems a sizable sum, it is paltry in comparison with the $10 million spent annually for the care of the syphilitic blind and the $32 million spent for the care of the syphilitic insane.

Vaughan, in 1936, while Commissioner of Health of the city of Detroit, requested from the city council an additional $200,000 per year for each of 5 years for early tuberculosis case finding and hospitalization. He was able to demonstrate successfully that the total extra appropriation of $1 million for this purpose would repay itself several times over by the end of that period. In 1930 only 15% of the new cases of tuberculosis were found while still in the minimal stage, 30% were moderately advanced, and 55% were far advanced. By 1943, as a result of the accelerated program for case finding and hospitalization, the figures for minimal and far-advanced cases were literally reversed so that 53% of newly diagnosed cases were in the minimal stage and only 17% had progressed to the far-advanced stage. When it is considered that the average hospital stay for minimal cases in Detroit was 9 months in contrast to 2 years or more for the far-advanced cases, the enormous saving to the taxpayers in terms of hospital costs alone becomes evident. In fact, at the time the program began it was calculated that the added annual expenditure of $200,000 saved about $1.4 million each year. The critical importance of careful health planning and appropriations to social and economic development has been emphasized by many, especially in relation to the developing areas of the world,[9-12] as well as in our own society. Several examples have also been presented in the chapters "World Health Problems" and "Planning and Evaluation." Most who address themselves to this question, however, stress the importance of health improvement measures in such situations being accompanied by advances in as broad as possible social and economic fronts in order to avoid a rapid increase in dependent people.

To further illustrate the magnitude of the savings that have been effected by pub-

Table 7-4. Estimated saving in lives during 1960 as a result of public health measures taken against certain diseases, United States*

Causes of death	Death rates†		Deaths		Lives saved
	1900	*1960*	*Theoretical*	*Observed*	
All causes	1,719.1	954.7	3,082,745	1,711,982	1,370,763
Infant mortality	99.9‡	25.7	425,359	108,800	316,559
Maternal mortality	6.1‡	3.2	25,973	1,360	24,613
Typhoid and paratyphoid	31.3	0.0	56,128	29	56,099
Dysentery	12.0	0.1	21,519	153	21,366
Diarrhea and enteritis	139.9	4.4	250,873	8,002	242,871
Smallpox	0.3	0.0	538	0	538
Measles	13.3	0.2	23,850	380	23,470
Diphtheria	40.3	0.0	72,267	69	72,198
Whooping cough	12.2	0.1	21,877	118	21,759
Scarlet fever and streptococcal sore throat	9.6	0.1	17,215	108	17,107
Erysipelas	5.4	0.0	9,683	22	9,661
Tuberculosis	194.4	6.1	348,604	10,866	337,738
Syphilis and its sequelae	17.7‡	1.6	31,740	2,945	28,795
Malaria	6.2	0.0	11,118	4	11,114

*Population 1960 = 179,323,175.
†Per 100,000 population, except infant and maternal mortality which are per 1,000 live births.
‡1915 rates.

lic health activities, Table 7-4 presents data on a number of causes of death, the major share of the reduction of which may justly be attributed to organized public health programs. For each cause there has been computed the number of deaths that would be expected to have occurred in 1960 if the rates of 1900 had been maintained. It is seen that by the reduction of these causes of death alone 1.33 million lives have been saved each year. Obviously these lives have some value. Even if the investment made in each of them were to be considered as merely $1,000, the total value saved to the nation would amount to more than $1 billion each year.

POTENTIAL SAVINGS BY PUBLIC HEALTH EXPENDITURES

In a sense, the previous discussion is an accounting of past successes. Consider in addition the potential savings in lives and money that could be made at the present time and in the future if all current knowledge were completely used. When this reasoning is applied to the total current picture of sickness and death in the United States, the results arrived at are staggering.

Slee,[13] in a study of public health problems of the aging population, has made a most interesting analysis along these lines. He considered the problem of the thousands of deaths that occur every year in the United States which could be prevented if the present body of existing knowledge were effectively applied. For each cause of death he estimated the potential percentage of reduction attainable at the present time, stating for each the major factors that would contribute to the reduction (Table 7-5). His figures have been modified to bring them up to date. Each of the theoretical percentage reductions was then applied to the number of deaths that were attributed during 1960 to each particular cause of death (Table 7-6). The difference between the resulting figures and the number of deaths that actually occurred indicates a total potential saving at the present time of over 500,000 lives per year. This saving, if it had been effected, would have reduced the crude death rate in the United States in 1960 by 30%, from 9.5 to 6.6 per 1,000 population. That this is not a fantastic concept is given testimony by the fact that some American communities and

Table 7-5. Postulated percentage reductions in deaths, by cause, if all available knowledge were used*

Cause of death	Reduction (%)	Suggested action
Typhoid and paratyphoid	100	Environmental measures Immunization Epidemiologic control
Meningococcal infections	100	Control of epidemics Adequate and early chemotherapy Antibiotics
Streptococcal infections	100	Chemotherapy Antibiotics Antitoxin
Whooping cough	100	Early and thorough immunization Hyperimmune serum, chemotherapy, and antibiotics for secondary infections
Diphtheria	100	Early immunization and adequate antitoxin
Tuberculosis—all forms	100	Intensive early case finding Hospitalization and treatment Adequate diet and housing
Dysenteries	100	Environmental control Chemotherapy
Malaria	100	Environmental control Chemotherapy
Syphilis	100	Intensive early case finding Treatment Epidemiologic control
Measles	100	Immunization Chemotherapy Antibiotics
Poliomyelitis	100	Immunization
Neoplasms	50	Early cancer detection and treatment centers Best possible physician and surgeon Chemotherapy Radiation therapy Surgery Circumcision Elimination of smoking

*Where chemotherapy and/or antibiotics have been listed as the explanations for the reductions in deaths, objection on the basis of the development of drug-resistant organisms will no doubt be raised. Gains possible today might be much less in a few years. It is felt that research will be able to remain one or two drugs, at least, ahead of the organisms.

With the one exception (all other causes) no variation of effectiveness of therapy and other control measures with age of the individual has been postulated. Since any scheme of correction would probably have been as liable to criticism as no correction, the latter course was followed.

Continued.

Table 7-5. Postulated percentage reductions in deaths, by cause, if all available knowledge were used—cont'd

Cause of death	Reduction (%)	Suggested action
Rheumatic fever	95	Best possible physician Prophylactic antibiotics
Diabetes mellitus	60	Best possible physician Intensive early case finding Diet Insulin Applied genetics
Diseases of thyroid gland	100	Best possible physician Newer drugs Surgery Iodization of all salt
Nutritional diseases	100	Adequate diet Diagnosis and treatment
Alcoholism and addictions	25	Psychiatry Nutritional therapy Sociology Education
Intracranial vascular lesions	10	Best possible physician Antihypertensive drugs and diet Anticoagulants Avoidance of infections Antibiotics
Diseases of the heart	10	Best possible physician Surgery
Pneumonia, broncho-	75	Chemotherapy Antibiotics
Pneumonia, lobar	90	Chemotherapy Antibiotics
Pneumonia, unspecified	75	Chemotherapy Antibiotics
Influenza	85	Immunization Chemotherapy and antibiotics for complications
Peptic ulcer—stomach and duodenum	50	Psychiatry Best possible physician
Diarrhea, enteritis, etc.	95	Environmental controls Chemotherapy Antibiotics

Table 7-5. Postulated percentage reductions in deaths, by cause, if all available knowledge were used—cont'd

Cause of death	Reduction (%)	Suggested action
Appendicitis	100	Surgery Chemotherapy Antibiotics
Hernia, intestinal obstruction	95	Best possible physician and surgeon
Cirrhosis of the liver	25	Newer nutritional knowledge
Biliary calculi	25	Best possible physician and surgeon
Nephritis and nephrosis	25	Chemotherapy Antibiotics Best possible physician
Diseases of the prostate	50	Best possible physician and surgeon
Complications of pregnancy	87	Complete elimination of deaths from toxemia and sepsis, and reduction of deaths from hemorrhage by 50%
Congenital malformations	10	Diet during pregnancy Avoidance of viral infections during pregnancy Surgery (as in recent heart and blood vessel operations)
Premature births	70	Adequate prenatal care and diet
Suicide	50	Psychiatry Sociology
Homicide	50	Psychiatry Sociology
Accidents—motor vehicle	50	Education Psychiatry Engineering Traffic planning and control Safety measures
Accidents—other	50	Education Psychiatry Safety measures Engineering
All other causes	50	Better medical care (except for under 1 year, where deaths from congenital debility, birth injury, and others peculiar to the first year of life could be reduced by 75%), adequate prenatal care and diet, and adequate care during first year of life

Table 7-6. Theoretical savings of lives, United States, 1960, had all available knowledge been effectively applied

Cause of death	Total deaths 1960	Theoretical reduction (%)	Theoretical deaths	Theoretical saving
Typhoid and paratyphoid	29	100		29
Meningococcal infections	644	100		644
Streptococcal infections	2,050	100		2,050
Whooping cough	118	100		118
Diphtheria	69	100		69
Tuberculosis—all forms	10,866	100		10,866
Dysenteries	355	100		355
Malaria	4	100		4
Syphilis	2,945	100		2,945
Measles	380	100		380
Poliomyelitis	378	100		378
Neoplasms	272,520	50	136,260	136,260
Rheumatic fever	734	95	37	697
Diabetes mellitus	29,971	60	11,948	17,923
Diseases of thyroid gland	958	100		958
Avitaminoses	3,857	100		3,857
Alcoholism and addictions	2,425	25	1,819	606
Intracranial vascular lesions	193,588	10	174,229	19,359
Diseases of the heart	660,978	10	594,880	66,098
Pneumonia, broncho-	34,405	75	8,601	25,804
Pneumonia, lobar	10,032	90	1,003	9,029
Pneumonia, other and unspecified	9,163	75	2,291	6,872
Peptic ulcer—stomach and duodenum	11,682	50	5,841	5,841
Diarrhea, enteritis, etc.	8,002	95	400	7,602
Appendicitis	1,871	100		1,871
Hernia, intestinal obstruction	9,081	95	454	8,627
Cirrhosis of the liver	20,296	25	15,222	5,074
Biliary calculi, etc.	5,757	25	4,318	1,439
Nephritis and nephrosis	13,684	25	10,263	3,421
Diseases of the prostate	8,774	50	2,939	2,438
Deliveries and complications of pregnancy	1,579	87	205	1,374
Congenital malformations	21,860	10	19,674	2,186
Premature births	19,460	70	5,838	13,622
Suicide	19,031	50	9,516	9,515
Homicide	8,446	50	4,223	4,223
Accidents—motor vehicle	38,137	50	19,069	19,068
Accidents—other	53,847	50	26,924	26,923
All other causes	237,903	50	118,952	118,951
Totals	1,715,879	31.4	1,174,906	537,476
Population 1960	179,323,175		179,323,175	
Death rate (per 1,000 population)	9.5		6.6	
Percentage reduction of death rate (actual to theoretical)			30.5	

several nations have actually reduced their rates close to that level. If the lives that could theoretically be saved are distributed appropriately by age groups, it is seen that benefits are possible at every point in the life-span. The greatest savings, however, would occur in the adolescent and young adult age groups, where a death involves the greatest possible economic loss. If this analysis were to be pursued further by applying estimated monetary values to each of the 500,000 deaths potentially preventable, the magnitude of the economic loss entailed would indeed appear to be stupendous. Thus, if again each life saved was considered to represent an investment of merely $2,000, the total value the nation could save annually would be more than $1 billion.

It often seems to be fashionable in the United States to complain of high taxes and governmental costs. On the other hand, the average American does tend to be a rather practical individual. When it is demonstrated to him that fundamentally the public health program is a matter of common sense and of true economy, he will readily subscribe in most instances to the necessary financial support. To an ever increasing extent the American public is realizing that attempted frugality in public health matters is penny-wise and pound-foolish.

REFERENCES

1. Fuchs, V. R.: The contribution of health services to the American economy, Milbank Mem. Fund Quart. 44:65, Oct. 1966.
2. Hanlon, J. J.: Can accounting sell health? In Economic benefits from public health services, Washington, 1964, Public Health Service Pub. No. 1178.
3. Linnenberg, C. C.: How shall we measure economic benefits from public health services? In Economic benefits from public health services, Washington, 1964, Public Health Service Pub. No. 1178.
4. Petty, Sir W.: Political arithmetic or a discourse concerning the extent and value of lands, people, buildings, etc., ed. 3, London, 1699, Robert Clavel.
5. Dublin, L. I., and Lotka, A. J.: Length of life: a study of the life table, New York, 1936, The Ronald Press Co.
6. Dublin, L. I., Lotka, A. J., and Spiegelman, M.: The money value of a man, ed. 2, New York, 1946, The Ronald Press Co.
7. Weisbrod, B. A.: Economics of public health, Philadelphia, 1961, University of Pennsylvania Press.
8. Bolduan, C. F., and Bolduan, N. W.: Public health and hygiene: a student's manual, ed. 3, Philadelphia, 1941, W. B. Saunders Co.
9. Horwitz, A.: Health—a basic component of economic development, Washington, 1961, Pan American Health Organization Misc. Pub. No. 66.
10. Fein, R.: Health programs and economic development. In The economics of health and medical care, Ann Arbor, 1964, University of Michigan Press.
11. Perlman, M.: Some economic aspects of public health programs in underdeveloped areas. In The economics of health and medical care, Ann Arbor, 1964, University of Michigan Press.
12. Ruderman, A. P.: The epidemiologist's place in planning for economic development, Public Health Rep. 81:615, July 1966.
13. Slee, V. N.: Public health and old people (unpublished study), School of Public Health, University of Michigan, June 1947.

Chapter 8

Government and public health

INTRODUCTION

Public health work, by definition, determines that it be carried on mainly under governmental auspices. The particular political system that exists determines the role of government in relation to health. Public health programs are financed and the broad organizational patterns for implementation of these programs are outlined according to basic policy decisions. In general a governmental system in a democratic society performs two distinct functions. The first is political function. The governmental system must provide a forum for debate on issues that exist in a given area and an appropriate instrumentality for their solution. It must provide a political structure that allows for the development of a concept of the good life to be formulated. It must also provide leadership and citizenship if self-government is to continue to exist. The definition of the role of government in relation to health is therefore an important part of the political function of government. The second general category is the service and regulatory function of a governmental system. Services necessary to a complex society which cannot be provided by individuals or private enterprise must be provided by government. Rules and regulations concerning individual behavior in relation to personal, group, and environmental hygiene must be formulated and enforced by government.[1]

Individuals involved in public health work are knowledgeable about the service function of government for this is their field of expertise. They have had, however, little opportunity in their formal educational experience in the past to gain an understanding of the political function of government. Because the political and service functions of government cannot be separated, it is imperative that those who work in public health administration possess an understanding of the political function of government and its relationship to the service function. This is the major theme of this chapter.

POLITICAL SYSTEM

Political science until recent years was for the most part a description of formal organizational structures such as legislatures or political parties along with normative political theory. In recent years political scientists have conceptualized politics as a system. Easton[2] defines the political system as "constituted by the multiplicity of social interactions involved in the policy making process oriented toward the authoritative allocation of values for society." Political scientists, therefore, have attempted to describe the system in terms of interactions and goals. Political activity is viewed as the interaction among governmental institutions and groups.[2] Governmental institutions are the vehicles through which the political process operates and therefore constitute one of the variables that must be studied in order to gain an understanding of the political process. The basic outline of governmental structure in the United States is contained in the Constitution. It is a federal system which is defined as "one where the governmental powers are divided by terms of a written constitution between a general government and the governments of territorial subdivisions, each government supreme within a sphere marked out in the Constitution."[3]

In this case the states are territorial units. In this country there has been a traditional fear of the powers of the general or central unit of government. This may be understood in the light of historical background. Some of the states actually spent part of their existence as distinct entities. For example, the present state of Vermont was an independent nation between 1777 and 1791. The eastern part of the present state of Tennessee was a separate country, Franklin, between 1784 and 1789. Texas was an independent republic from 1836 to 1845 and consequently had its own government that exchanged diplomats with the government of the United States. Hawaii, prior to becoming a territory of the United States in 1900 and subsequently a state in 1959, also existed as an independent nation.

It is often overlooked that not until the American Revolution was almost won did the original 13 colonies begin to think seriously about union; during the formative period numerous influential people insisted that each colony should be a distinct and separate nation similar to the situation on the European continent. In fact, several colonies had plans for importing members of European royal families in order to form the nucleus of American royal ruling classes. The Continental Congress ultimately solved the problem by settling upon the idea of a union of states. The decision, incidentally, was made by a narrow margin of votes.

The politically dominant state

In so joining themselves into a union the colonies, which were now called states, by no means surrendered their individual rights and prerogatives of which they were already intensely jealous and proud. Instead they took the attitude that most governmental problems would continue to be met and solved best on a separate and independent basis, with only a relatively few matters of common interest and concern

requiring reference to the joint overall federal government established by their union.

They recognized, for example, that "in union there is strength," that they had mutual interests in matters of defense against aggression, and that therefore a single national army and navy should be established and made up of men from all the states. Each state, however, organized and still maintained its own militia. The expediency of a single agency to deal with matters of international diplomacy was similarly realized, and a federal department of State was organized. In order to finance these activities of common concern a national treasury and taxing system were instituted. Subsequently as additional common problems developed or were recognized, appropriate federal agencies were established.

From the beginning the states were explicit with regard to functions and authorities delegated to the federal government, specifying them, fortunately, in relatively broad terms in the federal Constitution and subsequent amendments. All other activities and powers not so specified were retained by the states. This influenced the development of public health in America to a considerable degree since no specific mention is made of public health in the Constitution or its amendments. Accordingly, until recently the federal government has had no explicit authority to establish a federal health department. Furthermore, it was in no way mandatory that the individual states establish state public health agencies unless they wished of their own accord to do so. However, a time was reached when each state recognized the need.

Theoretically the states are fundamental units of government from which the federal and local governments derive. Article X of the Constitution of the United States provides that "The powers not delegated to the United States by the Constitution, nor prohibited by it to the States, are reserved to the States respectively, or to the people." One of the residual powers retained by the states is what is commonly called the police power. The police power may be defined in general terms as the power to protect and promote the health, safety, and welfare of the state and its people.[3] This concept is discussed in some detail in the following chapter, which deals with law and public health.

CHANGING CONCEPTS OF FEDERALISM

Operationally federalism has not remained static. The interpretation of the responsibilities of state and national government under the Constitution has changed considerably throughout our history. Many people today are accustomed to regarding the federal government as the ultimate source of power and money. While they do so with increasing justification, this was by no means always the case. The original concept of state supremacy has been briefly discussed. Suffice to say that in spite of recent trends the principle is not yet dead and it is doubtful that its complete demise is inevitable. For a considerable period of our history the federal government was a somewhat distant or mythical creature to the average citizen. This early relationship has been vividly described by Brogan[4] in the following way:

> It should be remembered that it was quite easy for the settler in the Middle West to have no dealings at all with the government of the United States. He paid no direct taxes; he very often wrote no letters and received none, for the good reason that he and his friends could not write. Yet the only ubiquitous federal officials and federal service were the Postmasters and the Post Office. There were no soldiers except in the Indian country; there were federal courts doing comparatively little business. True, the new union had built the National Road, down which creaked the Conestoga wagons with their cargo of immigrants' chattels. It fought the Indians from time to time and it had at its disposal vast areas of public lands to be sold on easy terms and finally given away to settlers. But no government that had any claim to be a government at all has had less direct power over the people it ruled. Politics was bound, in these conditions, to be rhetorical, moralizing, emotionally diverting, either a form of sport or a form of religion. The political barbecue, the joint debates between great political leaders were secular equivalents of the camp meeting and the hell-fire sermon.

Even the inhabitants of the older seaboard states shared this relationship. As Brogan continues:

> Few things, on consideration, prove less surprising than the evaporation of federal authority over the South once secession was adopted. Almost the only federal institution that meant anything to the common man was the Post Office—and by a statesmanlike turning of the blind eye, the new Southern Confederacy continued to allow the federal government to deliver the mail even after the seceding states had formally broken with the Union.

As time passed, with increasing urbanization, mechanization, travel, industrialization, and interstate and international problems, the national government came more and more into focus in the citizens' eyes. It appears that at the same time there began to develop a blurring of the image of local and particularly of state government. There was a period when local governments were in a very real sense self-sufficient, but gradually, as the demands made upon them increased, they looked more frequently to the state governments for assistance. Up to a point these appeals for help were within the financial ability of the states, but gradually they too became inadequate to meet many of the newer, more complex, and more expensive problems. White[5] discusses this accordingly:

> The states as instruments of progress are definitely losing ground. Their leadership, with rare exceptions, is mediocre; their administrative organization, again with occasional exception, is inadequate. . . . It seems possible indeed that the future structure of the American administrative system will rest primarily on the national government and the cities, at least so far as the urban population (now approaching 60 per cent) is concerned.

White points out that as early as 1918, Charles E. Merriman made the following suggestion:

> Those interested in preserving the balance of powers between the national and local governments might find the urban community a more effective counter weight . . . than the feebly struggling states . . . A city would not be obliged to climb far to go beyond a state. Already there are seventeen cities of a population over 500,000; nine states with less population than that, and if economic resources and cultural prestige are added to numbers, the contrast is more striking.

In this regard there are (in 1968) 29 cities with populations greater than 500,000, and a significant number of them contain and serve more people than do many of the states.

Originally the powers of the federal government were limited quite strictly to affairs of interstate and international concern. So intense was the desire to restrict the scope of these powers that they were referred to explicitly in the Constitution and its subsequent amendments. Innumerable aspects of our social, scientific, industrial, and political development have led in a direction that makes an increasing degree of centralization necessary if not also desirable for survival. To allow for this change and to still maintain the basic principles of our form of government presents a difficult problem indeed.

In order to accomplish both purposes federal agencies in recent years, with the tacit assent of the states, have increasingly resorted to indirect but constitutionally permissible techniques that have resulted in increased centralization of power in state governments themselves and more significantly in federal agencies. This movement received great acceleration during the 1930's, when the widespread economic depression dealt a devastating blow to local and, to a considerable extent, state finances, rendering them incapable of meeting the demands placed upon them. A procession of local governments, having fruitlessly appealed to their state capitals for assistance, turned to Washington as the only source of relief. In light of the underlying social and economic causes, these trends toward centralization are certain to continue and increase.

There are many methods short of total assumption of power and function that may be resorted to in order to achieve a practical measure of centralization. Perhaps the simplest is the offering of advice and information by a federal agency to the states or by the states to the local governments. This is so common in the field of public health as to have become one of the prime activities of state and federal health agencies. It takes but a short step to move from the transmission of printed advice and information to occasional visits of state and federal consultants, followed by the loaning of personnel to serve as resident consultants. This occurs especially in the face of local shortages in personnel. Increasingly, officers of federal agencies originally intended as consultants are assigned on a semipermanent basis to serve as directors of divisions of a state health department. Field technical units, developed by state health departments for the purpose of assisting the local units, in many instances assume the position of supervising and even determining the programs of local health departments. Thus we see activities designed for the purpose of rendering advice and information develop into programs of cooperative or outright centralized administration. A variation is a program of inspection and advice, often without authority, to bring about compliance with recommendations made. The inspecting and advising officials, for example, may merely report their findings to the central authorities, who may then promote additional legislation that often gives them increased supervisory powers. This has occurred, for example, in matters of hospital construction and inspection of sanitary installations.

On the surface the requirement of periodic fiscal and service reports may appear innocuous, and it is certainly justifiable in order to obtain and share information concerning the general welfare. However, even this may have an indirect centralizing influence of considerable impact. Theoretically a state or local health department has the right to organize its records and reports any way it sees fit to serve its purposes. However, after the right to require certain reports is obtained, the next step is to standardize them. Beyond this, in more than one instance the requiring of a certain type of report has resulted in an actual change in the local program itself, the local personnel following the path of least resistance, especially if financial grants are involved. This has occurred in varying degrees as a result of requirements for birth and death records, reports of communicable disease, and the standardized fiscal reports of health departments to federal health agencies. An accelerating technique that may be employed is to give the local official a nominal appointment as the local representative of state or federal agency. Thus we find many local health officers with appointments as collaborating epidemiologists of the Public Health Service.

In some areas local activities are subject to direct supervision and review by the higher government. For example, local assessments often must be reviewed and approved by a state board of equalization or by state tax commissioners. Prior permission may be required and is especially effective when the higher level of government participates in financing. It is rapidly becoming accepted practice to require that plans for city, county, and state hospitals be approved by state boards of health and national health agencies before allowing contracts to be consummated.

Of a similar nature are approval requirements for the appointment and removal of local officers. While in most states it is theoretically the prerogative of local governments to select their own health officer, in practice this is often not followed for various reasons discussed elsewhere. Not only is approval by the state health officer usually required but often selection is limited to lists prepared by the state health department. In some states local health officers are appointed and removed directly by the state board of health. In Ohio, employees of health districts are appointed from state civil service lists and, if no eligible individuals are available, from the register of local commissions. The requirement of prior permission is sometimes rendered unnecessary by the determination of standards by a state or federal agency.

The extent to which the average county health officer is affected by these influences may be pictured somewhat as follows: In the first instance he may be recruited by and trained under the auspices of the state health department, using federal funds. His appointment, if not made directly by the state health officer, will probably require his approval. Monthly reports of his activities and those of his staff will have to be made to the state health department on standard forms and a record of all work kept in a form book prescribed by the latter agency. By virtue of his probable designation as registrar he will have to report

births and deaths to the state health department on forms, this time prescribed by the National Center for Vital Statistics. Since in most instances he is appointed a collaborating epidemiologist, it becomes necessary to send weekly reports of outbreaks of communicable diseases to the Public Health Service as well as to the state health department. His maternal and child health program may necessitate operation, inspection, and approval of clinics and hospitalization facilities, using standards developed and required by the Children's Bureau, which will also ask for reports on standard forms. Arrangement for the use of x-ray equipment and for hospitalization of persons with tuberculosis will in most instances be made by him with the state agency. Finally, he will probably find it convenient if not necessary to obtain education materials, biologics, and even office forms and supplies through the state health department.

While all this may appear on the surface to result in an effective emasculation of the position of the local health officer, to be fair and practical it should be pointed out that all of these various relationships actually represent effective resources to which he may turn for assistance in order to develop and conduct a much more effective and satisfying program than he otherwise could. Considering the limited resources on a local level, one might with justification answer those who disclaim any concurrent limitation of local autonomy with the saw, "You can't have your cake and eat it too."

Details of contracts and design of hospitals and health centers have been specified as conditions for approval of plans by state and federal agencies in order to obtain federal funds. More and more types of licenses are being placed within the jurisdiction of state health departments and through them the Public Health Service and the Children's Bureau. The provision of the Emergency Maternity and Infant Care Program administered by the Children's Bureau through the state health departments during World War II and the many programs authorized by recent legislation such as the Social Security Amendments of 1965 (Medicare, Medicaid, Comprehensive Child Health Services, etc.) present many examples of the centralizing influence of the right to determine standards. The central agency may be vested with the right to issue general regulations that are binding on the locality or orders that result in a single centralized authority. Both measures are widely resorted to in public health work. Here the initiative passes from the local to the central agency. While common within states, this type of control is rare in federal-state relationships. The financial aspects of the grant-in-aid program will be discussed later in this chapter.

The federal government cannot dictate to the states the manner in which they should organize their governmental structure, establish their policies, or conduct their programs. However, actual dictation of these matters is not necessary in order for federal agencies to play a part in the improvement and expansion of public health and other services throughout the nation. The significance of holding the purse strings is well understood by all. "He who pays the piper calls the tune."

Sums of money transferred may be granted either conditionally or unconditionally; federal grants are usually of the former type, state grants more often of the latter. Because of this, federal grants are more apt to act as catalyzers than are state grants. In the ideal situation the local taxpayers would constantly exert whatever control might be necessary for the ensurance of the proper use of funds and it would be unnecessary to attach conditions to grants. When revenue is raised locally, this is more apt to occur than when funds come unfettered from without. By inserting limitations in the form of conditions to grants, therefore, the higher unit of government is in effect substituting for the controls that should ordinarily be exercised by the citizens themselves. There is danger, however, that conditions and standards may become too detailed or rigid to suit the diverse situations existing in a complex nation such as this. As Maxwell[6] points out:

Regional heterogeneity is of the essence of federalism, and . . . would seem to indicate that federal grants should be conditioned and closely policed. In practical fact, however, this would be an impairment of state sovereignty. Moreover, any detailed and uniform set of conditions would be unsuited to the diversity of regional and state needs. In a federalism, variation in standards of many governmental functions is common, and therefore the federal government is likely to get into difficulties if it attempts to prescribe common standards in grant programs . . . to surround federal grants with numerous conditions is to assume a homogeneity in state governmental needs which does not exist; to prescribe uniformity where there are deepseated reasons for diversity is an error. Here, then, is a dilemma of federalism.

Usually, conditional federal grants-in-aid require adherence to certain steps. First, the state must formally accept the terms of the grant, sometimes by means of legislation. Preparation for use of the grant must next be made by preparing and submitting sepcific plans and by establishing whatever organizations or agencies are indicated for their fulfillment. Plans are approved centrally by a national administrative agency. Usually, but not always, federal grants must be matched by the state or local government. The program or project itself is carried out by state or local agencies but is subject to central as well as local inspection and audit. Often, payment is made to the state only on satisfactory completion of the project or an agreed-upon part of it. Sometimes partial payment is made in advance.

A number of means of central influence and control are evident from the steps just outlined. The federal agency may refuse to approve plans or to cooperate financially in a state program because of unsatisfactory state organization or procedure. Payments may be withheld if conditions of agreement are not observed. Furthermore, the state has little or no recourse beyond the federal agency administering the grant. The application of central influences such as these has occurred frequently in the field of public health. In order to benefit from grants-in-aid administered by both the Children's Bureau and the Public Health Service the states have found it necessary to establish or remodel their personnel standards and merit systems to the satisfaction of these federal agencies. Record systems, auditing procedures, clinic and hospital construction and maintenance standards, and many other factors have been similarly affected.

The tendency toward centralization has been most evident in the fields of highway construction, education, and social security. It is interesting to study the similarities in the patterns followed in these three areas of public administration. Of particular interest to those engaged in public health work may be a comparison of the history of federal interest in public roads and in maternal and child welfare. The national government first became concerned with highways in 1893, when it established the Office of Road Inquiry, later the Bureau of Public Roads. The original bill establishing this agency included the following statement: ". . . it is not the province of this department to seek to control or influence said action [in building highways] except in so far as advice and wise suggestions shall contribute toward it. . . . The department is to furnish information, not to direct and formulate any system of organization, however efficient or desirable it may be." From the date of its establishment until 1912 the Bureau of Public Roads restricted itself to experimentation, advice to state and local highway officials, dissemination of information, and construction of demonstration roads.

In 1912 an act was passed authorizing construction of post roads, followed in 1916 by a more potent Federal Highway Act that set up a system of grants to the states to assist them in meeting the increased demand for good roads and the increased cost of building better types of roads. Where originally the local county governments had the chief responsibility for the construction and maintenance of highways, this major responsibility and its accompanying authority passed first to the state and then to the federal government. States now receive a large proportion of their highway funds through federal grants-in-aid, and the Bureau of Public Roads, the federal administering agent, establishes the standards, approves plans, audits the accounts, and inspects the completed work. The effectiveness of these indirect forms of control is indicated by the fact that in 1916, when the Federal Highway Act was passed, 15 states had no highway departments. By the following year every state had a recognized highway department acceptable to the Bureau of Public Roads.

Compare with this the act of 1912 which established the Children's Bureau, directing it to investigate and report ". . . upon all matters pertaining to the welfare of children and child life, among all classes of people . . ." It was designated as a clearing house for information on child health and was authorized to carry on research and also field studies. During the first 7 years of its existence the Children's Bureau adhered strictly to these specified functions. In 1921, with the passage of the Sheppard-Towner Act, the Bureau was authorized to participate in the promotion of maternity and infancy programs throughout the nation by means of federal grants to the states. Here the Bureau received its first major administrative responsibilities. As in the case of highways, some states anticipated the passage of the Maternity and Infancy Bill and created maternal and child health bureaus or divisions to administer the funds they would obtain if and when the bill became law. Accordingly, by the beginning of 1921 33 such state agencies had been established, and during the following 2 years 14 more were created. By 1929 maternal and child hygiene bureaus or divisions had been formed and were functioning in the territory of Hawaii and in all the states except Vermont, where the work was carried on under the immediate supervision of the state health officer.[7] In administering the act the Children's Bureau, as had the Bureau of Public Roads, set standards, approved projects, inspected work within states, and audited accounts. Although the functions involved in the Sheppard-Towner Act came to a halt in 1929, they were essentially reestablished in an expanded degree by the provision of Title V of the Social Security Act of 1935 and by subsequent legislation.

Further comparison is possible by considering the passage in 1942 of the Emergency Maternity and Infant Care Program for wives and children of men in the Armed

Forces. This program, administered by the Children's Bureau through the state health agencies, made possible and paid for personal medical care of patients. Although that program was temporary, the principles under discussion were subsequently applied to other program responsibilities of the Children's Bureau.

Concerning roads, White[5] has made the following statement:

Related expenditures on highways were thrown out of balance in 1933 and the latter years of the depression as a result of the huge emergency expenditures for public works and the resulting grants and loans to the states. From the fiscal point of view the national government has emerged in the crisis as the senior partner in the firm.

Perhaps this statement was prophetic with regard to the ultimate effect of the grant-in-aid programs on the functional relationship between the local, state, and federal governments. A large part of the considerable opposition to the maternity and infancy program, some of the other grant-in-aid programs, and the various medical care bills has been on this basis.

The foregoing may make those who plan and administer grants-in-aid appear as power thirsty annelids increasingly draining off the lifeblood of local self-initiative and independence. Somewhat the same viewpoint is expressed by Mustard.[8]

Directly, through broad interpretations of the Federal Constitution, and by new laws, or indirectly through grants-in-aid, parity payments, benefits, and rewards, the Federal Government is assuming prerogatives and accepting obligations, particularly in the field of social security, that a quarter-century ago were regarded as lying exclusively within the jurisdiction of the states. Pertinent in this connection is the fact that public health activities are more and more being considered as an integral part of the developing social security program and are receiving increasing federal attention. Thus the Federal Government is at present a potent influence in public health. Perhaps it is more virile than any other area of government for . . . many state governments are static in this field, and leadership has focused in the United States Public Health Service. The policy of federal grants-in-aid for state and local health work is becoming increasingly popular, and apparently will be continued in spite of what the opponents of this principle believe it implies sociologically and in terms of state and local autonomy.

However, in fairness to the administering agencies two considerations should be pointed out. First, it is doubtful that the promotion of bills to provide subsidies for highways, education, and public health programs represented at any stage determined premeditated attempts to transfer power to a central agency. When all aspects of the questions involved are reviewed, it would appear that the acts were passed and the programs developed to meet public demands and needs that could not possibly be fulfilled by the state government, much less by the local government. In other words, they evolved out of social necessity. Maxwell[6] explains this is the following terms:

Local governments have an administrative ability for performance of functions which is greatly in excess of their administrative ability for the collection of revenues. The case of the national government is the other way around: it has an ability to make efficient collection of taxes which is greater than its ability to handle expenditure. . . . It will not be necessary to suppose that all governmental functions are handled by the national government. Local government will have tasks to perform, not because of any defect in the national power, but for the sake of administrative efficiency.

The second consideration is that it must be conceded that these programs have resulted in a considerable improvement of service and facilities for all the people. Speaking of highways, for example, White[5] comments:

It is no exaggeration to state that in the . . . years since the first federal highway act a national highway system has been established at the direction of Congress by the Bureau of Public Roads, and that the standards of construction and maintenance by the states, and their subdivisions have been greatly improved as a direct result of national intervention through the grants-in-aid device. It is impossible to conceive that the transportation needs of the present could be met without coordination, guidance and supervision furnished by the national administration and the support of national funds.

Certainly no one would deny that the same conclusions could be drawn with reference to the extensive developments in public health over the past several decades.

An interpretation of grants-in-aid quite different from that ordinarily made was presented in a study of state aid in New York by Pond,[9] who stated:

American government involves a system of checks and balances unique among the societies of the world. A persistent effort to retain the maximum independence to the individual and preserve to him the minimum of interference on the part of government is clearly discernible. Every state has two opposite evils to avoid, on the one hand over-centralization and on the other, local autonomy run riot. It is often taken for granted that efficiency can be secured by excessive control over localities which largely eliminates the citizen's participation in local affairs. On the other hand, it is quite as frequently believed that local autonomy is something sacrosanct, even when it results in much greater evils than those arising from centralization. Many competent observers believe that England stands alone in achieving both efficiency and a large measure of local self-government. This has undoubtedly been the result of grants-in-aid. And this is a political mechanism which may fit in perfectly with our own system of checks and balances.

A more complete method of centralization is the partial or total assumption of function. In some states the state health department has direct control of local water and sewage facilities. The department of agriculture in some states has complete responsibility for food inspection. In one state the department of conservation has authority over hotels, resort areas, taverns, and other similar places, including their sanitation. Not infrequently clinics and even complete programs dealing with tuberculosis and venereal and other diseases are maintained and operated directly by the state health department.

A key factor in intergovernmental relations and especially the trend toward dominance by the federal government is the matter of fiscal resources available to or controlled by the respective levels. According to Snider,[3] "The increasing affluence of the national government in matters of policy cannot be seriously questioned. Furthermore, as to its major functions, the national government is free to set up its own complete administration. Its regulation can be made to override states. By its control of the field of taxation and to satisfy its own tremendous needs, it might force the states into progressive diminution of their own revenues and a reduction of their own activities."

Despite the foregoing qualifications and limitations the states today are performing more functions than in the past and are increasing expenditures for domestic programs at a rate actually greater than that of the federal government. Today the United States is essentially an urban society with a population of more than 200 million, 64% of which reside in the 212 Standard Metropolitan Statistical Areas as constituted in 1960. The process of urbanization which is occurring at an increasing rate demands that the relationships among the levels of government be redefined. A strict demarcation between the responsibilities of the state and national governments is no longer possible. Today the relationships are unclear and often confused. Meanwhile creative federalism is in the process of being operationally defined. Whether changes in our federal structure can occur rapidly enough to allow the governmental system to perform its two functions adequately in the future is undoubtedly one of the most crucial problems facing American government today.

ORGANIZATIONAL STRUCTURE
State and national government
Similarity exists between the organizational structure of the state and national governments. Very early in our history a system of checks and balances was devised which became an important part of our political tradition. Three branches of both the national and state governments exist: the executive or administrative, the legislative or policy making, and the judicial. On the national and, with one exception, on the state level legislatures are divided into two houses. A recent significant decision of the Supreme Court has held that the districts of both houses of a bicameral state legislature must be apportioned only on the basis of population.[10]

Local government
All local governmental units are creations of the state. As a result the character of the various local units varies from one section of the country to another.[11] The state-local government relationship is defined as a unitary system, i.e., powers are conferred upon subdivisional governments by the legislature of the state government. In other words the state legislature creates units of government and delegates to them.

The primary units of local government are the city, village, township, county, and special purpose districts. In addition to these units many special authorities, intergovernmental compacts, and cooperative service arrangements might be considered components of today's local governmental structure. According to the most recent available data there are 91,186 units of local government in the United States. Included are 3,043 official counties, 18,000 municipalities, 17,142 townships, 34,678 school districts, and 18,323 special districts other than school districts.[11] The expenditures of state and local government in 1965 were $74.95 billion, of which approximately $11.03 billion was received from the national government.[12]

Municipal government

Municipal units are incorporated, i.e., they are granted separate legal existence by the state to perform functions other than those resulting from state policies. Cities are governed under special charters, general laws, optional laws, or home rule charters.[11] Before incorporation an area is part of the sovereign state and shares in the benefits and legal exemptions of its sovereignty. On receiving a charter the municipality becomes a corporation and as such can have a corporate name and seal; own and convey real and personal property; raise monies by taxation, borrowing, or issuing bonds; make and enforce its own local laws; and sue or be sued under its corporate name. It differs, however, from other corporations in that it has two kinds of functions. There are, on the one hand, certain public functions in which the municipality acts for the sovereign state and concerning which cannot be sued without its consent. In most states fire and police protection and public health activities are considered public functions. There are, on the other hand, many activities in which a municipality is engaged primarily or exclusively for its own interests. Examples of these are the construction and maintenance of pavements, municipally owned and operated street railways, and water, gas, and electricity plants. In most instances a municipality is considered subject to suit concerning these activities.

The distinctions between private and public functions are varied. For example, while county highways are considered public, city streets are usually considered a private function. The construction of sewers is usually considered a public function in contrast to their maintenance, which is usually considered a private function. Very often the deciding factor is whether or not the individual citizen makes a payment for maintenance such as sewers or for a commodity such as water. The trend has been to make the municipality liable in case of doubt. Even with regard to their so-called public functions, municipalities are being held liable with increasing frequency.

Since the state government creates the municipality, it may also change or abolish it. Certain legal restrictions are involved, however, the complexity and significance of which are well illustrated by the case of Mobile v. Watson.[13] The city of Mobile, Ala., was incorporated by the grant of a charter from the state of Alabama. The city subsequently became financially bankrupt. Chartered private corporations are protected by the federal Constitution against subsequent alteration by a state, but a city charter, as has been pointed out, forms a public corporation that may be abolished or changed by the state. Accordingly, the legislature of the state of Alabama rescinded the city charter of Mobile, substituted the name "Port of Mobile," and then announced that claims against the former incorporated city were not collectable since the corporation no longer existed. The United States Supreme Court considered otherwise, however, and ruled that although the city was a state-created corporation with public functions it also carried out private functions concerning which it could be sued and held liable and, although the state had a right to abolish the city corporation, such an act in no way relieved the citizens of their debts.

Considering cities as the most prominent example of incorporated areas, their governments may take one of several forms. The oldest type is what has been termed the weak mayor-council plan. In this plan the citizens elect by popular vote a mayor and usually a bicameral council of considerable size consisting of councilmen-at-large, plus a number of aldermen from each ward or district of the city. The latter, because of the customary partisanship, usually become designated as ward bosses. The mayor in such instances often holds what might be considered an honorary social office, serving essentially as the officiating representative of the community and very little else. Although it is the oldest type of municipal government in America, it is rapidly becoming outmoded because it has been fraught with inefficiency and chicanery, and more efficient plans are being substituted for it. The strong mayor plan of local government is an adaptation of the older form. Here the legislative branch is reduced to a single councilmanic chamber, usually with far fewer members, all of whom are elected at large. The mayor is still elected for a limited term but is given greater executive powers and prerogatives, including increased power of appointment of departmental heads and other officials and greater control over the budget. In most instances the council may reduce budget items proposed by the mayor but may not add or increase items.

The early years of the twentieth century saw the development of two new forms of city government which have attempted to approach the management of civic affairs on a more businesslike basis. The first of these, the commission plan, came about as a result of the devastating earthquake and flood of 1900 at Galveston, Tex. The corrupt and inefficient weak mayor-council government found itself completely incapable of coping with the emergency situation and literally collapsed. Through the efforts of prominent citizens a substitute form of government was established on the basis of the essential services and activities required by the community. Civic affairs were organized in a small number of service departments (such as public safety, public works, public health and finance) and a legal department. Under this plan a functional commissioner was elected by popular vote for each department. In lieu of a mayor and council the commis-

sioners ran the city government somewhat like the board of directors of a business corporation. Although numerous communities have adopted this form of government, experience has subsequently indicated that, while theoretically an excellent plan, it has practical disadvantages. In many instances, for example, agreement among the several commissioners has become impossible, and often competitive departmental cliques have developed, jeopardizing the effectiveness of the total government. In other instances the commissioners in charge of public finance or of the legal department have found themselves in a position to thwart or control the activities and plans of the other departments. As a result the past three decades have seen a gradual rejection of the commission plan of government.

Interestingly enough the fourth or city manager type of government also developed as an aftermath of another catastrophic flood, this time in Dayton, O., in 1913. The experience of Galveston was duplicated, and in the place of the ineffective weak mayor-council system was substituted a plan whereby only a relatively small council was elected. This council of perhaps 20 to 25 laymen had no administrative duties, technical qualifications being therefore unnecessary. Their meetings usually required little time, their chief functions being the determination of general community policies and the employment of a salaried city manager whose tenure usually depended on satisfactory service. Again this was an attempt to operate a city government like a business corporation, with the employed city manager acting in an administrative capacity similar to that of the general manager of a private corporation. In many ways his position reminds one of the German burgomaster. As with the commission plan of government, the use of this plan has been confined almost entirely to small and intermediate sized cities. The extent of its adoption, however, has continued to increase, and already some counties, particularly on the West Coast, have adopted it.

In a few instances an attempt has been made to achieve a mixed or compromise type of approach. Thus the city of Philadelphia has a strong mayor-council form of government, but a key individual in the conduct of the city's services and affairs is a managing director, selected and employed by the mayor with the approval of the council. A certain amount of two-way or even three-way conflict is inherent to such a system in most situations.

County government

The county is the one almost universal unit of American government.[14] County government has been called "the dark continent of American politics."[15] To some it is anachronistic. However, counties are more or less convenient areas of administration laid out by the states for the decentralized local performance of certain governmental functions, regarded as primarily of state concern. It is important to recognize that a significant renaissance has been underway in an increasing number of counties during recent years. This was stimulated in large measure by a grant from the Ford Foundation in 1958 to expand and revitalize the National Association of County Officials, which has since been fortunate to enjoy exceptionally able and aggressive leadership. The role of the county is described by Snider[3] as having "greater functional importance today than it had a generation ago." He predicts that further expansion of the services provided by county governments is likely to continue in the future.

The boundaries of counties originally were determined, to a considerable extent, in terms of the distance a constituent could ride on horseback or in a buggy from his home to the county seat and back again within 1 day. While at the present time it is possible to traverse several states in 1 day by automobile, these old established county boundaries are still jealously adhered to.

The entire land area of the United States is divided into counties, 3,043 of them, with spectacular variation in size and population. They vary in size from Kalawao, Hawaii, with a mere 14 square miles, to the 20,131 square miles of San Bernardino County, Calif., which is larger than the states of New Hampshire, Vermont, Massachusetts, Rhode Island, and Connecticut

combined. The average county contains about 1,000 square miles. In terms of population, at one end of the scale is Loving County, Tex., with only 226 people, and at the other extreme is Los Angeles County, bulging with over 6 million. The average county has from 10,000 to 25,000 people. Several states, e.g., Georgia, Illinois, Kentucky, Kansas, Missouri, North Carolina, and Virginia, have 100 or more active county governments, while the state of Texas possesses 254. Delaware has only three county governments, and Rhode Island has five, from which all powers have been removed. In the other New England states county government is of secondary importance. The five counties of New York City are relatively unimportant, having given way to the single city government. City and county governments are merged in Baton Rouge, Denver, Philadelphia, Boston, New Orleans, and San Francisco. This is also true in 34 smaller cities in Virginia. In addition, two legally organized metropolitan governments, Miami-Dade County and Nashville-Davidson County, are essentially reorganized county governments. In South Dakota five county areas are attached to other counties for governmental purposes. Alaska, one of the newer states, hopes to overcome some of the organizational difficulties of the older states. By specific mandate of its constitution there are no counties in Alaska at the present time.[16] Of the counties with independent functional significance, four fifths lack incorporated areas of 10,000 people or more.[17] It is substantially correct, therefore, to say that the typical county is rural and that its government deals with the government of farmers.

Certain legal differences exist between rural and municipal governments. County governments are regarded in most instances as quasi corporations. This term has little definite meaning. It indicates, however, that while the county may for some purposes have an independent existence it is primarily an agent of the state and has no private functions. All its functions are public in nature, having been delegated to it by the sovereign state. Accordingly, the rules that govern its negligence or the torts of its officials are those that apply to the state rather than to city governments or to private corporations. A county, therefore, cannot be sued in the absence of permission from the state. In recent years, however, there has developed a tendency to hold counties liable for contracts or negligence of their officials. At any time a state may extend the degree of county liability by constitution or statute.

County administration has been handicapped by its legal relationships with the state. The flexibility that generally makes it possible for a city to frame a charter and determine its form of government and policies in line with its needs has not usually existed for counties. Instead they have had to accept whatever pattern of government the state legislature allowed, often without regard for the limited financial resources of the counties. As a result larger counties often must operate through a governmental structure that has long since been outgrown, while small counties are burdened by law with a system they do not need and cannot afford. However, county home rule is now provided for in some states. This allows counties to frame, adopt, and change their own charters. County home rule as a general principle has been concerned only with allowing the county to establish its governmental structure and has not increased its ability or freedom to enter fields of activities that have generally been forbidden the county and retained by the state. Often the freedom in determining structure has also been limited since states constitutionally or legislatively have required that certain county officials be elected even in a county home rule system. At present only 16 counties have framed and adopted charters, and most of these are in California.[18]

Problems of rural areas are simpler than those of an urban area. The economic and social life is geared primarily to agriculture. Life and behavior are more uniform, with less demand for luxury items, although recent trends have been effecting much change in this regard. Improved roads, automobiles everywhere, more convenient shopping centers, and television and radio have tended to make yesterday's luxuries com-

monplace in many rural areas. Except for the Southern states, in most although not all rural situations there are no complex nationality or racial problems, and the customs and inherited attitudes of thought present less variation. This is not meant to imply that the rural population is homogeneous. During the past few decades there has occurred widespread economic depression in the 1930's, World War II in the 1940's, and conflicts in Korea and Vietnam with their concomitant industrial, social, political, and economic effects in the 1950's and 1960's. These have brought about considerable equalizing among the regions. Nevertheless, distinct and evident regional differences still exist.

With a lesser density of population, people living further apart attend for the most part to their own affairs and self-maintenance, and there is development of considerably less social friction. They have little in the nature of private local interests. Social and economic as well as governmental activities are more in the nature of fractions of larger areas of the state as a whole. For example, while city streets exist primarily for the inhabitants of the city, roads in rural areas are necessary for all travelers as well as for those residing locally. True, the difference is one of degree, but it is nevertheless so great as to have received recognition in the courts.

Beyond the problems of the individual household and farm, the county seat commands most of the attention of the rural population. To most, it represents the prime social, recreational, educational, governmental, economic, and shopping center. The last is perhaps the most significant. Galpin,[19] in his studies of life in rural Wisconsin, summarizes, "It is difficult, if not impossible, to avoid the conclusion that the trade zone about one of these agricultural civic centers forms the boundary of an actual, if not legal, community, within which the apparent entanglement of human life is resolved into a fairly unitary system of interrelatedness. The fundamental community is a composite of many expanding and contracting feature communities possessing the characteristic pulsating instability of all real life." Beyond this, except in unusual circumstances, state and national affairs are of decidedly secondary import except insofar as they affect the county itself.

The results of these differences between rural and urban areas are reflected in the form of local government. Rural governmental machinery is simpler. Fewer officials, boards, and commissions are needed to enforce the simpler local regulations, to carry on the limited administrative work, and to conduct the small number of social welfare activities. Incidentally the officials, boards, and commissions that do exist are usually subject to little or no supervision. Since counties really require for the most part state functions on a smaller scale, much of the administrative work is either performed or supervised by state officials. The interest of the state in local rural affairs differs from its interests in municipal affairs. County boundaries are laid out by the state government with its own administrative convenience in mind and without regard to the special interests, wishes, or needs of any single area or group. The powers of local rural communities likewise are delegated by the state as a parceling out of its own administrative functions and not, as in the case of an incorporated municipality, with the idea of creating an independent political entity.

The functions of the county are, therefore, colored strictly by the circumstances of its origin. In the political field it conducts elections to provide the basis for local representation in the state legislature. Its own legislative powers are practically nonexistent, except for a quite limited authority to enact certain local ordinances. In the fields of administration and service it serves as the basis for the state financial levy, assessment, and collection, administers public welfare and relief to the poor, directs many school affairs, constructs and maintains roads and bridges, provides public health service, engages in licensing, the letting of local contracts, and the making of local appropriations, and determines salaries of local officials. As will be brought out subsequently, many of these functions are grad-

ually being assumed by the state governments themselves. Reasons for this include the increase in cost of road construction and the increasing professionalization, expansion, and improvement in public health, public welfare, and public school services. In terms of judicial functions the county, through its court, probates wills and registers deeds. It presents a convenient unit of area for the local administration of the state law. As pointed out elsewhere, the local justice of the peace is actually the lowest rung on the state judicial ladder. Counties also serve as the territorial units for the establishment of courthouses, penal institutions, and for the federal post offices.

Perhaps the greatest of all deterrents to good county administration is the almost universal lack of centralized administration. In all but rare instances there is no chief executive to correspond with a mayor or a governor, and the local supply of individuals qualified to serve in the various political capacities is exceedingly limited. Thus Phillips[20] refers to it as the "no executive" form of local government. As he points out:

There are, in general, two principal types of county governmental systems, but modifications are so numerous and sometimes so extensive that generalization is dangerous. The first . . . has a small board of from three to five commissioners or supervisors, which has considerable administrative authority and limited legislative or ordinance-making power. The second . . . has a relatively large board of from fifteen to one hundred and fifty members, with authority somewhat similar to that of smaller boards. The average size of the larger boards is approximately twenty-five members.

The "no executive" type of local government is so called because the board of commissioners or supervisors must share administrative authority with a comparatively large number of separately elected officers, such as the sheriff, coroner, treasurer, clerk, attorney, assessor, surveyor, recorder of deeds, registrar of wills, superintendent of schools, and in a number of cases, auditors, and other officials. Since these officials are elected and are thus directly responsible to the electorate, and since they derive their authority from constitutional or statutory provisions, they are subject to very limited control, if any at all, by the board of commissioners or supervisors.

The voter therefore is faced with the demoralizing task of choosing from a roster of miscellaneous public officials so lengthy that he can hardly know the names of them all, much less their qualifications. The result is an authority and responsibility so diffused and uncoordinated as to make efficient administration difficult or impossible. To a very real degree an official may administer his office simply within the limitations of his own conscience, often with disastrous effects for the public as a whole. This being the case, it is not surprising that partisan politics, inefficiency, and corruption are so rampant in American county government. All too often, appreciable sums of money appropriated for public benefits have found their way into private pockets rather than into their intended purposes.

The basis of county government is a large number of individuals elected from small subdivisions of the county, variously referred to as judicial districts, magisterial districts, militia districts, townships, and hundreds. As might be expected, the majority of those elected are farmers with no legal training or background in government. When meeting together at the county seat, they constitute a body of very local governmental representatives referred to as the county board of supervisors (e.g., Michigan), the county board of commissioners (e.g., New Mexico), the county court (e.g., Tennessee), the police jury (e.g., Louisiana), and other designations. Within the limitations imposed by the state they have the authority to levy and collect taxes and to borrow money for the construction and maintenance of county roads, bridges, a courthouse, a jail, and other public property. They have the responsibility of providing relief for the poor and establishing and operating polling places and canvassing the returns. They appoint certain local officials, impanel juries, and carry out numerous other miscellaneous activities. All local executive and legislative functions are in the hands of the county boards, some of which exercise a few judicial functions as well. Except for some counties in New Jersey that have administrative supervisors, the county judge in Arkansas, the ordinary in Georgia, and a few counties with qualified county managers or county administra-

tors (notably in California), it cannot be said that the American county has a chief executive comparable in position to the mayor of a municipality.

The types of other elected county officials vary somewhat in different parts of the country, but certain ones are found in practically all instances. The county sheriff is elected to protect life, liberty, and property and to carry out the judgments of the court. He has the authority to appoint deputies as needed. The office of county coroner involves the performance of autopsies and the holding of inquests concerning persons who have died suddenly or violently, without medical attention, or under suspicious circumstances. A most important official is the county clerk, whose function it is to collect and safeguard public records (including in many instances vital statistics), to issue licenses, to open and adjourn court sessions, and to keep a record of court proceedings and the proceedings of meetings of various county boards. If any elected county official is necessary and worthy of his salt, it is the county clerk. In some places a separate recorder of deeds is elected to keep a record of land titles.

A prosecuting attorney is usually elected to prepare evidence for the juries and to prosecute accused persons on behalf of the county. The county treasurer has the responsibility for receiving, recording, and disbursing all funds expended by the county, usually regardless of their source. An assessor is necessary to list taxable persons and property and to assess them at a fair evaluation. In a few states a special tax collector is elected, and in many states a county auditor is chosen to periodically audit county funds and expenditures. In some states this latter function is carried out by the county board itself or by its financial committee. The invitation to fiscal folly involved in the election of an auditor or the execution of this important function by any group of elected officials should be obvious. School boards are usually elected either at large or by district representation separately from the rest of the county government. The superintendent of schools is generally elected by popular vote, although in some states he is appointed either by state authorities or by the county school board. In not a few instances he is the highest paid and most influential official in the county. Many miscellaneous officers may be elected because of provincial need or tradition; among these are county surveyors, fence viewers, engineers, road commissioners, and poor commissioners.

Last but not least among the county officials is the county health officer. In most instances he is unique in not being locally elected. The tendency has been to consider this position the most professional of all local public positions and one that can be entrusted only to a specially trained and well-qualified person. Frequently local governments experience considerable difficulty in filling this position and increasing turn of necessity to outside agencies such as state health departments, civil service commissions, or schools of public health for assistance. As a result of this and other factors there has developed a tendency for many local health officers to feel more responsible to the state than to the county government which they serve.

Township government
Discussion of local government would be incomplete without mention of township government as found in the New England states.[21] This last remaining epitome of democracy functions around the town meeting, which consists of all the citizens entitled to vote. The citizens themselves constitute the true local legislative group. The nominal administrative agents are the selectmen or the township board of supervisors chosen by popular vote at the town meeting. In some places where no regular township meeting is held they serve also as the legislative agent. The functions and activities of the township and its officers are quite similar to those carried out elsewhere by county governments. As a result of the vast changes in the forms of transportation and communication there appears little if any justification for the continued existence of township government.

Within townships are found the governments of smaller urban groups such as vil-
lages and boroughs. These are usually organized by means of groups of elected representatives, variously termed councils, burgesses, and boards, that serve as legislative agents. In addition, they usually elect a single executive, who may be designated as mayor, president, burgess, superintendent, or chairman, to serve as the administrative agent. The functions of these governments are those of an embryonic urban community.

Special districts
Special districts are the most varied of all local units of government. They usually are established to deal with a particular problem such as education, water, sewerage, air pollution, and the like. In order to finance the specific undertaking, special districts have recourse to taxation, assessment, or charging rates based on service costs.[11] Due primarily to the trend of consolidation of school districts the number of special districts has declined in recent years.

Apportionment and local government
The question of whether the apportionment standard of populations will be applied to local units of government has not yet been resolved. The basis of representation to a county board was first challenged in a Michigan case, Brouwer v. Bronkema, in 1964.[22] Registered voters of the city of Grand Rapids challenged the apportionment of the members of the Kent County Board of Supervisors among the several townships and the city. It was concluded that "a part of the legislative power of the state is delegated to and exercised by the County Board of Supervisors. That Board, like its parent body, the State Legislature, must be apportioned on a population basis. . . ." The question of apportionment of county boards has been appealed to the United States Supreme Court. In May 1967 the Supreme Court approved unequal districting in the selection of a school board in Michigan and a city council in Virginia. It did not rule on the question of counties.[23] County home rule and reapportionment of county boards may make it possible to establish an organizational structure that would allow county government to function effectively and therefore be the unit of pri-

mary importance in the operation of creative federalism.

Metropolitan government

From the foregoing it is evident that many reforms are indicated in local government. One of the most pressing is the need for consolidation. It is inevitable that this should come about, and symptoms are already evident in certain fields of public service and in certain parts of the country. The provision of public health services in many areas on a multicounty basis furnishes one example of this trend. Another is the growing interest in the analysis and attack of social problems on a regional basis. The leading role in this latter movement has been taken by the Committee on Southern Regional Studies and Education, with permanent headquarters at the University of North Carolina. Strow[24] has defined the region as "a large area with natural boundaries wherein there are many resemblances among the inhabitants and their culture." Health regions may be considered to be "major areas with distinct health conditions identifiable with the areal limits and caused by the natural and human factors operating within the natural boundaries." The regional approach may be of considerable value in defining and locating public health problems, in revealing causal factors, in creating public consciousness concerning them, and in arriving at methods for their solution.

Attempts have been made to provide a governmental structure for metropolitan areas through a number of mechanisms. In one, intergovernmental agreements and contracts that allow for the provision of a single service on a regional basis are negotiated.[25] Another, which has not been used widely, consolidates county and city services that are performed under the same administration. In another type of city-county consolidation the limits of the city are extended to the county boundaries. This also results in the elimination of one unit of government.

Possibly the most effective structure for metropolitan government so far is the metropolitan federation. Municipalities in the metropolitan area continue their separate existence. Functions of regional interest, however, are transferred to a new central federated government. Examples of federated government include the Municipality of Metropolitan Toronto, Miami-Dade County, Nashville-Davidson County, and the Metropolitan Corporation of Greater Winnipeg. Since the formal legal mechanisms for metropolitan government in most areas have been lacking, informal voluntary bodies such as councils of governments have been formed. The membership on bodies such as these includes representatives who participate on a voluntary basis from the various governing units. The weakness of voluntary associations is that they have access to authority only through their member bodies.

Another mechanism that only very recently has begun to be utilized in an attempt to resolve the problem of a multiplicity of political jurisdictions in relation to one service area is the nonprofit corporation. Nonprofit corporations, with their boards of directors selected on a regional basis, in a variety of ways may assume effective and efficient administration of publicly financed projects. The result of an increase in the number of such corporations, however, could be a loss of control, manageability, and public accountability. The effect that the utilization of these nonprofit corporations in the implementation of public service programs has on government at all levels is an area that demands the attention of all concerned about government.[26]

It now appears evident that a type of local governmental structure that can adequately meet the needs and demands of an urban society does not exist in the United States today. The incremental changes that have occurred facilitate the performance of the service function of government but hinder the performance of the political function. They do not provide a structure in which regional issues can be debated and resolved. Progress along these lines is necessarily slow. Consolidation of local governmental units presents a most difficult political task with many factions ever alert to oppose it. County voters and county lines as they now exist are important to office holders, local merchants and bankers, political party workers, many property owners, and local newspapers; for patronage purposes they are important to local, state, and federal political factions. Today the inability of the governmental system to respond to demands made of it as a result of outmoded structure contributes in a large degree to the inability of the public health agency to solve health problems with the scientific expertise and knowledge that presently is available.

THE POLITICAL PROCESS

Political scientists have begun to study politics as a process. Utilizing the new methodologies of social science research, they analyze the political process in a systematic manner in terms of human and group behavior and its social and psychologic determinants.

The role of groups as they affect public policy decisions has been an area of particular interest. Banfield and Wilson[1] discuss city politics in terms of (1) the press, (2) business firms, (3) bureaucracies, (4) civic organizations, and (5) labor unions—the organizational groups which they view as playing a continual role in decision making.*

Another political scientist, David Truman,[27] advances the thesis that everything in the political process can be analyzed in terms of group action. He states, "Even in its nascent stages government functions to establish order in the relationship among groups for various purposes. What a particular government is under these circumstances, its forms, and its methods depends upon the character of the groups and purposes it serves." The electoral process and the role of political parties are specialized areas of this type of research.

Other political scientists[28] are currently studying voting behavior. "In casting a vote an individual acts toward the world of politics as he perceives the personalities [and] issues . . . . measuring perceptions and evaluations of the elements of politics is a

first charge in our energies in an explanation of the voting act." The premise of this type of research is that if voting decisions of the national electorate can be understood, one aspect of the total political process will be understood.* It would be helpful to public health administrators in understanding politics to become familiar with this type of current research in political science.

THEORIES OF COMMUNITY POWER STRUCTURE

An increasing number of studies have been carried out in an attempt to describe empirically the decision-making process in a community and thereby provide a model for the American political system. One of the earlier attempts is that of Floyd Hunter[29] in his study of decision making in Atlanta. The conclusion drawn from his study is that an elite, although not monolithic, body does control political decision making. The elitist model of politics which has been formulated by political philosophers such as Pareto and Mosca seems to be substantiated by Hunter's investigation.

The alternative model describes what prevails as a "dynamic system of power interrelationships, involving the interaction of many groups in a contest with each other with policies resulting from their conflict and compromise . . ." Dahl's[30] famous study of decision making in New Haven advances the thesis of pluralism. By studying three separate decisions on unrelated matters he has found little overlap in the groups of people promoting important programs in the city.

Many criticisms as to the validity of conclusions about the political process that might be drawn from community decision-making studies can be raised on methodologic and theoretical bases.[31] However, these studies, although they may not produce a model of the political system, do provide insights into the political process. As political scientists develop more sophisticated research techniques, more undoubtedly will

*For a more detailed discussion, see *City Politics* by Banfield and Wilson.[1]

*See *American Voter* by Campbell, Converse, Miller, and Stokes.[28]

be done in developing models of political action.

GOVERNMENTAL REVENUES AND EXPENDITURES

The relative needs of the different levels of government for funds vary considerably. In 1965-1966, for example, the federal government was responsible for approximately $129.9 billion, or 57.8% of the $224.8 billion for direct government expenditures. The 50 states accounted for about $34.2 billion, or 15.2%, and the 91,183 (1962) units of local government expended $60.7 billion, or 27%.[32] Total governmental ex-

penditures were $19.3 billion more than the previous year. These figures present only a partial picture, however. If spending is treated in terms of financing rather than in terms of direct final spending, the federal government was responsible for roughly $143 billion, or 63.6%, state government for $39.1 billion, or 17.4%, and local government for $42.68 billion, or 19%.[32] Increases in governmental expenditures for the period 1913-1961 are shown in Table 8-1. Expenditures by level of government during the 1965-1966 fiscal year are shown in Table 8-2.

The latest figures available of a break-

Table 8-1. Increases in all governmental expenditures, 1913-1961

	Amount (in millions of dollars)			
Item	1913	1941	1952	1961
Payrolls	$1,500	$7,400	$29,800	$50,215
Other current operations	391	9,000	26,300	91,723
Capital outlays	722	6,200	24,900	32,320
Public to private cash transfers	185	2,500	13,900	31,122
Interest on debt			6,600	9,710

Table 8-2. Governmental expenditure, by source and object, 1965-1966*

Item	Amount (millions of dollars)				Percent			
	All govern-ments	Federal govern-ment	State govern-ments	Local govern-ments	All govern-ments	Federal govern-ment	State govern-ments	Local govern-ments
Total expenditure	$224,813†	$143,022	$51,043	$60,994†	100.0	100.0	100.0	100.0
Intergovernmental expenditure	(†)	13,115	16,848	283†	—	9.2	33.0	0.5
Direct expenditure	224,813	129,907	34,195	60,711	100.0	90.8	67.0	99.5
Current operation	130,488	70,276	16,855	43,357	58.0	49.1	33.0	71.1
Capital outlay	39,981	17,652	10,193	12,137	17.8	12.3	20.0	19.9
Assistance and sub-sidies	13,363	9,048	2,301	2,014	5.9	6.3	4.5	3.3
Interest on debt	12,857	9,589	894	2,374	5.7	6.7	1.8	3.9
Insurance benefits repayments	28,126	23,342	3,952	830	12.5	16.3	7.7	1.4
Exhibit: Expenditure for personal services	72,963	32,904	10,561	29,498	32.5	23.0	20.7	48.4

*From U. S. Bureau of the Census: Governmental finances in 1965-1966, Series GF, No. 13, Washington, 1967, U. S. Government Printing Office.
†Net of duplicative intergovernmental transactions.
NOTE: Because of rounding, detail may not add to totals.

down of expenditures by the various units of local government are those for 1962. Expenditures of local government in that year totaled approximately $45.28 million (duplicative intergovernmental transactions excluded); counties, $8.88 billion; municipalities, $17.3 billion; townships and New England towns, $1.7 billion; school districts, $14.9 billion; and special districts, $3.15 billion.[33]

The amounts of money required are influenced chiefly by two somewhat related trends in public administration: first, the changing relationships among and emphasis upon different levels of government as previously discussed and, second, the greatly increased demands by the public for more and new types of service.

Most of the increase throughout the period can be attributed to increases in general government expenditures and national defense, with government utilities and other similar enterprises accounting for the remainder. Public to private cash transfers refer to public assistance, veterans' pensions, old age and unemployment benefits, and public employee pensions.

In order to meet these increasing fiscal demands, units of government on all levels are engaged in a constant search and struggle for additional sources of revenue. Each unit of government, maintaining its own taxation system, finds itself increasingly in conflict with other units of government.

In the early days of our history the most lucrative, stable, and accessible form of taxation was on general property. Since originally most governmental functions and services took place on the local level and because of early fears of federalism, the general property tax was reserved largely for use by local governments. As a result, even today the general property tax represents the major source of income for local governments, accounting in 1965 for about 87.1% of the total revenue obtained by local governments.[32]

With the great changes that have occurred in our social structure and means of earning a living, many new taxable items and activities have appeared. The shift to salaried income by a large proportion of

the nation's wage earners has made a tax on earned income practical. The federal government relies primarily on income taxes for the major share of its revenue. No one type of tax is so predominant for state governments, however. Sales and gross receipt taxes, including selective taxes on sales of motor oil, liquor, tobacco products, or other services, provide more than half of all state tax revenues.[32]

Beyond the general property tax, cities and counties have access locally only to fees from licenses, permits, assessments, fines and forfeitures, and institutional funds and earnings. For some time the tendency has been for local governments, both city and county, to give way to the state and federal governments when new revenue sources are discovered or in cases of tax conflict. Tax revenue by type of tax and level of government in fiscal year 1964-1965 is shown in Fig. 8-1.

This dilemma in which local governments now find themselves would not be so acute if the general property tax had remained as useful as it once was. Unfortunately, however, this tax has become increasingly difficult to administer, has been repeatedly subject to personal and political manipulation, and even if correctly applied may sometimes jeopardize individual property owners upon whom it is levied. To assess the value of personal property honestly and accurately is in itself a difficult and costly procedure. Added to this is the fact that most tax assessors are local individuals who by virtue of their local election are subject to feelings of indebtedness and favoritism. It is not surprising that the administration of the general property tax not only has been lax and inefficient but often has been used as a political tool.

Since ordinarily the need for revenue increases during periods of economic stress, local governments are faced with the dilemma of having to increase assessments, taxes, and collections on essentially the same people who because of general economic stress need the most help. Thus there occurs the very real possibility of taking from the right hand to pay the left and the possibility that because of decreased ability to meet

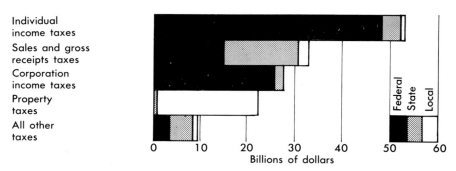

Individual income taxes
Sales and gross receipts taxes
Corporation income taxes
Property taxes
All other taxes

Federal
State
Local

0   10   20   30   40   50   60
Billions of dollars

Fig. 8-1. Tax revenue based on type of tax and level of government (1964-1965).

Table 8-3. Trend of tax delinquency, 1930-1944, median year-end delinquency, 150 cities over 50,000 population

Years	Percent	Years	Percent
1930	10.15	1938	10.70
1931	14.60	1939	9.25
1932	19.95	1940	8.70
1933	26.35	1941	6.80
1934	23.05	1942	6.00
1935	18.00	1943	4.70
1936	13.90	1944	3.90
1937	11.30		

tax demands a considerable share of private property will be turned over to government itself by default, thereby eliminating it as a source of tax revenue. As a result, when local tax monies are most needed, collection becomes more difficult. A striking example of this is the state of Georgia, where in 1936 over one third of county taxes were uncollectable. This problem, when it occurs, is not peculiar to rural areas or to the economically unfavored Southeastern states. Table 8-3 presents the extent of tax delinquency that occurred in the 150 cities of over 50,000 population during the period of economic depression between 1930 and 1944.[34]

Another factor to be considered with regard to the general property tax is that much property is exempt from taxes. Using Georgia again as an example, the following are not subject to taxation: public property, places of religious worship and burial, charitable institutions, educational institutions, funds or property held or used as endow-

ment by such institutions, real and personal estate of any public library and of any literary association connected with such a library, books, philosophic apparatus, paintings and statuary of any company and association kept in a public hall and not held as merchandise or for sale or gain, farm products grown in the state and remaining in the hands of the producer during the year following their production, and personal property up to the value of $300 and of a $2,000 homestead upon application of the taxpayer. In Georgia these account for about one quarter of all real and personal property.[35] As a result the bulk of real property tax is paid by farmers and small-home owners who as individuals are not organized as are other groups and are therefore unable to exert influence on tax determination bodies.

The concept of tax sharing has been discussed frequently in recent years. Basically those individuals who support tax sharing argue that the federal government, which

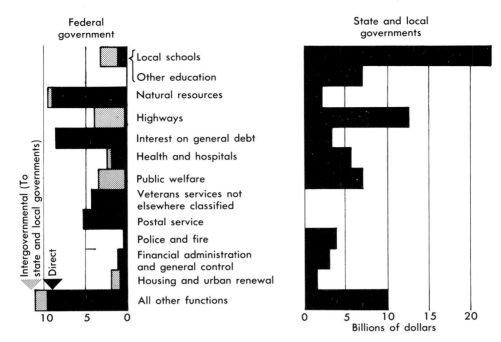

Fig. 8-2. General expenditure, excluding funds for national defense and international relations, based on level of government and function (1964-1965).

has an expanding base from which to draw revenue and a highly developed tax-collecting system, should return a small percentage to the states. Walter Heller, economic advisor to the President in 1960, proposed that federal revenues be returned to states with few or no strings. Many questions are raised as to exactly how tax sharing should be implemented: How much money should be shared? On what basis? What should be the relationship of the states to metropolitan areas and metropolitan areas to the federal government in any tax sharing scheme? Therefore it will probably be some time before taxing authorities and procedures are changed.

The growing public demand for government services and the resulting increase in expenditures have been previously referred to. A cursory study over a period of years of itemized expenditures for various specific activities makes evident the fact that the greatest increases have occurred in relation to public service and construction for public use. Looming large among the increased

items are those related to social security, including the prevention of illness and the promotion of health, insurance against unemployment and illness, and other similar social prophylactic measures (Fig. 8-2). As a matter of fact, merely over the 25-year period 1940 to 1965 total expenditures on all levels of government for health and medical services multiplied more than tenfold, from $803.9 million to $9.22 billion (Table 8-4).

In order to overcome the inadequacies of state and local tax systems it has been necessary to resort increasingly to intergovernmental transfers in the form of grants-in-aid, shared revenues, payments for services, and other types of transfers. Thus in 1965 not only was a total of $11.6 billion transferred from the federal to the state governments but an additional $1.5 billion was transferred by the federal government directly to local governments.[32] In addition, local governments received $16.85 billion from state governments. Health and hospitals represent public services in which

Table 8-4. Public expenditures for health and medical care, by type of expenditure, United States, selected fiscal years 1928-1929 through 1964-1965*

Type of expenditure	Amount (in millions of dollars)											
	1928-1929	1934-1935	1939-1940	1944-1945	1949-1950	1954-1955	1959-1960	1960-1961	1961-1962	1962-1963	1963-1964	1964-1965
Total public expenditures	$509.5	$558.5	$858.4	$2,571.0	$3,086.0	$4,358.2	$6,359.3	$7,035.1	$7,619.3	$8,286.3	$8,997.5	$9,949.3
Health and medical services	410.5	517.3	803.9	2,504.8	2,561.0	3,947.7	5,784.9	6,476.5	7,046.1	7,668.0	8,333.4	9,216.3
General medical and hospital care	216.6	231.8	340.5	354.7	914.5	1,217.3	1,952.2	2,202.8	2,136.4	2,274.9	2,446.8	2,670.3
Defense Department facilities	29.2	28.0	99.5	1,631.0	315.6	763.4	804.7	848.7	909.9	883.7	963.7	1,038.9
Medicare	—	—	—	—	—	—	60.1	61.0	73.2	75.0	75.4	81.3
Veterans' hospital and medical care	30.0	56.0	72.1	98.3	585.9	722.6	884.5	953.8	968.0	1,020.3	1,069.3	1,138.9
Public assistance (vendor medical payments)	—	—	—	—	51.3	211.9	492.5	588.6	812.4	1,000.7	1,147.6	1,375.0
Workmen's compensation (medical benefits)†	25.0	65.0	90.0	122.0	193.0	315.0	415.0	450.0	475.0	505.0	540.0	575.0
Temporary disability insurance (medical benefits)‡	—	—	—	—	1.4	6.0	15.6	19.6	21.5	25.7	29.3	23.0
Medical vocational rehabilitation	—	—	.4	1.4	7.4	9.2	17.7	20.4	22.5	26.0	31.2	39.8
Maternal and child health services	5.0	6.7	13.8	62.1	29.8	92.9	138.8	151.8	173.3	185.2	208.3	230.1
School health (educational agencies)	9.0	9.9	17.9	23.3	30.6	65.9	101.0	115.0	129.0	130.5	132.0	133.5
Medical research	—	—	3.1	17.0	72.9	138.9	471.2	603.9	819.1	964.0	1,101.7	1,235.2
Other public health activities	95.7	119.7	166.6	195.0	358.6	404.6	431.6	460.9	505.8	577.0	588.1	675.3
Medical facilities construction, total	99.0	41.2	54.5	66.2	525.0	410.5	574.4	558.6	573.2	618.3	664.1	733.0
Veterans Administration	4.0	2.9	14.1	16.2	156.2	33.0	57.5	53.7	52.1	69.8	76.4	84.4
Defense Department	(§)	(§)	(§)	(§)	(§)	33.0	40.0	44.0	24.0	23.0	42.9	34.3
Other	95.0	38.3	40.4	50.0	368.8	344.5	476.9	460.0	497.1	525.5	544.8	614.3

*Adapted from Social Security Administration: Social welfare expenditures, 1964-65, Social Security Bulletin **28:**10, Oct. 1965.
†Includes medical benefits paid under public law by private insurance carriers and self-insurers.
‡Excludes medical benefits paid under public law in California and New York by private insured and self-insured plans; such benefits included in insurance benefits under private expenditures.
§Data not available.
Note: Totals may not add due to rounding.

significant amounts are transferred ($684 million). The total expenditure for health, hospitals, and sanitation after intergovernmental transfers in 1965-1966 amounted to $10.9 billion, of which $2.45 billion was spent by federal agencies, $2.97 billion by state governments, and the remaining $5.52 billion by local units of government.[32]

GRANTS-IN-AID

In recent years social problems (one portion of which are health problems) of increasing scope and complexity have developed. Concurrently the attitude of the public toward the role of government in the solution to these problems has changed. The public believes that health is a basic human right, that high levels of health are possible, and that health services must be expanded accordingly.[36] The response of government to this demand has been primarily at the federal level. Many factors are relevant in this development, but of particular significance is the previously discussed imbalance of revenue sources among governments. The primary responsibility for the initiation and implementation of health programs, however, still remains at the local level. The mechanism that allows for federal financing and local implementation has been the grants-in-aid. These have been defined as "sums of money assigned by a superior to an inferior governmental authority."[37] Grants-in-aid represent one form of transfer of public funds for the purpose of equalizing revenue among the several levels of government and among the states and their contained local areas. They are intended to improve the quality and expand the quantity of governmental programs in less affluent areas and areas of special need by augmenting their revenue with legal transfers of funds from more wealthy regions. No reasonable person would sanction the continuance, for want of adequate funds, of insanitary conditions and inadequate public health programs in some areas that might adversely affect others. This being the case, it becomes necessary to provide some method for assisting the smaller or less favored units of government to meet their obligations. Another justification of the in-

creasing use of grants-in-aid may be found in the situation previously discussed, i.e., the local government units are more restricted as to types of revenue and are administratively in a disadvantageous position for levying and collecting some of the more lucrative sources of funds. Few would deny the right of local governments to share in the fiscal benefits of automobile excise taxes since the local areas must share in the building and maintenance of the roads over which vehicles travel. It would be confusing, however, to say the least, should each locality attempt to apply and collect its own automobile excise tax. A revenue such as this is obviously applied most efficiently by a higher level of government.

Another purpose of grants-in-aid, as was indicated in the discussion of centralization, is to provide some measure of supervision or control over the activities of the lower units of government. Snavely[38] comments that on an intrastate basis, "State authorities, more frequently specialized in their fields and free from local prejudices, can offer valuable suggestions and advice to the communities. Advice, however, even of an official character, is often unwelcome unless an immediate gain can be realized by its acceptance or a loss sustained from its refusal. A double-barrelled gun of this nature, loaded with a reward for compliant counties and with a penalty for recalcitrant districts is available for the central governments in the form of State subventions." What is said here with regard to state and local relationships applies perhaps even more in the federal and state relationship.

Related to this, and arising as a result of it, is a fourth purpose of grants-in-aid: the enforcement of minimum standards upon the recipient of the grant. Undoubtedly, few things have been as influential in promoting the employment of qualified local public health personnel, for example, as have been the conditions attached to grants by both state and federal health agencies.

The idea of grants-in-aid is by no means new, having been first applied in this country in New York State in 1795 for the improvement of schools in the poorer, particularly rural, areas of that state. Federal grants to states began as early as 1808, when Congress instituted an annual appropriation to assist the states in the development of their respective militia.[39] No conditions were attached to these grants, and no federal supervision was exercised. Perhaps the next development of significance was the passage in 1862 of the Morrill Act, which entitled each state to a grant of public lands based upon the total number of its members of Congress. States not containing public land were given scrip. The only condition was that not less than 90% of the gross proceeds was to be used for the establishment, endowment, and maintenance of agricultural and mechanical colleges. Subsequent acts added to the original provisions an annual grant of cash to each state. In 1887 the Hatch Act was passed, which provided $15,000 per year to each state for the establishment of agricultural experiment stations. With this act there was instituted the condition of submission of an annual financial report, followed 8 years later by provision for a federal audit. This established a pattern that has never since been altered.

The rising tide of federal influence in state and local affairs is well illustrated by another phase of social security, relief for dependents. Traditionally the care of such individuals in America has been a local and often a private affair. The economic depression of the 1930's changed all this, when, because of lack of funds, first private charity, then local governments, and in turn state governments found themselves quite incapable of meeting the tremendously increased demands. Only one other source of assistance remained—the national government. As a result numerous federal agencies which provided for the first time a basis for a broad system of federal social security were established. These agencies concerned themselves with dependent children, the unemployed, the handicapped, and the aged. This soon crystalized into a permanent legally established program. Again it should be pointed out that this represented not a premeditated design or plan of federal officials but a response to the increasing incapabilities of lower levels of governmental

units to meet problems that essentially were those of the nation as a whole. Some writers have pointed out that even if the federal government were to withdraw from this field of activity a definite change in attitude on the part of the public has occurred and the psychologic loss of prestige by the states is practically irreparable.

The changes that have occurred in the relationship between the federal and state governments have also resulted in some change in the relationship between state and local governments and local and federal governments. Theoretically the national government has no relations with cities. However, even antedating the depression there had appeared signs to indicate closer contacts between national and municipal authorities. As early as 1925, Anderson[40] pointed to numerous instances in which national agencies played a significant role in the determination and management of municipal affairs. A more detailed study of federal service to cities was made in 1931 by Betters,[41] who commented: "The wide range of activities of the national government which touch intimately on current problems of municipal administration may surprise many." He pointed out that federal agencies had already developed standards in weights and measures, traffic and safety, zoning and building, highway construction, and milk sanitation, and had carried out studies and surveys on local education, finances, crime, vital statistics, and public health. In addition, federal agencies were actively engaged in a cooperative sense in food and drug control, municipal water supplies, sewage disposal, and other fields. Again the economic depression of the 1930's and subsequently World War II accelerated the intimacies of these relationships. Although the federal agencies operated for the most part through the state governments as an intermediary, they did in some instances deal directly with cities. The possible revolutionary consequences of this caused White[5] to comment:

The extent to which actual control of municipal affairs was lodged in Washington as a result of these emergency measures is not easy to define. The federal government did not attempt to weaken the control of the state over its political subdivision, and no change in the legal status of the city was imposed . . . contacts between cities and the national government were broad and in their extent spectacular; but the states were not dispossessed of their traditional constitutional position as guardians of municipal government. The change has been a change in climate rather than a change in topography. Future lines of development are not clear, but it seems likely that the research and advisory services of the national government to cities are destined to increase in importance. So far as the cities enter into debtor-creditor relations with Washington, an element of fiscal supervision may appear. . . . Movement has been rapid since 1933, and a federal bureau of municipal relations is much more within the realm of the practical than it was before the events of the depression. Here is an aspect of central tendencies which in the case of the great urban centers may be of special significance, for they have little to derive from the state capitols as they have much to gain from in Washington.

The rural areas of America were not absent from this scene of changing governmental relations. Except for the financing of the county agent program and aid to rural education and agricultural research, contact between the federal government and the rural areas was lacking until the establishment of the Agricultural Adjustment Administration in 1933. The federal government entered into cooperative programs with the farm population, involving the adjustment of farm production to nationally established quotas and the direct payment to individual farmers for compliance with contracts regarding certain crops. County production control associations were established, covering practically all parts of the rural area of America and including several million cooperating farmers. In the process the state governments were largely ignored. Associated with this program were activities such as the national nutrition program, which had a direct bearing on the health not only of the farm families but of the nation's population as a whole.

Federal grants-in-aid for public health work began with the passage of the Chamberlain-Kahn Act of 1918. Stimulated by the increased threat of venereal diseases during World War I, Congress provided an appropriation of $1 million for each of 2 years to be distributed to the states on the basis of population. The program was administered, not by the Public Health Service but

by an interdepartmental social hygiene board. After the second year the appropriation was cut and then finally eliminated. As a result little of a lasting nature continued in any but the wealthier states.

The next use of federal grants for public health purposes was in the field of maternal and child health. Again as a result of increased interest during the war the Sheppard-Towner Act of 1921 was passed. It provided grants of $1.24 million per year to the states for 5 years "for the promotion of the welfare and hygiene of infancy." Contingent upon certain conditions, chiefly the existence of a bureau of maternal and child health, each state was eligible for a flat sum of $10,000 and a share of the remainder on the basis of its proportionate population. The share of the remainder and one half of the flat grant had to be matched by the state. This act was the subject of strenuous opposition, not only on the part of states' rightists but also of the American Medical Association, which, as it did later in relation to the Emergency Maternity and Infant Care Program of World War II, viewed it as an entering wedge toward state medicine. Since some professional jealousy existed between the administering Children's Bureau and the Public Health Service, some criticism of the Sheppard-Towner Act was also forthcoming from the latter. After extending the provisions of the act for 2 years, Congress terminated the grants in 1929.

Thus the second venture in federal grants for public health programs was short lived and relatively unsuccessful. Despite this, many authorities[38] consider the need for federal and state initiative and aid to be greater in public health than in any other governmental function:

Experience has shown that local governments of rural communities in general will not appropriate sufficient funds for the support of full time health units unless some assistance is forthcoming from outside agencies. Since it is in the rural sections that unsafe water supplies, unsanitary sewage disposal, inadequate medical attention and malnutrition combine to spread disease, it is in these communities that the greatest expenditures should be made. Despite the existing needs, the rural districts, even when aid is offered them, frequently hesitate or refuse to expend their revenue for the protection of health.

Grants-in-aid are intended to promote progress and improvement in lower governmental units by making it possible for them to provide better services and facilities than they can from their own unaided resources. Sometimes, however, this purpose is defeated by the system of distribution. Injudicious methods of subsidization may demoralize a community by fostering overreliance on the higher unit of government with loss of local initiative and sense of responsibility, by causing them to indulge in lavish expenditures, or by allowing them to use the grants as an excuse for unwarranted reductions in local tax rates. Similarly there is a risk of pauperizing communities that happen to be poor in the first instance by enticing them into increasing local taxation and even indebtedness in order to raise funds for matching purposes. Or there is risk of encouraging them to inaugurate programs and raise public expectancies that cannot be sustained on a long-range basis. Another serious objection has been the tendency for categorical grants to lead to unbalanced state and local programs based in large measure upon financial expediency.

The sound, effective, and equitable distribution of subventions, therefore, presents a difficult problem indeed. Not infrequently plans have resulted in proportionately and absolutely more aid being allotted to wealthier communities than to those most in need. By distributing grants on the basis of taxable capacity either directly or indirectly through complete matching requirements, by granting equal amounts to all communities, or even by granting on the basis of population alone there is a tendency, if anything, to increase the inequities rather than to solve the problem.

The great increase in the numbers and types of grant-in-aid programs in the health and health-related fields in the last several years has created very serious problems of manageability. The Eighty-ninth Congress alone passed acts which created 21 new health programs, 17 new educational programs, 15 new economic development programs, 12 new programs for cities, 17 new resource development programs, and 4 new manpower programs.[42] Over 170 different federal aid programs exist, financed by over 400 separate appropriations, 21 federal departments, 150 Washington bureaus, and 400 regional offices. The dispersement of responsibility for programs continues to exist on the state level. Funds for programs are channeled for different patterns under a variety of rules and regulations. Effective program implementation at the point where services are given to people (local) is almost impossible because of the administrative confusion which has been created because of the existing grant-in-aid system.

The critical situation that exists with reference to the proliferation of grant-in-aid programs having no effective mechanisms for their implementation has been recognized. Attempts are being made at all levels of government, particularly the federal level, to coordinate efforts. In the health field a significant step has been taken in this direction by the passage of P.L. 89-749, the Comprehensive Health Planning and Public Service Amendments of 1966, which will be discussed later.

The circumstances that cause increased needs and high governmental costs are the same as those that result in insufficient resources for meeting the needs and costs. States and communities with proportionately many children and elderly persons, inadequate sanitary facilities, high disease and death rates, and slum conditions have need of more extensive and costly public services than do other states and communities. However, these are the very places that find it less possible to provide them. In order to accomplish their fundamental purpose grants-in-aid must be provided, at least in part, in an inverse ratio to the wealth of the various recipient areas. In this way the proportionate amounts received by communities tend to be in accordance with their relative needs.

In distributing grants-in-aid there exists the possibility of taking funds from some areas and giving them to others that may be just as able to finance themselves as are those from which the funds were taken. One method of avoiding this involves correcting the apparent taxable capacity of communities to a true common denominator by determining equalized assessments, which is difficult to do, or by using assessment ratios to provide estimated true valuations.

A plan of distribution based on actual financial needs, supplemented by additional grants to encourage compliance with minimum standards, will provide some assistance to all communities and, in addition, will give consideration to those unable to raise funds enough of their own to supply the necessary services. If the superior governmental unit allots only a partial share of the maximum possible subsidy to those areas failing to raise the estimated amount of revenue as determined by the use of assessment ratios, this will act as a powerful incentive to provide local funds more in keeping with local financial ability. A plan like this is admittedly more difficult and costly to administer but in the long run will justify itself in terms of greater general improvements, equity, and satisfaction.

The Social Security Act of 1935 provided for federal and state cooperation in public health matters on an increased and more or less permanent basis. It provided for annual grants "to assist states, counties, health districts and other political subdivisions of

Table 8-5. Amount (in thousands of dollars) of Public Health Service formula grants for health services*

Program	Fiscal year 1963	Fiscal year 1964	Fiscal year 1965
Cancer control	$ 3,500	$ 3,500	$ 3,500
Chronically ill and aged	13,000	13,000	11,750
Dental health	—	—	520
General health	15,000	14,000	10,000
Heart disease control	7,000	7,000	7,000
Mental health	10,950	10,950	6,750
Radiological health	1,500	2,000	2,500
Tuberculosis control	3,250	2,900	3,000
Water pollution control	5,000	5,000	5,000
Total	$59,200	$58,350	$50,020

*From Public Health Rep. **82:**132, Feb. 1967.

Table 8-6. Number and amount (in thousands of dollars) of Public Health Service project grants for health services*

Program	Fiscal year 1963		Fiscal year 1964		Fiscal year 1965	
	Number of awards	Amount of grants	Number of awards	Amount of grants	Number of awards	Amount of grants
Air pollution	—	—	—	—	108	$ 4,945.0
Cancer demonstration	69	$ 2,559.6	83	$ 2,618.5	118	3,459.0
Community health services	106	5,628.1	50	1,541.4	145	7,446.8
Hospital and medical facility planning	—	—	—	—	32	1,879.4
Mental retardation planning	—	—	136	7,066.0	46	1,831.5
Migrant health	30	750.0	35	1,050.0	65	2,808.9
Neurological and sensory disease services	43	1,464.2	58	1,703.1	85	2,503.1
Tuberculosis control	37	1,369.9	41	1,791.2	72	5,106.6
Vaccination assistance	1	243.6	93	9,570.7	124	16,859.6
Venereal disease control	96	4,578.8	76	6,421.0	71	7,240.2
Water pollution control	14	521.5	22	645.8	31	1,175.6
Total	396	$17,115.7	594	$32,407.7	897	$55,255.7

*From Public Health Rep. **82:**132, Feb. 1967.

States in establishing and maintaining adequate public health services." The annual sum of $8 million, which was subsequently increased ($38,879,300 for 1952), was to be distributed among the states by the Surgeon General of the United States Public Health Service on the basis of three factors: population, special health problems, and financial need. The relative weight given these factors was left to the discretion of the Surgeon General after "consultation with a conference of the State and Territorial health authorities."[43] Grants-in-aid by the Public Health Service for fiscal year 1965 are shown in Tables 8-5 and 8-6.

The failure to specify more exactly the method of distribution of funds appropriated by legislatures has given cause for objection from many quarters. A report of the Municipal Finance Officers Association[44] states as follows:

The federal government has never had a continuing relief policy. The total amount of grants available has hinged primarily upon vacillating concepts of necessity. In addition, allocation of individual grants has been based upon wide administrative discretion. Such a procedure has hardly contributed to predictable municipal budgets. . . . . The financial aid of the upper levels of government has undoubtedly saved many localities from complete disaster. Yet the unstable aid policies which have accompanied the greater reliance upon state-collected, locally shared taxes and grants-in-aid have served to accentuate revenue fluctuations for many local governments.

In like manner, many health officers have complained of the difficulty involved in attempting long-range programs due to the uncertainty surrounding the amount of both federal and state funds that might be depended upon for budget planning.

Prior to the passage of P.L. 89-749, which entirely alters the grant-in-aid program as it relates to health, an attempt was made by the Public Health Service to determine indices of financial need and of special health problems, but the results have not been completely satisfactory and the relative bases of distribution have been somewhat variable. Thus in the first year, 1936, 57.5% was distributed on the basis of population, 22.5% on the basis of special health problems (judged by the number of deaths from all infectious and parasitic diseases and from pneumonia but not including venereal disease, for which a separate grant was made), and 20% on the basis of financial need. But for the year 1941 funds were distributed on the basis of 29.4% for population, 41.2% for special health problems, and 29.4% for financial need.

The Public Health Service has tried to consider other factors such as the relative cost of rendering health services in each state and the existence of special programs in particular states. Of the amount distributed on the basis of special health problems, one half has been based on mortality, one fourth according to relative costs of services, and one fourth as a remainder. Financial need has been based essentially on per capita income as computed by the United States Department of Commerce.

Matching requirements have been a result of administrative decision rather than of legal specification. Under Section 314d of P.L. 89-749 requirements for state matching are being formulated. The requirements for hospital construction funds are variable. In any case the federal share must be not more than two thirds or less than one third. The conditions under which states make grants-in-aid to localities vary considerably from no specific predictable basis of distribution to the use of complex mathematical formulas, which, incidentally, are admittedly sidestepped more often than not. No standard formula is applicable to all the states, and each works out its own solution to its own satisfaction. A summary of several state plans that have been used may be of illustrative interest:

Florida

Per capita grant varied by population size, with required per capita local contribution (50 cents considered basic) and system of bonus for excess local contribution and penalties for deficiencies in local contributions. One percent is added to or deducted from basic state contribution for each cent above or below 50 cents per capita from the county—not to exceed more than 50% of original basic state contribution. The state retains the right to add or subtract 5% or less of this.

Allocations may be made for special needs not subject to formula.

Georgia

Percentage of state participation varies with population with most populous areas receiving 30% and least populous receiving 75%.

Illinois

One dollar subsidy for $3 local money or 30 cents per capita, whichever is less. Special need subsidy added in poorer counties to equalize available resources to approximate $1.20 per capita statewide.

Louisiana

Total amount available for allocation to local departments is divided by population—this per capita amount is used as general basis and then modified by past progress and health and financial need of area.

New York

In counties and cities over 50,000 population on basis of 50% of cost of public health services, except where a county health department is established in which event state aid is given in amount of 75% on first $100,000 expended and 50% on balance of expenditure.

North Carolina

Based on population, financial needs, and specific program needs.

The most progressive state action in this regard is the Public Health Assistance Law passed by California. This law, which became effective September 19, 1947, provides an annual sum for local health services that is allocated according to a formula written into the law. Each county receives either a basic allotment or a capitation, whichever is less. The remainder, after subtraction of 7.5% of the total for administrative and consultative services and training, is allocated to health departments that meet standards on a straight per capita basis.[45]

It is of further interest to note that this act officially provides for a California Conference of Local Health Officers which, among other things, must approve standards relating to local health service before they can be established by the State Department of Public Health. This plan warrants close study by the federal agencies responsible for the distribution of grants to state and local governments since it appears to go far in eliminating many causes for dissatisfaction.

In Michigan a committee appointed by the governor has proposed a formula that attempts to take into consideration population, rate of growth, special need or problems, local tax base, and an indication of local determination.

COMPREHENSIVE HEALTH PLANNING AND PUBLIC HEALTH SERVICE AMENDMENTS OF 1966

This very significant piece of legislation, signed into law November 3, 1967, provides for comprehensive planning for health services, health manpower, and health facilities on the state and local level. It broadens and increases the flexibility of support for health services in the community and provides for the interchange of federal, state, and local health personnel.

P.L. 89-749 provides for the following types of planning grants: (1) state formula, (2) areawide project, and (3) training, studies, and demonstration, as well as formula and project grants. However, there are significant differences in how the formula and project grants are administered. Formula grant funds will be available to states and, through them, to local communities on a flexible basis. Until the present time, grants have been given according to defined disease or health problem categories. Under the act they are given to establish and maintain adequate public health services of all kinds, based upon a state plan for the planning and provision of public health services that has approval of the Surgeon General. Project grants are awarded to public or nonprofit private agencies and organizations to focus upon priority health targets. The goal of this legislation is to allow for the effective utilization of all available health resources. Under Section 314 of the act states must provide for the establishment of a single agency responsible for the administration and supervision of the state health planning function. For the most part states have designated the state health department; other states have created new interdepartmental agencies in the office of the governor. At this point, local and regional areas are struggling to create organizational structures through which comprehensive health planning can be implemented on that level. States and localities will be able to use health service money for the areas of highest priority according to their health needs.

The passage of this act has resulted in changes in agency organization at the federal and state levels. An office of comprehensive planning has been established in the office of the Surgeon General, and a major reorganization of the Regional Office structure of the Public Health Service has been necessary. Applications for grants under the law must pass through the appropriate regional office. The regional medical director is provided assistance through an Advisory and Review Council, the membership of which must be representative of wide interests, including industry, the medical profession, and universities.[46] Great responsibility rests on public health administrators in the implementation of P.L. 89-749, for this is the first instance of local and state agencies' being given authority and responsibility for the design and implementation of a comprehensive program to be financed federally. Whether local and state health professionals, government and nongovernment, will be able to meet this challenge successfully will undoubtedly affect the determination of whether this type of a block grant program will be utilized in other service areas. P.L. 89-749, therefore, presents a great challenge and opportunity in the development of effective creative federalism.

GOVERNMENT AND METROPOLITAN AREAS

As is evident from this brief discussion of government and public health, the critical problem is whether the governmental system can adapt itself in order to function effectively under dramatically changing circumstances. Urbanization has resulted in great concentrations of people living and working in what have become known as metropolitan areas and megalopolises. The basic patterns of American governmental structure were designed at a time when the urban phenomonen was nonexistent. A critical area of concern today is government for urban America. What type of governmental structure can be designed to assure the continuation of representativeness and

responsibility to the people yet allow for the financing of services for the burgeoning urban complexes that contain and indeed generate most of the health problems and needs?

Many groups of political scientists, governmental workers, and interested citizens have been formed to study and attempt to arrive at solutions to this perplexing problem. Among them are the National League of Cities, the National Conference of Mayors, Urban America, the National Commission on Intergovernmental Relations, the U. S. Conference of City Health Officers, and the Association of County Health Officers. It would now appear that the crucial test of the efficacy of the American governmental system in the late twentieth century will be its ability to operate in an urbanized society.

REFERENCES

1. Banfield, E. C., and Wilson, J. Q.: City politics, Cambridge, 1966, Harvard University Press.
2. Easton, D.: The political system, New York, 1953, Alfred A. Knopf, Inc.
3. Snider, C.: American state and local government, New York, 1965, Appleton-Century-Crofts.
4. Brogan, D. W.: The American character, New York, 1944, Alfred A. Knopf, Inc.
5. White, L. D.: Introduction to the study of public administration, New York, 1939, The Macmillan Co.
6. Maxwell, J. A.: The fiscal impact of federalism in the United States, Cambridge, 1946, Harvard University Press.
7. U. S. Children's Bureau: The seven years of the maternity and infancy act, Washington, 1931, U. S. Government Printing Office.
8. Mustard, H. S.: Government in public health, New York, 1945, Commonwealth Fund.
9. Pond, C. B.: Special report of the New York State Tax Commission, No. 3, Albany, 1931, New York State Tax Commission.
10. Reynolds v. Sim, U. S. 533 (1964).
11. Bromage, A. W.: Municipal government and administration, New York, 1957, Appleton-Century-Crofts.
12. U.S. Bureau of the Census: Statistical abstracts of the United States, 1966, Ed. 87 Washington, 1966, U. S. Government Printing Office.
13. Mobile v. Watson, 116 U.S. 289 (1886).
14. Duncombe, H. S.: County government in America, Washington, 1966, National Association of Counties Research Foundation.
15. Gilbertson, H. S.: The county, the dark continent of American politics, Chicago, 1917, The National Short Ballot Organization.

16. Local government under the Alaska Constitution—a survey report, Chicago, 1959, Public Administration Services.
17. U. S. Bureau of the Census: County and city data book, 1962, (A statistical abstract supplement) Washington, 1962, U. S. Government Printing Office.
18. Ross, R. M., and Millsop, K. F.: State and local government, New York, 1966, The Ronald Press Co.
19. Galpin, C. J.: The social anatomy of an agricultural community, Research Bulletin 34, University of Wisconsin Agricultural Experiment Station, Madison, University of Wisconsin Press.
20. Phillips, J. C.: State and local government in America. New York, 1954, American Book Co.
21. Gould, J.: New England town meeting, safeguard of democracy, Brattleboro, Vt., 1940, Stephan Daye Press, Inc.
22. Brouwer v. Bronkema, Mich., 1885 (1964).
23. Graham, F. P.: Supreme court limits one-man one-vote rule, The New York Times, May 23, 1967, p. 1.
24. Strow, C. W.: Regionalism in relation to the health of the public, Amer. J. Public Health 37:898, July 1947.
25. Dyckman, J. W.: Life in super city, Science, 138:1089, Dec. 7, 1962.
26. Smith, B. L. R.: The future of the not-for-profit corporation, The Public Interest 8:127, Summer 1967.
27. Truman, D. B.: The governmental process, New York, 1951, Alfred A. Knopf, Inc.
28. Campbell, A., Converse, E. P., Miller, W. E., and Stokes, E. D.: American voter, New York, 1964, John Wiley & Sons, Inc.
29. Lockard, D.: The politics of state and local government, New York, 1963, The Macmillan Co.
30. Dahl, R.: Who governs? New Haven, 1961, Yale University Press.
31. Polsby, N. W.: Community power and political theory, New Haven, 1963, Yale University Press.
32. U. S. Bureau of the Census: Governmental finances in 1965-1966, Series GF, No. 13, Washington, 1967, U. S. Government Printing Office.
33. U. S. Bureau of the Census: Census of government—1962, Compendium of government finances, Washington, 1962, U. S. Government Printing Office.
34. Bird, F. L.: The trend of tax delinquency, 1930-1944, New York, 1945, Dunn and Bradstreet, Inc.
35. Hughes, M. C.: County government in Georgia, Athens, 1944, University of Georgia Press.
36. Barns, E. M.: The role of government in the provision of health services, Bull. N. Y. Acad. Med. 41:7, July 1965.
37. Feiner, H.: Grants-in-aid, Encyclopedia of the Social Sciences 7:152, 1932.
38. Snavely, T. R., Hyde, D. C., and Biscoe, A. B.: State grants-in-aid in Virginia, New York, 1933, The Century Co.
39. Annals of Congress of the United States, Tenth Congress, First Session, 1808.
40. Anderson, W.: American city government, New York, 1925, Henry Holt & Co., Inc.
41. Betters, P. V.: Federal services to municipal governments, New York, 1931, Municipal Administrative Service Publication 24.
42. Reston, J.: Johnson's administrative monstrosity, The New York Times, Nov. 26, 1966.
43. Social Security Act of 1935, Section 602 (C).
44. Municipal Finance Officers Association: The support of local government, Chicago, 1939, The Association.
45. Halverson, W. L.: Fiscal relationships between the state and local health departments in California, Amer. J. Public Health 38:922, July 1948.
46. Cavanaugh, J., and McHiscock, W.: Comprehensive Health Planning and Public Health Service Act of 1966 (P.L. 89-749), Health, Education, and Welfare Indicators, Jan. 1967.

Chapter 9

Law and
public health

DEFINITION OF LAW*

Many books have been written dealing exclusively with the nature and definition of law. It is interesting that, although the average citizen probably considers law as an exact and strictly defined field, its mere definition presents the members of the legal profession with perhaps their most difficult problem. Law, at least in a democracy, depends in the last analysis on the collective wishes of the people, and the type and extent of their wishes vary through place and time. It should be realized that human behavior is subject to a never-ceasing process of evolution as are also the social factors determining or influencing it. However, law is not unique in this since definitions are not easily forthcoming in many other fields, e.g., literature, art, or from the point of view of our immediate interest public health. Perhaps under such circumstances the essential goal should be to arrive at some reasonably satisfactory definition that will serve as a point of departure for a practical pattern of behavior. An example might even be as simple as the immortal statement of some unknown character who said, "There is plenty of law at the end of a nightstick."

In order to guide our thinking it might be well to consider the definitions promulgated by some of the outstanding legal theorists in history. For example, Blackstone[3]

considered law as a "rule of civil conduct prescribed by the supreme power in a state, commanding what is right and forbidding what is wrong." It is to be noted in passing that this greatest of all jurists refrained from including in his definition the criteria involved in determining "right" or "wrong" at any particular time. Wilson[4] extended himself somewhat further in his definition by considering law as "that portion of established thought and habit which has gained distinct and formal recognition in the shape of uniform rule backed by the authority and power of government."

CHARACTERISTICS OF LAW

A law implies an actual or potential command; and a command signifies nothing more or less than a wish or desire. However, the commands and desires of law differ from ordinary personal commands and desires in that they (1) represent community desires or commands, (2) are applicable to all in the community, (3) are backed by the full power of the government, and (4) provide for all people the administration of justice under these laws. Wilson's definition might be considered to be more desirable since it either states or implies all of the characteristics mentioned.

PURPOSE OF LAW*

The primary purpose of law might be said to be the promotion of the general

---

*For a more detailed discussion, see *The Nature and Sources of Law* by Gray[1] and *The Nature of the Judicial Process* by Cardoza.[2]

*For a more detailed discussion, see *Sociology of Law* by Gurvitch.[5]

good by the regulation of human conduct in order to protect the individual from other individuals, groups, or the state, and vice versa. In order to effect such protection it must be possible for the individual, the group, and the state to predict within reasonable limits the probable course of judgment in the event of an infringement of the law. Therefore, another purpose of law is to assure, insofar as possible, uniformity of action in order to prevent errors of judgment or improper motives or actions on the part of judicial officers. It is often said that the wheels of justice turn slowly. The rate would be impossibly slow if the accumulative experience of earlier judges were not available to the people and to the courts. This also is a purpose of law.

The most fundamental means by which law endeavors to carry out its purposes is the definition of rights and duties existing between individuals or groups. Legal relationships form the essential subject matter of law, and rights and duties are the most important of legal relationships. A legal right is a power, privilege, or interest of an individual or group that is recognized and protected by law. Simultaneously the law imposes upon all others the obligation to refrain from violation of the right. Thus the possession of a right by one person always implies a corresponding duty on the part of some other person or persons to respect that right. For example, A and B enter into a contract. Their legal relationship may be expressed as either A has a right that B perform an act or B owes A a duty to perform an act.

Rights are of two kinds, primary and secondary. Primary rights are those that result merely from an individual's existence as a member of society. A citizen holds these primary rights against the entire community individually and collectively, and the community and each of its individuals owe him a corresponding duty to refrain from violating them. Thus a citizen's person and property are held to be inviolate; that is his primary right, and all others owe him a duty to respect it. Such rights exist not by virtue of any action taken or decision made but are the kind of rights

which were termed "natural rights" by eighteenth century legal theorists. They are sometimes spoken of as "rights in rem" and "rights of ownership." Their violation is considered a civil wrong (a tort) or a crime, depending upon their magnitude and upon whatever statutory law declares them to be. Libel, slander, trespass, negligence, and the like are civil wrongs or torts.

Secondary rights are those superimposed upon primary rights as a result of individual action and decision. They are not held against all other persons generally but only against a specified person or group. These rights arise as a result of contract. For example, A and B enter into a contractual agreement. Before the contract their legal relationship, consisting of rights and duties owed each other, was fixed and equal. Now due to the contract their legal relationships are quite different. A's previous primary rights are now increased by a secondary right that B carry out the action agreed upon in the contract. This new right differs in kind from primary rights, first, because it is not due simply to A's existence but results from a mutually agreed upon contract and, second, because it is a right held against B alone and no others.

Remedial rights are sometimes referred to as a third form of rights. They come into existence on the violation of the legal primary and secondary rights just discussed. In other words they are rights resulting from a personal injustice and are held against the individual committing the legal wrong. What they really amount to is a right of reparation, usually in terms of money damages. In other words all that is meant by saying that a person has a remedial right is that, if he appeals to the court, he will in all probability be rendered a favorable verdict. As Justice Holmes observed, a remedial right is in the nature of a prophecy.

SYSTEMS OF LAW
Development*
The concept of law has gone through many changes throughout the centuries of

---

*For a more detailed discussion, see *Growth of Law* by Cardoza[6] and *The Quest for Law* by Seagle.[7]

recorded history. With primitive man it apparently originated as a combination of gradually developing customs based on tradition and supposedly divine dictates. Perhaps the chief function of the patriarchs of a tribe was to define the practices evolved and followed by their predecessors, and these customs were gradually given the significance of established precedent and law. As to the meaning or reason for such laws, it was the theory of the Hindus and Chinese that laws were an essential necessity of human society; due to the innate depravity of man, as evidenced by his nature, laws were necessary to prevent violence and injustice. Therefore it became a primary duty first of the tribal leaders and ultimately of their successor, the state, to formulate and enforce rules of human behavior and conduct.

The Grecian theory of law was somewhat different and followed in general the basic philosophic pattern of their civilization. The Greeks argued that all necessary social laws really existed in nature and were merely waiting to be discovered, similar to the principles of physics. In fact, nature was thought of more or less as an expression of the total of all universal law. This concept that law exists perennially waiting to be discovered as natural truths held sway for over 1,700 years, passing through Stoic philosophy, Roman law, the principles of the Christian Church, and on through the medieval civilizations and governments. It is significant from our present point of view that the men who founded the American Republic and formulated the Declaration of Independence and the United States Constitution with its Bill of Rights had as their legal background the natural theory of law. It is noteworthy that the basic idea of the Declaration of Independence deals with the natural rights of men, which are to be secured rather than granted by government.

Since the establishment of the republic our concept or theory of law has undergone considerable change, especially since the beginning of the twentieth century, so that we now see legislation merely as a man-made device for the regulation and control of human conduct in order to assure the ultimate wishes of the greatest number or of the dominant groups in the community.

STATUTORY LAW

At the present time practically the entire Western world is governed by a combination of two distinct systems of law: (1) statutory law, based essentially on Roman civil law, and (2) the common law of England. Roman law began its development very early in the Roman state. The first authentic legal records were established in 450 B.C. as the Twelve Tables. To these were added innumerable unwritten laws that ultimately as a result of the Institutes of Justinian and others were codified into a system of written law so perfect that even today it operates as the basic law of most European countries. Its geographic adoption was related, of course, to the paths of Roman conquest, which brought the Roman legal code into practically all parts of the continent. Following the decline of the Roman Empire, the resulting daughter nations retained the Roman legal system since they had little other pattern to follow. Later, states such as the members of the American Republic provided legislatures to make whatever laws were necessary for government, and the resulting collections of legislative acts constituted the statutory law. For a time the attempt was made to adhere rather strictly to statutory law, but as societies became more complicated, especially as a result of urbanization and industrialization, innumerable additions had to be made in the form of specific interpretations, court decisions, and rules and regulations. The result is that at the present time, e.g., in the United States, written or statutory law constitutes only a small part (about 2%) of all existing laws.

COMMON LAW*

It was recognized at an early date that statutory law was in many cases too general to be directly applied to particular cases. As a result there followed the development of courts, the judges of which were expected to

---

*For a more detailed discussion, see *The Common Law* by Holmes.[5]

be guided in their specific decisions by the established customs of the community. England took particular strides in this direction. Essentially this recognition of the legal importance of custom represented a practical recognition of the rights of a people to take part in the making of the rules and laws governing their conduct and relationships. This was a great step toward liberty. A custom, in order to be entitled to consideration in law, must meet certain conditions. First, it must have existed for a long time or, as Blackstone put it, "have been used so long that the memory of man runneth not to the contrary." It must be followed continuously, i.e., constantly observed and respected whenever an occasion for its observance or respect arises. Second, it must have a peaceful purpose and be reasonable and not inconsistent with the general spirit of the law. Third, it must be definite rather than vague and must be considered binding on all people. Finally, it must be consistent with all other customs of society.

STARE DECISIS

With the gradual development and extension of use of the common law courts another practical procedure soon became indicated. The administration of justice would have become impossibly slow were it necessary to judge every particular controversy directly against existing written law and custom. There developed, therefore, the doctrine of stare decisis (the decision stands), whereby a rule of law, whether based upon custom or upon being recognized by the courts and thereby applied to the solution of a case, formed a precedent that should be followed in all similar cases thereafter unless subsequently deemed absurd or unjust or unless repealed by the legislature. As summarized by Kent,[9] "A solemn decision upon a point of law arising in any given case becomes an authority in a like case, because it is the highest evidence which we can have of the law applicable to the subject and the judges are bound to follow that decision unless it can be shown that the law was misunderstood or misapplied in that particular case. If a decision

has been made on solemn argument and mature deliberation the presumption is in favor of its correctness; and the community has a right to regard it as a just declaration or exposition of the law, and to regulate their actions and contracts by it. It would, therefore, be extremely inconvenient to the public, if precedents were not duly regarded and implicitly followed."

The American colonies, having been settled primarily by people of Anglo-Saxon origin, had as their original legal basis the written law existing in England at the time of their migration plus the vast volume of common law which had evolved in England up to that time. It naturally followed that there was superimposed upon this an additional and ever increasing amount of common law based upon the social customs that evolved on the new continent. For example, the law governing the state of Indiana consists of:

First. The Constitution of the United States and of this state.
Second. All statutes of the general assembly of the state in force, and not inconsistent with such constitutions.
Third. All statutes of the United States in force, and relating to subjects over which congress has power to legislate for the states, and not inconsistent with the Constitution of the United States.
Fourth. The common law of England, and statutes of the British Parliament made in aid thereof prior to the 4th year of the reign of James I (except the second section of sixth chapter of 43rd Elizabeth, the eighth chapter of 13th Elizabeth, and the ninth chapter of 37th Henry VIII) and which are of a general nature, not local to that kingdom and not inconsistent with the first, second and third specifications of this section.*

Added to this is all the common law evolved in Indiana since the inception of its statehood. Statements similar to this are to be found in the constitutions or statutes of each of the American states with the exception of Louisiana.

EQUITY OR CHANCERY

Up to the time of William the Conqueror (A.D. 1066) the administration of justice was

*Section 1-101 (244) Burns Indiana Statutes Annotated 1933.

limited to the application of existing laws. However, William the Conqueror assumed the doctrine that the sovereign was the ultimate source of all justice and that he himself was above the law. Hence the well-known saying, "The king can do no wrong," developed. Therefore he and the English rulers who followed him for a considerable period dispensed justice as they considered desirable or expeditious.

Thus if some wrong were committed for which the law offered no true remedy or if the plaintiff felt that the law had not given him complete justice, the king could be appealed to for assistance beyond the power of the courts. As common law courts came to depend more and more on precedents as guides in their dispensing of justice, they became more and more rigid. Accordingly, the king was appealed to with increasing frequency, so much so that the king's chancellor, who was otherwise spoken of as the "keeper of the king's conscience," was made responsible. This was eventually followed by the establishment of separate courts of chancery or equity, the essential purpose of which was to render as complete justice and restitution as possible, going beyond the dictates of existing laws if necessary. As time went on, such courts became strictly limited to situations for which no adequate remedy or solution was offered by the regular law courts. Eventually, however, as chancellors and their courts rendered more and more decisions and judgments, they too, as a matter of course, became more or less bound by precedents, sometimes defeating the original purpose of their existence.

This system of equity as a supplement to the written and common law was also brought to America and established as a part of our legal structure. Separate chancery or equity courts still exist in a few states along the Eastern Seaboard and in the Southeast. Otherwise, for practical purposes the same court now sits as a court of law, dispensing strictly legal judgments, and again as a court of equity, administering relief in cases for which the law as it exists offers no remedy. Equity serves as the basis for the proper administration of justice in many cases of public health concern, reference to a few examples of which will be made.

Certain principles have been laid down to define the natural sphere of interest and applicability of equity. They may be summarized as follows:

Equity will not suffer a wrong without a remedy. This is very fundamental, considering the reason for the development of equity.

Equity delights to do justice and not by halves. Thus it is the intention of equity that all interested parties be present in court and that there be rendered a complete judgment adjusting all rights for the plaintiff and preventing future litigation. An example of this is presented by a case* questioning an amendment to a Wisconsin statute relating to the licensing of restaurants. A subsection had been added providing that no permit should be issued to operate or maintain any food-serving business where any other type of business was conducted unless the facilities dealing with the preparation and serving of food were separated from such other business by substantial partitions extending from the floor to the ceiling and with self-closing doors. The provisions of the subsection were applicable only to restaurants commencing business after the effective date of the subsection. In a mandamus proceeding in which it was sought to compel the state board of health to grant a permit to conduct a restaurant, the complainant contended that the added subsection was void under the federal and state constitutions in that it denied due process and equality before the law. The basis for licensing the business involved, said the court, was for the protection of the public health and safety. "If protection of the public health and safety requires partitions in case of a business subsequently to be commenced, then by the same token it requires them in case of existing businesses; and if one operating an existing restaurant is not required to maintain the partition, and one about to establish a restaurant is required to maintain one, then manifestly the latter is denied equal protection with the former." On this basis the supreme court sustained the contention of the complainant, declared the amending subsection void but allowed the existing statute to remain in force, and instructed the board of health to grant the requested permit, thereby adjusting all rights and preventing future litigation.

Equity acts in personam. A law court may merely render a judgment against a person's property rather than against the person himself. For example, the court may command a sheriff to seize and sell enough of the unsuccessful defendant's goods and turn over to the plaintiff sufficient proceeds to meet the money judgment of the court. Equity, on the other hand, commands an indi-

---

*Wisconsin Supreme Court: State ex rel. F. W. Woolworth Co. v. Wisconsin State Board of Health et al., 298 N.W. 183 (1941).

vidual to perform or to refrain from performing whatever acts constitute the subject of the litigation. Such an action by a court of equity is known as injunction. Failure to obey the command of the court places the defendant in contempt of court and, thereby, subject to personal punishment. Thus if the sewage from the premises of one householder gives rise to an intolerable situation on the property of another, the ordinary court of law can merely render a judgment for money damages in favor of the offended property owner. This, however, does not solve the problem since the original nuisance still exists. In equity, however, not only may there be rendered a judgment of cash restitution for damages already done but, in addition, the court may issue an injunction directing the person responsible to abate and prevent the nuisance from recurring in the future.

Equity regards the intention rather than form. This constitutes a weapon against legal decision. Law concerns itself with a strict interpretation of a form of a law transaction, or contract, but equity considers also the intent. This is illustrated by a case* involving the question of whether common-law marriages, which do not necessitate a license, were included under a state law requiring premarital examinations as a prerequisite for marriage licenses. The superior court said that the act was clearly a public health measure designed to assist in the eradication of syphilis, to prevent transmission by a diseased spouse, and to prevent the birth of children with syphilitic weaknesses or deformities and should be construed so as to effectuate its purpose if at all possible. "Certainly," said the court, "the legislature never intended that such an important hygienic statute could be circumvented by the simple device of the parties entering into a common-law marriage without first obtaining a license."

Equity regards that as done which ought to be done. If a contract is broken, the court of law may render a money judgment for damages, whereas equity orders or commands (mandamus) that the contract be specifically performed. This is illustrated by the previously cited case of F. W. Woolworth Company v. Wisconsin State Board of Health et al.

Equity recognizes an intention to fulfill an obligation. If an individual promises or contracts to do a thing or if he has done anything that might be regarded as at least a partial fulfillment of the promise or contract, equity assumes that he intends to do it until the contrary is shown. This has sometimes served as a stumbling block to public health officials. For example, a person maintaining a public health nuisance may necessitate numerous fruitless visits and inspections on the part of public health workers. Finally, as a means of last resort the wrongdoer may be brought to court. If he can demonstrate to the satisfaction of the court that in some although inadequate manner he has followed the suggestions or commands of the public health official, the court may dismiss the case, saying in effect: "Why do you bring this man to court when he is taking steps to meet your requirements?"

Equity follows the law. In accordance with this maxim an equity court will observe existing laws and legal procedures, insofar as possible, without hindering its own function in the administration of justice.

Where there is equal equity, the law must prevail. If both parties to the litigation are judged to have equal rights, the case will be sent back to the law courts where the party with a right in law will have that right enforced.

The logic of this and the previous principle is obvious, considering the purpose for which equity was established. Equity is as an adjunct to law, not a substitute for it.

He who comes into equity must do so with clean hands. If an individual claims a wrong, he himself must be free from a related wrong or the equity court will not listen to him. This was a factor in the well-known Chicago drainage canal case,* in which a court of equity refused a judgment against the city of Chicago for the city of St. Louis, partly on the basis that St. Louis itself contaminated its own public source of water.

He who seeks equity must do equity. This is similar to the previous principle in that not only must the plaintiff have clean hands but he must be and have been willing to do all that is right and fair as a part of a transaction or a judgment.

Equity aids the vigilant, not the indolent. This is known as the doctrine of laches and calls into effect the statute of limitations that fixes definite intervals within which legal action may be instituted after the cause for action has occurred or becomes complete. These time intervals are not the same for all actions and vary further among the states. If a person wishes to receive relief from an equity court, he must be prompt in applying to it. In other words he must not "sleep on his rights."

ADMINISTRATIVE LAW

In the statutory legislation of an earlier day dealing with comparatively simple social and economic structures the understandable attempt was usually made to include in the written statutes a considerable amount of detail with reference to the problem at hand. However, in more recent times, with the accelerating complexity of our social and economic systems and with ever increasing knowledge in all fields, it has become obviously impossible to include

---

*Superior Court of the State of Pennsylvania: Fisher v. Sweet and McClain et al., 35 A 2nd 756 (1944).

*Missouri v. Illinois, 180 U.S. 208, 2 S. Ct. 331, 45 L. Ed. 497 (1901).

within the statutes sufficient detail to cover adequately all of the situations that might arise in the practical application of the true intent of the law. At the same time our governmental structure has become more and more complicated and has had more and more demands placed upon it in the form of public services and regulatory functions previously undreamed of. The relative recency of the modern public health program provides a good example of this. To meet the situation, there have been established by government, on a statutory basis, a considerable and increasing number of administrative agencies set up for the purpose of putting into effect the intent of legislation.

The procedure of passing enabling legislation written in more or less general terms was evolved. This legislation included clauses delegating administration and enforcement to a new or existing administrative agency, giving the agency the power and responsibility to formulate whatever rules, regulations, and standards were necessary for carrying out the purpose of the law. It naturally follows that such powers and responsibilities must be in conformity with all existing laws of the community, the state, and the nation. Thus, although the legislative branch of government is the only body that may actually formulate and enact a law and although this power cannot itself be delegated, the legislature may delegate the power to make whatever rules and regulations are necessary to carry out the intent of the law. (In some states even administrative rules and regulations must be reviewed and approved by the state attorney general.) All such administrative rules and regulations, when properly formulated and when not in conflict with existing laws of the state and nation, have all the force and effect of law even though they arise from an administrative agency and not from the legislature itself. However, their interpretation by the courts tends to be somewhat more rigid than the interpretation placed upon the enactments of the legislature itself.

CLASSIFICATION OF LAW

From the point of view of consolidation it might be desirable to include a few words on the classification of law. Perhaps the simplest method of classifying laws is (1) by origin and (2) by application.

From the point of view of origin law may be classified as follows:

Constitutional law—law developed by specially designated bodies or legislatures convened for the purpose of framing or amending a constitution
Statutory law—legislation which may arise from either representative assemblies or by the process of initiative and referendum
Decree or administrative law—rules, regulations, standards, orders, etc. issued by executive or administrative boards or officers within the sphere of their legal competence and responsibility in order to carry out the intent of statutory laws
Common law and equity—decisions made by courts in specific cases

From the point of view of application law may be classified as follows:

Public law—law concerned with the establishment, maintenance, and operation of government; the definition, relationships, and regulation of its various branches; and the relationship of the individual or of groups to the state
1. *Constitutional law*—deals with the basic nature, structure, and function of the state in relation to the powers of the various branches of government; sometimes includes a bill of rights
2. *Administrative law*—as discussed previously
3. *Criminal law*—concerned with offenses or acts against the public welfare and safety, such being considered as offenses against the state and varying from petty offenses and misdemeanors to felonies

Private law—law concerned with the rights and duties of individuals and groups in relation to each other; it was originally based largely on common law but is increasingly becoming subject to statutes.

COURTS

American government is based on the wise principle of the separation of powers. Accordingly, legislation can be formulated, considered, and ultimately enacted only by the legislative branch. After its enactment the legislature has no further concern with a law except for the possibility of subsequent amendment or repeal. On passage a law is referred to the executive branch of government for its administration and enforcement. However, the constitutionality of the law and the manner of its enforcement are subject to review at any time on the initiative of the citizenry by the third or judicial branch of government, which is manifest by the actions of the courts. It is the duty of the courts to pass upon the constitutionality of laws, to interpret them in the interest of justice and the public good, and to determine their validity whenever controversies related to them are brought before the court in the proper manner.

The jurisdiction of the court may be either original or appellate; i.e., the courts may be a place where the merits of a controversy are originally passed upon, or they may be a place to which an unsuccessful and dissatisfied litigant may appeal for a review of the action taken by a court of original jurisdiction. Using the judicial system of the states as a point of departure, their courts may be divided into three categories. At the top are the superior courts, including the state supreme court, the superior court, the court of appeal, or the court of civil appeals. Such courts usually have five to nine justices who hear appeal cases from the lower courts of the state and who have in some instances varying amounts of original jurisdiction. Appeals may be taken from here to the Supreme Court of the United States if the case involves the federal Constitution, federal laws, or treaties. Below the state superior courts are the intermediate courts, including the circuit courts, the district courts, the county courts, and the common pleas courts, the terminology differing in different states. These are courts of original jurisdiction and the first two hear appeals from lower courts in some states. In other states these functions are separated. It is to be noted that a county court, although locally elected and locally responsible for the administration of its verdicts, is actually part of the state judicial system. On the lowest or most local level are the locally elected justices of the peace, who in effect individually constitute the lowest rung on the state judicial ladder.

In addition, a state may set up certain special courts to deal with particular social problems such as juvenile delinquency, domestic relations, industrial relations, etc. On the municipal level of government, by virtue of a charter granted by a state government, an urban community may have the privilege of setting up certain courts of its own to administer justice in cases involving problems of concern limited to the municipality itself. Thus there are police courts with original jurisdiction in minor matters and municipal courts with original jurisdiction in more important cases and also serving as a place of appeal from the police court.

On the federal level is the Supreme Court of the United States, consisting of a chief justice and eight associates, to which cases may be appealed from the lower federal courts and state supreme courts in instances where the federal Constitution, laws, or treaties are considered to be involved. In addition it has some original jurisdiction in interstate, maritime, and some other matters (see Article III, Section 2, of the Constitution and the Eleventh Amendment). To expedite the federal judicial system a number of intermediate courts have been established. Thus there are 10 federal circuit courts with appellate jurisdiction and below them over 90 federal district courts, which are the principal federal courts of original jurisdiction. There are, in addition, federal courts for special purposes such as the Customs Courts and the Federal Court of Claims. There might also be mentioned the increasing number of federal administrative boards, e.g., the National Labor Relations Board, which have a certain amount of delegated original jurisdiction.

SOURCES OF PUBLIC HEALTH LAW

Public health law may be defined as that body of statutes, regulations, and precedents that has for its purpose the protection and promotion of individual and community health. While the term "public health" was not entirely unknown to contemporaries of the authors of the American Constitution, its present-day sense and significance were undreamed of. After all, there was no public health profession in existence, and science was not to enter the golden era of bacteriology until about 100 years later. Three quarters of a century were to pass before the need for establishment of the first state health department was to be felt. Still 40 years more were to pass before the formation of the first county health department. The founders of our country cannot be censured, therefore, for not considering public health functions specifically in their organization of the new government. They were so remarkably astute and farsighted, however, as to provide for future developments in many fields by the use of certain broad and general phrases that in subsequent periods were to make possible broad interpretations of the Constitution, thereby allowing the introduction and inclusion of certain public health activities in the functions of the federal government.

By far the most important of these broad phrases is that occurring in the Preamble to the Constitution, which includes among the fundamental purposes of the government the intent to "promote the general welfare." This recurs again in Section 8 of Article I, which, dealing with the functions of Congress, gives it power "to lay and collect taxes . . . and provide for the common defense and general welfare . . ." It is the generous interpretation of this by the Supreme Court which has made possible the activity of the Children's Bureau in maternal and child health and the subsidization by means of federal grants-in-aid of state and local health programs by the Public Health Service. In fact, these federal agencies owe their very existence in large part to the intent that has been read into the "general welfare" phrase.

In addition, the varied and widespread activities of the federal government in fields relating to health have as their legal basis the manner in which numerous other clauses of the Constitution have been interpreted. Thus the direction to Congress "to regulate commerce with foreign nations, and among the several states, and with the Indian tribes" has been construed to include such matters as international and interstate quarantine, sanitary supervision, vital statistics, and direct responsibility for the health of the American Indians. The provision for the establishment of "post offices and post roads" has led to the right of the federal government to bar from the mails material deleterious to the public health. The power "to raise and support armies" and to "provide and maintain a navy" logically placed responsibility for the health of the armed forces (in recent years a not inconsiderable fraction of the population) in the hands of federal agencies. Complete and exclusive jurisdiction over the inhabitants of the seat of the national government (the District of Columbia) is also specified.

The reader may be reminded at this point that the United States, far from being one nation, is in a very true sense a federation of 50 separate nations, called states, each with its own history, economic and social problems, and still somewhat jealously guarded intrastate interests. It will be recalled that the members of the constitutional convention carefully guarded the rights of their respective states, jointly turning over to the newly formed federal government only such powers and activities as they felt desirable and necessary for the common welfare and survival of all. Matters which they could adequately handle as individual states were retained by the states. Therefore the federal government truly was and is a creature of jointly concurred action of the several states. Since the beginning it has been inferred that all matters not specifically mentioned in the Constitution and its subsequent Amendments were questions to be dealt with primarily by the states. It is for this reason that we find the more complete and coordinated organization of public health activities on the state and local levels. Each state has developed its own characteristic body of legislation and judicial interpretation as well as its own characteristic type of organization for the implementation of its public health laws, being in a position to do very much as it wishes within the limitations of interstate and international conflict. Although we have these 50 differing sets of public health laws and organizations, certain fundamental legal principles, however, are involved in all. It is to a brief discussion of some of these fundamentals that we must now turn for further consideration of sources of public health powers.

EMINENT DOMAIN

The first of the basic powers of a state is that of eminent domain, sometimes referred to as the power of condemnation. This is the power or right of a sovereign state to summarily appropriate an individual's property or to limit his use of it if the best interest of the community makes such action desirable. In so doing, however, the state must provide an equitable compensation. In effect the state has the right to demand the sale or limitation of use of private property. The distinction between the exercise of the power of eminent domain and actions upon which legislatures may insist without compensation is not clear cut at any given time and varies from time to time. The history of zoning measures to control the height of buildings has been cited as a good example of this. At first the state attempted to control the height of buildings by purchasing from individuals their primary right to build on their own property above the height that was considered most desirable from the community standpoint. Since this action was upheld in the courts, it was resorted to by more and more people in more and more communities until it got to the point where, as one writer[10] aptly stated, it resembled the economy of the mythical village of Ballycannon, where everyone made his living by taking in his next door neighbor's washing. In other words, when resorted to on a wide scale, use of the power of eminent domain amounts to individuals' (as taxpayers) purchasing the exercise of a right from themselves as private citizens. Inevitably such a procedure becomes ineffective as a measure of control. Recognizing this, the public through its legislatures may finally say, "We shall forbid this particular action or use by the individual," and the courts more often than not will uphold the action.

In a certain sense the procedure followed by some health departments in the past of paying an allotment to chronic carriers of typhoid bacilli in order to make sure of their refraining from engaging in food-handling occupations represented the purchase by the state of an individual's primary right. The states in most instances finally simply forbade such activity by these persons.

As pointed out by Ascher,[10] it is interesting to note that those who attempted to bring about a form of building control that eliminated the necessity of compensation deliberately avoided a test case for about 10 years. Finally, when the Ambler Realty Company protested the restriction of its use of land by the village of Euclid,* the United States Supreme Court upheld this arbitrary use of the police power in a sweeping opinion that had as one of its basic contentions that over 900 cities were already subject to zoning and about one half of the urban dwellers of the nation lived under the benefits of zoning procedures. This is perhaps another way of saying that within a relatively short period of time the social concept of zoning had become part of the custom of American communities and that its requirement could be considered as having become part of the common law.

LAWS OF NUISANCES
(NOSCITUR AD SOCIIS)

Long before our nation and its government were conceived, the concept was developed by medieval legal theorists that, while "a man's home is his castle," an individual's use of his private property could be detrimental to others. The use of private property is unrestricted only so long as it does not injure another's person or property. If this occurred, a nuisance was considered to exist and the individual whose person or property was injured could seek assistance from the courts. Innumerable examples of this exist in the field of public health, especially with regard to the salubrity of the physical environment. For example, an individual property owner has the right to dispose of his sewage in any manner that he may see fit, provided that it cannot actually or potentially affect another. If he allows raw sewage to flow onto the land of another, a social injustice has obviously occurred and the health and well-being of others have been placed in jeopardy. Legal relief against nuisances may be obtained in the courts by means of (1) a suit of law for damages resulting or (2) a

---

*Village of Euclid v. Ambler Reality Co., 272 U.S. 365 (1926).

suit in equity to forbid or abate the nuisance.

It is perhaps unfortunate that a large proportion of public health officials still consider the use of the law of nuisances as one of their most important if not their chief legal recourse. The pursuit of this point of view eventually leads to many difficulties and dissatisfactions since the law of nuisances is subject to increasing limitations. Some of these limitations are discussed below.

In the first place there are many things or uses of things that do not intrinsically constitute a nuisance but are merely in the wrong place. An example of this is provided by the case of Benton et al. v. Pittard, Health Commissioner, et al.,* in which the plaintiff protested the establishment and operation by a health department of a venereal disease clinic in a residential district. The complaints were that the disease of the patients who would congregate in the neighborhood "were not only communicable but were offensive, obnoxious and disgusting; that the clinic operation would be offensive to the petitioners and that their sensibility would be injured; and that their dwelling would be rendered less valuable as a home and place of residence." The defending health officer and county commissioner filed an answer and a general demurrer, a form of pleading that, while admitting all the facts, challenged their legal sufficiency to constitute a cause of action. The judge, after hearing both sides, denied the plaintiff's request for an injunction and sustained the demurrer. On being appealed, however, the Georgia Supreme Court stated that the fact that the clinic was to be operated as a public institution would not alone prevent it from becoming a nuisance if located in a residential section and that the statutory provision requiring the care of venereally infected persons did not imply the right to perform such care in any location. "In other words, a nuisance may consist merely of the right thing in the wrong place regardless of other circumstances." On this basis the

judgment of the original trial court was reversed.

Another factor tending to limit the value of the law of nuisances is that a great many of the legal doctrines and decisions dealing with nuisances and their abatement were developed before the germ theory of disease became accepted scientific fact. During most of its development there existed no obvious factual or scientific data on which to base conclusions, and those appearing in court in such cases were merely pitting their opinions against the opinions of others. This left the court as its only final recourse the expression of its own opinion. As a result there has been built up a mass of unsound and unscientific decisions, which, because they are precedents, continue to influence the public health problems of present-day communities. This also explains in part why many supposedly modern health departments are required to expend much time, energy, and funds in activities that have little relationship to public health, e.g., garbage and refuse control.

Still another difficulty is caused by the fact that recourse to the law of nuisances does not overcome one of the rules of law. Decision by a law court that a nuisance exists may result in damages being paid to the plaintiff but does not necessarily effect the solution or abatement of the noisome circumstances. There is, of course, the possibility of resorting to a court of equity with the hope of obtaining complete justice. However, here again it is found that a rule of equity may provide a way out for the defendant in that if he can demonstrate to the court's satisfaction his intention or, better yet, partial action to abate the nuisance, the case in all probability will be dismissed from court. The thought might arise that the situation could be improved by trying to bring about more up-to-date judicial interpretations and judgments regarding nuisances. Although theoretically possible, the task involved in order to accomplish this would be enormous. Furthermore, even if modern present-day standards could be made the basis of definition, these standards and definitions might become outmoded with the passage of time.

---

*Georgia Supreme Court: Benton et al. v. Pittard, Health Commissioner, et al. 31 S.E. 2nd 6.

POLICE POWER*

There remains another means of legal recourse for the public health official to consider, i.e., the police power that the sovereign state possesses. As a matter of fact, public health law owes its true origin and only real effectiveness to this inherent right of the state. Police power originated in the so-called law of overruling necessity, which claims that in times of stress such as fire, pestilence, etc., the private property of an individual might be summarily appropriated, used, or even destroyed if the ultimate relief, protection, or safety of the group indicated such action as necessary. Through time this concept expanded to include even activities designed for the prevention of causes of social stress. The United States Supreme Court has on numerous occasions not only upheld the principle of the police power of the state but also has defined its scope in sweeping terms to include, as did Chief Justice Marshall, all types of public health laws and to acknowledge the power of the states to provide for the health of their citizens.† It should be noted, however, as Justice Brown stated, that ". . . its [legislature's] determination as to what is a proper exercise of its police powers is not final or conclusive but is subject to the supervision of the court."‡

One of the best definitions of the police power was given in the case of Miami County v. Dayton,§ in which the court defined it as "that inherent sovereignty which the government exercises whenever regulations are demanded by public policy for the benefit of the society at large in order to guard its morals, safety, health, order and the like in accordance with the needs of civilization."

Although the possession of police power is fundamentally that of the sovereign state, the legislature of the state may for practical purposes delegate it to an administrative agency acting as its functional agent. The

use of the police power is not a matter of choice when it has been delegated to a governmental agency. The agency has a definite and legal responsibility to use it and further is accountable for the manner in which it is used. When the means for action are made available to him, the public officer responsible may be compelled to exercise the police power delegated to him if the public interest indicates such action. Failure to do so makes the public official guilty of malfeasance of office. However, although application of the police power may be indicated and demanded, the manner in which it is employed is usually left to the discretion of the administrative officer; i.e., the public officer may select his own methods of enforcement, formulating rules, regulations, and standards as he deems necessary unless the statutes that made him responsible specifically prescribed the method of procedure.

The position of a public health officer in this regard, as related to the summary abatement of a nuisance, was well stated by the Iowa Supreme Court in a case* involving such action by a health department in enforcing an ordinance dealing with the improper and indiscriminate dumping of garbage. In upholding the action of the board of health the court stated that, although nothing in the statute granted to the officers immunity from the consequences of unfair or oppressive acts, "the particular form of procedure prescribed may vary from the customary procedure, but essential rights are not violated by granting to the board the right, in an emergency, to proceed in the abatement of a nuisance detrimental to public health, and it is safe to say that most cases calling for action on the part of boards of health are matters requiring immediate action." Of perhaps greater significance, the court went on to say that, even though the courts had not been uniform in their holdings, it believed that the weight of authority as well as reason and necessity prescribed that in cases involving the public health, where prompt and efficient action was neces-

*For a more detailed discussion, see *The Police Power* by Freund.[11]
†Perhaps the best known case is Gibbons v. Ogden, 9 Wheat. 1, 6 L. Ed. 23 (1824).
‡Lawton v. Steele, 152 U.S. 133 (1893).
§Miami County v. Dayton, 92 O.S. 215.

*Iowa Supreme Court: State v. Strayer, 299 N.W. 912 (1941).

sary, the state and its officers should not be subjected to the inevitable delays incident to a complete hearing before action could be taken.

The careful distinction between the power of inspection and the right of privacy has become increasingly important as a result of a recent ruling of the California District Court of Appeals.* The court held that the entry by a health inspector into a private residence for the purpose of a routine housing inspection at a reasonable time and on presentation of proper credentials was not a violation of the Fourth or Fourteenth Amendments of the United States Constitution. "The court reasoned that the ordinance in question was part of a general regulatory scheme which was civil in nature, limited in scope, and could not be exercised except under reasonable conditions." The court then defined the conditions in which privacy may be restrained. "In those areas of exercise of the police power where the chance of immediate tangible harm is present, such as in premises which might present fire or communicable disease hazards, the right of privacy most probably will be accorded only that constitutional protection that is given to property or economic rights. In intimate or personal activities not at all likely to cause immediate danger to life or limb, the right of privacy will approach the more protected constitutional position of freedom of expression."[12]

The right of a legislature to delegate rulemaking power to an administrative agency has been questioned many times, but only in one instance has such power been denied to a state or local board of health. This occurred in Wisconsin,† where it was held that the State Board of Health was simply an administrative agency and that no rulemaking powers could constitutionally be delegated to it. On the other hand, the Ohio Supreme Court stated "that the legislature in the exercise of its constitutional authority may lawfully confer on boards of health the power to enact sanitary ordinances having the force of law within the district over

which their jurisdiction extends, is not an open question."* The question was more or less settled by the United States Supreme Court, which held the following:

(1) That a State may, consistently with the Federal Constitution, delegate to a municipality authority to determine under what conditions health shall become operative.

(2) That the municipality may vest in its efficiency broad discretion in matters affecting the applicability and enforcement of a health law.

(3) That in the exercise of the police power reasonable classification may be freely applied and that regulation is not violative of the equal protection clause merely because it is not all-embracing.†

It is obvious and logical that a municipality or an administrative agency in dealing, for example, with questions concerning the public health can act only when it has been given specific authority for such actions and that the ordinances adopted by the legislative body of the municipality must not only be limited to the subject matter of the power delegated but also must not conflict with or attempt to set aside any provision of the Constitution, of the state law, or of any other sanitary regulations of the state. The same conditions apply to regulations adopted by local boards of health. They can apply only where the subject matter has been placed by law under the jurisdiction of the local board of health.

POLICE POWER, ADMINISTRATIVE LAW, AND JUDICIAL PRESUMPTION

The delegation to administrative agencies and officers of the right and power to formulate rules, regulations, and standards in order to implement the intent of legislation has given rise to a relatively new and increasingly important branch of law and source of enforcement powers. It is unfortunate that in the public health profession there are still many who do not adequately realize the great administrative possibilities presented by sound administrative

---

*Camara v. San Francisco, 277 A.C.A. 136 (1965).
†State v. Burdge, 95, Wis. 390, 70 N.W. 347 (1897).

*Exparte Co. 106 O.S. 50.
†Zucht v. King, 260 U.S. 174, 43 S. Ct. 24 (1922).

law.* There are many communities which, although sometimes possessing adequate enabling legislation for various public health activities, have only limited control because of the failure of their health officials to make the rules, regulations, and standards necessary for the proper and adequate implementation of the statutes. By failing to form a solid background based as much as possible on sound scientific criteria, the public health official by his own neglect places himself, his department, and the community at an unnecessary and unwarranted disadvantage. Mentioned in the discussion of the law of nuisances was the undesirable possibility of the public health official being in the position of pitting his mere opinion against that of the defendant. The court's only alternative in such a situation would be to express its own opinion regarding the desirability of the action rather than its legality. Ideally it is only the latter with which the courts are essentially concerned, and as much as possible it is preferable that they not have to make decisions regarding the sense or desirability of an action. When a scientist, a health officer, or another expert is in a position to provide the court with definite regulations and standards based on scientific criteria or group judgment, especially if they have been drawn up with the idea of administering legal advice, the judge of the court is no longer in the somewhat embarrassing position of having to balance what amounts to the personal opinion of the plaintiff against that of the defendant and then being himself forced to make a decision by expressing his own personal opinion. The very existence of sound rules, regulations, and standards serves to pass the burden of proof from the administrative agent to the defendant in the case so that the judge can avoid conflict and save time and face by saying, for example, that the defendant has not presented evidence to show that the health officer did not fairly apply the rules, regulations, or standards that by virtue of their development are more or less accepted without question. Thus there has been

established what is termed a judicial presumption in favor of the findings, conclusions, and recommendations of the enforcing administrative official.

In order to obtain the maximum amount of judicial presumption certain conditions are desirable and should be borne in mind. First, laws and ordinances should contain only broad principles with delegation of authority to the enforcing or administrative agency for the development of the necessary details. Second, such rules, regulations, and standards as may be indicated by the law or ordinance should be carefully formulated. Third, they should be based as much as possible on accepted scientific facts or authoritative group judgments. Fourth, it is desirable that they be written with the aid of an administrative lawyer. Fifth, advantage should be taken of the opportunity presented in the process of making the rules, regulations, and standards to lay the foundation for their ready acceptance by the public and the courts of the community. This is meant to imply that the process presents an important opportunity for education and persuasion as well as democratic participation. If those who are to be affected are consulted in the writing of a regulation, they will develop in the process an understanding which is a first step toward voluntary cooperation, acceptance, and self-enforcement. At the same time the public health administrator is provided an invaluable opportunity to determine in advance how far the community is willing to go.

LICENSING

A related method of legal enforcement and control is found in the technique of licensing. The legality of the principle of licensing as a method of control and enforcement as well as a source of revenue to meet the cost of the administration of a law has been well established and accepted for a long while. However, intent and methods of licensing are constantly subject to questioning in the courts as are all other methods of enforcement. Licenses may be granted or revoked under conditions imposed by public health authorities provided

*For a more detailed discussion, see *Administrative Law—Cases and Comments* by Gellhorn.[13]

that there is a statutory basis for the licensing and there is no oppressive, discriminatory, or arbitrary action involved in their application.

An example to illustrate the latter is that of a city board of health which voted that after a certain date no more milk distributor licenses would be granted to persons who were not residents of the city.* The plaintiff operated a well-qualified dairy 6 miles beyond the city limits and brought suit to compel the issuance of a license, charging that the regulation was discriminatory. The state law said, "Boards of health may grant licenses to sell milk to properly qualified persons." The court held that the word "may" in the state law should be construed as meaning "shall" so that a local board of health, existing by virtue of state law, had no alternative but to issue a license to any person who satisfied the sanitary requirements. More pertinent to the question at hand, it further held that the limitation on nonresidents was unreasonable and arbitrary and that if it had been included in a law instead of a resolution it would have been ruled unconstitutional.

On several occasions licensing has been found useful by health authorities in accomplishing a certain amount of indirect control and prevention of problems not obvious from the primary purpose of the licensing. Several communities, for instance, have found it necessary to institute the licensing of individuals engaged in certain personal service occupations such as masseurs and beauty parlor operators in an attempt to stop advertising by prostitutes operating under the guise of these occupations. This particular use has caused no difficulty since the right of health departments to maintain sanitary control over individuals engaged in personal services in order to prevent the spread of communicable diseases has been well established.

However, when an ordinance requiring permits or licenses can be shown to have no public health basis, it will probably be considered an infringement of personal

rights by the court and declared invalid. This is illustrated by the case* of a city board of health that passed a regulation providing that no person should engage in the business of undertaking unless he had been duly licensed as an embalmer by the board of health. The Massachusetts Supreme Court held the regulation unconstitutional and invalid, saying, "We can see no such connection between requiring all undertakers to be licensed embalmers and the promotion of the public health as to bring the making of this regulation by the board of registration in embalming or the refusal of a license by the board of health on account of the regulation within the exercise of the police power of the state."

NECESSITY OF BASIC PUBLIC HEALTH LAWS

In a DeLamar lecture given in 1920, Dr. Allen W. Freeman,[14] who was at that time Commissioner of Health of Ohio, said: "Every thoughtful sanitarian has in his mind the picture of that ideal system of health administration which would be founded on scientific principles, organized on the basis of administrative efficiency, and manned by a staff of trained workers filled with the spirit of public service. This ideal organization would have behind it a volume of law which, while fully recognizing the principles of individual liberty, would permit no man to offend against the health of his neighbor." Although Dr. Freeman added with considerable justification, "However thoughtfully a proposed measure may be prepared by its framers, it has by the time it is enacted into law usually been so altered by ill-considered, hasty or prejudiced amendment as to have lost all semblance of its original form," there may be considered to advantage some of the fields of public health activity in which fundamental legislation is desirable or necessary. The first of these is concerned with the registration or reporting of births and deaths. It is conceded by all to be well-nigh impossible to carry out a public health pro-

---

*Whitney v. Watson, 85 N.H. 238, 157 A. 78 (1931).

*Wyeth v. Cambridge Board of Health, 200 Mass. 474, 86 N.E. 295 (1909).

gram in the absence of basic information concerning the circumstances surrounding nativity and death. In most parts of this country it is the public health agency that is charged with the responsibility for assuring the collection of this information. In order to achieve this, it is necessary that each state have the necessary legislation and administrative machinery dealing with mandatory reporting of these biologic events by those in the best positions to submit such reports, the attendants at births and deaths. Related to this is the need for legislation requiring the reporting and control of cases of certain types of illnesses, especially those of a communicable nature. To accomplish this adequately requires careful and exact definition of certain terms such as cases, communicable, isolation, etc. and the listing of the morbid conditions to be included. In accord with what has been said elsewhere, such defining and listing is best accomplished by inclusion in the rules and regulations drawn up by the administrative agency rather than in the body of the statute, which should limit its concern to broad principles, responsibilities, and penalties. The desirability of this is particularly evident on considering the spectacular changes that have occurred in recent years in the areas of diagnosis, treatment, and social management of many of the communicable diseases. If details of reporting and control appear in the law, further scientific advances are certain to result either in the necessity of changing the law or allowing it to become hopelessly out of date.

In the field of food and milk control an enormous, confusing, and very often contradictory mass of legislation and regulation exists. Undesirable as this situation undoubtedly is, all will agree that certain types of legal control are necessary. It is obviously important for a community to exercise some control over those who produce and handle its food and milk supplies.* This has been repeatedly upheld in the courts. With reference to milk, the Con-

necticut Supreme Court explained in an opinion, "The State may determine the standard of quality, prohibit the production, sale, or distribution of milk not within the standard, divide it into classes, and regulate the manner of their use, so long as these standards, classes, and regulatory provisions be neither unreasonable nor oppressive. The many recorded instances in which the courts have sustained this power of regulation bear witness to the liberality of their viewpoint where the public health and safety are concerned."* Judicial prejudice in favor of rules, regulations, and standards dealing with the sanitary quality of food and milk supplies has been extended far beyond the actual product itself. It has long been accepted as proper for the responsible health authority to formulate rules, regulations, and standards dealing with the sources of food and milk, the health and sanitation practices of all who come in contact with them, the sanitary facilities provided such persons, and the sanitary nature of all machinery, instruments, or utensils involved in their transfer from the source to the ultimate consumer.

In the field of general sanitation, including the sanitary problems involved in housing and industry as well as the supervision of water supplies, sewage disposal, and the like, basic legislation is necessary in order to place responsibility in the hands of the public health agency and to give it such powers as are needed in order to activate the intent of the law. Licensing of certain trades and occupations has been mentioned briefly. It is obvious that before such a procedure can be put into effect the necessary legal justification must be brought into existence.

Perhaps the most fundamental of all is enabling legislation for the establishment and development of local work. It should go without saying that a local area being ultimately subject to the state must be granted the legal right to establish official activity dealing with the public health. The rapid expansion in recent years of local health work, especially on the county level,

*See *Legal Aspects of Milk Control* by Tobey[15] and *The Legal Phases of Milk Control*.[16]

*Shelton v. City of Shelton, 111 Conn. 433 (1930).

has developed increasing interest in the proper formulation of such enabling acts. In the first national conference on local health units held in 1946, Dr. Harry S. Mustard[17] summarized the essentials that should be included in enabling legislation for local health work. These essentials are included here for their conciseness and inclusiveness:

1. That this volume of law should provide assurance that there is a proper balance between local autonomy and state supervision.
2. That this volume of law should provide insurance that where a local unit of government is too small for effective public health administration, combinations of local jurisdictions may be made.
3. Insurance that health work locally will not be scattered among different elements of the local government.
4. Insurance that budgets for local health units be sufficient to meet at least a minimum in terms of funds, and to meet standards as to personnel.
5. No local jurisdiction will remain in want of health service, merely because of unfavorable financial position locally.
6. Supplementary to this insurance that even the poor areas will be included, there should be insurance that there will be adequate state aid.
7. Insurance that the whole state system of local health units will not be jeopardized by local option.

A valuable summary of recent state legal practice in this regard is available as a result of a study in 1952 by the Public Health Service.[18]

WRITING AND PASSAGE OF LAWS AND REGULATIONS

To complete the discussion of court actions, we should consider a statement by Tobey[19]: "These cases also demonstrate that the actions of public health authorities must be conducted in a strictly legal manner, with due guarantee of the constitutional rights of individual citizens and the people as a whole. If regulations or procedures are defective, the courts have no choice but to uphold the law as it should be, and this they will do despite their willingness to support all reasonable public health measures. Public health officials must bear in mind that prevention applies to law as well as to sanitary science, and they should see to it that legislation and law enforcement comply with adjudicated standards and modern jurisprudence."

In accord with this it might be well to consider briefly a few practical considerations with regard to the proper formulation of laws and regulations. Before doing so, it is worth repeating at least two important legislative handicaps to effective administration.* The first of these is that in the formulation and passage of statutes legislatures often attempt to do too much by writing into the law itself too much detail with regard to administrative responsibilities, organization, itemized appropriations, and procedure. In at least one state, for example, the salaries of the state health officer and others are specifically limited in the state constitution, ignoring economic changes, competition for good administrative personnel, and progress in general. As a result this particular state, during a period of high living costs and generally increased salaries, finds itself unable to obtain or hold qualified personnel for the administration of its public health program. The thought comes to mind that in the sound administration of a private corporation the board of directors, being somewhat analogous to a legislature, does not attempt to decide on details of procedure, operation, and the like.

The second legislative handicap is the sacrificing of long-term considerations to immediate, local, or personal advantage. It is possible to find many examples of this in the field of public health. In more than one place, legislation and appropriation have been passed supposedly for the control of tuberculosis or syphilis, but have emphasized the care of the chronic cases and ignored the all-important factor of early case finding and control of the early infectious phase in the individual. The logical solution to these handicaps may be found in the passage of legislation that considers general policy and leaves the details of procedure and operation to whatever ad-

---

*See *New Horizons in Public Administration* by White.[20]

ministrative agency the legislature may see fit to hold responsible. This, of course, requires that administrative agencies assume their full responsibility in carrying out the intent of the statutes by adequately and effectively formulating and enforcing whatever rules, regulations, and standards are indicated.

It is customary in the United States for responsibility for the public health to be vested in a board of health that is directed to employ as its agent a health officer and whatever other personnel are needed in order to carry out its policies. It is much better that rules, regulations, and standards be passed by someone other than the enforcement officer. The public then feels that it is being treated more fairly and that the enforcement officer is not grinding his own axe. In turn the health officer is relieved of the onus of enforcing his own regulations and the risk of repeated personal liability. This alone presents an important justification for the interposing of boards of health between the legislative body and the functioning agency. With these words of introduction the following suggestions are made concerning the formulation of rules and regulations by public health agencies:

1. First is the necessity that they be promulgated by a board of health or whatever other administrative agency in which this authority and responsibility is vested. Furthermore, the agency must have been properly created and legally existing in the eyes of the legislature. If any of its members have been improperly chosen, elected, or appointed, the entire board does not legally exist and all of its actions are considered invalid.

2. The actions of the board must arise by virtue of power and responsibility that has been expressly or impliedly delegated to it by the state legislature.

3. The pronouncements of the board must relate and be limited to its legal jurisdiction and not infringe upon the jurisdiction of another agency or another governmental entity.

4. The rules and regulations must not conflict with the Constitution and laws of the United States or with the constitution and laws of the state of which the agency is a part.

5. The rules and regulations must be reasonable and no more drastic than is necessary.

6. All rules, regulations, and standards must be adopted by a legally constituted board of health legally convened in an official session. No indi-

vidual member of a board has power to enact a regulation any more than an individual Congressman has power to enact a statute. Final enactment can result only by a vote at a properly called meeting of the board, notice of which has been given to each of the members of the board and at which a quorum is present. To attempt to act on a regulation by means of telephoning or visiting the office or home of each member individually does not constitute action by a legally convened meeting of the board.

7. Since a board of health regulation is in effect a law, it follows that the same care should be exercised in its formulation as is exercised in drawing up a state or federal statute. The first consideration in this regard is proper form (including a title and enacting clause), a series of consecutively numbered articles each related to one subject, a statement concerning the time when the regulation is to become effective, and a statement of penalties involved in instances of proved infraction.

8. The ordinance or regulation must be precise, definite, and certain in its expression and meaning. Complicated high-sounding phrases should be avoided, punctuation used sparingly, and parenthesis almost never. Foreign or technical terms should be avoided if possible. It has been often said that there can be a lawsuit for each extraneous or ill-chosen word and for every ill-advised punctuation.

9. If the legislature prescribes the manner in which regulations and ordinances should be passed, such prescription must be exactly adhered to. If, for example, it is specified in the state law that a proposed ordinance be read and voted upon favorably at three successive meetings of a legally constituted and convened board, this cannot be fulfilled as has been sometimes attempted by having the clerk stand and read the ordinance and call for a vote three times during the same meeting.

10. The ordinance or regulation must be enacted in good faith and in the public interest alone and designed to enable the board of health to carry out its legal responsibilities. It should therefore be impartial and nondiscriminatory, applying to all members of the community.

11. In some states it is necessary that actions of boards of health be approved by the attorney general of the state.

12. On legal passage the final step is proper and adequate publication of the rule or ordinance in order that those who are to be affected by it shall have ample opportunity to be informed concerning it.[21] This is usually carried out by means of publishing in the local newspapers.

Concerning this last requisite, Gellhorn[13] makes the following comment: "Regarding publication of administrative legislation the situation, especially in the states, is confusing almost to the extreme and eventual reform is certain to be demanded as a result of this disregard of the public interest in knowing what rules and orders they are subject to. Such lack of adequate publication has undoubtedly led to judicial hostility toward delegated legislation and authority."

A final caution might be given concerning frequent practice of adoption or incorporation of rules and regulations by reference. This procedure has the enticement of being convenient and easy but may give rise to legal difficulties in that only existing things can be legally incorporated by reference. Therefore each time the original regulation or law is changed, it is necessary to reincorporate by reference. Furthermore, it is legally impossible, although it is sometimes attempted, to adopt or incorporate a subject by reference on a blanket basis through time because such action amounts to committing the public to regulations that are not yet in existence. It is comparable to asking the public to sign a blank check.

This is not meant to entirely condemn the technique of reference since its convenience amply justifies its use. However, it should be used with full knowledge of its limitations and potential disadvantages, some of which are illustrated by the case* of a board of health that adopted a regulation dealing with the sale of milk and milk products in accordance with the unabridged form of the 1939 edition of the United States Public Health Service Milk Ordinance. The publication of the new regulation did not contain the ordinance but stated that a certified copy was on file in the office of the board of health. The Ohio Supreme Court in ruling on the case of a defendant charged with violating the regulation, stated: "The effectiveness of legislation by reference has been so generally recognized . . . that no very specific declaration appears in the reported cases." The court added, however, that "no by-law or ordinance, or section thereof, shall be revived or amended unless the new by-law or ordinance contains the entire by-law or ordinance, or section revived or amended,

and the by-law or ordinance, section or sections so amended shall be repealed." So long as there was no violation of this section, the court said that it saw no objection to the incorporation by reference in a regulation of a district board of health of a duly enacted statute or a duly enacted ordinance that had been theretofore properly published. However, the Supreme Court was of the view that the publication of a board of health regulation, which omitted the rules of conduct to be observed and merely referred those who might be affected to a copy of the terms on file in the office of the board of health, did not constitute proper publication as meant by the law and that until proper publication had been made any such regulation was not effective.

LIABILITY AND AGENCY*

In order to accomplish a desired purpose such as the completion of a contract or the rendering of a public service, practicality usually makes it necessary that the one (the principal) who is legally responsible for fulfilling the contract or for rendering the public service obtain an agent or agents to carry out the details involved. This relationship between a principal and his agents gives rise to an additional series of legal complications, especially in terms of those things for which the principal is liable and those for which the agent is liable. In public health work the citizens of a community as represented by their legally designated board of health may be considered the principal, whereas the health officer acts as the agent of the people and is responsible to the board.

This view has been held repeatedly by the courts, as illustrated by two cases[†] in which the courts observed that the authority for the appointment of a city health commissioner was precisely the same as for the appointment of nurses and other employees and that the health commissioner was not a public officer but an employee

---

*Ohio Supreme Court: State v. Waller, 55 N.E. 2nd 654 (1944).

*For a more detailed discussion, see *Public Health Law* by Tobey,[22] pp. 279-327.
†Ohio Supreme Court: Scofield v. Strain, Mayor, et al., State ex rel.; Reilly v. Hamrock, Mayor, et al., 51 N.E. 2nd 1012 (1943).

under the direction, supervision, and control of the board of health.

The fundamental rule governing the relationship of principal to agent is that the principal is liable for contractual agreements or other acts of an agent, provided that the agent has acted within the real or apparent scope of his authority. It should be noted from this that the principal is not vested with a blanket liability for all contracts or all acts that might be carried out in his name but is liable only for those acts for which the agent has been given power by him. The most important and difficult problem is to define or determine the meaning and extent of the agent's real and apparent authority and power.

The powers of an agent have been divided into real and apparent. An agent's real power consists of the authority expressly or impliedly delegated to him by the principal. Expressed powers are given usually in the form of actual and explicit instructions. Thus a board of health may instruct a health officer to control the spread through the community of a communicable disease.

Added to this expressed authority, the agent also has certain implied powers in order to find it possible to do whatever is reasonably necessary to carry out the instructions given. The health officer, therefore, on being instructed to control the spread of communicable disease may correctly assume the implied power and authority to include whatever administrative procedures are reasonably indicated, e.g., quarantine, contact examination, etc., in order to accomplish the responsibility given him in relation to the expressed powers.

Over and above his real authority, expressed or implied, the agent has certain so-called apparent powers. In the use of these, the agent really exceeds his actual power and he would be considered liable in many instances were it not for the concept that other persons under certain circumstances are correct in believing that the agent has power to act. The use of apparent power is involved in major part in the solution of individual problems, each with its own peculiar circumstances, and

the test of its correct use is the determination of whether or not a reasonably prudent person in similar circumstances would have been justified in acting as did the agent on the behalf of his principal. This may be illustrated by the case of a health officer* who in the face of a smallpox outbreak hospitalized an individual erroneously considered to have smallpox with the result that the patient became infected with smallpox while in the isolation hospital. The erroneous diagnosis having been made in good faith by the attending private physician and similarly confirmed by the health department diagnostician after exercising due and customary care and judgment, neither the private physician nor the community through its authorized public health agents were held liable. As the court stated, "To hold otherwise would not only invite indifference at the expense of society, but the fear of liability would well-nigh destroy the efforts of officials to protect the public health."

This emphasizes that an agent owes to his principal the exercise of a degree of care and skill which a reasonably qualified and prudent person in terms of the community involved at the time would be expected to exercise under similar circumstances. Therefore the professional agent, in terms of our particular interest a health officer, owes to his principal (the community) the exercise of a reasonable degree of care and skill as judged by the time and place. It should be noted that, except where a contract exists to the contrary, there is involved no guarantee that a certain result will be effected. All that is required by the law is the exercise of that degree of skill, knowledge, and care usually displayed by similar members of the profession under similar circumstances.

In the absence of malice or corruption or a statutory provision imposing the liability, health officers generally are not liable for errors or mistakes in judgment in the performance of acts within the scope of their authority where they are empowered to ex-

---

*Dillon's Municipal Corporations 771, as quoted in *Public Health Law* by Tobey,[22] p. 294.

ercise judgment and discretion. Personal liability therefore depends on proof of bad faith which "may be shown by evidence that official action was so arbitrary and unreasonable that it could not have been taken in good faith."[23] While obviously difficult to ascertain, bad faith has been demonstrated to the satisfaction of the courts, as in the case* of a smallpox patient who was forcibly transferred from her home to a dirty, insanitary cabin, for which action a health officer was understandably held liable.

It logically follows, however, that if reasonable and legal instructions have been given to an agent by his principal it is the agent's duty to obey them even though he may disagree with them or think that he knows a better way in which to accomplish the purpose desired. In such an instance, should the agent willfully disobey the principal's instructions or laws, and injury or any other undesirable result follow, the agent is liable for whatever damages have been sustained as a result of his disobedience.

With regard to liability of the principal if it is a government it must first be reemphasized that the state is sovereign and as such cannot be sued or held liable by its individual citizens except where it grants permission. Since county governments are essentially local administrative and political units of the sovereign state, the same rule tends to be applied to them. However, there is an increasing tendency on the part of states to allow counties to be sued and to hold them liable whenever there is question or doubt. Municipalities are somewhat different in that they are corporations carrying on various functions and services. Some of these functions, e.g., the operation of a transportation system or a water works, are considered private, and the city may be sued concerning them; however, other functions and services such as the maintenance of police and fire departments are public functions, and concerning these the city cannot be readily sued. Public health activities fall into this category. Some states

have been very specific in this regard, as evidenced by a Michigan Supreme Court decision which said, "The matter of public health is not local; it concerns the State. In matters relating to public health the city acts as an arm of the State, and the property whose use is devoted to the public health is used in the discharge of a governmental function."*

EXTENT OF USE OF LAW IN PUBLIC HEALTH

Seen in its proper relationship, legal enforcement represents only one of several ways by which an administrator acting as an agent of the community may bring about desirable results and effect conformity to the socially desired standards of the community. In effect, the administrator has three main tools or methods of approach at his disposal—education, persuasion, and coercion—and the extent to which he successfully blends and balances them is one of the best measures of true administrative ability. As Tobey[22] has stated, "A health officer who is constantly involved in court actions, either as plaintiff or prosecutor or as defendant, would hardly be classed as an efficient public officer since he should be able to administer the public health of his community or State and enforce the public health laws in the great majority of cases by means of persuasion and education and by suitable action before the board of health." The efficient and reasonable health officer must be ready to recognize sincere and honest attempts to meet the standards set up by society when such attempts are within the range of social tolerance, and he must be able to explain the tolerance point to the average citizen, the legislature, and the courts.

The reader should not infer that [legal and regulatory] restrictions are the basis of all public health activities. Such a conclusion would be unfortunate, although it might represent the philosophy of a group of health officers that is now rapidly disappearing. Many of the most important achievements of public health have had the support of laws and ordinances requiring conformity to speci-

---

*Moody v. Wickersham, 111 Kan. 770 (1922).

*Michigan Supreme Court: Curry v. City of Highland Park et al., 219 N.W. 745 (1928).

fied sanitary standards. Without this support movements for the extension of public health work would have evolved more slowly and would still be far from their present state of development. Informed public opinion would have brought about great improvement, but more slowly. The coercive power must, therefore, be considered a powerful factor in the development of effective public health work, but it has definite limitations.[24]

The early history of public health in America might be characterized by almost complete dependence on legislation and its enforcement.

During the past generation the student of public health has witnessed a rapid shift in emphasis away from the doctrine of direct control toward that of education. This change has been due in no sense to the failure of the regulatory theory but rather to the broadening scope of public health that now includes problems of personal hygiene. . . . Even the exercise of the regulatory authority must rest on education, for an uninformed legislative body will not enact proper laws or appropriate funds for their enforcement, and an uninformed public will not tolerate regulations it does not understand or appreciate.[24]

In many if not most instances social legislation is framed by persons who are somewhat more advanced in their social thinking than is the average citizen. Only relatively recently has the realization come about that legislation dealing with social concepts that are too far ahead of the citizenry as a whole is almost inevitably doomed to failure. Many tragic examples of this nature may be found in the history of public health; one of the best known is the fate of the General Board of Health of England, established in 1848, that failed as a result of overenthusiasm due to Edwin Chadwick's social thinking and planning, which was too far ahead of the people of England at the time. At least one local health officer in America was literally tarred and feathered because of his persistent attempts to institute complete pasteurization of milk when the strongly opinionated citizens of his area were not intellectually prepared or ready for it.

As a result of the relatively recent realization that social progress of all types must be based on an understanding and acceptance by the majority of those involved, leaders in the field of public health administration have turned to the more practical procedure of concerted educational and persuasive action, minimizing the legal and enforcement approach. Boyd[25] pointed out that permissive legislation for the establishment of local health units in Illinois existed for 25 years, but as a result of the legislation alone only six county health departments came into being. As a result of subsequent public educational methods, however, the citizens in most parts of the state expressed their desire for local health departments with practically no opposition. The place of legal enforcement in present-day public health activity has been well stated by Lade[26] in discussing the control of venereal disease:

Now compulsion is not the only recourse in these cases—not even the first recourse. A substantial number of contacts resistant to examination and patients delinquent from treatment will respond to information, reassurance, persuasion, or assistance when unable to pay for examination or treatment. Indeed, the extent to which these measures are successful is to a degree a measure of the efficiency of a health department, and a demonstration of the superiority of our democratic government over a dictatorship. But there will always be a residue of cases resistant to all of these measures who are the kernel of the venereal disease problem. Here a show of force is frequently all that is necessary. Nevertheless, behind the facade there must be a solid structure of duly constituted authority, lest we have government by the whim of officialdom. Hence, law is necessary as an expression of sound medicolegal thinking in a problem which concerns all the people.

COURT PROCEDURE

Since despite all wishes to the contrary every active health officer will sooner or later find himself in court, it may be well to include a few words concerning court procedure. When court action appears to be necessary, all other efforts for the conformance to social standards and for the enforcement of a law or ordinance relating to them having failed, the first step is to bring charges against the offender. The party who initiates the action is called in law the plaintiff and in equity the complainant. The individual against whom action is brought is known as the defendant in both law and equity. In bringing charges against the defendant the first step is to determine which court has jurisdiction. The same action may be interpreted as constituting any one of several different criminal acts, depending on the intent, the circumstances, the existing laws, and the consequences. Thus to give dangerous, contaminated material to an individual is considered an assault, to make it available to the public at large results in a criminal nuisance, and if sent through the mails, it is a breach of the postal regulations. The first two offenses are crimes under the common law or statutes of a state; the third is a crime under the acts of the Congress of the United States. As pointed out previously, violations of public health laws or regulations usually are considered misdemeanors. In any case infractions of these laws constitute a criminal act so the case is within the jurisdiction of a criminal court such as a police court.

The plaintiff then files with the court a complaint (sometimes referred to as a declaration, information, petition, bill, or statement of claim) that he has drawn up himself or preferably with the aid of a municipal, county, or state attorney. This should consist of a detailed statement by, let us say the health officer, of the facts and circumstances leading up to the controversy and including the terms of any regulation or ordinance violated, the plaintiff expecting to prove the facts and circumstances beyond reasonable doubt in court with the aid of creditable witnesses in order to obtain a favorable judgment. The magistrate of the court then issues a summons ordering the defendant to appear in the particular court on a certain stated day and hour, and the summons is served in person to the defendant by an officer of the court. The purpose of the summons is to give actual written notice to the defendant that legal action has been instituted against him. Its personal service is essential since a court is powerless to render a judgment against a defendant who has not been so notified. Each individual is entitled to his day in court in order to have the opportunity to bring out whatever defense he may find possible. The defendant now has a choice of six procedures:

1. He may ignore the proceedings, placing himself in default and inviting judgment against himself.
2. He may confess to the accusation of the plaintiff and again invite a judgment against himself.
3. He may enter a plea in abatement, questioning whether the court has power or jurisdiction to act against him and whether proper procedure has been followed.
4. He may file a demurrer, stating in effect that, while he admits the truth of what the plaintiff states as a matter of law, the facts do not entitle him to recover.
5. He may file an answer or a plea consisting of a denial of the facts stated in the plaintiff's declaration.
6. Again the defendant may admit the facts brought out by plaintiff but bring out still other facts in avoidance or in excuse of those alleged by the plaintiff. Pleading continues until one side denies the facts claimed by the other, thereby raising an issue calling for a decision and the case is then ready to go to trial.

Most public health legal controversies do not take place before a jury, although either side is entitled to a trial by jury if it so wishes. The first step in such instances is the impaneling of a jury, consisting of the calling of prospective jurors from an approved list and questioning them individually concerning prejudices for or against either litigant. The function of the jury is to decide questions of fact, in contrast to the judge's function of deciding questions of law. When the court proceeding gets under way, counsel for each side may make an opening statement that explains briefly what he expects to prove. Following this, each side introduces its evidence.

All offenses consist of two factors, i.e., the criminal act and the criminal intent, and both must be proved beyond reasonable doubt in order to demonstrate the commission of a crime. A criminal act is an action or omission that the law forbids. To be considered criminal the act must be defined by a law or regulation forbidding its commission. The rule of law is strictly interpreted in favor of the accused so that the act is not considered criminal unless it corresponds exactly with the definition contained in the law. The criminal intent is the state of mind of the accused at the time when the criminal act was committed. It involves a conscious recognition of the unlawful nature of the act, followed by a determination to perform the act. The courts presume the existence of criminal intent on the basis of the actual commission of the act and it is usually unnecessary to produce evidence of criminal intent unless the accused attempts to prove that at the time the criminal act was committed he was incapable of determining or understanding its nature and unlawfulness or that the act was involuntary. Such proof must be based on (1) infancy, (2) insanity, (3) mistake of fact, (4) accident, (5) necessity, or (6) compulsion. If he is able to do so to the satisfaction of the court, although the commission of a criminal act is recognized, the proved lack of criminal intent causes the court to consider that he did not perpetrate a crime and he will be declared innocent.

When all evidence has been brought forth, the judge instructs the jury concerning the law involved in the issues raised and the jury then retires to decide upon a verdict. When the jury renders its verdict but before the court pronounces judgment, the losing party may make a motion for a new trial. This may be granted if the court feels that there has been made an erroneous ruling concerning the admission or rejection of evidence, if an erroneous instruction has been given to the jury, or if the verdict is obviously contrary to the weight of the evidence given. If the motion for a new trial is refused, the court renders its judgment. If the losing party still feels that there was a substantial error in the conduct of the trial, he may thereupon take the case on appeal to a superior court of appeal, in which case he is termed the appellant and the other side is the appellee. The court of review or appeal is exactly what its name implies since it does not conduct a new trial. It simply considers the record of the proceeding that took place be-fore the inferior trial court, the exceptions taken to ruling of the trial judge with regard to procedure, pleading, admission of evidence, instructions, etc. If the court of review or appeals decides that a substantial error prejudicial to the losing side was made by the lower trial court, the judgment of the lower court is reversed and the case is remanded for a new trial.

EXPERT WITNESS

Occasionally the public health worker takes part in a court proceeding, not as a plaintiff or defendant but as an expert witness for either side or for the court itself. Whereas ordinary witnesses are restricted in their testimony to exact statement of facts, expert witnesses are called upon to give opinion testimony. Before being considered an expert witness, evidence of competency must be presented to the satisfaction of both sides. In general any licensed physician is considered to qualify as an expert witness in controversies dealing with medical questions. Specialization is not necessary, and the expert witness may give an opinion even if he never before saw either litigant and even if he never before observed a similar case. Expert witnesses are customarily compensated for their services, but compensation can never be contingent on the winning of the suit by the side for whom the individual appears as a witness.

Courts in general tend to be suspicious of any opinion or expert testimony, and its acceptance by the court depends largely on the manner in which it is given. With this in mind the expert witness should prepare himself well for whatever questions he might anticipate will be presented to him. He should be serious and unassuming and present an attitude of wanting to assist an intelligent jury in their rendering of a verdict by offering whatever special knowledge he may possess. The expert witness should be free of partiality and bias, frankly and honestly admitting a fact even if it injures the side that employed him as a witness and honestly admitting lack of knowledge on a particular item if he does not have it. He should listen carefully to all questions and answer clearly, directly, and concisely in language understandable to the jury (with a simple yes or no whenever possible). The wise witness never volunteers information when on the stand, assuming that, if significant, counsel will bring it out. Finally, perhaps the most fatal mistake that might be made by an expert witness or any witness for that matter is to allow himself to be successfully prodded into losing his temper.

REFERENCES

1. Gray, J. C.: The nature and sources of law, New York, 1909, Columbia University Press.
2. Cardoza, B. N.: The nature of the judicial process, New Haven, 1921, Yale University Press.
3. Blackstone, W. In Lewis, W. D., editor: Commentaries, Philadelphia, 1897, Rees, Welsh & Co.
4. Wilson, W.: The state, elements of historical and practical politics, Boston, 1918, D. C. Heath & Co.
5. Gurvitch, G.: Sociology of law, New York, 1942, Alliance Book Corp.
6. Cardoza, B. N.: The growth of law, New Haven, 1942, Yale University Press.
7. Seagle, W.: The quest for law, New York, 1941, Alfred A. Knopf, Inc.
8. Holmes, O. W.: The common law, Boston, 1881, Little, Brown & Co.
9. Kent's Commentaries, Lecture 21.
10. Ascher, C. S.: The regulation of housing, Amer. J. Pub. Health 37:507, May 1947.
11. Freund, E.: The police power, Chicago, 1904, Callahan.
12. Forgotson, E. H.: 1965; the turning point in health law—1966 reflections, Amer. J. Public Health 57:934, June 1967.
13. Gellhorn, W.: Administrative law—cases and comments, Chicago, 1940, Foundation Press, Inc.
14. Freeman, A. W.: Public health administration in Ohio, DeLamar Lectures, Johns Hopkins University School of Hygiene and Public Health, Baltimore, 1921, The Williams & Wilkins Co.
15. Tobey, J. A.: Legal aspects of milk control, Reprint 939, United States Public Health Service, 1924.
16. The legal phases of milk control, Reprint 1343, United States Public Health Service, 1929.
17. Mustard, H. S.: Legal aspects of planning for local health units, Amer. J. Public Health (supp.) 37:20, Jan. 1947.
18. State laws governing local health departments, Washington, 1953, Public Health Service Pub. No. 299.
19. Tobey, J. A.: Recent court decisions on milk control, 1933, Reprint 1555, United States Public Health Service.
20. White, L. D.: New horizons in public administration, Tuscaloosa, 1945, University of Alabama Press.
21. Joffey, L. A.: Publication of administrative rules and orders, American Bar Association Journal 24:393, 397, 1938.
22. Tobey, J. A.: Public health law, ed. 3, New York, 1947, Commonwealth Fund.
23. Kirk v. Aiken Board of Health, 83 S.C. 372 (1909).
24. Anderson, G. W. In Graham, G. A., and Reining, H., editors: Regulatory administration, New York, 1943, John Wiley & Sons, Inc.
25. Boyd, R. F.: Legal aspects (of local health units) from viewpoint of a state health department, Amer. J. Public Health (supp.) 37:31, Jan. 1947.
26. Lade, J. H.: The legal basis for venereal disease control, Amer. J. Public Health 35:1041, Oct. 1945.

Part III

Administration
of
public health

The knowledge and abilities expected in modern public health work are many and varied. Ordinarily the basic professional training prepares the individual for only a small part of the duties he must perform. Society and its health problems have become increasingly so complex that the functions of the health officer and of many of his staff are now primarily those of public administrators and are only secondarily related to their original professions.

A department of health is a public agency created to perform several types of public tasks. Like most other public agencies, its functions may be categorized as (1) service, e.g., the operation of a tuberculosis clinic or of a laboratory; (2) control of certain human activities, e.g., the isolation of communicable disease cases or supervision of food and industrial establishments; (3) education of the public concerning healthful behaviorial patterns, e.g., immunization, diet, and proper care of infants; and (4) guardianship, e.g., the collection and safeguarding of certain public records, especially those relating to birth, illness, and death.

To perform these functions successfully requires the adequate application of all facets of administrative practice. Gulick[1] invented the acronym "posdcorb" to indicate the component functions or activities involved in administration. The meaning of this word may be explained as follows:

*P*lanning the things that need to be done

*O*rganizing the formal structure of the agency

*S*taffing the agency

*D*irecting the work of the agency and making decisions relating thereto

*C*oordinating all staff activities

*R*eporting to the executive and through him to those to whom he is responsible

*B*udgeting and all other aspects of fiscal management and control

In a similar sense Litchfield[2] characterizes the administrative process as a cycle that includes (1) decision making, (2) programming, (3) communicating, (4) controlling, and (5) reappraising.

Considerable progress has been made in all phases of administration during recent decades. Public health organizations have contributed to and benefited from these changes significantly. In this relatively short period of time there has occurred a considerable amount of long-range planning in public health. This may be exemplified by the White House Conferences on Child Health, the Emerson Report on Local Health Units for the Nation,[3] The Arden House Conference,[4] and the National and World Health Assemblies. Of particular importance is the recent enactment of The Extended Comprehensive Health Planning and Public Health Amendments (P.L. 89-

749). With regard to structural organization there is much interest and activity in the consolidation of public health agencies and the integration of internal administrative responsibility. This has brought about a new interpretation of the function of executive personnel of health agencies. In the field of agency staffing there have been developed techniques of job classification and examination of prospective employees, increasing adoption of merit systems, and preservice and in-service training programs. These have resulted in a notable decline in patronage appointment and an increasing employment of professionally qualified individuals for executive as well as technical positions.

The internal organization of many agencies has undergone constant experimental change, and administrative analysts, functioning first as consultants and later as employees of health agencies, have accelerated the development and acceptance of greatly improved procedures. These changes have also brought about better coordination of staff activities within organizations and, in addition, have resulted in markedly expanded interagency coordination. This incidentally has been one of the many factors involved in the expansion of national administrative power and influence at the expense of the states, and of the states at the expense of the local governmental units. During this same period there has come about a more practical attitude toward the establishment and use of budgetary procedures. Administrative and service functions of health departments have expanded greatly. In this category are included responsibility for hospital construction and standards for and operation of facilities for maternal and child care, tuberculosis, and venereal disease treatment. There has been a steady shift away from law enforcement by court action to law enforcement by administrative regulation, with further concurrent shift away from the use of laws and regulations for health promotion to the more basically sound educational approach. Each of these many factors has placed increasing burdens upon public health officials and has forced them to adopt a broader view of their responsibilities and functions. The important developments in this field have led to an emphasis on preservice and in-service training in the various aspects of administration by schools of public health, health agencies, and the Joint Committee on Executive Development of the American Public Health Association and the Association of Management in Public Health. Discussed in the chapters of this section are the organizational, personnel, fiscal, planning, evaluative, and public relational aspects of public health work.

REFERENCES

1. Gulick, L.: Notes on the theory of organization. In Gulick, L., and Urwick, L., editors: Papers on the science of administration, New York, 1937, Institute of Public Administration.
2. Litchfield, E. H.: Notes on a general theory of administration, Admin. Sci. Quart. 1:12, June, 1956.
3. Emerson, H.: Local health units for the nation, Camden, N.J., 1951. Thomas Nelson & Sons.
4. Report of the American Public Health Association Task Force, Arden House Conference, Oct. 12-16, 1956, Amer. J. Public Health 47:218, Feb. 1957.

Chapter 10

Organizational principles

PURPOSES OF ORGANIZATION

The field of administration consists essentially of two parts: (1) administrative organization, which deals with the internal structure and disposition of the personnel and resources of the agency, and (2) administrative management, which is concerned with the direction of the personnel, fiscal control, and other techniques related to operation. It is the former with which we are concerned at this point. Subsequent chapters will take up the various phases of administrative management. A certain amount of overlapping, however, is unavoidable. Generally speaking, the aim of organization is to arrange people into working groups, associating those with similar functions or purposes in order to more efficiently obtain a desired result from their group action. Gaus, White, and Dimock[1] state this in more detail, "Organization is the arrangement of personnel for facilitating the accomplishment of some agreed upon purpose through the allocation of function and responsibilities. It is the relating of the efforts and capacities of individuals and groups engaged upon a common task in such a way as to secure the desired objective with the least friction and with the most satisfaction for those for whom the task is done and those engaged in the enterprise." Although illustrating the difference between organization and management, this definition also points out the relationship between the two, indicating that organization consists of more than the placement of groups of personnel as if they were building blocks. The process of organization, by virtue of the

nature of those involved, is forced to consider personalities to a certain degree. However, the extent to which this is allowed should best be limited as much as possible. It should be remembered that in the long run the organization is expected to outlast any individual in it, and, accordingly, it is better to fit the personnel to a sound structure rather than to sacrifice sound structure to individual whims of personality.

GENERAL PRINCIPLES OF ORGANIZATION

In launching an organization there are certain basic questions that must be asked by the person who finds himself in the responsible executive position: What is expected of him? In what direction are he and the organization headed? What is the logical order of initiating activities? There is likely to be great temptation to try to develop simultaneously on all fronts. To avoid this requires self-control, careful and continuous analysis, a sense of timing and strategy, patience, and deliberateness. Unless this is done the executive soon finds himself and his organization involved in a confusing, meaningless series of uncoordinated moves.

The steps involved in the development of an organization or a program have been well and succinctly described by Dimock[2] as follows:

First, you must know what the job of your agency is—if in business what the product and the market are to be; if in government, what the statutory authority and the executive mandate indicate. Second, you must select and appoint at least two or three key men to your staff so that the organization may begin to unfold. You can now formulate your plans somewhat more in detail because you have additional principle power on which to draw. Third, recognizing the size of the task, you intepret your plans into financial terms which means budget and work planning. You can now begin to fill in the gaps in your organization with the necessary personnel, thus continuing the biological process of cell division already started when you picked your right hand man. And finally, you must prepare to expand, to gear your enterprise in such a way that you can take on new functions, new activities and emphasis without losing your stride.

Many executives of new organizations feel themselves torn between two extremes: a wish just referred to, to start immediately on all fronts regardless of possible inadequacy of preparation, personnel, or facilities and a wish to defer any action on a program until all desirable, adequate personnel and facilities are available. Both approaches, of course, are unwise. Every organization, including the new ones, must function and must produce to some extent and in some direction even at the start. However, it is far better to engage in one or a few activities that offer a reasonable chance of acceptance and success than to move inadequately in all directions at once. Careful study of any community will reveal certain problems that are sensitive and others that are not controversial. Thus an attempt by a new health department or executive to push an effective industrial hygiene program in a mining community may bring about disastrous consequences. Both labor and management may regard the activity with suspicion and do everything possible to prevent its acceptance and success. Under ordinary circumstances neither faction will have any objection to a maternal and child health program or efforts to secure protection against disease. In the long run it may be advisable for the public health agency to establish a foothold and to gain community acceptance and support by beginning along these lines with the hope of subsequently moving on to other fields. In other words, the planning and organization of the public health program may often best be done on a gradual selective basis even when this involves the sacrifice of immediate benefits for long-range progress. Both the new and the well-established organization must continually move and grow. Stasis actually represents retrogression in these dynamic times, and a program based solely on the status quo has already begun to decay and die.

In his classic *Organization as Affected by Purpose and Conditions,* Robb[3] emphasizes the following:

> Most organizations have grown gradually, and the conditions surrounding this growth often influence greatly the form that the final organization takes. Long existence of customs and methods, and the consequent knowledge of the plan throughout the organization, may be of more importance than the features that might be secured by a theoretically better structure.

This concept is emphasized even more dramatically by Frank[4] in his thesis that there are three ideal types of administrative organization rather than merely one. He lists them as " (1) *under-defined,* in which role expectations of administrative behavior are not well spelled out; (2) *well-defined,* in which administrative roles are explicitly and coherently defined; and (3) *over-defined,* in which role expectation cannot be satisfied by role incumbents." In his discussion of how these three types of organization differ in their implications for vitality and change he points out the desirability and advantages of the first or under-defined type of organization in fluid or changing circumstances. It provides the greatest opportunity to exercise imagination, initiative, and innovation on the part of employees rather than to fix or freeze them and their abilities. He tops this with a statement that should be rethought frequently by all public health workers:

> All of us who have ever been clients of an organization, bureaucratic or otherwise, which resembles the (so-called) ideal type of well-defined roles, have noticed and I venture to say suffered and denounced the conformity and ritualism in role performances to which type 2 organization gives rise.

To a considerable extent, organizational theory stems from military experience because of its example of the value of discipline, the exact definition of functions, and the clear placement of responsibility. Early attempts to transfer these principles to government, business, and industry and later to public service appeared initially to be appropriate and successful. Eventually, however, they were found to result in problems and mistakes when the ends sought were quite different from military victory, requiring acquiescent obedience. Nevertheless, some type of organization is necessary and, as has been indicated, the problem is which type. The choice depends much upon purpose and circumstance. As Sayre[5] points out, "Organization theory in public administration is a problem in political strategy; a choice of structure is a choice of which interest or which value will have preferred access or greater emphasis. Organization is, therefore, a determinant in bargaining."

The approaches to organization theory, according to Sayre, may be identified as "(1) organization as a technological problem in scientific management; (2) organization as a social process emphasizing human relations, informal organization, face-to-face relationships, etc.; (3) organization as the anatomy of decision-making, explored by an analysis of formal and informal decision-making patterns; and (4) organization as the concept of an entity which can and should be held accountable for something and responsible to someone."

There are certain well-established principles of organization that are applicable equally to public and to private enterprise. In the final analysis they consist essentially of the application of common sense to the management of a group of people working toward a common goal: the maintenance of a balance between responsibility and authority, a consideration of the limits of human capability, and the relationship between ultimate productive action and the supplementary needs related to it. The outstanding principles may be summarized in the following adaptation of an outline by Pfiffner and Preshus[6]:

1. An organization should have a hierarchy, sometimes referred to as the "scalar process," wherein lines of authority and responsibility run upward and downward through several levels with a broad functional base at the bottom and a single executive head at the apex.
2. Every unit and person in the organization without exception should be answerable ulti-mately to the chief executive officer who occupies the supreme position in the hierarchy.
3. The principal subdivisions on the level immediately under the chief executive officer ordinarily should consist of activities grouped into divisions or bureaus on the basis of function or general purpose.
4. The number of these departments should be small enough to permit the chief executive to have an effective "span of control," yet large enough to provide effective contact with all of the major functions of the organization.
5. Each of these departments should be self-contained insofar as this does not interfere with the necessity of integration and coordination.
6. Provisions should be made for staff services, both general and auxiliary in nature, to facilitate overall management of the organization as a whole and coordination and function of its component divisions.
7. In organizations large enough to warrant it, certain auxiliary activities, such as personnel and finances, should be directly under the chief executive officer and should work closely with similar units in each of the line departments.
8. The distinction between staff and line activities and personnel should be recognized as an operating principle and be made clearly understood to all concerned.

LEVELS OF ORGANIZATION
Policy making
From the standpoint of organization public agencies such as those dealing with public health may be divided into three distinct levels: policy making, administrative, and functional. Policy making is primarily a function of legislative bodies concerned essentially with the overall or broad aspects of public responsibilities and programs. Thus the legislative branch of government determines the areas in which a public agency must act and the boundaries that limit that action. The details of policy are usually left or delegated to boards, the members of which are usually appointed rather than elected. Thus it is customary in the United States for the public health law to be promulgated by the legislature and for the detailed rules and regulations necessary for the practical implementation of the mandate of the law to be stated by a board of health. The actions of both the legislature and the board are of course subject to adjudication by the courts.

Boards

Boards of health preferably consist of an odd number of members, neither too many nor too few (usually five or seven), appointed by the executive head of the government, the chairman of the county board of supervisors, the mayor, or the governor for overlapping terms. Thus members of a committee of five may serve for 5 years each, with one appointment expiring each year. In practice there is considerable variation in the manner of appointment of board members, in their characteristics, and in their constituent number. Using state boards of health as an example, the number of members appointed varies from three in several instances to fourteen in one state. With but a few exceptions, members of state boards of health are appointed by the governor, whose selections are subject to senate approval in about a dozen states. In several states the appointment must be made from a list of nominees submitted to the governor by the state medical association, and in one state members actually are appointed directly by the state medical association. In another state it is specified that the "Medical Association together with the Comptroller General shall be known as the State Board of Health." In this case the executive committee of the state board of health (seven members of the medical association) performs the functions usually delegated to state boards of health. The usual period of service on boards varies from 2 to 7 years, with 6 years being the most common. In about three fourths of the states the terms of the members of the state board of health are overlapping.

Referring for descriptive purposes to state boards of health, few states specifically require lay representation. The majority of states stipulate that a certain number (and in a few instances all) of the members must be physicians. Other specifications include a dentist, a civil or sanitary engineer, a pharmacist, an attorney, a veterinarian, an osteopath, and a woman. In one state the board of health consists of three ex officio members: the governor, the attorney general, and the superintendent of health, who in this instance is appointed by the governor. The inappropriateness of such an arrangement as well as of a completely medical board is obvious. It is desirable that there be represented on a board of health the interests and points of view of certain key groups in the community. The most important of these but the most commonly overlooked is the public itself.

Elling and Lee[7] provide an interesting and provocative analysis of community leadership and health board membership. They classify community leaders into three occupational types: (1) economic dominants—business executives and men of wealth; (2) elective leaders—elected labor officials, politicians, and government officials (all of whom depend for their position on some kind of popular support); and (3) knowledge specialists—professionals and executives of community organizations, e.g., religious, civic, educational, law, etc. They note that voluntary health agencies and hospitals, as might be expected for fund-raising purposes, have a predominance of the first category (business executives and men of wealth) on their boards. This is in contrast with governmental health boards, the majority of whose membership is drawn from elective leaders and knowledge specialists. Perhaps of greater significance is the authors' observation that in neither case does the leadership tend to be representative of the population. They maintain, "This situation may not be bad if the leadership for whatever reason . . . has pursued a benevolent policy and sought to raise the level of living in the community. This is a matter of personal judgment. Extensive benefits have apparently derived from the leadership's decision to focus on and rejuvenate the local community. Those who have not fared well in the process and those who have not yet had their turn at 'the table'— for example, the deprived Negro and other families in Pittsburgh's notorious 'Hill District'—will perhaps judge otherwise." Goodenough[8] also points to this as a major error in representation at the policy level. As he indicates, the higher levels of the health organization have their closest associations with the *sponsoring public* (those who provide the financing) and some of its *entailed publics* (those whose interests are apt to be affected by the agency's activities). They tend to have the least association with the *target public* (the object of the sponsoring public's and the agency's program). By contrast, the agency's field staff has its closest association with the target public but has limited power or incentive when major decisions are made regarding the agency's programs. As a result the target public—the one for which the agency is supposed to exist—is relatively unrepresented in problem analysis and policy decisions. This pattern now appears to be undergoing rapid change largely as a result of insistence by various civil rights groups, the Office of Economic Opportunity, the labor unions, and some other organizations. Increasingly there is pressure and action to seat representatives of those to be served on various types of boards and committees that deal with health and other social questions. This trend will hopefully improve the heretofore undesirable and untenable situation.

Certain objections to the policy of having boards consist of ex officio members should be indicated. Sometimes this is done as a means of reducing or avoiding administrative costs. Although it is true, as claimed by some, that ex officio membership provides contact and understanding between several agencies of government and government officials, such members are usually appointed to the board without any consideration of their ability to be of service. Furthermore, this added responsibility, if taken seriously, consumes either much personal time or time that might better be devoted to the duties of the individual's primary office. Not infrequently the health officer is added as an ex officio member of the board of health. This defeats some of the basic purposes of the board, which will be discussed later. No objection is raised, however, to the health officer's meeting with the board as a nonvoting participant and perhaps acting as its secretary.

Generally speaking, therefore, boards of health should be more equitably representative than ordinarily is found. There are many advantages to this. Policies will be developed with a better understanding of the opinions and preferences of those most directly concerned and affected and of the probable receptivity and results. Policies are thereby more apt to be realistic and acceptable and therefore more easily enforced. When the primary groups affected are represented on the board, there is provided an opportunity for them to be educated and to understand the viewpoints of others in the community and of the responsible public authority. Opinions that tend to be hidden or overlooked are brought out into the open and given a fair opportunity to be heard. Finally, the determination of policy by a reasonably representative board is a much more democratic procedure than is administrative dictation by either an elected or appointed official.

A legally established board has still other advantages for the health officer and his department. It provides for a nonpolitical method of appointment and removal of the executive health officer, who should be a professionally trained career person and as such protected from political interference. By virtue of its delegated responsibility a board also protects the health officer from many legal involvements. Finally, if provision is made for overlapping terms, the board provides for continuity of community public health thought, direction, and action from one political administration to another or when a change of health officers occurs.

It is only fair to state that under certain circumstances boards may have disadvantages that arise in either or both of two ways: conflict among the members of the board itself or conflict between the board and its executive officer. Although it is generally desirable for boards to be representative of the constituency they serve and of outstanding interested parties and groups therein, conflict within boards is more likely to occur when the membership represents many diverse groups. Occasionally, board members may choose sides, with the result that agreements can seldom be reached; as a consequence effective administrative action by the executive officer is weakened or paralyzed. The actions of the board in instances such as this may consist of a series of majority or minority decisions and bitter charges that one side or the other is attempting to steamroll policies through or to capture impartial members. In such situations what real progress may be made depends largely upon the joint action of any impartial board members and a wise executive officer. Working together for commonsense mediation, they may sometimes bring about conciliation or at least effective compromise.

Conflict between the board members and the executive officer may develop in several ways. The executive officer, either because of dogmatic personal forcefulness or preoccupation with his daily work, may ignore his board, fail to consult or give it work to do, or disregard its recommendations. If the board and its traditions are weak, he may get away with it. Not infrequently, on the other hand, there may be one or more particularly active and forceful board members who because of overenthusiasm or a wish to express power and influence may step beyond their prerogatives and attempt to enter the field of operations. In doing this they encroach upon the functions and responsibilities of the executive personnel. In addition to these situations there is the type of executive who because of personal weakness or of particular confidence in his board may try to pass his responsibilities to it. Fortunately this is observed relatively infrequently. From the foregoing it is seen that the ideal relationship between an executive officer and his board is a delicate one wherein each party must be constantly alert to his own responsibilities and prerogatives and those of the other party. Board members must always bear in mind that the field of operation belongs to the administrative or executive officer, who in turn must respect the functions and responsibilities of the board by keeping them informed, asking their advice, and including them in his professional plans.

Boards have certain specified responsibilities and functions. In a very real sense a board of health should be the health conscience of the community. In the final analysis the board of health is the legal representative of the community's public

health program and agency. As such it has certain semilegislative powers, particularly with regard to the promulgation of rules and regulations that may be deemed advisable for the community. Related to the semilegislative powers are certain limited semijudicial powers in that a board of health may hold hearings on some matters relating to the public health. Perhaps the most important administrative responsibility of a board of health is its customary power to appoint the executive health officer and if necessary to dismiss him. Boards of health sometimes have responsibilities relating to determination of general administrative and program policy, approval of major appointments, and budget review and approval. Except in very unusual circumstances, such involvement in the details of operation are generally considered undesirable. A board of health should meet at regular intervals, at least once each month, at the request of the health officer, and at times of emergency. Board members should be free to advise the executive officer either on his request or on their own initiative. They are entitled to be kept informed, should have access to all health department records, and, when their suggestions and recommendations are not followed, are entitled to an explanation.

It cannot be denied that an organizational pattern that includes a board of health may sometimes appear to be less efficient and slower in action than one operated along more dogmatic, bureaucratic, or dictatorial lines. The design of an organization is necessarily of great importance in the search for an efficient instrument of action. In a democratic society, however, the organizational mechanism must correspond, at least in its fundamental form, to a pattern that is acceptable to the people who are to be served. It is often necessary to sacrifice some measure of efficiency in deference to the public wish for freedom of action and even to their prejudices and lack of understanding. A realization of this serves to emphasize the basic importance of public education in the public health program, which in the final analysis bears the most satisfying and lasting fruits.

Advisory committees

A few comments should be made with regard to advisory committees. Because of the numbers involved, complete interest representation is impossible to achieve on the policy-making board of health. To offset this, many public health agencies have formed advisory councils or committees as an additional means of obtaining broader community contact and participation. Many times the existence of advisory committees enables civic-minded individuals and citizens with specialized knowledge or interest to render services of great value to the community.

Advisory committees are of two general types—constituent and technical. Members of constituent advisory committees may be chosen for their personal qualifications or because they represent social, professional, or other groups in the community. The chief advantage and use of constituent advisory committees is to act as a channel through which the community, on the one hand, and the health department, on the other, are kept aware of each other's thoughts, plans, and action. They are of considerable value in the health education program as well as occasionally serving as a line of defense for the functional public health agency. Members of technical advisory committees assist the administrative officers of the public health agency in the formulation of plans and in the development and application of various techniques of value in the public health program. Naturally the larger and more complex the community, the greater the number of technical advisory committees that might be indicated. Thus a large city or state health department may have advisory committees dealing with problems of pediatrics, maternity, engineering, law, and the like. Advisory committees should, of course, have no powers, and the executive officer must be constantly on guard to thwart the assumption of power by overenthusiastic advisory committee members. A mitigating technique in this regard is for advisory committees to be established on a temporary basis, the need to be determined by the executive officer of the health department. This is generally considered to be good practice since it is pointless to have a permanent committee for needs that arise only occasionally.

Administrative level

On the executive or administrative level of organization is what is often referred to as the hierarchy, built upon a scalar plan. At the apex of the pyramid is the chief executive who, for our purpose, is the health officer or health commissioner. Although an employee, he is in a somewhat different position from the rest of the employed personnel of the agency. It is he who is responsible for the overall management of the agency and for the planning and implementation of its program 24 hours of every day. Whereas the remainder of the personnel may be subject to civil service or merit system status, he usually is not. The activities of the chief executive are usually defined and limited by the terms of the corporate charter or state law. He has the privileges of what has been called an economic royalist, which means that he has been entrusted with a considerable sum of other people's money and is expected to find ways to put it to as profitable use as the law allows and his board approves. On the other hand, his position differs from that of a private executive or administrator in that, while the latter may do anything except what the law forbids, the public administrator may do only those things that the law specifically allows.

The functions of a chief executive are threefold: political leadership, administrative management, and ceremonial representation. It is with the second of these that we are chiefly concerned. In fulfilling his managerial duties the health officer should first acquaint himself thoroughly with the most minute details of certain aspects of his position. The first of these are his rights, prerogatives, and responsibilities. This becoming acquainted involves a careful study and analysis of the public health law and sanitary code under which he is to operate. Next he must familiarize himself with the facilities actually and potentially available to him, including finances, personnel, and materiel. In order to exercise his rights, meet his responsibilities, and properly use the resources available to him the health officer must next perform a careful and thoroughgoing analysis of all his evident and potential problems. These problems are not necessarily restricted to matters requiring professional or technical knowledge. Many of them may be in the realm of personnel management, public relations, or finances.

Beyond this initial stocktaking, which of course should be frequently repeated, the public health administrator has a number of duties of a managerial nature. Some of these are imposed by charter, constitution, or statute, some are defined in executive orders, while others may be merely customary or attributable to the administrator's personal wishes and interests. The most important of these is the determination of the basic administrative policy of the agency. It is the health officer's right and duty to decide in what direction the program should move, when each move should be made, and the manner in which progression is best achieved. Next he must issue the necessary oral or written orders, directions, and commands to his subordinates in order to put his administrative policy into effect. This necessitates that he work out the details of organization of the agency and its internal structure, subordinate leadership and responsibilities, and organize whatever committees are needed to solve controversies, adjust relationships, or establish policies and techniques to meet emergencies. This leads to the need for coordinating the activities of the subdivisions of the agency. Most of this is best accomplished at lower levels, but the chief executive has a clear responsibility for overall coordination. He must arbitrate claims of conflicting action and overlapping jurisdictions. Within the agency he serves as the court of last resort.

In the financial field he must develop a fiscal program for the agency, prepare and submit a budget, and supervise the expenditure of the appropriations. He should have direct responsibility for the appointment, supervision, and discharge of all personnel in the level immediately below him, usually consisting of division and bureau heads and certain staff and auxiliary personnel. Discharge, however, should be subject to review and approval of a civil service board. Although in large agencies choice and supervision of line personnel should be a prerogative of the appropriate division or bureau chief, decisions should be subject to the approval of the chief executive. The executive health officer by virtue of his position bears the ultimate responsibility for supervision, facilitation, and control of administrative operations. He is not expected to perform all or even part of the many jobs or services of the agency, but it is his responsibility to see that they are done properly and effectively. This means that in order to be effective he must pass down or delegate some of his authority and responsibility. This frequently ignored fact will be later discussed in more detail. Another duty of the chief executive relates to public relations, the subject of Chapter 16. In addition, general policies must be established and disseminated throughout the structure of the organization. Management planning must be carried on continually and must include job analyses, organizational studies, budget planning, work flow studies, and insofar as possible standardization of systems, techniques, and procedures. Internal checks must be established to automatically show danger signals when responsibilities are not met or when authority is overstepped. Finally, provision must be made to assure this flow of management up, down, and across the hierarchy of the organization.

Even though the foregoing rules are sound and are based upon many experiences, one of the easiest organizational mistakes that can be made is to assume that a position or function can be established according to hard-and-fast specifications and that any one of a number of people can be found to fill it satisfactorily and equally well. Human beings are not made to fit into precise patterns. According to Pfiffner and Preshus,[6] "The functions delegated to each man can be performed only within the limits of his individual capabilities. The best procedure for preparing an outline of responsibilities is first to draft an ideal organizational chart, then to sit down with the individuals whose names appear on the chart, discuss specific responsibilities with them at length and with infinite patience, and then to allocate responsibilities wherever common agreement dictates."

GENESIS OF THE PUBLIC HEALTH ADMINISTRATOR

At this point it may be of value to consider the nature of the public health administrator in order to obtain a better understanding of him and his function. Is he merely the individual in nominal charge of the organization or program component thereof? It is not necessarily that simple. It is unfortunately true that some public health administrators are little more than the individual whom circumstance happens to have placed in the top position in an organization. In a real sense, however, the term "public health administrator" may be a misnomer. Although it is true that those who are called upon to direct public health programs have usually come up through the ranks, accumulating in the process experience in many program aspects of public health activity, by the time they reach the point of being placed in a position of high authority and responsibility they are often no longer primarily public health workers. By this time they may be only secondarily public health workers and have become primarily public administrators with special interests in and responsibilities for the management of activities related to the public's health.

This is not meant to imply that such individuals need not have a solid background in public health work. In fact, it is difficult to think of anyone's successfully understanding and directing a group of public health specialists without knowing, through past training and experience, what kinds of people they are, their abilities, their potential contributions, and what it is that they are attempting to do. The essential point is that the individual commonly referred to as a public health administrator typically finds himself called upon to make fewer and fewer decisions in the technical, professional, and scientific aspects of public health since he is too busy, or should be,

with broader policy matters. Besides, he has or should have working for him many other experts who are better able to handle the strictly technical details. To the contrary, more and more of the public health administrator's time must be devoted to strictly administrative and managerial problems—how to obtain funds, how to get people to work together, how to deal with other parts of the government and with the public, and similar nonpublic health or nonmedical matters. It should be noted that all these activities in one way or another involve *relationships*. Indeed, executive or administrative work is essentially a relationship type of work. The executive or administrator is always relating to someone else. If he is not, he is wasting his time on something that a clerk could do much better.

The genesis and fate of individuals in such positions are interesting. The term "spiralist" has been suggested by some British writers to depict the shift in role that certain individuals such as public health administrators and similar managerial officials undergo. Their development or evolution is somewhat as follows. An individual obtains some very specific education. He begins to put his acquired specialized knowledge to work in a particular field. At that point he is at the direct center of a potential spiral. If he succeeds, he acquires in the process more knowledge and experience not only in the area of his original specialized interest and its efficient application but also in related fields. His concepts, imagination, and interests begin to move laterally outward in ever widening circles. Because of this, he becomes more ambitious and more valuable to his organization. Therefore, he begins to progress upward as well as laterally into positions of greater and greater responsibility. Each of these in turn widens his horizons even more. Up to a certain point, as he progresses outward and upward in this spiral, he still continues to work in his original field. However, he may eventually reach a point where his interests and value have become so broad as to cause the centrifugal force of the outward and upward movement to throw him out of the orbit of the spiral in whose center he originated. In such an eventuality he is by no means lost to his original field. He has, in fact, become part of a much larger enterprise of which his original spiral was but one of several parts. When this happens, therefore, although he does not cast off the influences of his original field of interest, they become somewhat secondary to an even greater and more significant interest.

Thus it is with the public health administrator who begins (perhaps as a clinic physician, field nurse, or field engineer) performing some specialized service, then progresses to become the chief of a particular specialized program, later becomes perhaps the director of a small generalized health unit from which he may be called into a central office for broader program planning and direction, and eventually is placed in charge of all the many activities involved in a broad-based, multidisciplinary public health program. In the medical field he may even progress to appointment as a health officer, commissioner of health, surgeon general or a minister of cabinet rank with overall responsibility for the conduct and representation of all aspects of his chosen field of interest. By this time he has progressed far from the specialized clinic physician that he originally was, and the demands upon his time and energy are such as to preclude involvement in the minutiae of clinical or specialized affairs. He has now passed out of the orbit of the specialized public health spiral and has entered the larger orbit of public administration. He has become a public administrator with particular interest in health matters.

Despite this, not infrequently one sees individuals who have achieved or have been appointed to positions of high managerial and administrative responsibility who apparently cannot overcome their nostalgia for their initial specialized interest. They continually want to crawl back into their original professional womb. Although they may have working under their direction individuals with great competence and more current specialized knowledge, they find it impossible to believe that anyone can handle the detail as well as themselves. They erroneously consider it a sign of weakness

to behave otherwise. They simply cannot keep their fingers out of the minutiae of the specialized activity. Such individuals can never be good administrators. One cannot have it both ways no matter how sincere or capable. If the individual in high authority insists upon personal involvement in detailed specialized decision and activities, obviously he will have insufficient time or energy for the requirements of his administrative and managerial duties and responsibilities. If he cannot think and act differently, he had better vacate his top policy and administrative position in order to allow someone else to function in it more adequately. On the other hand, if he remains and attempts to play both roles, the price will be chronic exhaustion and the loss of good personnel.

It is appropriate to ask why many public health administrators concentrate on professional and technical matters rather than on their administrative and managerial responsibilities. It is perhaps because, having begun as professionals, they feel competent, comfortable, and secure in the former, whereas they are not quite sure that they know how to do the latter and are therefore really afraid of the job.

THE ADMINISTRATOR'S ORGANIZATIONAL ROLE

What then are the roles of the public health administrator? They are many. The public health administrator may be regarded in a variety of ways by a variety of people or groups, depending upon the circumstances of the contact or relationship. There are the viewpoints of his family and friends, the members of his board of health, the political hierarchy, his subordinates and superiors, the private practitioners of medicine and other healing arts, the irate citizen, the businessman and industrialist, and his own viewpoint of himself. Sometimes in the privacy of his own thoughts he can feel very lonely, confused, disillusioned, and sorry for himself. *But,* he must never show it. This is perhaps the first and most important lesson to be learned.

In general, however, his roles may be considered as fourfold: (1) a technical professional specialist, (2) a public official, (3) an administrator, and (4) a community leader.

With regard to the first, his role as a technical professional specialist, it has already been indicated that by the time he gets into his administrative position his personal expertise is already somewhat diluted by his broader responsibilities, not to mention the passage of time and scientific advances. Accordingly, perhaps his wisest and most practical recourse is to be thoroughly aware of sources of technical and professional expertise around him and not to be too proud or afraid to use them. After all, no one can expect him to be all things to all men.

As far as his role as a public official is concerned, he has certain commonly expected responsibilities. Predominant among these are (1) to represent the community's overall interests and leadership in all matters relating to health in its broadest terms, (2) to engage in certain ceremonial activities, both as a figurehead and as a personality, (3) to assure that the laws governing his jurisdiction and organization are faithfully and equitably enforced and complied with, and (4) to make known to his superiors changes in goals, laws, and resources that in his judgment are desirable or necessary.

In his role as an administrator he must be a program planner, a program builder, a program organizer, a program staffer, a program leader, and, finally, a father image. He must develop a capacity for making things happen, for getting things done through his organization and the efforts of those who are involved.

To paraphrase the words of the American Management Association, he must become adept at guiding human and physical resources in the form of dynamic units of organization to the satisfaction of those served and with a high sense of morale, achievement, and satisfaction on the part of those who render the service.

Attention should be directed to a few personal details. In filling this administrative role the public health administrator should have three outstanding characteristics: (1) a genuine inherent interest in and affection for people (including his staff), (2) a strength or power of personality which gives an impression of considerable reserve force power and ability (i.e., a sense of determination and sincerity), and (3) a scientific and analytic type of mind which aims at winning or achieving by means of prevention rather than by means of remedying health or administrative errors that have been allowed to occur.

To assist him in the demonstration of these, the good administrator should consciously develop and exercise certain important personal traits:

For staff stimulation—enthusiasm, cheerfulness, unselfishness, resoluteness

For organizational stability—calmness, consistency

For efficiency and time saving—receptivity, simplicity, directness, and frankness

For conformity—firmness, tact, toleration, patience

For restraint—dignity (to assure that responsibility is not regarded lightly)

For staff loyalty—courtesy, consideration, kindness

By virtue of his role as a community leader, the considerable power and resources at his disposal, and the fact that he is now part of a larger sociopolitical spiral or galaxy, the public health administrator at this point has become an *agent of social change*. Unfortunately, many public health administrators do not appear to recognize this fact, much less to realize the full significance of it. All too many administrators of public health programs seem content to drift along from day to day and year to year merely attempting to solve problems as they arise by the forces of chance and circumstance rather than to plan and function forcefully in order to determine or to circumvent chance. They are content to ride in or even to follow the wagon instead of driving or leading it down the road they think it should follow. They are content to be passive participants rather than deliberate contributors to the determination of public health and social progress. They do not recognize the great challenges presented to them for the achievement of broad social and economic progress.

THE SCALAR PRINCIPLE

The term "scalar principle" has been referred to in the preceding discussion of the hierarchy and the executive officer. It consists of the administrative arrangement of the functional groups or units in steps as in a scale (Fig. 10-1).

This involves the three considerations of leadership, delegation, and functional definition. There must be a single supreme leader of the organization, but, as has been discussed, in order to exercise his leadership effectively it is necessary that he delegate both authority and responsibility to subleaders on the various subordinate steps in the organization. Each of the primary steps, usually referred to as divisions or sections, is determined on the basis of secondary constituent purpose or function, such as water control, food control, or milk control. The looseness of and the resulting confusion from different terminologies are somewhat unfortunate; department, division, bureau, service, and office often are used interchangeably if not haphazardly in the structural plans of many organizations. Actually it matters relatively little how the terms are used so long as they are used in a consistent manner and are understood.

The fundamental concept of the scalar principle is unity of command, with lines of authority and responsibility going both up and down so that every individual in the organization is directly responsible to only one superior and through him ultimately answerable to the head of the organization. These lines are sometimes referred to as organization lines or channels. In theory all intraagency communications and actions are supposed to follow these lines and should never cross or short-circuit them. Daily practice tends to produce many exceptions to this rule. While some kind of formal organization with its hierarchy is obviously required and while employees are accustomed to working within it, such organization is not necessarily well liked. Many employees, professional as well as otherwise, are in a constant state of conscious or subconscious rebellion against it. Rebellion may not be overt or manifest by subversive action. Usually it consists of subtle resistance such as refusing or being unable to meet officially established performance standards.[9]

Under any circumstance lines of authority and responsibility should never be considered permanent since good organization, as well as progress, depends partly on the skills and personalities of the individuals involved and partly on the nature of the functions to be performed. "If the organization doesn't permit a man to go directly to anyone who can help him with a problem, it may retard rather than help him. If you insist that a man must always follow a strict

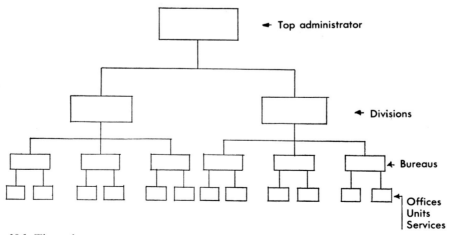

Fig. 10-1. The scalar process.

organizational hierarchy, you may have simply installed red tape. To put it another way, you have set up an obstacle to action."[10] Clarence B. Randall,[11] former president of Inland Steel Corporation and Special Advisor on Foreign Economic Policy to President Eisenhower, has dealt with this practical issue in his fascinating book *The Folklore of Management*. He stresses the importance of flexibility of mind and method in order to achieve good administration, pointing to the infinite variety of changing circumstances. An organization or organization chart which may be precise today may be of little use tomorrow. Then he makes the following statement:

> There is one further difficulty with overemphasis on the formalizing of relationships, which is this: a chart which suits one group of persons will need revision just as often as there are personnel changes. Jobs have no vitality of their own. . . .Take the man away and the job will never be quite the same again. A relationship which functions smoothly under a particular chart and the one set of job descriptions, so long as the original incumbents remain, will begin to show stress when promotion, death, resignation, or retirement intervene. No two individuals will ever bring successively to one job the same complex of strengths and weaknesses, and when a new teammate arrives, some compensating adjustments must be made by those around him. No chart can ever do this for them.

The wise administrator, therefore, "will remember that the organization chart is a useful scaffold with which to build a house but will know that it is not the house."

An organization, in other words, is a living thing which continually grows and changes, and its structure, accordingly, must be adaptable. The administrator must set up the best structure possible but should never hesitate to change it for a good reason. The units to be headed by subleaders should be established or differentiated on the basis of functional definition. The trend has been to provide a small number of relatively large major divisions, each with a single major purpose or function and each further subdivided into bureaus, if necessary, on the basis of subfunctions.

While sound in theory, this is often more easily said than accomplished since many instances arise in which two or even more departments or other organizational units

are involved and appear to have valid claims. Should the industrial hygiene program be placed in a state health department or in a state labor and industry department? If the former is decided upon, should responsibility for the program be delegated to the division of environmental health or the division of medical services; or should it be set up as an entity in itself? Should the school health program be in the department of health or in the department of education? Whether assigned to one or the other, the school health program involves safety, sanitation, medical services, and education, each of which extends into other fields. With these problems in mind White[12] asks the question, "When is a function of sufficient major importance to warrant organization as a division rather than as a bureau with other related functions in a broader unit? Decisions on such cases usually flow from other considerations than abstract plan, the pressure of interest groups, the capacity of those who possess to resist change, bureaucratic and political bargaining. The concept of function itself is not entirely precise although it is a genuine guide. The very fact that no division can be functionally self-sufficient and must inevitably have frontier problems with its neighbors is itself a further guide to the necessity for general staff and strong overhead management."

While it is best for the individual division or bureau to be concerned with a particular function, each should contribute to an overall major purpose of the department as a whole and not be allocated to the department as a result of a search for a roosting place. At least one department on the federal level, the Department of the Interior, has been referred to as a federation of unrelated bureaus rather than a department. Occasionally it is found expeditious and practical to form administrative units on bases other than functional. Thus they may be determined by geographic area, such as the Tennessee Valley Authority, or by type of clientele, such as the Department of Public Welfare or the Children's Bureau.

The question frequently arises in relation to public service organizations such as health departments whether the unit of organization should conform geographically to already existing boundaries, such as corporate limits and county lines, or whether altogether new boundaries should be established based entirely on the nature of the problem to be met or the distribution of the public to be served. This latter concept is what the British refer to as problem or service "catchment areas." Theoretically at least there is much that can be said in favor of this type of administrative district. The size and limits of an administrative district, being divorced if necessary from political boundaries, may be determined on the basis of groups of population, trading or economic areas, topographic considerations, or convenience of officials and citizens. They are relatively easy to readjust with little or no friction, in contrast with service areas whose boundaries conform to those of established political units. The effect of the latter is commonly seen when attempts are made for purposes of efficiency to expand the jurisdictions of local health departments either by combining a city with its surrounding county or by combining two or more counties for health service purposes. Vested political interests are

disturbed. Conflict arises between city and suburb and between village and farm.

Nevertheless, the administrative district based upon problem or service needs has limited governmental status, no independent existence, and usually no power to raise revenue in its own right and by its own action. Hence, public health units in the United States are based on well-established politically defined units of government: municipalities, counties, combinations of counties or combinations of counties and municipalities, and states. The characteristics of such units of government have been outlined by Anderson[13] in the following manner:

1. The unit has its own separate continuing governmental organization, either a board or a council, or in some cases a single elective or appointive official.

2. This governing body has the power year after year to provide some governmental service, or some quasi-governmental service like a public utility on its own responsibility and subject to its own control.

3. This governing body is independent of other local governments and is not a mere board handling some function on behalf of, or as a department of, another local corporation.

4. The area covered by a unit of local govern-

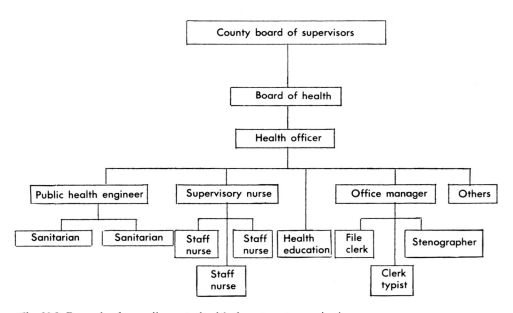

Fig. 10-2. Example of a small county health department organization.

ment may or may not coincide with the area of some other local government. If the areas coincide, the test is whether the corporate existence is separate for the two or more units occupying the same area. There can be separate public corporations in the same area, of course, if they are organized for different purposes.

5. Among the important powers of any unit of local government the power to raise revenue by taxation, or by special assessment, or by fixing rates for service rendered must be considered one of the most important. When other tests fail, this test may decide the case.

Returning for a moment to the internal structure of the organization, it is not possible to make a single rule concerning the number of subdivisions or bureaus that should be established. The decision varies with individuals, time, place, and circumstances. Some agencies, such as health departments, with many professional types (engineers, physicians, nurses, veterinarians, health educators, etc.) may justify a larger number of subdivisions than will an agency with a more or less homogeneous personnel, such as a fire department. Furthermore, some executives feel that they must have, and are capable of maintaining, more effective and frequent contact with the workers of their organization through many division chiefs.

The smaller the organization, the greater are the tendency and reason for the chief executive to have personal contact with all phases of activities. This is most completely seen in the small county health unit where the limited staff makes much subdivision unnecessary. The typical result is a structure such as illustrated in Fig. 10-2.

In this situation the health officer, in addition to performing the medical activities of the agency, personally carries out all the staff and auxiliary functions and directly supervises the rest of the personnel, except in the case of staff nurses, who, when sufficient in number, are supervised directly by a chief nurse and indirectly by the health officer.

ORGANIZATIONAL STRUCTURE

The problem of structural organization is an important one because upon its solution depends whether the chief executive is actually in command of or at the mercy of his organization. The more widely dispersed his direct organizational contact, the further away he gets from the functions of top administration. Generally speaking, a small number of divisions is desirable, giving a quantitatively limited but qualitatively strong span of control. Too fine a structural breakdown tends to bring about a number of undesirable effects. The number of fields or directions upon which the average capable human being can effectively focus attention is limited and has been estimated to be not more than six to eight. The type of structure unfortunately found so frequently in large health departments with a dozen or more divisions strung out across the line makes it impossible for the administrative health officer to grasp and to hold in his span of attention and control all phases of the program. He finds it difficult to see the activity of each division in relation to all the others, and this results in unbalanced decisions and a field day for pressure groups or a few forceful division chiefs.[14]

An example of this horizontal type of administration is shown in Fig. 10-3, which presents the structure of the health department of a moderate sized state with a relatively small and homogeneous, predominantly rural population (State A). Interpreting the organization chart literally, it appears as if 17 division directors report directly to the chief executive officer. That an arrangement of this nature could actually function as depicted is improbable. In practice, in most instances of this type, there is usually some division of responsibility and authority between the state health officer and his one or several deputies.

Fig. 10-4, which presents the plan of organization followed for many years by the health department of State B, illustrates a particularly poor structure. The Commissioner had a dual responsibility to the Governor and to the Public Health Council, the members of which were also appointed by the Governor. Directly responsible to the Commissioner in turn were the directors of nine separate divisions, a number considered somewhat excessive for effective span

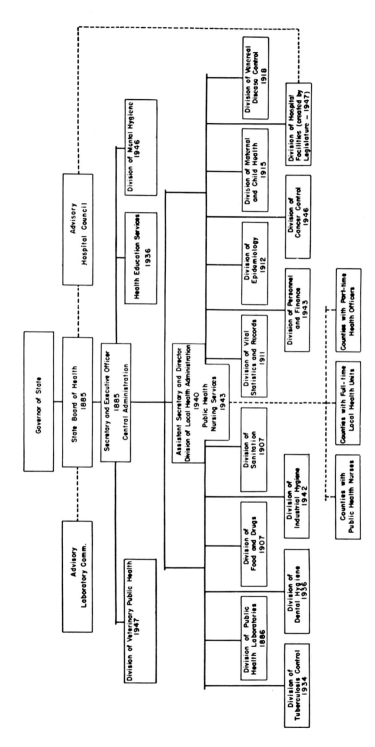

Fig. 10-3. Organization of State A health department.

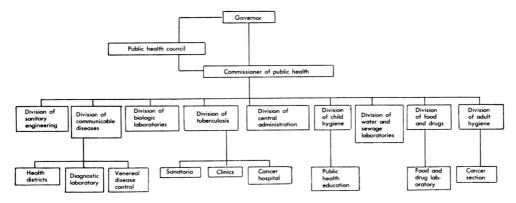

Fig. 10-4. Former organization of State B health department.

of control. Attention should be called further to a number of incongruities within the line structure. Altogether there were four separate laboratories, not counting those which for good reason were located in and served the hospitals. The laboratory designed to serve the Division of Sanitary Engineering was itself set up as a divisional entity. While the Cancer Section was within the Division of Adult Hygiene, the Cancer Hospital was placed in the Division of Tuberculosis. Public Health Education was effectively provincialized in the Division of Child Hygiene. A final point of wonder was the placement of responsibility for Health Districts in the Division of Communicable Diseases. Interestingly enough this particular state health department had a long and honorable record of effective service, perhaps, one might say, despite its form of organization. Recently it has been reorganized into five sections: general services, preventive medical services, hospital and medical services, environmental sanitation, and local health service. Each contains a reasonable number of logically related divisions, the directors of which are responsible to a deputy of the Commissioner. Since being reorganized it has operated even more effectively and with greater coordination and smoothness.

A particularly satisfactory and workable arrangement is presented in Fig. 10-5, which shows the structure of the health department of one of the largest and most complex states. In this organization the span of control for the chief executive and for each of those directly responsible to him has been limited to a reasonable practical number. Furthermore, services and functions have been combined in as logical a manner as possible. Lines of direct responsibility and reciprocal relationships are clearly indicated.

There are three types of organization charts: skeleton, personnel, and functional. Skeleton charts, of which the foregoing are examples, merely present the major units of the organization. Personnel charts show, in addition, the major positions and often the names of those persons occupying them. Functional charts not only depict the major units but also describe briefly the functions, purposes, duties, and activities of each.

A small number of divisions does not necessarily free the chief executive from details since there may easily develop several layers of administration which block him off from the rest of the organization, as illustrated in Fig. 10-6.

A final warning with regard to number and type of divisions or bureaus relates to the danger of statutory definition of an organization's internal structure and the functions of each division or bureau. When this is done, as has occurred in a number of instances in public health, there invariably develops a group of inflexible and unmanageable principalities.

The bureau is the basic functional unit

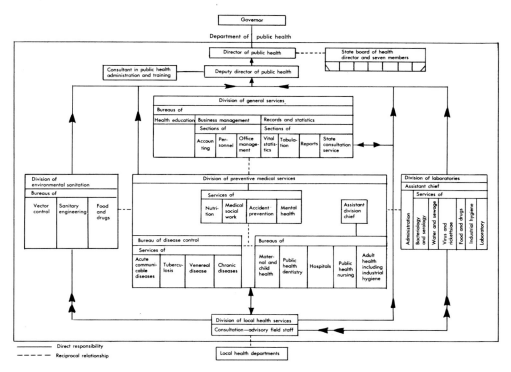

Fig. 10-5. Organization of State C health department showing lines of responsibility and relationship.

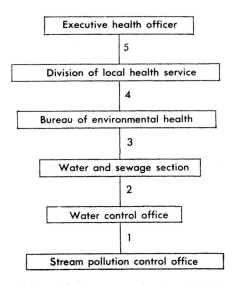

Fig. 10-6. Undesirable organizational stratification.

of the department. Generally speaking, it has a homogeneous structure intended to perform a particular task or a series of closely related tasks, in contrast with the division, whose function it is to coordinate, to maintain effective working contact between the functional bureaus, and to channel the basic functional units communicating with the chief executive. Ordinarily the bureau is a very stable unit of organization. It may be moved within or even without the total organization into new relationships with others of its kind, but it is seldom torn apart or abolished. While the direction of a bureau involves some problems of general management, the outstanding problems are usually technical in nature, dealing with the most effective manner in which to perform the specific task at hand. Work is assigned to divisions and bureaus usually on the basis of the character of the work itself. Not infrequently, however, other circumstances, such as an unfilled supervisory position or the personality of a particular bureau chief, may affect the distribution of activities. A particularly aggressive bureau or division chief, wishing to become a minor empire builder, may extend his jurisdiction in as many directions as possible, usually along the lines of least resistance. The units of organization supervised by less forceful persons, thereby tend to lose their functions and in the long run to pass into oblivion.

Even within the functional bureau the workers are grouped unofficially if not officially. Interestingly enough, even if management should fail to do so, the workers will eventually arrange themselves into the ultimate functional units of activity. Naturally it is best for all concerned if such arrangements are a matter of organizational policy and planning. In order that this may be so, each employee in each position should be characterized from several points of view. Gulick[15] suggests that proper grouping must be based on a consideration of five factors, which for our purposes may be illustrated as follows:

1. Major *purpose* or service, such as milk control, operating a treatment clinic, or education
2. *Process* used, such as laboratory analysis, administration of therapy, or home visits
3. *Persons* or *things* dealt with or served, such as expectant mothers, tuberculosis patients, or restaurants
4. *Place* where service is rendered, such as the Eastern Health District, Macomb County, or Central High School
5. Knowledge, skill, and facilities available and procedural convenience

STAFF SERVICES

Until relatively recently almost all bureaus and divisions of public agencies were more or less self-contained units performing all of the activities and functions necessary for their operation and maintenance. Beginning about 1900, with the expansion of public service and its increased specialization, there developed the trend of splitting off from the various functional units of organization all operations of a staff or housekeeping nature. Activities of this type were then brought together to form what

are referred to as staff and auxiliary services. They are usually aligned structurally in close relationship with the chief executive officer of the organization. Still more recent has been the tendency to develop these staff agencies into a combination of service and control units.

Staff agencies do much more than study, plan, and advise. Their ultimate purpose is to facilitate the work of administration. They frequently are called upon to assist the line or functional units by working with them but without infringing on their authority or responsibility. The executive staff agency is not in the direct line of the administrative hierarchy. Lines of authority, command, and responsibility should not pass through them. Instead, they are situated somewhat apart, on the sidelines so to speak, as adjuncts to the office of the chief executive. Because of this rather special status, their purpose and value often tend to be misunderstood. Occasionally the staff person may have a certain amount of specially delegated authority, but when this is so, it must be made clear to all concerned that the authority has been delegated and that it is definitely limited as to time and extent.

Staff agencies are of three types: administrative, service or auxiliary, and technical. General or administrative staff functions are usually concerned with problems of overall management, such as budgeting, program planning, personnel management, and structural organization. They are designed to assist the chief executive in handling important management matters without his becoming entangled in a mass of details. This is accomplished through personal secretaries and in larger organizations through administrative assistants and economic advisors. The functions of administrative staff personnel vary considerably. The staff officers in most instances receive reports and investigate the efficiency and administration of the units making up the organization; they look for duplication of work, formulate and suggest plans for the coordination of the units, and handle the route work of the executive. In collecting documents and information and in planning a course of action they advise the chief executive with reference to problems and proposals, and, when a decision is made, they may transmit and explain the orders to the line officers concerned and follow up by observing and reporting the results. In theory they have no independent power or authority apart from the chief.

An administrative staff officer usually finds himself in the peculiar situation of having an interesting, important, and fruitful job but one in which his intentions are frequently misunderstood. He therefore must possess certain peculiar characteristics in order to carry out his duties properly. First of all, he must have negotiating ability rather than a highly developed capacity to command. This requires great patience and persistence rather than a tendency toward making quick and fixed decisions. He needs a broad range of practical knowledge rather than extensive specialized or technical expertness in one or a few fields. He must be loyal to the policies and views of his superior rather than concerned with the promotion of his own plans or recommendations. Finally, he must have an honest willingness to remain more or less in the background rather than a wish for personal prominence and publicity. As aptly stated in the report of President Roosevelt's Committee on Administrative Management, "He must be possessed of high competence, great physical vigor and a passion for anonymity."

Service or auxiliary staff functions usually deal with the more strictly housekeeping activities of the organization, including the facilitation of office services such as the operation of a stenographic pool, statistical services, legal aid, central purchasing and supplies, and accounting. While usually referred to in terms of services, many of these activities relate, at least in part, to control of line units.

One of the auxiliary services that sometimes gives rise to controversy is that of central purchasing and supplies. While this office is intended to assist the line or functional units in the most efficient and economical manner possible, there is an implied division of responsibility and authority between the unit which uses and that which purchases. Theoretically the procedure should operate in about the following manner: The functional or line unit, perhaps a bureau or a division, takes the first step. It decides upon the articles or material needed and describes them on a standard form, specifying the quantity required, the desired time and place of delivery, and any special considerations of the purchase in question. This requisition may even include the names of preferred manufacturers when one commercial product is considered superior to those of other companies. The requisition is sent to the central purchasing office usually after it has been examined by the comptroller or fiscal officer in order to be certain that sufficient funds are available. Actual purchase may then be made by the central purchasing officer, if possible on the basis of open competitive bids. The authority to purchase is vested solely in him. Upon delivery, inspection and maybe even laboratory tests are carried out to ascertain the proper quality and quantity of the materials supplied.

The point of possible controversy revolves primarily around whether the purchasing officer should have the right to modify a requisition either quantitatively or qualitatively. The extent to which he has this right depends essentially upon the policy of the particular organization and occasionally upon legally specified authority. Another objection concerns the delay encountered in obtaining the materials. Functional units not infrequently complain that by the time delivery is made the need has passed. Many organizations have attempted to solve this problem by allowing direct purchase of emergency material and specialized equipment under specified circumstances.

Technical staff service, as the term implies, is primarily concerned with methods, planning, and technical aspects of the operation. The technical personnel are functional specialists, such as are found in technical field staffs of state health departments, and skilled specialists loaned to states and localities by the Public Health Service, the Children's Bureau, or other similar agencies. Whenever such technical specialists are loaned to work in line units, they should be answerable to the director of those line units rather than to some technical headquarters or to the top executive.

The relationship of the technical field staff to the functional line unit poses a number of problems. The situation in which they are perhaps most clearly seen is the functioning of a technical field staff of a division of local health service in a state department of health. The objective, of course, is to provide a smooth effective channel along which the knowledge and facilities of the central organization can flow to and through local units without destroying the initiative of the local personnel or impairing the authority which the director of the local unit must possess if he is to administer his program successfully.

Complete autonomy of the local units tends to inhibit the flow of technical service and advice from specialists in the central office to their counterparts on the local level. On the other hand, for central office specialists to have directing authority over corresponding specialists or technicians on the local level interferes with or destroys

the proper coordination of the various activities of the local organization. When this occurs, the director of the local unit is reduced to little more than an administrative clerk. This is an unfortunate occurrence since the local health officer is the only person with local personnel and facilities who is in a position to know where, when, how, and to whom local service should be rendered.[9]

As in the case of the administrative staff, care must be taken on the top level to assure complete understanding, both on the state and on the local level, of the purpose and function of the technical field staff. In turn the members of the field staff must do everything possible to deserve and gain the trust and confidence of the local personnel. The first and perhaps most important step toward this goal is for the top executive of the state or central agency to choose the members of the field staff as much on a personality basis as for their technical knowledge and ability.

Much depends on the organizational arrangement by which the aid of the technical experts of the central agency is channeled to the local unit. A mistake that has

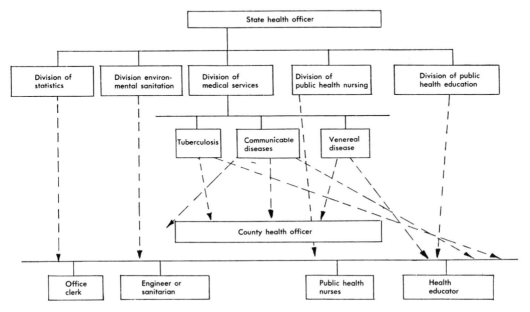

Fig. 10-7. Unsatisfactory organization of technical field staff.

been made occasionally is to follow the pattern illustrated in Fig. 10-7. In this situation each functional division of the state agency independently sends its expert consultant directly to the personnel of the local agency. Even if this pattern is improved to the extent of channeling all the state technical field consultants through the county health officer, confusion and annoyance will still result. Coordination of the policies, activities, and methods of approach is extremely difficult, if not impossible, to attain. A given worker on the local level is apt to have several consultants from the state agency on his hands during the same period. In fact, the meeting of the state consultants in the field may be quite unexpected to them. The waste and inefficiency inherent in such a situation is obvious.

Experience has indicated that a much better approach to the problem is that illustrated in Fig. 10-8. By this pattern all technical field consultants who go into the local units originate from a single coordinating division or headquarters. Duplication of efforts and multiplicity of visitors are avoided. All requests or plans for field consultation are channeled through the director of the local unit, on the one hand, and the director of the division of local health service, on the other, the latter usually designated as Deputy State Health Officer.

One of the potential dangers involved in the use of staff agencies is that the chief executive may become overenthusiastic or impatient with his functional subordinates and direct a staff assistant in whom he may have personal confidence to take a line situation in hand and straighten it out. Invariably this results in divided responsibility, with the personnel in general not knowing exactly whose orders they are expected to follow. Naturally this tends to cause resentment on the part of the division or bureau head. Furthermore, the personnel of the unit frequently adopt an interesting protective attitude toward their division or

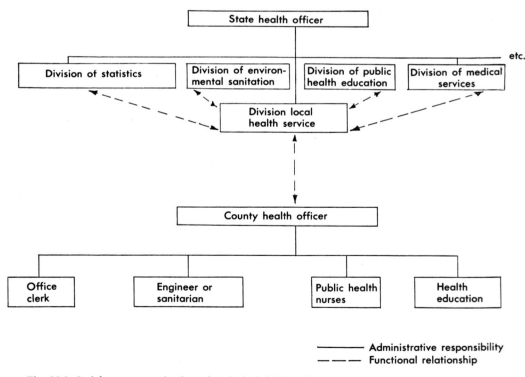

Fig. 10-8. Satisfactory organization of technical field staff.

bureau chief even if they know him to be weak or to have other faults. The staff officer more than anyone else then finds himself in the unenviable middle position between the chief executive, on the one hand, and the functional personnel, on the other. Operating units are understandably jealous of their integrity and authority and resist any interference by an outside person, whom they may consider an administrative spy, stooge, or snoop. In any case they can easily thwart the work of a staff officer by following a policy of noncooperation and passive resistance of a degree short of insubordination. The staff officer in such cases must move warily, taking the time to win over not only the director of the operating division but also his personnel, demonstrating that he is there to assist rather than to criticize or undermine. The most desirable approach is to study the situation in cooperation with the division and with its assistance to seek a remedy. New findings or recommendations should be reported to the chief executive, preferably in company with the head of the operating unit involved, to whom should fall the responsibility for issuing whatever orders or taking whatever steps are considered necessary for correction or improvement of the particular situation.

DECENTRALIZATION

A problem somewhat similar to the relationships between a county health department and the technical field staff of a state department of health exists when an agency attempts to decentralize its operations for purposes of greater efficiency and service. As has been said elsewhere, one of the chief characteristics of public health work is that it deals essentially with people rather than with things. Even in the sanitary control of inanimate material such as food, milk, or water it is the attitude, understanding, and cooperation of the producer, the handler, and the purveyor that are the important factors. Most of a health department's budget is devoted to the salaries of professional workers who work with or serve the public or groups thereof. Nothing is manufactured. Practically speaking, the sole product is in-

terpersonal relationships. This being the case, it is only good sense to attempt the delivery of these personal services and interpersonal relationships as close to and as convenient for the consumer as possible.

In a very real sense no one really lives in a city, state, or nation. As far as actual living is concerned, it occurs in neighborhoods. This is particularly true of large cities, wherein only a relatively few blocks are meaningful in the daily life of the average individual, i.e., the area around the home, the school, the church, the shopping and recreational centers, and for the breadwinner the area around the place of employment. Certainly a city hall or a state capital building is relatively meaningless to the average person, and, if he has any feeling for them at all, the chances are that they are not particularly friendly. Attempts have been made in some places to carry out public health programs from city halls or state capitals. None have really succeeded. Increasingly, therefore, attention has been given to the decentralization of personnel, activities and services to the maximum extent practical and possible.

In such situations, large cities for example, it is customary to divide the total area into districts each with a population of from 100,000 to 200,000 persons. In defining the district boundaries attention should be given to factors that may limit movement, such as streams, ridges, or railroad tracks, to concentrations of industries, to socioeconomic concentrations, to public transportation facilities, to boundaries of other departments and agencies, and to numerous other considerations. A district health center is usually established in each district, with perhaps a number of satellite clinic facilities, preferably near shopping centers, serviced from the district health centers. The health centers serve as the headquarters of the district health staffs and as the location of the more important activities of the district health program.

Mere physical decentralization alone, however, does not result in a decentralized program. It must be recognized and accepted that the public health personnel who work in a particular district are in the best position to be familiar with the problems, needs, and resources within that district. Therefore, insofar as that district is concerned, the district personnel should have the responsibility and the authority for determining and carrying out the details of the daily operations and activities, consistent, of course, with the overall policies and goals of the organization as a whole. Furthermore, in order to assure a well-coordinated district program, all personnel assigned to a district should work under the administrative or *operational* direction of a district health officer. Some measure of administrative authority and responsibility must also be decentralized, or the intent will be defeated by red tape and delayed communications or starved by bureaucratic anemia. An important consideration therefore is to obtain capable individuals for the positions of administrative leadership in the decentralized units, and to allow them, organizationally and functionally, to determine and carry out their local programs to the maximum extent feasible. So that they can do so, of course, provision must be made for obtaining and dispensing funds,

personnel, and materiel. Also a communications system must exist among the decentralized units and between them and the central offices. These are management functions which can only be carried out centrally. In addition, the central administration's program divisions must be concerned with the establishment of standards and qualifications, with performance or quality control, and with the *professional* and *technical* aspects of program conception, planning, supervision, and evaluation.

It would appear therefore that, except in very small agencies, organizational activities and responsibilities divide themselves naturally into three functional areas: management, field operations, and professional or technical direction. One of the most difficult administrative problems is to bring about a method of organization and a degree of personnel understanding that will allow each of these three functional areas to perform adequately and satisfactorily both unto itself and in relation to the other two. Fig. 10-9 illustrates an example of this type of organization which has proved to be successful.

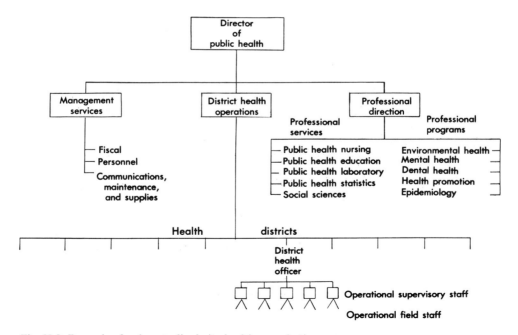

Fig. 10-9. Example of a decentralized city health organization.

COORDINATION AND CONTROL MEASURES

To devise a sound organizational structure and to staff that structure with qualified personnel under a capable chief executive does not necessarily guarantee continued successful function. There must be put into operation and constantly maintained certain measures and techniques in order to make sure that the principles and policies set down are adhered to, that the plan which has been adopted is followed, that the responsibility delegated has been met, and that the orders and work which have been assigned have been fulfilled. The general purposes of these measures are (1) to keep the activities of the total organization and each of its component parts in line with established policies, (2) to maintain a proper balance among the various divisions and bureaus of the organization, (3) to maintain efficient work standards and performance, (4) to assure consistency of action, and (5) to prevent the development of personnel stresses and strains through the promotion of harmonious and satisfactory work relationships.

The tendency for certain aggressive subexecutives to magnify the importance of their work and to become empire builders has been referred to. Usually every unit in an organization is imbued with the essential value of its work and can present arguments to justify its expansion in terms of jurisdiction, appropriations, and personnel. However, the resources available to the total organization are limited and must be carefully and logically distributed among all the functional units on a basis determined by the overall purpose and program of the organization. To accomplish this successfully involves continuous efforts for the coordination of all parts of the organization.

Coordination has been spoken of as the dynamics of organization. It is a broad term that includes a wide variety of activities, the aim of which is to have related workers or groups of workers function harmoniously and effectively together where and when they are needed to avoid duplication and conflict. Pfiffner[6] has presented an excellent example of automatic administrative coordination in terms of what occurs when a fire alarm is sounded. When the police and firemen answer the call, "upon their arrival they are likely to meet repair crews from the telephone company, the gas company, and the electrical company. The high pressure pumps of the water company are already in action. All of these coordinated activities have been set in motion through the alarm system." In public health work this type of situation can be observed perhaps most dramatically in the teamwork of a well-trained epidemiologic staff working to control an outbreak of a communicable disease. Diagnosis and control of the problem requires the smooth, well-coordinated interaction of many types of personnel. Medical and nursing personnel provide care for those already afflicted in order to speed their recovery and to prevent the further spread of disease from them. Field investigators obtain personal histories and make whatever other inquiries and examinations are necessary in order to trace the original source of the epidemic. Here the sanitarian and the engineer may play a most important role. Working with them may be a staff of laboratory workers. Meanwhile the cooperation of the public and the professions is solicited through the efforts of health educators.

There are many techniques that may be used to assure effective control of the activities and program of an organization. Much could be written about each, and the following is intended as merely a brief outline. The most elementary step that can be taken is the development of an organization chart. Several aspects of this have already been discussed, and little more will be added at this point. Suffice to say, the very concept of the use of organization charts has been a subject of controversy. Some authorities in administration have warned of danger in the mere existence of charts since there may easily develop a tendency to tie the future of the program to the chart, thereby hampering growth and development, rather than to constantly adjust the chart to the program. True as this potentiality may be, it is felt that to attempt to administer a program and to supervise an agency of any but the smallest size without some form of organization chart showing channels, responsibilities, and authority is like trying to steer a ship blind without a chart to show passages, reefs, and shoals, on the one hand, and without established connections with the engine room, on the other.

Once the structure is established, many methods of overall management and control of the activities of the agency become possible. Various types of manuals have been found to be of value even in small agencies. Worthy of particular mention are administrative manuals which present the legal and other policies to be followed and technical or work manuals which describe in detail the steps to be taken in the performance of particular functions. Standing orders for the nursing personnel may be considered a special example of this category. Manuals are especially useful for the orientation of new personnel and are indicated particularly in larger organizations. As is the case with many similar types of materials, they must not be allowed to become stale but must constantly be reviewed and brought up to date. Of like nature are written executive and administrative orders, information circulars, and special instructions and directives. These should be numbered, codified, indexed, and routinely channeled throughout the organization.

One of the chief means of administrative contact with and therefore control of the functional units of the organization is through written records and reports that may be required to flow upward. Generally speaking, these are of two types: financial and service. In the typical large health department, for example, the staff nurses routinely submit daily or weekly reports of visits and services with costs of transportation or mileage noted. These are summarized, first, for the individual nurse's service and payment records and, second, for the monthly and annual report of the nursing division. When correlated with salaries, overhead, and transportation costs, the ingredients of service cost accounting become available. Records and reports should not be relied upon entirely for contact with the functional units. Those in executive posi-

tions do well to get out occasionally to the level where the work is being done and the service is being rendered.

It is important to review at least periodically the purpose of and need for each record or report. Two examples in my experience may serve to illustrate the point. In one large health department the request was made for a review of certain office procedures. It was found that one clerk-typist was devoting her entire time to the compilation and typing of a very detailed monthly report, referred to as Dr. X's report. When each report was completed, it was sent to another office, where it was immediately and permanently filed. Inquiry brought out that, while Dr. X had once asked for the information, he had left the organization about 8 years before. A similar instance was discovered in the progress of a community health survey. Here a certain record flowed through a small office with a single typist, who carefully made a copy of each record before sending it on its way. The copy was filed by her with equal care, but in response to questioning she stated that to her knowledge no one had ever referred to her file of copies. The origin of this strange ritual was never discovered.

To a considerable extent the program and activities of a health department are implemented by means of correspondence. The handling and routing of correspondence, therefore, becomes important. One occasionally finds chief executives, such as health commissioners of even large cities and states, who for reasons of vanity, distrust, or uncertainty insist that all incoming and outgoing mail pass through their hands. This procedure, of course, is foolish and wasteful and is indicative of questionable administrative ability. A practical screening procedure should be developed in order to conserve the time and energy of those in the hierarchy of the organization. Thus bureau chiefs may read or scan most or all of the dictated correspondence arising within their units, and division chiefs may read a great deal, whereas the chief executive may limit himself to letters involving complex issues, controversial cases, new policy, or important persons.

Before the close of this discussion on the higher level of the organization mention should be made of staff conferences and special committees. Staff conferences serve the dual purpose of administrative control and promotion of good personnel relations. They are best held at definitely stated intervals, neither too long nor too short. Some health departments find it advantageous to have staff meetings weekly, others biweekly, and still others monthly. In times of emergency or when developing a special program, they may, of course, be held more frequently. While the chief executive should preside and steer the meetings, he should not monopolize the discussion. Each division and bureau head should be provided with an opportunity to present his problems or contributions. The designation of a staff secretary and the keeping of minutes are sound policies to be strongly recommended. Pro tem staff committees often serve important purposes. They may be formed for the purposes of inspection, survey, investigation, planning, coordination, or technical study. Usually they should include one or several representatives from whatever unit or service is involved, and they should report back to the executive or to the staff.

Closer to the functional line employees are a number of procedures that facilitate control. Important among those that might be mentioned are work-flow charts, cross-checks, job analyses, and descriptions and standardization of methods and procedures. The use of internal cross-checks is frequently possible. These are arrangements for checking the work of one employee, unit, or agency against that of another. Examples which may be cited in the field of public health are the routine or spot check of reports of inspections against related laboratory reports and the check of supplies of biologics furnished against therapeutic or immunologic services rendered.

The classification of positions is important but merely as a first step. There is great need at this time in the field of public health for extensive job analyses and revisions of job descriptions. Not only would they make possible more logical employ-

ment standards, qualifications, and placement policies, but they could help to improve the training curricula in schools of public health. The public health profession has progressed considerably with regard to the establishment of standards, particularly when the relatively brief existence of the field is considered. Standards have been formulated for both the quality and quantity of various professional types of personnel, for basic or minimum programs, for utimate goals, and for many technical procedures. This has been the result largely of committees of the American Public Health Association, especially those concerned with laboratory methods and administrative practice. Out of them have come, for example, the widely accepted and used reports on Standard Methods of Water and Milk Analysis, Control of Communicable Diseases, and Evaluation of Health Practices.

REFERENCES

1. Gaus, J. M., White, L. D., and Dimock, M. E.: The frontiers of public administration, Chicago, 1936, University of Chicago Press.
2. Dimock, M. E.: The executive in action, New York, 1945, Harper & Brothers.
3. Robb, R.: Organization as affected by purpose and conditions. In Merrill, H. F., editor: Classics in management, New York, 1960, American Management Association.
4. Frank, A. G.: Administrative role definition and social change, Human Organization 22:238, Winter, 1963-1964.
5. Sayre, W. S. In Sweeney, S. B., and Davy, T. J., editors: Education for administrative careers in government service, Philadelphia, 1958, University of Pennsylvania Press.
6. Pfiffner, J. McD., and Preshus, R.: Public administration, New York, 1967, The Ronald Press Co.
7. Elling, R. H., and Lee, O. J.: Formal connections of community leadership to the health system, Milbank Mem. Fund Quart. 44:294, July 1966.
8. Goodenough, W. H.: Agency structure as a major source of human problems in the conduct of public health programs, Amer. J. Public Health 55:1067, July 1965.
9. Weber, M.: The theory of social and economic organization, New York, 1947, Oxford University Press, Inc.
10. Schleh, E. C.: Successful executive action, Englewood Cliffs, N. J., 1962, Prentice-Hall, Inc.
11. Randall, C. B.: The folklore of management, New York, 1962, Mentor Executive Library Books.
12. White, L. D.: Introduction to the study of pub-

lic administration, New York, 1955, The Macmillan Co.

13. Anderson, W.: The units of government in the United States, Public Administration Service Pub. No. 42, 1934.

14. Editorial: Vertical versus horizontal administration, Amer. J. Public Health **32**:86, Jan. 1942.

15. Gulick, L.: Notes on the theory of organization. In Gulick, L., and Urwick, L., editors: Papers on the science of administration, New York, 1937, Institute of Public Administration

Chapter 11

Organization
of
official public health agencies

INTRODUCTION

It is probably an understatement to say that official public health programs in the United States are organized along rather complex lines. That this should be found in a nation with a reputation for organizational ability is frequently puzzling not only to visitors from other countries but also to citizens of this country whose activities and occupations bring them only occasionally into personal contact with public health agencies. This complexity of organization is attributable chiefly to the form and structure of government as it was established in the nation and shows the influence of democratic and more or less decentralized development. One of the clearest overall pictures yet presented is that devised by Mountin and Flook to illustrate their concise and valuable *Guide to Health Organization in the United States.*[1]

Generally speaking, official public health activities may be considered on four levels: local, state, national, and international. The first is often subdivided into municipal programs and those of rural areas although, increasingly, core cities and the areas surrounding them are merging their health resources and providing common services under a united administration. As in the case of the government as a whole, while each political level has its own public health structure, no one of them is by any means completely independent of the others. Quite to the contrary, and increas-

ingly there is a melding of local public health functions and responsibilites with those of the state and in turn of state functions and responsibilities with those of the federal government. This interrelationship is implied in Fig. 11-1, which depicts the levels of governmental health activity.

LOCAL HEALTH ORGANIZATION

On the lowest or local level, where in the last analysis most service to the public is actually rendered, there are a number of agencies with varying degrees of official concern for the public health. It is here that direct person-to-person contact is made between the individuals comprising the public and their locally employed public health personnel. While the most personal of all health services are rendered by private practitioners of medicine, dentistry, and nursing, their place in the picture will not be presented at this point other than to include them in the diagrams. Similarly the part played by the voluntary agencies is included diagrammatically here and discussed in Chapter 12. Local health departments, therefore, are designed to render on-the-spot, direct service to the people of a local governmental jurisdiction. The units of local governments may be municipalities, towns, townships, counties, or combinations of them. Organizations concerned with the health of towns and cities were established relatively early in our history. In an attempt to serve the more rural areas town-

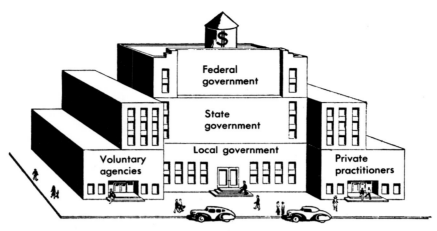

Fig. 11-1. Levels of health organization. The complete health structure. (From Mountin, J. W., and Flook, E.: Guide to health organization in the United States, Washington, 1953, Public Health Service Pub. No. 196.)

ships or civil districts have been used extensively in the past. With the development of good roads and rapid transportation, however, this makeshift has been undergoing a process of abandonment in favor of the establishment of countywide health departments. Of additional significance, as has been mentioned, is the recent trend toward the formation of joint city-county health departments.

The establishment of public health organizations on the basis of these larger units of government or combinations of them has been necessitated by a consideration of the number of people and the size of area adequate to raise enough public tax funds to support at least a minimum staff of qualified public health workers. In most instances it is recommended that an area should contain at least 50,000 people before it considers the establishment of a health unit of its own. Exceptions exist, of course, depending essentially upon wealth, density, health problems, and geography. As of 1960, there were in the United States 1,557 full-time local health departments of one type or another which served 2,425 counties, including 307 cities, and covering areas with a combined population of approximately 167 million people or 94.4% of the population. Areas not served by local health depart-

ments were limited to 647 counties, or about 21% of the 3,072 counties in the nation, which included nearly 10 million people or about 6% of the nation's population.[2,3] Since then, although exact information is not available, it is known that additional areas have been included in county or district health units to bring the population served even closer to 100%.

It is interesting to consider the characteristics of the counties which have no organized health services. Haldeman[4] has summarized them as follows:

1. They are located in 27 states, primarily in the western Great Plains and Rocky Mountain areas.
2. They have small total populations and are sparsely inhabited.
3. The median age of their population is relatively high.
4. Generally they have lost population in recent years.
5. A high proportion of the population is employed in agriculture and relatively few in manufacturing.
6. They have a significantly smaller percentage of non-white inhabitants than the country as a whole.
7. They have a relatively high family income and educational level.
8. They have a higher percentage of occupant-owned dwellings than the rest of the country.

Returning to areas which have organized full-time health services, the pattern throughout the nation is by no means uniform. Tremendous variation may be observed with regard to numbers and qualifications of personnel, types of programs, and financing. Personnel and finances, hence programs, are especially thin in areas where local health services are provided by state district health units.

As a consequence of these inadequacies and inequities and because of the general broadening scope of the field of public health, the 1940's saw the development of a forceful movement to achieve complete coverage of the nation with adequate and practical full-time local health units. It was keynoted by the Emerson report, *Local Health Units for the Nation*,[5] and promoted by a series of national, regional, and state conferences. The movement culminated in attempts to obtain legislation to provide federal subsidization of local health units through state health departments. Emerson and his committee suggested as a goal the establishment of a total of 1,197 units to include 318 single-county units, 821 multi-county units, 36 county-district units, and 22 city units including the District of Columbia and one unit of three cities. The populations of these units ranged at the time from 10,200 to 7.5 million, with an average of 110,000; 86% had populations of 45,000 or more; 171 of the county or district units contained a total of 198 cities of 50,000 or more people. There were 154 units with 1 city each, and 44 cities in the remaining 17 units.

Despite these extensive efforts, only few additional full-time local health units were created. In 1947 there were 1,284 units covering 1,874 counties, and by 1960 they had increased to only 1,557 units covering 2,425 counties. This, in conjunction with a recognition of the nature of the uncovered areas just presented, has led to a reexamination of the bases upon which full-time local health units should be established—or might conceivably not be practical or needed. In reflecting upon the saturation point that seems to have been reached in the establishment of such units, Haldeman[4] states:

This may stem from the many changes in health problems which have occurred over the years. It may be that new and additional resources such as voluntary health agencies, industrial health programs, insurance schemes and other prepayment plans are now providing, more acceptably, some services which in the past were supplied by the health department. Or perhaps the greater interest of private physicians in preventive medicine coupled with better methods of communication and transportation and increased public enlightment regarding the individual's own responsibility for his personal health have reduced the need for organized health departments.

Another not necessarily conflicting viewpoint might hold that the reason for the plateau in organizational development is temporary and is only a reflection of the transition between (1) a period of public attitude and professional programming based essentially on communicability and (2) such a period based essentially on the complexities of the control of chronic disease and the provision of comprehensive medical care. The ultimate effect of the many medical care programs begun in the second half of the 1960's will be interesting to watch.

The usual pattern of organizational interrelationships involved in the provision of health services on the local level is shown in Fig. 11-2. Necessarily a health department on the local or any other level cannot be expected to include within its organization personnel and facilities for the solution of every phase of the public health problems of the community. Many other persons and agencies play important roles. In rural areas county farm agents and home demonstration agents are active in nutrition and health education. The department of public works has a most important responsibility for sanitary waste disposal. Departments of education, welfare, police, and others all contribute in some degree to the community health program. Nevertheless, the local health department should be the focal point, the catalyst, and the leader in activities in this field.

On three occasions, 1940, 1950, and 1963, the American Public Health Association has issued official policy statements concerned with services and responsibilities of local health departments. In the most recent[6] it emphasizes that the fundamental responsibility of a local health department is (1) to determine the health status and

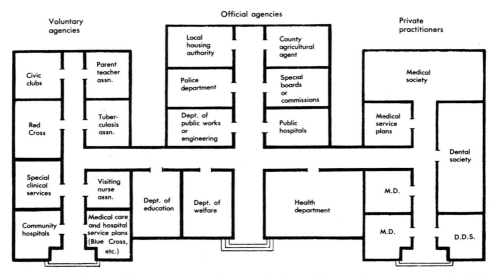

Fig. 11-2. Levels of health organization. The ground floor of the health structure—local official and voluntary agencies and private practitioners. (From Mountin, J. W., and Flook, E.: Guide to health organization in the United States, Washington, 1953, Public Health Service Pub. No. 196.)

health needs of the people within its jurisdiction, (2) to determine the extent to which these needs are being met by effective measures currently available, and (3) to take steps to see that the unmet needs are satisfied. It also places emphasis on the role of the local health department in social planning, particularly in the areas of medical care, regional planning of health services, effective use of natural resources, and efficient delivery of traditional services. With reference to specific functions of local health departments those listed in the 1950 policy statement were considered as still valid, with the recognition of the need to be constantly alert to new emerging problems. The following, therefore, may be regarded as appropriate and necessary functions of a local health department[7]:

I. Recording and analysis of health data
  A. Recording and analysis of reports of births, deaths, marriages, divorces, and notifiable diseases
  B. Maintenance of registers of individuals known to have certain specific long-term diseases and impairments
  C. Conduct of special surveys to determine the prevalence and resultant disability from various diseases

  D. Collection and interpretation of morbidity data from such sources as clinics, hospitals, organized nursing services, prepayment plans, industry, and workmen's compensation and disability insurance programs
  E. Maintenance of continuing records on the number and qualifications of all types of health personnel, the quantitative and qualitative resources of available facilities, and the types and extent of health services provided through various voluntary and public programs
  F. Periodic evaluation of community health needs and services

II. Health education and information
  A. Stimulation of the public to recognize health problems that exist, to study the resources available for meeting the problems, and to develop and put into action programs designed to solve them
  B. Cooperation with and assistance of official and voluntary organizations such as departments of education and civic, youth, and other community groups in the development of their health programs
  C. Provision of individual instruction by public health nurses and other personnel, as in the case of families in which communicable disease has occurred, of mothers attending well-baby conferences, or of diabetic and other patients who are

taught to follow the regimen prescribed by the family physician

D. Organization of lectures, classes, and courses, such as parents' classes, courses for food-handlers, classes for diabetics, and lectures to community groups

E. Use of mass educational and informational media such as newspapers, magazines, pamphlets, movies, radio, and television

F. Development of a well-rounded program of professional education, designed to assist the local health professions to maintain and improve the quality of service

III. Supervision and regulation

A. Protection of food, water, and milk supplies

B. Control of nuisances, sanitary disposal of wastes, and control of water and air pollution

C. Prevention of occupational diseases and accidents

D. Control of human and animal sources of infection

E. Regulation of housing

F. Inspection of hospitals, nursing homes, and other health facilities by means of
   1. Public education and individual instruction
   2. Issuance of regulations
   3. Laboratory control
   4. Inspection and licensure
   5. Revocation of permits and, as a last resort, court action

IV. Provision of environmental health services (as necessary)

A. Construction of pit privies

B. Drainage and larvicidal treatment of mosquito-breeding areas and residual spraying of homes for insect control

C. Rat proofing of buildings and other rodent and insect control measures

V. Administration of personal health services

A. Immunization against infectious diseases and other preventive measures such as the application of fluoride to children's teeth

B. Advisory health maintenance service, as in child health conferences, prenatal clinics, parents' classes, and public health nursing visits

C. Case finding surveys of the general population, such as chest x-ray surveys, serologic tests for syphilis, cancer detection programs, and school health examination (adult health inventories and "multiphasic" surveys for the detection of various groups of diseases may also be included)

D. Provision of diagnostic aids to physicians, such as laboratory services and crippled children's, cancer, cardiac, and other diagnostic and consultation clinics

E. Provision of diagnostic and treatment services for specific diseases such as syphilis, tuberculosis, dental defects in children and expectant mothers, and orthopedic, cardiac, and other crippling impairments in children

VI. Operation of health facilities

A. Operation of health centers and clinics

B. Operation of general or special hospitals (as necessary)

VII. Coordination of activities and resources

A. Provision of effective leadership in meeting community health needs

B. Encouragement of coordination of various official and voluntary agencies to avoid duplication and overlapping and to assure efficient and economical administration

C. Participation on interdepartmental or regional boards dealing with public water supplies, sewage and refuse disposal, control of atmospheric pollution, housing, city planning, hospital planning, zoning regulation, development of recreational areas, and other public programs which have significant implications for community health

In order to carry out its mandate the official public health agency in rural or small urban situations requires only a relatively simple type of organizational structure. Legal responsibility for the public's health is commonly placed in a local board of health, the members of which are appointed by the locally elected officials, i.e., in cities by mayors and in counties by boards of supervisors or their equivalent. The board of health usually appoints and employs a county health officer, frequently subject to approval by the state health department. Increasingly, state health departments have been establishing standards and qualifications that must be met by those appointed to local public health positions. This particular type of state supervision has met with relatively little local resistance since in most instances local units of government have found it necessary to turn to the state health department for assistance in finding capable candidates for the position. While assistant medical personnel are occasionally found in county health departments, the nationwide shortage of personnel and the general inadequacy of local funds have served to preclude the employment of more than one physician in a great many county health departments.

The employment of all other personnel is customarily a prerogative of the local health officer but is subject to civil service regulations if they exist. This, of course, is as it should be. His staff usually consists of one or several workers in environmental sanitation, public health nursing, and office management as well as an occasional health educator and a laboratory worker. Infrequently encountered as yet, except in larger units, are nutritionists, public health dentists, and representatives of other professions. The workers in environmental sanitation may consist of any combination of engineers, professionally trained sanitarians, or sanitary inspectors trained on the job. The preferred situation for most county health departments would probably be a sanitary engineer supervising an adequate number of professionally trained sanitarians. Ordinarily, approximately one half the funds and one half the positions of the local health department are devoted to public health nursing. This means that, of the various professions, nursing will be most represented. Even the smallest local health unit will or should have several nurses on its staff. This being the case, while an actual division of public health nursing may not exist structurally, one of the nurses, selected on the basis of training, experience, and personality, should be appointed as supervising nurse. Where several office workers are employed, one should be designated to serve as office manager and to supervise the work of the others. In this way responsibilities are much more apt to be clear cut and understood by those concerned. All members of the staff, as indicated in Fig. 10-2, should be ultimately responsible to the county health officer, who in turn is responsible to the board.

Current standards suggest the employment of the following types and numbers of professional personnel in order to provide the minimum desirable services to a community:

Medical personnel—1 per 50,000 population (the best qualified to serve as health officer, the others preferably to direct the school health program, the maternal and child health program, and the epidemiology program)

Sanitary personnel—1 per 15,000 population (one preferably a public health engineer)

Staff nursing personnel—1 per 5,000 population (one per 2,500 population if bedside nursing is included)

Supervisory nursing personnel—1 per 6 to 8 staff nurses

Office personnel—1 per 15,000 population

Other specialized personnel—as problems demand and funds make possible

When funds and candidates are not available to make possible the employment of other types of personnel that may be needed or when full-time employees are not practical, as is sometimes the case in staffing clinics, the gap may be filled by the part-time employment of private practitioners or the use of services of district or state agencies. Wherever possible, however, the employment of full-time personnel is recommended.

In the larger local units of government, particularly municipalities or combinations of them with their surrounding county areas, more extensive personnel and organization obviously are required. In general the distribution of types of personnel per unit of population is similar to that followed in the smaller areas with various numbers of different types of specialists added to meet the problems and demands inherent in the particular situation. The increased total number of employees naturally leads to the formation of a more formalized organizational structure with the bringing together of similar and related functions into divisions and bureaus. The general pattern still holds with the same basic principles of organization followed. Although there is no standard organizational structure, certain functional divisions are nevertheless almost universally encountered. Thus there usually exist divisions of vital statistics and records; sanitation, sanitary engineering, or environmental health; maternal and child health; public health nursing, either as an entity or integrated into the activities of several of the other divisions; laboratory service; epidemiologic service or communicable disease control; and health education. Increasingly one also finds a division of adult health and/or chronic disease. Each functional category, now large enough to comprise a unit, should have its director and possibly subdirectors. The direct professional service activities of those in the top administrative positions become greatly minimized, giving way to functions of a managerial and supervisory nature. An example of a more extensive agency is presented in Fig. 10-9.

STATE HEALTH ORGANIZATION

Still more varied is the pattern of public health organization on the state level. In each instance more than one agency has responsibility for activities in this field. A study[8] made by the Public Health Service in 1950 indicated a total of 60 different types of state agencies which contributed in some way to state health programs. The diversity of these agencies may be seen from the following consolidated tabulation:

Department of health
Department of welfare, social security, emergency relief, general assistance, etc.
Department of agriculture
Department of labor, labor and industry, labor and immigration, etc.
Department of education, public instruction, etc.
Special boards, commissions, or independent offices established specifically for the activity indicated (tuberculosis board or commission, cancer commission, workmen's compensation commission or bureau, industrial accident board, dairy and food commission, hotel commission, livestock sanitary board, water resources board, commission for the blind, crippled children's commission, mental disease commission or department, state toxicologist, state veterinarian, etc.)
Board of control of affairs, department of state institutions, etc.
Independent state hospital, independent state laboratory
Department of conservation
State university or college
Department of mines and minerals
Department of engineering, department of public utilities
State experiment station
Independent licensing and examining boards
Department of motor vehicles, department of public safety
Department of civil service and registration, department of registration and education
Other departments or offices of state government

The variety of state agencies participating in health activities is not measured alone by the aggregate count. Dispersion of health responsibility is also extreme and varied when viewed within individual states. The number of agencies performing health activities in a single state ranges from 10 to 32 . . . The variation among states in assignment of responsibility for health functions is due in great measure to two main factors: Complexity of state governmental organization and extent of health services provided by the state. The former is probably the more important in determining the total number of agencies. . . .

Numerous agencies are often responsible for a single activity within a state. As many as 13 separate agencies are engaged in accident prevention work in one state, while a total of 12 participate in some form of health education in another. Other programs in which 7 or more individual agencies participate in at least one of the States are mental hygiene, crippled children's services, prevention and treatment of blindness, licensure for health reasons, medical care, vocational rehabilitation (restorative measures) maternal and child health, hygiene of housing, and school health services. With this multiplicity of agencies concerned with a single health program within a state, it is easy to imagine some of the difficulties encountered in developing uniform standards of performance and achieving common goals.

It should be noted that this complex and diffuse situation on the state level has not clarified appreciably since the survey was conducted. However, in every state without exception some one agency is invested with primary responsibility for the public health program. Usually this is a state department of public health, although in one instance, the state of Maine, public health is a subdivision of a department of welfare. As on the local level, the state health department should provide the leadership on its governmental level in public health matters, all other agencies acting in this field as contributory or auxiliary agencies. This relationship of a state department of public health with other agencies on its level has been illustrated by Mountin and Flook as in Fig. 11-3.

In all except a few states the direct personal service functions of state health departments are decidedly few and are limited largely to the provision of traveling specialized personnel and mobile equipment to local areas unable to afford them. Many state health departments, for example, staff, equip, and maintain mobile chest x-ray

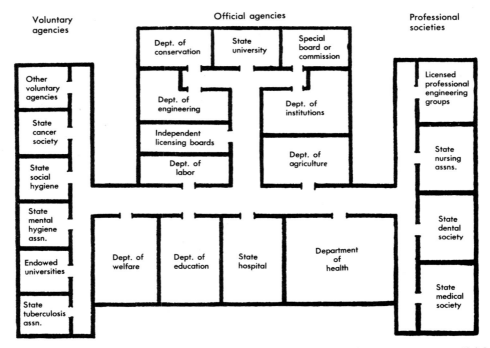

Fig. 11-3. Levels of health organization. The second floor of the health structure—state official and voluntary agencies and professional societies. (From Mountin, J. W., and Flook, E.: Guide to health organization in the United States, Washington, 1953, Public Health Service Pub. No. 196.)

units, dental clinics, and facilities for the examination and treatment of the venereal diseases. In general the functions of a state health department are the following[9]:

1. To represent the public health interests and goals of the state to the elected governing body of the state
2. To promulgate and enforce public health rules and regulations applicable throughout the state
3. To determine state public health policy and to provide a state-wide coordinated public health program with clear objectives for the guidance of local health departments
4. To promote the establishment of full-time local health units
5. To develop an appropriate plan for the co-ordination of local health services with related hospital and medical programs which may be developed on a regional basis
6. To provide financial assistance to supplement the resources of local health departments
7. To make consultation and other special services available
8. To assist localities to set up demonstrations on a temporary basis

9. To establish minimum and stimulate optimum standards of performance
10. To develop a recruitment and training program for local health department personnel
11. To delegate certain legal responsibilities of the state health agency, insofar as feasible and practical, to well-organized and adequately staffed local health departments
12. To carry on all relationships with local citizens and groups through the medium of or in cooperation with the local health departments
13. To carry on a statewide program of health education
14. To evaluate continually or periodically existing state and local programs

From this list it is possible to summarize state health department functions into the few categories of statewide planning, state and federal relations, interstate agency relations, and certain statewide regulatory functions. But above all else the chief raison d'être for a state health department is the extent to which it stimulates and assists local departments to do a satisfactory job.

Table 11-1. Frequency of activities in 50 state health departments*

Activity	Frequency	Activity	Frequency
1. Abattoirs	1	53. Local health services	42
2. Accident prevention	8	54. Machine tabulation	2
3. Administrative services	9	55. Masseur license	1
4. Adult health	3	56. Maternal and child health	50
5. Air pollution	10	57. Meat and poultry inspection	1
6. Alcoholism	9	58. Medical and/or hospital care	5
7. Bacteriology	15	59. Mental care	1
8. Barbers and beauticians	6	60. Mental health	27
9. Bedding and upholstery	6	61. Mental retardation program	4
10. Biologics	6	62. Merit system—local	1
11. Blood bank	1	63. Merit system—state agency	3
12. Branch laboratories	10	64. Milk sanitation	14
13. Building maintenance	1	65. Narcotics control	2
14. Camp sanitation	2	66. Nursing	50
15. Cancer control	31	67. Nursing homes	6
16. Canning and bottling plants	1	68. Nutrition	29
17. Central files	1	69. Oil field pollution	1
18. Chest x-ray survey	3	70. Orthopedic program	1
19. Child guidance	2	71. Payroll	1
20. Chronic diseases control	30	72. Pedodontics	1
21. Civil defense	7	73. Personnel	34
22. Communicable diseases	45	74. Plumbing	6
23. Crime detection laboratory	1	75. Pneumotherapy stations	1
24. Crippled children's services	26	76. Poison information	2
25. Dairy products	2	77. Polio control	1
26. Dental health	46	78. Professional registration and license	3
27. Diabetes control	1	79. Program planning, development, and evaluation	7
28. Diagnostic services	4	80. Property control	3
29. Engineering	43	81. Public relations	1
30. Environmental health	50	82. Publications	4
31. Epidemiology	11	83. Rabies control	1
32. Examining boards	2	84. Radiologic health	11
33. Film library	1	85. Regional offices	18
34. Finance, fiscal, accounting, etc.	13	86. Research	5
35. Food and drug control	24	87. Rheumatic fever	2
36. Funeral director licensure	1	88. Sanitarian local services	1
37. Geriatrics	3	89. School health services	11
38. General sanitation	19	90. Shellfish sanitation	5
39. Grants-in-aid administration	1	91. Social services	6
40. Health education	50	92. Staff health services	1
41. Hearing and vision	4	93. Statistical services	6
42. Heart disease control	25	94. Training	8
43. Hospital survey, planning, and construction licensure	42	95. Tuberculosis control	43
44. Hospitals and sanatoria adm.	16	96. Typhus control	1
45. Hotel sanitation	3	97. Vector control	12
46. Housing	1	98. Venereal disease control	30
47. Industrial health	36	99. Veterinary medicine	13
48. Institutional sanitation	1	100. Vital statistics	49
49. Laboratories	47	101. Water and sewage	23
50. Legal services	4	102. Water pollution	19
51. Library	4	103. Well drilling	1
52. Local health administration	4		

*Included are all activities on the 50 organizational charts phrased to have a fairly clear meaning. About 40 other activities are not included because of varying degrees of ambiguity or lack of definition. None thus deleted occurred in more than 10% of the 50 charts reviewed.

This is reflected in a recent analysis of the health structures of state governments[10] which indicates that most activities are distributed under five most common major units of organization: administration, preventive medicine, environmental health, local health services, and laboratories. In performing the details of work within each of these the several states engage in a wide variety of activities as shown in Table 11-1. It should be noted that different terms are frequently used for activities which represent or include the same or similar activities. Thus, while only one state lists grant-in-aid administration as an activity per se, this function is performed elsewhere in the organization as part of local health administration (4 states) and local health services (42 states).

In attempting to carry out the many activities listed, each of the 50 states has developed its own unique pattern. Some have constructed strongly centralized organizations, in contrast with others with activities decentralized insofar as possible. As discussed and illustrated in Chapter 10, the subdivisions or functional units within the structure of state health departments vary extensively both in number and in manner of emphasis and arrangement. No two state patterns are identical, but similarities are to be noted. Thus a recent analysis by the Association of Management in Public Health indicates in two thirds of the instances the state health commissioner with a span of control of seven divisions or bureaus comprised of: (1) administration (including finance, personnel, hospital administration, vital statistics, and health education), (2) local health services (usually including public health nursing), (3) preventive medicine (usually including chronic diseases and adult health and sometimes mental health), (4) maternal and child health (usually including nutrition and crippled children's services), (5) dental health, (6) environmental health (including industrial hygiene and sanitary engineering), and (7) laboratories.

In summary, the trend has been for state health departments to restrict direct services as much as possible, to limit the number of major organizational units to about 6 in order to make possible an effective executive span of control, and to decentralize activities, particularly in larger states.

FEDERAL HEALTH ORGANIZATION
General
The most complex organizational picture of public health in the United States is found on the federal level. The history and development of some of the federal public health agencies have been discussed in Chapter 2. The purpose at this point is merely to describe briefly the more important of them and to bring out their interrelationships. Until recently, in place of a federal department of health there existed an illogical maze of miscellaneous departments, bureaus, offices, agencies, commissions, services, and authorities, each responsible for one or several aspects of the federal government's concern with health. This situation came about through a pyramiding of special legislation, often originating from executive requests, bureaucratic expansion, or the pressure of special interest groups. Once an agency is formed or designated to deal with a particular interest, that interest and the independence of the agency involved are jealousy guarded. An extreme result of such a procedure is well illustrated by the fact that the responsibility for the health of the inhabitants of the Pribilof Islands is vested in the Fish and Wildlife Service of the Department of the Interior. Recent years have seen several attempts to consolidate this perplexing and mushrooming group of federal agencies, but at best, consolidation of governmental affairs is a slow process. In the health and social services field, progress was gradually made, resulting first in the formation of the Federal Security Agency in 1939 and eventually in the establishment on April 11, 1953, of a Department of Health, Education, and Welfare.

The many federal agencies that have been established up to now, dealing with one or more aspects of public health, may be separated into four primary categories. The first is more or less concerned with broad general interests. Its only example is the Public Health Service. The second is concerned with the welfare of special groups

Text continued on p. 231.

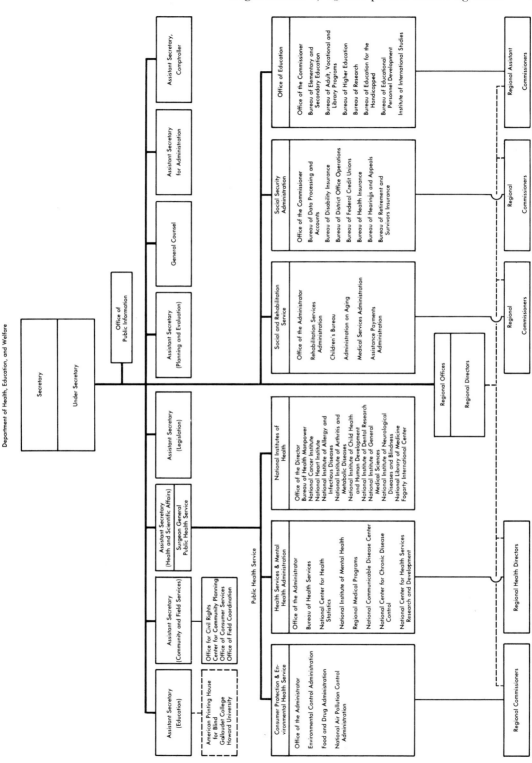

Fig. 11-4. Organization of the Department of Health, Education, and Welfare.

Table 11-2. Federal agencies engaged in health work*

Participating agency	Health activities	Method of administration†
Department of Health, Education, and Welfare:		
Public Health Service	Maintenance of research laboratories for study of cause, prevention, and treatment of disease	Direct service; research
	Assistance to states in establishing and maintaining proper sanitation facilities, general public health services—including dental health, occupational health, training of personnel, and extension and strengthening of full-time local health organizations—and special programs for the control of the venereal diseases, tuberculosis, mental health disorders, cancer, heart disease, water pollution, air pollution, radiation, and noise and for development of hospitalization plans and construction of hospital facilities	Grants-in-aid; studies and demonstrations; advisory service; loan of personnel; regulation
	Provision of hospitalization, general medical and dental care, and preventive health services for American merchant seamen, members of the United States Coast Guard, Coast and Geodetic Survey, and other legal beneficiaries of the Service	Direct service
	Provision of care and treatment for certain civilian beneficiaries of the federal government and for residents of the District of Columbia suffering from mental disorders	Direct service; research
	Operation of special hospitals (leprosarium and narcotic hospitals)	Do
	Provision of treatment for general and allied special illnesses of Negroes in the District of Columbia and surrounding areas	Do
	Establishment and operation of federal employee health service programs to promote and maintain the physical and mental fitness of government employees	Direct service; advisory service; loan of personnel
	Conduct of studies of mental diseases and drug addiction, and investigation of needs for narcotic drugs for medical and scientific purposes	Studies and demonstrations
	Assistance to institutions and to competent research workers for research in medical and related sciences	Research grants
	Assistance to medical institutions for treatment of cancer	Loan of radium
	Cooperation with official and nonofficial national organizations and institutions on health matters	Advisory service
	Estimation of requirements of controlled materials for civilian health, and arrangement for allocation of materials for this purpose during an emergency	Direct service; advisory service
	Collection and publication of vital and public health statistics, including epidemiologic data	Do
	Control of the spread of communicable diseases in interstate traffic	Direct service; regulation
	Assistance to states, municipalities or interstate agencies for defraying expenses in connection with plans for construction of waste treatment works	Grants-in-aid; advisory service
	Assistance to states, municipalities, or interstate agencies for construction of necessary waste treatment works	Advisory service; loans
	Supervision of milk, food, and water used on interstate carriers	Direct service; regulation
	Stabilization of the quality of foods and drugs through inspection, analysis, and control of labeling	Direct service; regulation research; advisory service
	Training of public health workers	Grants-in-aid; direct service

*Adapted from Mountin, J. W., and Flook, E.: Guide to health organization in the United States, Washington, 1953, Public Health Service Pub. No. 196, pp. 6-13 (subsequent changes made).
†As used here, "direct service" refers to services actually performed or directly purchased by the designated federal agency; "grants in-aid" are funds allotted by the federal agency to state or local agencies for performance of service; "advisory service" is limited to the giving of advice and setting of standards.

Table 11-2. Federal agencies engaged in health work—cont'd

Participating agency	Health activities	Method of administration†
Department of Health, Education, and Welfare—*cont'd* Public Health Service—*cont'd*		
	Production and dissemination of health information and education materials	Direct service
	Protection of this country from the importation of communicable diseases from abroad	Direct service; regulation
	Supervisory control and licensure of biologic products used in the prevention and treatment of diseases	Do
	Control of diseases in the event of epidemics and disasters	Direct service; regulation; advisory service
	Administration of medical care and public health among Indian wards of the government and Alaskan Eskimos	Direct service
	Assistance to other federal agencies in the discharge of their health functions	Advisory service; loan of personnel
	Collaboration with foreign governments and with international organizations on world health matters	Advisory service; loan of personnel; studies; information
Social Security Administration	Administration of federal health insurance programs; disability insurance	Direct payment of social security to individuals; provision of health insurance funds to states; standard setting; studies; advice and consultation
Social and Rehabilitation Service: Children's Bureau	Assistance to states in extending and improving maternal and child health and crippled children's services	Grants-in-aid; studies; advisory service
	Cooperation with official and nonofficial national organizations and institutions on maternal and child health and crippled children's matters	Advisory service
	Collaboration with foreign governments and with international organizations on maternal and child health and crippled children's programs	Studies; advisory service; information; loan of personnel
	Collection and dissemination of information in the field of child life and maternal health, and results of research studies under way in universities, schools, child welfare institutes, and other public and private agencies	Studies; information and education
Medical Services Administration	Assistance to states for public assistance payments (which may include provision for medical care) to dependent children, to the blind, and to the permanently and totally disabled	Grants-in-aid; studies; advisory service; standard setting
Rehabilitation Services Administration	Assistance to states in rehabilitating persons who are vocationally handicapped because of a mental or physical disability	Grants-in-aid; advisory service
	Rehabilitation of disabled residents of the District of Columbia	Direct service
Administration on Aging	Oversight of standards for social services by state and local agencies; guidance in administration of federal and state programs for the aged	Grants-in-aid; studies; standard setting; advice and consultation
Office of Education	Stimulation of education in the fields of public health, school health, and physical education	Studies and demonstrations; advisory service; information
	Assistance to states for vocational education which includes training in health fields	Grants-in-aid; advisory service
	Collaboration with national and international groups in fields of school health and physical education	Advisory service; information
Department of Agriculture: Agricultural Research Administration	Direction and coordination of physical and biologic research activities, many of which have a direct bearing on health	Direct service; advisory service

Continued.

Table 11-2. Federal agencies engaged in health work—cont'd

Participating agency	Health activities	Method of administration†
Department of Agriculture—*cont'd*		
Bureau of Animal Industry	Investigation of the cause, prevention, treatment, and control of diseases affecting both man and animals	Direct service; payment of indemnities; studies; regulation; research; advisory service; information
Bureau of Human Nutrition and Home Economics	Control of sanitation and wholesomeness of meat or meat-food products sold in interstate and foreign commerce	Regulation; direct service
	Conduct of research on food and other goods essential to healthful everyday living, studies of housing and equipment, and dissemination of information obtained	Studies; research; information
Bureau of Agricultural and Industrial Chemistry	Investigation of the properties and industrial utilization of farm products for foods, feeds, drugs and other products of health significance	Research
Office of Experiment Stations	Assistance to states in cooperative research in agriculture, rural health, nutrition, and diseases affecting man and animals	Grants-in-aid; advisory service
Bureau of Dairy Industry	Promotion of dairy industry and development of sanitary methods of handling milk and the processing of milk products	Direct service; studies and demonstrations
	Control of the manufacturing or processing of renovated butter	Regulation
Bureau of Entomology and Plant Quarantine	Investigation and control of insects affecting the health and well-being of man, and collaboration with state, foreign, and other organizations on control of such injurious pests	Direct service; regulation research; advisory service
Bureau of Plant Industry, Soils, and Agricultural Engineering	Promotion of improvement of design and sanitary aspects of farm homes, buildings, and storage facilities	Research
Farmers Home Administration	Provision of supervised credit and loans to farmers for construction or repair of houses and farm buildings, and for meeting the needs for family living, including health services, sanitary facilities, and insect pest control	Direct service; credit and loans
Extension Service	Promotion of rural health and better farm living, environmental sanitation, and improved farm housing	Grants-in-aid; advisory service; information
Forest Service	Provision of sanitary facilities in the national forests and supervision of general sanitation of forest areas	Direct service
Rural Electrification Administration	Improvement of rural sanitation facilities and water supplies	Direct service; advisory service
Production and Marketing Administration	Assistance, through state agencies, to schools having nonprofit school lunch programs in the interest of better nutrition and health for children	Direct service; grants-in-aid
	Establishment and enforcement of standards of purity and wholesomeness of various food products and control of the manufacture and sale of insecticides, fungicides, rodenticides, and disinfectants to prevent injury to man and other animals	Direct service; regulation; advisory service
	Administration of defense functions with respect to availability of farm equipment, fertilizer, and the supply and allocation of foods for proper nutrition	Direct service; advisory service
Bureau of Agricultural Economics	Collection, analysis, and distribution of statistics of health significance such as farm accidents, incidence of disease, and patterns of health care	Direct service; surveys and studies; advisory service; information
Office of Foreign Agricultural Relations	Cooperation with Food and Agriculture Organization of the United Nations and with federal agencies on international programs to raise the level of nutrition and standards of living, and to improve conditions of rural populations	Advisory service; information
Department of Commerce:		
Bureau of the Census	Collection and publication of basic statistics of population, housing, agriculture, industry, and other data for use by other agencies in planning health programs and services	Direct service; advisory service

Table 11-2. Federal agencies engaged in health work—cont'd

Participating agency	*Health activities*	*Method of administration†*
Department of Commerce—*cont'd*		
Maritime Administration	Provision of medical and dental care for enrollees of the United States Maritime Service and for Cadet-Midshipmen of the United States Merchant Marine Cadet Corps; operation of health and sanitation program at merchant marine training stations	Direct service
Business and Defense Services Administration	Distribution of controlled materials needed to meet the needs for civilian health requirements and coordination of other federal, state, and local agencies in obtaining such materials	Direct service; advisory service
Coast and Geodetic Survey	Insurance of safe navigation of coastal and intracoastal waters by means of surveys and charts of coastal areas; provision of emergency health and medical services to shipwrecked and destitute persons in Alaska and other remote localities	Direct service
Department of Defense:	Provision of basic policies, plans and programs in the medical and health fields as will provide guidance for the several military services in safeguarding the health of military personnel and their dependents	Do
	Operation of health and medical care programs for military personnel and their dependents	Do
	Provision of pure water for military posts and the District of Columbia, and improvement of navigable rivers, harbors, and waterways in the interest of flood control, maintenance of water supply, abatement of water pollution, and other use of water	Do
	Training of personnel for health work	Do
	Cooperation with other federal agencies on health and medical problems	Direct service; advisory service
	Direction of research, in and out of the Department, toward solving health problems arising out of military operations	Research
Department of the Interior:		
Bureau of Mines	Investigation of causes of mine accidents, inspection of mines, training in mine rescue and recovery work	Direct service; studies and demonstrations; information
	Production of lightweight, noninflammable gas helium used in nonexplosive anesthetics and in the treatment of some respiratory diseases	Direct service
Federal Water Pollution Control Administration	Prevention, control and abatement of water pollution	Direct service; research and demonstrations; grants-in-aid; training; assistance to states in enforcement
Fish and Wildlife Service	Promotion of programs for control or destruction of wild animals that endanger man or domestic animals through the transmission of diseases	Do
	Detection and elimination of stream pollution hazards	Do
	Conduct of research on methods of canning or processing of fishery products to ensure a sanitary and wholesome food	Research
Office of Territories	Provision of medical and health services for the inhabitants of territories and trust territories	Direct service
National Park Service	Provision of safe water and sanitary camp facilities in national parks	Direct service
Department of Justice:		
Immigration and Naturalization Service	Provision of physical and mental examinations of immigrants, and medical care of quarantined aliens	Direct service; regulation
Bureau of Prisons	Provision of medical, psychiatric, dental, and nursing services to inmates in federal prisons and correctional institutions	Direct service
Department of Labor:		
Bureau of Labor Standards	Promotion of industrial health and safety	Direct service; studies and demonstrations

Continued.

Table 11-2. Federal agencies engaged in health work—cont'd

Participating agency	*Health activities*	*Method of administration†*
Department of Labor—*cont'd*		
Bureau of Labor Standards—*cont'd*		
	Coordination of enforcement of wage, hour, industrial home work, child labor, and safety and health laws	Direct service; advisory service
	Training of state and foreign personnel in health and safety	Direct service
Women's Bureau	Promotion of the welfare of wage earning women and conduct of studies on health and working conditions of women in industry	Studies; advisory service
Bureau of Labor Statistics	Collection and analyses of data on environmental conditions in industry significant to health and publication of reports	Direct service; investigations and studies; information
Wage and Hour and Public Contracts Divisions	Administration of Fair Labor Standards Act to ensure minimum wage rates and the proper use of child labor in the production of goods for interstate commerce	Regulation
Bureau of Employees' Compensation	Administration of health and safety standards in industries under government supply contracts in excess of $10,000	Direct service
	Administration of benefit payments to injured workers for necessary medical and hospital services and compensation for disability and death	Direct payments of benefits
Bureau of Employment Security	Provision of medical and health services for migratory farm laborers at reception centers and while enroute to and from work contractor and reception centers	Direct service
Department of the Treasury:		
United States Coast Guard	Enforcement of regulations to ensure safety of life and property on the high seas and navigable waters under jurisdiction of the United States	Direct service; regulation
	Provision of medical and surgical aid to crews of United States vessels, and to shipwrecked and destitute persons in Alaska and other remote localities	Direct service
Bureau of Narcotics	Enforcement of federal narcotic laws and regulation of quantities of narcotic drugs to be imported, manufactured, or exported for medical purposes	Direct service; regulation
Office of Economic Opportunity	Assistance to state and local governments in the establishment and operation of a variety of programs to raise health, educational and other social levels of the socially and economically underprivileged; Head Start; comprehensive medical centers	Grants-in-aid; advice and consultation
Department of Housing and Urban Development	Assistance to local public housing authorities for planning, financing and construction of safe, sanitary, and adequate dwellings for low-income families; demonstration cities	Grants-in-aid; advisory service; loans; studies
	Assistance to state and local governments for repair of damages and rehabilitation of disaster-stricken areas	Grants-in-aid; advisory service
Atomic Energy Commission	Production and distribution of radioactive materials used in medical research	Direct service; advisory service
	Conduct of medical and clinical research at field installations and hospitals, and provision of research guidance in the physical and biologic sciences	Direct service; grants-in-aid; research; advisor; service; information
	Training in radiologic safety in the interest of civil defense	Direct service; research grants
	Control of distribution of information regarding the use and safety of radioactive materials	Direct service; advisory service; information
Defense Production Administration	Establishment of policies regarding health manpower needs and the expansion of production and general allotment of strategic materials used in meeting civilian and military health needs	Direct service; advisory service; loans
Federal Civil Defense Administration	Assistance to states for protective equipment and facilities	Grants-in-aid
	Provision of a coordinated plan for the protection of civilian life and property from enemy attack	Direct service; advisory service; public education

Table 11-2. Federal agencies engaged in health work—cont'd

Participating agency	Health activities	Method of administration†
Federal Trade Commission	Control of unfair or deceptive advertisements of food, drugs, devices, or cosmetics in interstate commerce	Regulation
Agency for International Development	Assistance to foreign countries to promote health and economic development	Direct service; grants-in-aid; studies and demonstrations; advisory service; information
Peace Corps	Training of foreign students in public health and other fields through educational exchange programs	Direct service; advisory service education
Interstate Commerce Commission	Promotion and enforcement of health and safety standards in the railroad industries and in the operation of railroads and motor carriers in interstate traffic	Investigations; regulations advisory service
National Science Foundation	Development and strengthening of a national policy of basic research in the medical, biologic, physical, and other health sciences, awarding of scholarships and graduate fellowships in these fields	Direct service; advisory service
National Security Resources	Coordination of activities of federal agencies with respect to manpower and natural resources as they affect national health and security; provision of advice to the President on the coordination of these resources	Direct service; advisory service
Selective Service System	Provision of health data of draftees examined for military service	Direct service
Tennessee Valley Authority	Maintenance of medical and public health service for employees	Do
	Cooperation with state and local health authorities in the control of insects, water pollution, general sanitation, and other public health services for the area	Direct service; advisory service
Veterans Administration	Provision of authorized health and medical services, including hospitalization and rehabilitation to former members of the armed forces	Direct service; research
	Administration of training benefits for veterans of the armed services; through this program more trained personnel will be made available for health work	Training grants
	Training of personnel in health work	Direct service

in the population. Included here are the Children's Bureau, the Women's Bureau, the Administration on Aging, the Farmer's Home Administration, the Agricultural Extension Service, the Office of Indian Affairs, the Medical Divisions of the Army and the Navy, and the Veterans Administration. The third category includes agencies concerned with special problems or programs, such as the Office of Education, the Social and Rehabilitation Service, the Food and Drug Administration, the Federal Trade Commission, the Bureau of Labor Standards, the Bureau of Labor Statistics, many bureaus within the Department of Agriculture (animal industry, entomology and plant quarantine, dairy industry, production and marketing, human nutrition and home economics, etc.), the Bureau of Mines, the Maritime Commission, and the Tennessee Valley Authority. The Social Security Administration and the Bureau of Employee's Compensation may also be included in this category in the sense that they provide medical care to special groups. The fourth category may be considered to be made up of certain quasi-independent institutions such as St. Elizabeth's Hospital and the Freedmen's Hospital. A fifth category might be considered to handle the international health interests of the government of the United States. The functions of all these agencies vary from direct personal service to regulation, consultation, demonstration, research, education, and financial grants-in-aid. Table 11-2 presents a summary of the federal agencies engaged in health work with their health functions and methods of administration.

As just stated, the most important of the federal agencies dealing with public health matters in 1953 were brought together to form the Department of Health, Education, and Welfare, the organization of which is shown in Fig. 11-4. This agency was created with the purpose of grouping under one administration those agencies of the government whose major functions are to promote social and economic security, educational opportunity, and the health of the citizens of the nation.

Public Health Service

From the broad overall point of view of public health the principal organization included in the Department of Health, Education, and Welfare is the United States Public Health Service. Most of the functions of the Public Health Service take the form of research, demonstrations, interstate and international quarantine, advice on technical matters and loan of officers to state and local health departments, and other federal agencies with particular health interests. Probably its most significant contribution is made through financial grants-in-aid to state and territorial health agencies for the expansion and improvement of their programs and those of the local jurisdictions they include. The functions of the Service may be summarized as follows:

1. Study of the causes and means of propagation and spread of the diseases of mankind and development of methods of prevention and control

    In this work the Public Health Service maintains several research laboratories, chief among which are those of the National Institutes of Health, the Communicable Disease Center, and the National Environmental Health Center. In addition to investigations carried on at the Institutes and their field stations, financial assistance is given through research grants to universities, laboratories, and other public and private institutions for research projects upon recommendation of Service advisory councils. Funds are also available for research fellowships, both in the Institutes and in various university medical schools.

2. Maritime quarantine and inspection of pas-

sengers and crews of vessels and airplanes arriving from foreign ports for protection of the country from the importation of quarantinable diseases from other countries

    Examination of immigrants for detection and isolation of persons suffering from mandatorily excludable disease. Medical inspection of aliens is performed in collaboration with the Immigration and Naturalization Service of the Department of Justice.

3. Interstate quarantine for prevention of the spread of diseases from state to state

    The federal health agency prescribes conditions under which persons and things may move in interstate commerce. It assists states in controlling epidemics and may, on request, take complete charge of serious outbreaks. Regulation of conditions existing within the boundaries of a particular state is a duty that remains under state jurisdiction.

4. Dissemination of public health information, including collection and publication of reports of disease prevalence in the United States and foreign countries, and other pertinent information regarding conservation of the public health

5. Assistance, through grants to states, counties, cities, and health districts, in establishing and maintaining proper sanitation facilities, general public health services—including industrial hygiene, mental hygiene, and cancer control—and special programs for the control of the venereal diseases and tuberculosis

    Grants made under this authority represent the actual transfer of funds from federal to state treasuries for employment and training of personnel for state and local health work, purchase of supplies and equipment, provision of appropriate facilities for care and treatment of designated illnesses, and payment of general operating expenses. Services include the loan of personnel for temporary duty and the provision of consultation and advice to state and local health departments. Assistance is also furnished states in the development of hospitalization plans and construction of hospital and allied health facilities.

6. Supervisory control and licensure of the manufacturers of biologic products—vaccines, serums, toxins, antitoxins, arsenicals, and similar preparations—used in the prevention and treatment of diseases

    This control has been established to ensure safe and standard products.

7. Study of mental diseases and drug addiction and investigation of legitimate needs for narcotic drugs

8. Provision of hospitalization, general medical and dental care, and preventive health services for American merchant seamen, members of the United States Coast Guard and

the Coast and Geodetic Survey, and for other legal beneficiaries of the Service

In this connection the Service operates 16 hospitals and 25 outpatient clinics and contracts for service in over 100 other places not served by Public Health Service hospitals. It assigns medical and dental officers to ship duty to provide medical and dental care at sea for the Coast Guard and the Coast and Geodetic Survey. The Public Health Service, in cooperation with the Bureau of Prisons, maintains a medical and health program in federal prisons. The Public Health Service also provides medical care and public health services to Indian wards of the government and Alaskan Eskimos.

9. Operation of special hospitals—the National Leprosarium and two hospitals specifically for the care of mental patients and persons addicted to the use of narcotics
10. Cooperation with other federal agencies in discharging their various health functions through assignment of personnel for assistance
11. Collaboration with and participation in the functioning of international health organizations

In carrying out this service particular attention is given to the direction of programs for the exchange of international health and related personnel.
12. Collection and publication of data on vital statistics, which are basic materials for public health programs and give valuable information concerning public health trends

Through measurement of death rates from different causes the progress of health programs directed toward reduction of particular diseases or conditions can be evaluated.
13. Administration of St. Elizabeth's Hospital, the principal hospital for treatment of mentally ill civilian beneficiaries of the federal government, and Freedmen's Hospital, a general hospital with specialized departments affiliated with the Howard University Medical School

Both of these hospitals are under the direction of the Surgeon General of the United States Public Health Service.

The work of the Public Health Service is directed by a Surgeon General appointed by the President. It is organized into three administrative units: the National Institutes of Health (including the National Library of Medicine), the Health Services and Mental Health Administration, and the Consumer Protection and Environmental Health Service. The last consists of the Environmental Control Administration, the Food and Drug Administration, and the Air Pollution Control Administration (Fig. 11-4). For decentralization of services and assistance to states, nine regional offices are maintained in Boston, New York, Charlottesville, Chicago, Atlanta, Kansas City, Dallas, Denver, and San Francisco. At the present time, in addition to a National Advisory Health Council, there are advisory councils for cancer, mental health, heart disease, dental research, arthritis and metabolic diseases, neurologic diseases and blindness, allergy and infectious diseases, general medical sciences, child health and human development, health research facilities, radiation, and training. The Federal Hospital Council, with both advisory and operational duties, is responsible to the Surgeon General for the administration of the Hill-Burton Hospital Survey and Construction Act. The Surgeon General also calls an annual conference of state and territorial health officers and whatever special conferences or committees as may appear indicated.

Children's Bureau

Next in importance to the Public Health Service is the Children's Bureau, formerly located in the Department of Labor, but now in the Social and Rehabilitation Service of the Department of Health, Education, and Welfare. From a functional viewpoint the separate existence of the Children's Bureau has always appeared somewhat illogical. Its justification has been linked to the two arguments that the needs of children must be considered as a whole and that they form a population group unable to organize and to speak for themselves. A chief function of the Bureau is to enable each state to extend and improve the health services for mothers and children. This is accomplished through assistance to states in the support of prenatal, postnatal, and well-child clinics, of demonstrations of delivery and other services, and of public health nursing services for maternal and child health supervision. The Bureau has played an important role in the promotion and development of divisions of maternal and child health in all of the state health departments. It also sponsors a cooperative federal and state program of services for crippled children. The programs of the

Children's Bureau are carried on in a manner similar to the Bureau of Health Services of the Public Health Service, primarily through grants-in-aid to the states and through consultative services. During World War II the Bureau served as the administrative agency for the Emergency Maternity and Infant Care Program for the wives and infants of servicemen. By early 1949, when the program was terminated, close to one and a half million expectant mothers and about one third of a million infants had been provided with care by private physicians of their choice, paid through the program. As discussed elsewhere, this program not only represented a nationwide experiment in medical care but also provided invaluable experience in administration for many public health workers. The Maternal and Child Health Amendments of 1963 made it possible for the Children's Bureau to provide grants to state and local health agencies for comprehensive maternity care of high risk mothers. With the passage of the Social Security Amendments of 1965, the Children's Bureau has had the responsibility for the administration of Section 532 of Title V, Part 4, which provides for the development of high quality comprehensive health services to children and youth.

By collecting and distributing information the Children's Bureau maintains a clearinghouse on research in progress in the total field of child life both inside and outside the federal government. It conducts surveys and studies on the nature and extent of child health problems and analyzes and reports statistics on maternal and child health and crippled children's services provided under grant-in-aid programs. It provides federal financial aid for specialized training projects in services to children, to students and workers in child health, and to teaching institutions.

Individually or as a team of specialists in maternal and child health, consultants of the Bureau visit state health and crippled children's agencies to advise on the operation of state programs, standards of service, and ways of extending and improving health services to mothers and children.

In carrying out its responsibilities the Children's Bureau cooperates with official and nonofficial national organizations and institutions; it stimulates interest, participation, and cooperation on the part of educational, social, and welfare agencies for the coordination of resources and services; and it participates in a broad program of international cooperation.

Other federal agencies

The United States Office of Education of the Department of Health, Education, and Welfare is engaged in several activities related to health. It promotes programs of health education and school health and safety, engages in investigations relating to medical examination of school children and their teachers, promotes school lunch programs, and administers a grant-in-aid program for vocational education in health.

The Food and Drug Administration is a federal organization, now located in the Department of Health, Education, and Welfare, chiefly concerned with the quality of foods and drugs. Its efforts are directed toward the promotion of purity, standard potency, and accurate labeling of substances within its jurisdiction, which include food, drugs, cosmetics, tea, certain milk products, and poisons.

Outside the Department of Health, Education, and Welfare are a number of branches of the Department of Agriculture which engage in programs concerned with health. The Bureau of Animal Industry inquires into the cause, prevention, and treatment of diseases of domestic animals, which naturally have an influence upon many phases of human health. Federal meat inspection services are administered by the Production and Marketing Administration, which also administers the Insecticide Act. The labor branch of this office finances medical care and health services for migrant farm workers. The Bureau of Dairy Industry is active in investigations and education relating to the sanitary production and handling of milk. The Bureau of Entomology and Plant Quarantine, while primarily concerned with the protection of crops from parasitic insects, necessarily contributes much knowledge and service to the control of insects affecting man. Active in research and service relating to foods, nutrition, and dietary habits is the

Bureau of Human Nutrition and Home Economics, which with the agricultural extension service in cooperation with state land grant colleges has accomplished much in the improvement of rural health and nutrition. Of importance and interest in assistance for medical and dental care is the Farmer's Home Administration within the Department of Agriculture. Its beneficiaries are chiefly low-income farm groups. Needed medical and dental care is made available through provision of supervised credit and loans.

In the Department of the Interior are a number of agencies with specialized interests in public health problems. The Bureau of Mines conducts an important health, sanitation, and safety program in relation to the mining and quarrying industry. In company with the Fish and Wildlife Service it is concerned with certain phases of the problem of stream pollution. The latter agency also contributes to health protection by promoting rodent control programs. Originally the Department of the Interior through its Office of Indian Affairs had responsibility for the operation of hospitals and programs for the general improvement of health and sanitation on Indian reservations. In 1953 this responsibility was transferred to the Public Health Service.

Federal agencies in international health affairs

Originally the interests of the United States Government in international health affairs were limited to measures designed to prevent the introduction of certain diseases. Developments in world history, economics, and methods of transportation, however, have made it necessary to adopt a broader viewpoint and to assume responsibilities of great significance to international public health. These newer responsibilities are of two types: first, participation in development of public health programs in other specific nations and, second, participation as one of a number of partners in the promotion of worldwide health. The most important federal agencies involved in these activities are the Office of International Health of the Public Health Service, the Agency for International Development of

the Department of State, and the Peace Corps.

The Office of International Health of the Public Health Service was established to coordinate and give general direction to all Service activities in the international health field; to maintain liaison with agencies in this field; to represent the Service in international health conferences; to direct a program on international exchange of health personnel and educational material; to draft sanitary conventions and regulations and health reports required by international agreements; to collect and distribute data relating to foreign medical and health institutions; to supervise special health missions to foreign countries; to advise the State Department regarding development of plans, programs, and policies for consideration by the World Health Organization; and to advise the Surgeon General on international health matters.

In relation to the foregoing the United States Government has representation in the World Health Organization, the Pan-American Health Organization, and the Anglo-American Caribbean Commission.

The bilateral international health activities of the United States Government are centered in the Agency for International Development of the Department of State. In the planning, staffing, and conduct of its health programs it relates intimately not only to the Office of International Health of the Public Health Service and to other significant parts of the federal government, especially the Peace Corps, but also to several state health departments and to a number of universities, schools of public health, and schools of medicine. Its activities and those of the multilateral international health agencies are described in more detail in the following section.

INTERNATIONAL HEALTH ORGANIZATION*

Introduction

A consideration of the field of international health may be approached from several direction: first, from the standpoint of

---

*See Chapter 3, which discusses certain aspects of world and international health problems.

the specific preventable diseases and health problems that exist under various local, national, or regional circumstances; second, from the standpoint of the various organizations that are or have been active in the field; and, third, from the standpoint of the relationship to present or potential public health organizations or structures in the various political units of the world. In the final analysis it is this latter which is the most important. It must always be borne in mind that effective, fruitful, lasting action can occur only on the local level where the people, their problems, their communities, and their governmental structures are found. Therefore, international health work cannot be thought of as a field unto itself. It has meaning only in its relation to the many national and local components of the total world health picture. It is with this reservation that certain aspects of international health activities are presented.

World Health Organization[11]

Before World War II various activities had occurred in the international health arena. Most notable of these was the development of the Pan-American Sanitary Bureau in 1902, the International Office of Public Health in 1907, and the Health Organization of the League of Nations in 1921. In 1923 the International Office was absorbed into the Health Organization of the League, which continued to function, as did the Pan-American Sanitary Bureau, through the period of World War II.

In 1944, while the war was still in progress and Paris was occupied by the Nazis, an international conference was held in Montreal to discuss the fate of the Health Organization of the League. Stemming from this and culminating at a further conference in New York in 1946, a constitution for a World Health Organization was signed by 61 nations. The organization began official existence on September 1, 1948. The duties and powers of the Health Organization of the League of Nations and the health functions of the temporary United Nations Relief and Rehabilitation Administration were transferred to the new agency. Subsequently the Pan-American Sanitary Bureau (now the Pan-American Health Organization), while retaining a separate identity, became the World Health Organization's regional office for the Americas.

By September 1968 the World Health Organization had an enrollment of 125 member and 3 associate member nations, which makes it the largest of the specialized agencies of the United Nations. The United States has been an active member since its formation in 1948 under authorization of P. L. 80-643.

The constitution of the World Health Organization, particularly in view of its definition of health as "a state of complete physical, mental, and social well-being and not merely the absence of disease or infirmity," has been aptly referred to as the Magna Charta of health because of its affirmation that health is "one of the fundamental rights of every human being, without distinction of race, religion, political belief, economic or social condition" and because of its recognition that "the health of all peoples is fundamental to the attainment of peace and security."

The headquarters of the World Health Organization is in Geneva, Switzerland. Regional offices are located at Brazzaville, for Africa; Washington, for the Americas (Pan-American Health Organization); New Delhi, for Southeast Asia; Copenhagen, for Europe; Alexandria, for the Eastern Mediterranean; and Manila, for the Western Pacific. It is financed by prorated and special contributions from active member nations and from the United Nations Technical Assistance Board. In 1967 its regular budget was approximately $51.5 million. An annual World Health Assembly, which determines international health policy and program, is the agency's legislative body. Each member nation is allowed three delegates but only one vote at the Assemblies. An executive board has the responsibility of putting into effect the decisions and policies of the Assembly and deals with emergency situations in the name of the Assembly. Normally this technical nonpolitical group of 24 health experts, who are elected at the Assembly, meets twice a year. A secretariat, headed by a director-general, includes a technical and an administrative staff of more than 3,000 persons located at the Geneva headquarters and in the regional offices. It is responsible for the day-to-day work of the organization. The World Health Organization avoids one of the basic errors of the health office of the former League of Nations, that of overcentralization, in that it provides for 6 regional committees comprised of representatives of the member states in each region. These regional committees formulate regional policies and supervise the activities of the regional offices. In addition, 44 expert panels and committees, which involve more than 12,000 experts in various fields, have been established to advise the World Health Organization on technical aspects of its activities and to keep it up to date on current scientific research.

The functions of the World Health Organization have been summarized as follows:

1. It is the one directing and coordinating authority on international health work. It is not a supranational ministry of health but rather a worldwide cooperative through which the nations help each other to help themselves in raising health standards.
2. It provides to member countries various central technical services, i.e., epidemiology, statistics, standardization of drugs and procedures, a wide range of technical publications, etc.
3. Its most important function is to help countries to strengthen and improve their own health service. Upon request it provides advisory and consulting services through public health experts, demonstration teams for disease control, visiting specialists, etc.

The World Health Assembly has given top priority to six major problems, malaria, maternal and child health, control of tuberculosis, control of venereal diseases, environmental sanitation, and nutrition. Special attention is also given to programs for the control of parasitic and virus diseases, activities in the field of mental health, and family planning. Technical assistance in the field of public health administration, originally placed in the second priority group,

has been receiving ever increasing attention.

There are two important distinctions between the health office of the League of Nations and the World Health Organization, which replaced it. First, the functions and activities of the latter are very broad. For the first time in international affairs emphasis is placed not upon quarantine, checking epidemics, and other defensive measures but upon positive aggressive action toward health in its broadest sense. Second, whereas the former organization was an integral part of a political body, the World Health Organization, although related to the United Nations, is nevertheless a separate independent agency with its own constitution, membership, and sources of funds. As yet it is too early to determine with assurance what the future holds for this organization. Much depends upon the ability of the nations of the world to live with one another in peace and cooperation. It has been commonly said that, despite its political affiliation, the old health office was the most successful part of the League of Nations. In view of this fact one might hope with reason that the new organization has an even greater chance of success, effectiveness, and permanency.

Pan-American Health Organization

The turn of the century saw the establishment in 1902 at the Second Inter-American Pan-American Conference in Mexico City of the Pan-American Sanitary Bureau, more recently renamed the Pan-American Health Organization. Its headquarters is in Washington, D. C. This was the first permanent international health agency and the longest lived up to the present. It was organized to be governed by an elected directing council and a director-general. It is supported by annual financial quotas contributed by each of the American Republics. Under the provisions of the Pan-American Sanitary Code, which was ratified by all 21 of the American Republics in 1924, it became the center of coordination of international action and information in the field of public health in the Western Hemisphere. It holds an annual conference of high quality which is attended by delegates from all member nations. Through its development it has been given the responsibility and authority to receive and disseminate epidemiologic information, to furnish technical assistance upon request to member countries, to finance fellowships, and to promote cooperation in medical research. It has done much to promote professional education in Latin America. It also serves as the regional office and agent in the Americas of the World Health Organization, while nevertheless maintaining its own identity.

United Nations Children's Fund

The United Nations Children's Fund is an agency whose history and activities have been intimately related to those of the World Health Organization. At the demise of the United Nations Relief and Rehabilitation Administration in 1946 certain of its funds were transferred to a newly formed agency organized to assist especially the children of war-torn countries. The program gradually expanded to include other activities and other areas, particularly underdeveloped countries. Over the past few years as an emergency agency the Fund has spent large sums of money, especially on food and supplies, for child and maternal welfare activities throughout the world and particularly in war-torn areas. Beyond this, however, and usually through partnership with the World Health Organization it has been carrying out large and significant programs of BCG vaccination, yaws control, and malaria control demonstrations. Organized originally as a temporary emergency agency, it has filled such a need and attracted such support that in 1953 it was given permanent status, and its name was changed to the United Nation's Children's Fund.

United States bilateral
health programs

So far we have been considering the development of what have been commonly referred to as the multilateral organizations in public health, i.e., organizations whose financing, staffing, policy making, and operations are entered into and shared by more than two and usually many nations. In addition, there exists another type of international health cooperation which is carried out by what are now referred to as

bilateral agreements and organizations. This comes about when two nations for reasons of mutual interest agree to work together on certain matters dealing with public health.

The United States Government became significantly involved in bilateral international public health activities as a result of World War II. In January 1942 the Foreign Ministers of the American Republics, concerned over the turn of world events, considered areas wherein cooperation among the republics of the Western Hemisphere was necessary for the common good and survival. Health needs were placed high on the list. They recommended that through bilateral and other agreements the necessary steps be taken to solve the environmental sanitation and health problems of the Americas and that to this end, according to capacity, each country contribute raw material, services, and funds. The United States was asked to accept the responsibility of leadership, and an Office of the Coordinator of Inter-American Affairs was established. Originally it was attached to the office of the President of the United States but later assumed a governmental corporate structure with the name Institute of Inter-American Affairs. It was given the responsibility of initiating and conducting bilateral technical assistance programs in health, agriculture, education, and other fields.

Promptly, in intimate relation with each of the other republics involved, 18 cooperative health programs were established. The activities of each program were financed by contributions from both the United States and the other governments concerned, and the programs were determined jointly by an official of the host government, usually the minister or director of health, and the chief of the group of technicians assigned by the United States to the host country.

From the beginning the program has had four chief areas of emphasis: (1) the development of local health services through health centers; (2) the sanitation of the environment, with particular emphasis on water supply, sewage disposal, and insect control; (3) the training and full-time employment of professional public health workers; and (4) the education of the public in health matters. It has stressed complete community health development under full-time trained direction with active community participation.

Stimulated by the tremendous needs for rehabilitation throughout the world, by requests of newly formed nations for assistance, and by the proved value of the programs of the Institute of Inter-American Affairs, the United States has organized since the end of World War II a succession of agencies each to serve certain problem or areal needs. Predominant among these were the Mutual Security Administration and the Foreign Operations Administration. In July 1955 these and the Institute of Inter-American Affairs were all joined to form the International Cooperation Administration. In 1961 it was further reorganized to become the Agency for International Development. While organizationally in the Department of State, it is in effect a semi-autonomous agency of the government in that its funds are appropriated separately by an annual Mutual Security Act.

The Agency for International Development cooperates with other nations by providing military, economic, and technical assistance. A significant component of the last is assistance in public health matters. At the present time the public health personnel of the Agency for International Development is actively engaged in numerous types of cooperative health programs in various countries throughout the world. Many public health and related workers from the United States, representing a wide spectrum of professional disciplines are involved in its programs. One of the most significant contributions of the Agency for International Development and of its predecessors has been in the field of training. Fellowships for advanced training in the United States and elsewhere have been granted to several thousand professional health workers of other countries, and many thousands more have been given in-service training in connection with ongoing cooperative health programs.

During the 5 years 1961 through 1965, AID expenditures for health purposes (not including loans for water supply and waste disposal) totalled $515.76 million. For fiscal year 1965 expenditures in millions of dollars were as follows: control of specific diseases, $9.2; environmental sanitation, $15.4; operation of health facilities, $5.0; health training of professional personnel, $2.2; construction, remodeling, and equipping of health facilities, $1.8; and other miscellaneous health activities, $6.4.[12]

Peace Corps

Mention should also be made of the Peace Corps, which is related organizationally to the Office of the President of the United States. This organization sends large numbers of mostly young volunteers to work on request in socially and economically underprivileged areas of the world. In many instances they augment significantly the technical assistance provided by the Agency for International Development.

Nongovernmental agencies

No summary of international health cooperation would be complete without emphasizing, though briefly, the great contribution which has been made by nongovernmental agencies. As far as shirt-sleeve technical assistance is concerned, undoubtedly the earliest endeavors were those of the various church missions and medical missionaries. In addition, there have been certain philanthropic foundations with interest in international health based upon the highest altruistic motives. Outstanding among these organizations have been the Unitarian Service Committee, the American Friends Service Committee, the various Catholic Mission groups, the American Bureau for Medical Aid to China, the Foreign Mission Agencies of the Baptist and Methodist churches, the Near East Relief Agency, and many others. Representatives of all these have performed yeoman service, working hand in hand with the people of villages and farms in many lands on a basis of true friendship and equality.

Among the foundations, the Rockefeller Foundation is the best known in the field of international assistance in health. It has operated in almost all countries of the world in the five decades of its existence. Its contributions and successes are many and great and include such activities as the control of malaria and yellow fever, the development of recognized centers of learning in medicine and public health, the provision of postgraduate fellowships to many individuals, and the demonstration of sound methods of organization and operation of health programs. More recently it has been joined by several other foundations, notably the Kellogg Foundation, which is especially interested at the present time in further improving professional education in the Latin American countries.

Conclusion

To some it may appear as if the programs of international health are too many, too varied, too dispersed, and too confusing. While this may be true to some degree, it has been by no means unexpected or undesirable. The field of international cooperation for mutual development is rather new. It has been necessary and logical to approach it somewhat on the basis of caution and trial and error, rather than to attempt at some premature date to establish a fixed pattern which might have stifled future growth and thought. The last few years have seen the beginning of a process of pulling the pieces together both in the multilateral and in the bilateral areas, and it is to be expected that the future will see an ever more .logical and fruitful organizational approach to the tremendous problems which still exist in public health throughout the world. The names of some organizations may have changed frequently. If so, it should be borne in mind that only results count and that titles are incidental.

Finally, it must be realized that there will always be an important place for all three types of international health work, i.e., the multilateral, the bilateral, and the nongov-ernmental. Each in its way provides support to the others. Sound, effective, and cooperative correlation of all of their activities may result in the ultimate achievement of the universally desired goal of world health and through it indirectly in world peace.

REFERENCES

1. Mountin, J. W., and Flook, E.: Guide to health organization in the United States, Washington, 1953, Public Health Service Pub. No. 196 (subsequent changes made).
2. Sanders, B. S.: Local health departments, growth or illusion, Public Health Rep. **74:**13, Jan. 1959.
3. Organization and staffing for local health services, Washington, 1961, Public Health Service Pub. No. 682.
4. Haldeman, J. C.: Unpublished data presented at Annual Meeting of the National Advisory Committee on Local Health Departments, March 18, 1958.
5. Local health units for the nation, Report of Sub-Committee on Administration Practice, American Public Health Association, New York, 1945, Commonwealth Fund.
6. The local health department—services and responsibilities. An official statement of the American Public Health Association, adopted Nov. 10, 1963.
7. The local health department—services and responsibilities, An Official Statement of the American Public Health Association, adopted Nov. 1, 1950.
8. Distribution of health services in the structure of state government, 1950, Washington, 1952, Public Health Service Pub. No. 184, Part 1.
9. The state public health agency; an official statement of the American Public Health Association, Amer. J. Public Health **55:**2011, Dec. 1965.
10. Shubick, H. J., and Wright, E. O.: Composite study of fifty health department organizational charts representing forty-nine states and the District of Columbia, unpublished report, 1961.
11. The World Health Organization, Geneva, 1967, Division of Information, WHO.
12. American Association for World Health: American review of world health, New York, 1966, The Association, Vol. 14, No. 3.

Chapter 12

Voluntary
health agencies

INTRODUCTION

Voluntary health agencies are organizations supported by private or nontax funds and directed by privately employed individuals who often lack public health training. They have no legal powers. While by no means unique to the United States, they are especially numerous in this country. This may be due to certain characteristics that were important in our historical and social development: goodwill, friendliness, sympathy for the fellow who is down, a desire to improve the human race, a penchant for carrying out studies and reforms, and a tendency to form and join organizations of all sorts for many purposes. It might be said that one aspect of the democratic philosophy as developed in America was a widespread concern for the welfare of one's neighbor or fellowman.

The voluntary health movement began with the Anti-Tuberculosis Society of Philadelphia in 1892. Its development epitomizes the voluntary health movement as a whole. Encouraged by the formation of the earlier Philadelphia society, a group of unusually intelligent and enthusiastic private citizens banded together in 1904 to organize the National Association for the Study and Prevention of Tuberculosis. The membership of the group is worthy of special mention. It included Trudeau as president, William Osler, Bowditch, Bates, Janeway, Welch, Billings, Victor Vaughan, and other individuals of like quality. Among the six lay members of the board were Homer Folks, Samuel Gompers, and Edward T. Devine, who were most prominent in the develop-

ment of social welfare in the United States. At that time tuberculosis caused one tenth of all deaths and was the leading cause of destitution and orphanhood. From the start it was decided that eventually the job was one for government since voluntary funds could never hope to meet the total bill. It was recognized, however, that government action in a democracy does not necessarily precede or preclude public opinion and that the public and the government needed to be educated. This the association believed it could do, and it proceeded with the eventual organization of 50 state associations and approximately 3,000 local affiliates.

At first the financing of the National Association posed a difficult problem. It was temporarily solved during a transition by the Russell Sage Foundation, which assumed the responsibility for the 10 years from 1907 to 1917. Meanwhile the Tuberculosis Christmas Seal idea had been developed in Denmark. This was considered an especially desirable fund-raising technique since it gave individual citizens a personal interest in the fight against tuberculosis. The idea was quickly adopted in this country, and by 1914 it provided the bulk of the funds not only of the national but also of the state and local associations. As an indication of its wide appeal, about $35 million to $40 million are raised each year by the sale of penny Christmas Seals. The pattern of distribution of proceeds for most publicly supported voluntary health agencies was set from the beginning by the National Association, which decided to leave the bulk of funds raised, 95%, to the state and local associations while the national agency retained only 5%.

NUMBER AND TYPE

Since the establishment of the Anti-Tuberculosis Society of Philadelphia in 1892 a confusing number of separate voluntary health agencies (approximately 100,000) have been formed that draw their support from literally millions of persons and serve millions of others in various ways. These agencies have been both effective and ineffective, efficient and inefficient, blessed and belittled, intelligent and unreasonable, cooperative and uncooperative. These are but a few of the possible and inevitable outcomes of rapid development of a large number of independent undertakings. They have, however, one characteristic in common—they seldom die. Hochbaum[1] has summarized the typical sequence very well. "In a young organization, almost all its activities are geared to deal with the very objectives and purposes for which it was created —nothing matters as much as its self-avowed mission. Later, however, increasingly strong concerns develop to maintain and strengthen the organization for its own sake, to expand its activities, to stake out a scope of goals and activities, and to protect this domain against intrusion by other agencies."

Voluntary health agencies involve the time and often the money of at least 500,000 rather exceptional men and women who serve on boards or committees as well as the time and effort of over 1 million other voluntary workers. According to the American Association of Fund-Raising Counsel, private philanthropy accounted for $1.4 billion in health expenditures for the year 1964-1965. These figures exclude not only the American Red Cross but also the large philanthropic foundations, industrial health services, and a large number of agencies that only incidentally furnish health services. The American Red Cross is in a class by itself; it had a peacetime membership of about 5 million, which increased during the war years to 36 million people. There are now about 4,000 chapters and 6,000 branches. During the $3\frac{1}{2}$ years from the Pearl Harbor bombing to May 1945, contributions amounting to $654 million were raised. The American Red Cross is the only voluntary agency with quasi-official status; the President of the United States serves as its president, and the organization is considered the official disaster relief agency of the nation.

As early as the close of World War I concern had developed about the growing number of fund-raising agencies. In 1918 the National Information Bureau that had been established laid down the following eight precepts to guide philanthropic agencies that might wish approval by that agency. So well were they stated that they have remained unchanged and useful ever since[2]:

1. Board—An active and responsible governing body (must maintain direction of the agency), serving without compensation, holding regular meetings, and with effective administrative control.
2. Purpose—A legitimate purpose with no avoidable duplication of the work of other sound organizations.
3. Program—Reasonable efficiency in program management, and reasonable adequacy of resources, both material and personnel.
4. Cooperation—Evidence of consultation and cooperation with established agencies in the same or related fields.
5. Ethical promotion—Ethical methods of publicity, promotion and solicitation of funds.
6. Fund-raising practice—In fund-raising:
   (a) No payment of commissions for fund-raising.
   (b) No mailing of unordered tickets or merchandise with a request for money in return.
   (c) No general telephone solicitation of the public.
7. Audit—Annual audit, prepared by an independent certified public accountant or trust company, showing all income and disbursements, in reasonable detail. New organizations should provide a certified public accountant's statement that a proper financial system has been installed.
8. Budget—Detailed annual budget, translating program plans into financial terms.

Voluntary agencies concerned with health may be considered to fall into several categories. First and most important is a large group of agencies supported by citizen contributions and donations. These are subdivisible into the following four types, which demonstrate a remarkable degree of specialization:

1. Agencies that are concerned with specific diseases, e.g., the American Cancer Society, the National Tuberculosis and Respiratory Disease Association, the National Foundation, the American Social Hygiene Association, and the American Diabetic Society.
2. Agencies that are concerned with certain organs or structures of the body, e.g., the National Society for the Prevention of Blindness, the American Society for the Hard of Hearing, the National Society for Crippled Children, and the American Heart Association.
3. Agencies that are concerned with the health and welfare of special groups in society, e.g., the American Child Health Association (now extinct), the Maternity Center Association, and the American Negro Health Association.
4. Agencies that are concerned with particular phases of health and welfare, e.g., the National Safety Council and the Planned Parenthood Federation of America.

The second large group of voluntary agencies engaged in health work is composed of foundations established and financed by private philanthropy. Prominent among the many that might be mentioned are the Rockefeller Foundation, the W. K. Kellogg Foundation, the Commonwealth Fund, the Milbank Memorial Fund, the Children's Fund of Michigan, the Rosenwald Fund, and the Markle Foundation. Organizations of this type have functioned in a variety of ways, particularly by promoting and subsidizing local health departments, especially those in rural areas, and by supporting basic research as well as public and professional education.

The third main group of voluntary health agencies is made up of professional associations such as the American Public Health Association, the American Medical Association, the National League for Nursing, and their state and local affiliates. In addition to providing a meeting ground for professional workers in their respective fields these associations do much to establish and improve standards and qualifications, encourage research, further health education, and promote programs.

Integrating agencies such as health councils and community chests and councils constitute what may be considered a fourth group. There are now more than 1,000 of these multiple interest organizations. They are found on local, state, and national levels; their purpose is the coordination of the activities of the many specialized voluntary agencies.

A fifth group of nonofficial agencies that may be considered to have some interest in the public health consists of an increasing number of commercial organizations that have found it worth while for one reason or another to participate in the promotion of sanitary and hygienic habits and programs. Predominant among these are several of the large insurance companies that have carried out very extensive and valuable educational programs and demonstrations. Some activities have also been engaged in by industries concerned with the manufacture and sale of soap, sugar, milk, meat, eating and drinking utensils, and other products. Generally speaking, this latter group must be dealt with cautiously since their programs are based primarily upon a desire for increased profits and improved public relations.

FUNCTIONS AND ACTIVITIES

The Gunn and Platt study and analysis[3] of voluntary health agencies listed eight basic functions of voluntary health agencies. These are described briefly in the following paragraphs.

Pioneering. This involves exploring or surveying for needs not being served and for new methods of dealing with needs already recognized.

Demonstration. Voluntary health agencies have rendered particularly significant service by carrying out or subsidizing experimental projects designed to demonstrate practical methods for improvement of public health and for the wider application of proved methods by official and other agencies. Projects have ranged from the demonstration of the value of full-time local health departments, to home delivery service, visiting nursing service, nutrition programs, and business and record procedures.

Education. This is probably the single most important function of voluntary health agencies. In fact it might be said that all other functions have education as their goal. Although activities in this field have been designed primarily for the public, many of the agencies have made provisions for or have engaged in all types of professional training by means of fellowships, in-service training courses, and the maintenance or subsidizations of field training areas.

Supplementation of official activities. With no legislative restrictions to encumber them, the voluntary health agencies have very frequently found themselves in a position to augment the activities of official health departments. Often official health agencies have been unable to enter new fields of service and action because of political restrictions or public reservation. In such instances the voluntary agencies have rendered yeoman service by stepping in to fill the gap between currently accepted practice and more advanced scientific knowledge. Usually when this is done, the custom has been to provide the new service for a limited period of time, at the end of which the official agency is expected to carry on.

Guarding citizen interest in health. Voluntary health agencies, because of their nature, representation, and support, have often been in a position to guard the public interest not only by promoting the official health program but also by defending it against political and other interference. By like token they have sometimes found it necessary to subject official health agencies, programs, and officials to study and criticism. This has occasionally given rise to ill feeling, and some health officials have looked upon voluntary agencies as presumptuous and interfering. Health departments, however, being official, tax-supported agencies, should expect to be subject to scrutiny and if necessary criticism by the citizenry and the various groups that represent them. It has been exceedingly rare that such criti-

cism has not been to the ultimate good not only of the community but of the official health agency itself. More than one unqualified, politically sponsored individual has been barred from health officership, and more than one qualified health officer has been supported in his program and maintained in his position by vigorous public support stemming from the voluntary health agencies.

Promotion of health legislation. In every state and community there is a constant stream of proposed legislation of concern to the public health. It is of course a responsibility of the health officer to provide leadership in the support or condemnation of each one. In many instances his voice alone is of little avail and attracts scant attention from the legislative body. A great source of strength in this regard is the group of cooperative voluntary health agencies that are active and influential in his community. With a prime interest in health matters and representing large numbers of voting citizens, their opinions carry much weight. In addition these agencies have played an active part in the initial formulation and promotion of desirable health legislation.

Group planning and coordination. These functions have been particular concerns of health federations and councils and of health divisions of councils of social agencies. With the development of many voluntary agencies in a community and their potential or actual overlapping and conflict, there has resulted a great need for action in this field. Related to this is the need for increased coordination between the programs of the voluntary agencies and those of the official agencies in the community.

Development of well-balanced community health programs. This is really not a function in itself, but rather the total cumulative result of the successful accomplishment of the several foregoing purposes and functions. By protecting and promoting the official health department, by increasing the hygienic consciousness of the community, and by providing funds and facilities where gaps exist, the voluntary health agency may make the difference between a mediocre community health program and one that is truly effective.

FINANCING

Important to the understanding and evaluation of voluntary health agencies is the manner in which they are financed. The professional associations are supported by membership dues, whereas the health activities of commercial agencies are usually financed by budgetary items designated for education or public relations. The philanthropic foundations of course owe their existence essentially to large bequests from wealthy individuals. This source of funds, however, is significantly decreasing in importance with the breaking up of large personal fortunes. The most important group to be discussed is that made up of agencies supported by relatively small contributions or donations from large numbers of individuals. A number of techniques have been developed by these organizations, each tending to be jealously guarded by whatever agency first devised and used them. Some of these techniques have been spectacularly successful, depending in many instances upon emotional rather than intellectual appeal, carefully developed and conducted by promotional agencies that specialize in the business of fund raising.

The first and still one of the most successful methods is the Tuberculosis Christmas Seal, previously referred to. Their cost of only a penny each has appeared to be insignificant to most economic or social groups, and, while most sales are in the form of several sheets of 100 each, it is by no means unusual to find children in poor districts purchasing at least one or a few separate stamps. Although to some this may be a point of criticism, the fact that it is done represents at least a certain amount of educational impact upon all classes of society, thereby making the fight against tuberculosis truly a people's fight. An important additional incentive has been the identification of the Tuberculosis Christmas Seal with Christmas greeting cards. This campaign has been so successful that several other agencies have adopted the technique, e.g., the Easter Seal, inaugurated in 1934 by

the National Society for Crippled Children.

Another effective technique was developed by the National Foundation for Infantile Paralysis. Associated with the name of a great national leader, Franklin Delano Roosevelt, who was himself stricken with that disease, there developed a custom of annual drives involving very careful planning, organization, and promotional activities. A gala ball to raise funds was held in the nation's capital and was attended by many dignitaries. Similar events were held in cities, towns, and even small villages throughout the nation. Concurrently, the public was deluged on the streets, in their homes, and in places of amusement such as theaters with requests for contributions to the March of Dimes. These techniques have been amazingly fruitful and have brought in large sums of money. In 1958 this organization changed its name to the National Foundation and expanded its scope of interest to include arthritis, birth defects, and disorders of the central nervous system.

Other methods used to raise money are dues for nominal membership, the sale of educational literature, fees for services, personal solicitations, and direct mail appeal. Another innovation is the radio or television quiz program, which has benefited several voluntary health agencies very considerably. Certain of the techniques have caused not a little public resentment, particularly when pressure or embarrassment potentially enters into the appeal. Examples of this nature are the passage of contribution boxes in a lighted theater and the use of neighbors for personal door-to-door solicitation.

Recent years have seen an increasing trend toward joint fund-raising efforts. This is epitomized by the United Fund approach, which once each year by major community effort raises funds for a large number of member organizations, the local, state, and national offices of which receive appropriate amounts. At present there are about 1,500 United Fund agencies and about the same number of Community Chests. The latter, unlike the United Fund agencies, primarily collect money only for local agencies. Also, United Fund agencies are increasingly allocating a certain proportion of the funds they raise to the United Health Foundations, Inc., which in turn supports a broad range of research and demonstration projects at universities, health departments, and other agencies. Unfortunately not only have some agencies refused to affiliate with the United Fund but also inevitably a number of new voluntary agencies appear that add their separate appeals to that of the Community Chest or United Fund and thereby again create confusion. Recognition must also be given to the very natural wish of many people to contribute to one or a few causes in which they are personally interested rather than to what may appear as a large, vague, and indefinite fund. This problem came to a head toward the end of the 1950's, when a number of the large national foundations, notably those concerned with cancer, poliomyelitis, tuberculosis, and crippled children, forbade their local units to participate in United Fund campaigns or Community Chests. As stated by Ray R. Eppert, Vice President of United Community Funds and Councils: "These agencies who seem determined to wage a trade war for the contributors' dollars have thrown down the gauntlet to federation." He grimly warned them to "Change their policies" or "suffer the consequences."[4] That this warning may not be inevitably idle is indicated by a growing tide of questioning and criticism in the public press as well as in professional journals.[5-8]

An important consideration in connection with the fund-raising activities of voluntary health agencies is the cost of the fund-raising campaign itself. An analysis of seven national organizations in 1945 showed a variation of from 6 cents to about 38 cents per $1 collected.[3] An analysis of the annual report of one agency led to the conclusion that 68% of the income was spent for agency office maintenance and fund raising. This, however, was somewhat extreme. The average cost of raising a "voluntary" dollar at that time was reported as 5.9 cents by Community Chests and Councils, Inc. A much more recent study by Hamlin[7] brought out a discouraging lack of improvement. While 10 of the large national agencies claimed a cost of from 7 cents to 15

cents for each $1 raised, an auditor found the figures to vary from 12.5 cents to 36.2 cents. Some of these high costs, however, were claimed to be due to inclusion of some educational costs in the fund-raising costs. One of the strongest recommendations of both the National Health Council study by Gunn and Platt and of the recent Rockefeller Foundation study by Hamlin has been for the establishment of a uniform accounting system and a standard chart of accounts. There has been little evidence over the years to indicate any great interest in this on the part of the individual voluntary health agencies. Hamlin found the situation so confused and discouraging that he even urged the President of the United States to establish a permanent national commission on voluntary health and welfare agencies.

DESIRABLE AND UNDESIRABLE CHARACTERISTICS

From the foregoing it is apparent that voluntary health agencies have both desirable and undesirable features. On the favorable side is the fact that these agencies have developed as a result of spontaneous reaction on the part of groups of citizens. Their leadership usually consists of devoted, personally disinterested, intelligent, nonpartisan individuals. Usually the agencies have been established to meet a real and commonly felt need. Without question, public health in America could never have reached its present high level in the absence of the voluntary health agencies. They are unrestricted by statutory or program limitations or by partisan politics. Because they are so relatively unhampered, they can adapt their programs rather readily to changing needs and conditions, thereby often shortening the lag between the acquisition of new scientific knowledge and its application. Much that has been accomplished in improved professional education, standardization of techniques and procedures, and research can be placed to their cerdit.

On the other hand, voluntary health agencies have certain undesirable features or disadvantages. Not a few official health departments have been placed in the position of having to conduct poorly balanced programs because of pressure from voluntary agencies. This may come about in two ways: a voluntary agency may exert pressure upon the health department to overemphasize its particular interest or, contrariwise, some voluntary agencies have caused health departments to underemphasize certain programs because the voluntary agencies have wanted to monopolize activities in those fields. Such tactics may serve to jeopardize appropriations for official health agencies. Similarly, despite the avowed purpose of leading the way until an activity is officially adopted, many voluntary agencies are reluctant to surrender any parts of their programs. In fact, it is rare to find a voluntary agency closing up shop as did the American Child Health Association when it felt is had accomplished its purpose. With the multiplicity of existing organizations, overlapping of function and high administrative costs are certain to result. Reference has been made to the growing confusion of the public. This results from overlapping functions as well as from multiplicity of appeals. Thus one still finds many communities in which several groups of nurses operate out of an equal number of agencies, visiting homes and working in clinics. Certain of the voluntary agencies do not accede to the policy of affiliating or even coordinating their activities with each other, much less with those of local official health organizations. Finally, and one of the most serious objections, the public tends to contribute on an emotional basis and to the organization that makes the loudest and most prolonged appeal and then feels that it has done its part toward the support of the entire public health program. An interesting example is that in recent years the agencies concerned with tuberculosis and with poliomyelitis have each raised about the same amount annually, despite the fact that there are many more cases and deaths from tuberculosis each year than there are cases and deaths from poliomyelitis.

CURRENT TRENDS AND THE FUTURE

Twenty years ago, in an article entitled "Is the Private Health Agency on the Way Out?," Marquette[8] called attention to three major developments that he felt were certain to have an important effect on the future of voluntary health agencies. First was the trend toward the allotment of federal Social Security funds to the United States Public Health Service and other agencies for the categorical approach to important health problems such as venereal disease, tuberculosis, cancer, mental health, heart disease, and dental health. These allotments of federal funds intended for state and local as well as for national use were already making it possible for official health agencies to enter into territory previously occupied almost exclusively by the private health agency. The second development, which grew largely out of the National Health Conferences, was the increased appropriation of tax monies for hospital and medical services. Related to this was the support, albeit often reluctant, by the American Medical Association of moves for more government participation in public health, mental hygiene, health education, the care of mental patients, the support of tuberculosis hospitals, facilities for convalescent care and rehabilitation, group hospitalization, and cash indemnity against sickness. A third development of great impact was the economic depression of the 1930's, followed by the trend toward higher taxes during and since World War II. Working together, these two factors served to eliminate some large fortunes and to reduce somewhat the inclination of many people to contribute to what they increasingly considered to be governmental responsibilities.

In light of what has occurred since, Marquette's observations were accurate. Previously the respective traditional roles of public and voluntary health agencies were more clearly defined. Education, experimentation, demonstration, and the provision of direct personal services were regarded as the strengths and proper domain of voluntary agencies. The expansion of governmental services has brought about a shift in the traditional roles. While the fundamental distinction between the freedom of the voluntary agency and the statutory requirements imposed upon governmental agencies remain, that distinction is becoming increasingly hazy. Community sanctions tend increasingly to limit the freedom of action of voluntary agencies, while a plethora of special grants now provide governmental agencies with greater program flexibility. As a result, today there are many areas in which both types of agencies are in a position to render essentially the same types of services for the same kinds of individuals.[9] Related to such factors as the nation's economic growth, the population increase, the changes in age distribution, and the remarkable mobility and urbanization of our society, a number of other developments have contributed to the shift from voluntarism to official agency action. Among these are (1) the spectacular advances in medical science, (2) a growing demand by the public for health services now possible as a result of these advances, (3) an affluent society that can and is increasingly willing to support these services through taxes, (4) a considerable improvement in the educational level of most of our citizenry, and (5) the development of a national social philosophy that regards health as a fundamental human right to be guaranteed by the government.

The voluntary health agencies are now faced with the problem of what to do about these trends. Some have already accepted the policy that when a tax-supported agency develops to the point where it can take over the work, the private agency should either leave that field or cease its operation entirely. In order to decide logically upon a sound future course it has been recognized as desirable that these agencies subject themselves and their communities to careful scrutiny in order to reevaluate problems that do or may exist and their relationship to them. Reevaluation is further indicated for bringing up to date the position occupied by the voluntary agency in the community and its relation to all other official and nonofficial organizations. Accordingly, recent years have seen the establishment of appraisal or evaluation committees in an increasing number of voluntary health agencies. The United Fund and Community Chests and Councils, Inc., have played an important role in the encouragement of this procedure. In speaking of agency appraisal,

the National Health Council suggests that the following be set up by the board of each voluntary health agency[3]:

. . . machinery for the periodical appraisal of the agency, at intervals of perhaps five years, by qualified experts with wide knowledge of the field of activity as well as of agency and community organization. This is particularly needed in the swiftly changing trends that are ahead. Valuable as is self-analysis, the outside and objective approach reduces the likelihood that smugness or self-satisfaction will establish itself. Such an appraisal should consider (a) adequacy and effectiveness of program; (b) financial status and future; (c) cooperative relationships; (d) adequacy of staff and executive direction; and (e) future opportunities and functions. Properly planned and carried out with the full cooperation of board and staff, such an appraisal will be worth more than it costs. Funds should be set aside and gradually accumulated for such an accounting and future planning. No agency would think of omitting its yearly financial audit merely to save the cost. It is even more important to have an audit of the organization itself made at intervals in order to determine how wisely it expends its money.

In addition to the evaluations sponsored by voluntary agencies themselves, the past decade has seen the development of communitywide surveys performed by outside experts. Many of these have been sponsored by Community Chests and Councils, Inc., financial support coming from any one of a number of sources: the local community fund, the council of social agencies, private subsidies, or the local government itself. With the passage of the Partners in Health Act (P.L. 89-749) in 1966, it is anticipated that an even more searching evaluation of voluntary as well as of official health programs will take place. Certainly this would be fundamental to any comprehensive health planning.

Reference has been made to the National Health Council. In a sense its organization represents an attempt to adapt voluntary health agencies to the changing times. At the time of its organization in 1920 it was hailed as one of the most important steps taken in the field of public health up to that time. Its avowed goals included consolidation of funds and facilities, increased efficiency of action through joint planning, housing, and programming, and the provision of services and conferences conducive to evaluation. Its program has not been as successful as had been originally hoped because of, among other reasons, resistance on the part of many agencies to the idea of unification for fear of loss of agency integrity.

A number of other steps worthy of mention have been taken to keep voluntary health agencies up to date and to increase their community value. Until relatively recently many agencies have been directed by interested lay persons. At first they served without pay, but that policy was soon recognized as being administratively unsound. Accompanying the increased employment of full-time agency directors has been a recognition of the need for some type of training. As a result in-service training courses and other types of programs designed to fill the need have been established and conducted. Recognition of the need for training has grown to the point where at the present time not only are curricula presented (usually during the summer months) for executives of voluntary health agencies but also educational qualifications for this type of personnel have been developed by the Committee on Professional Education of the American Public Health Association.[10]

That voluntary health agencies should find themselves in the position of having to give way here and tighten up there is neither surprising nor undesirable. Nor do these trends necessarily indicate their approaching demise. As aptly stated by Marquette[8]:

There is really no occasion for leaders outside the tax supported health field to have any concern as to the continued importance of their work. It is rather a matter of elasticity and adjustment. Everybody in the public health field knows that so much remains to be done and that we fall so far short of using effectively the instruments that medical science has placed at our disposal for combating disease, that the combined public and volunteer health forces will be needed for years to come. It must all be properly integrated and the private agency must see the changing picture and be ready to modify its role.

However, as the Hamlin report[7] stated:

"If the unstinting philanthropic spirit of the American people is to be translated into the greatest public good and their confidence in the agencies maintained, the structure and objectives of voluntary agencies should be reviewed and modernized." The study committee believed that five major steps were available to voluntary agencies.

1. Stronger voluntary agency leadership.
2. Higher standards for local affiliates.
3. Increased participation in organized planning.
4. Better reporting of programs and accomplishments.
5. Greater emphasis on research and the application of new knowledge.

In the interest of objectivity we must observe that the need for increased attention to each of these five items applies equally to official health agencies. Furthermore, if voluntary and official health agencies not only both did these things but did them in concert, the health of the public would be the better for it.

REFERENCES

1. Hochbaum, G. M.: Health agencies and the Tower of Babel, Public Health Rep. **80**:331, Apr. 1965.
2. Lear, J.: The business of giving, Sat. Review, Vol. 63, Dec. 2, 1961.
3. Gunn, S. M., and Platt, P. S.: Voluntary health agencies: an interpretative study, New York, 1945, The Ronald Press Co.
4. United funds battle health agencies which aim to go it alone, The Wall Street Journal, XXXVIII, No. 195, p. 1, July 18, 1958.
5. Editorial: The giver's dilemma, Amer. J. Public Health **46**:1336, Oct. 1956.
6. Carter, R.: The gentle legions, New York, 1961, Doubleday & Co., Inc.
7. Hamlin, R. H.: Voluntary health and welfare agencies in the United States, New York, 1961, Schoolmaster's Press.
8. Marquette, B.: Is the private health agency on the way out? Amer. J. Public Health **29**:46, Jan. 1939.
9. Levine, S., White, P. E., and Paul, B. D.: Community interorganizational problems in providing medical care and social services, Amer. J. Public Health **53**:1183, Aug. 1963.
10. Committee on Professional Education of the American Public Health Association: Educational qualifications of executives of voluntary health agencies, Amer. J. Public Health **35**:499, May 1945.

Chapter 13

Personnel

INTRODUCTION

Parran,[1] former Surgeon General of the United States Public Health Service, once stated: "The tripod upon which the public health structure of any country rests is (1) a force of well-trained personnel, (2) the appointment, promotion and retention of personnel on a merit basis, and (3) adequate financial support, evidencing public understanding of the problems involved." It is significant that the first two of these deal directly with questions of personnel. The third is partly so concerned since financial support of public health programs is manifest chiefly in the payment of salaries. These considerations plus the fact that the management of personnel and their problems is one of the health officer's first, continuing, and most difficult tasks make it important to give attention to this field.

In order to discuss the subject intelligently certain phases of the background of public health in America must be considered. First, it must be recognized that public health work in the modern sense is of relatively recent origin. Thus the first state health department was established only 100 years ago, and we were well into the twentieth century when the first county health departments were organized.

A second significant factor was the decision to carry out most public health work within the framework of government. This necessitates frank recognition of some of the traditional American attitudes toward public service, such as acceptance if not support of the ideas of political patronage and of the spoils system, a tendency to expect and to tolerate some degree of inefficiency in public affairs, and a heritage of relatively

low salaries. Fortunately all of these factors are well on their way to disappearance. It should be recognized, however, that the word politics often is misunderstood or misinterpreted. What is meant most often is a type of selfish, pernicious partisanism. This is passing out of the American scene as a result of a greatly broadened educational base, the growth in demand for good and efficient public services, and the appearance of a more dedicated and sophisticated type of political leader.[2] Furthermore, it should be realized that there may be many forms of pernicious politics other than those stemming from political parties and that all of them are deterrents to efficient service. The public health administrator by virtue of his contacts and activities may find himself involved in personal politics, fraternal politics, racial politics, religious politics, professional politics, labor politics, economic and social politics, and politics of many other types. It must be realized that political activity is a necessary part of our system of representative government and indeed of sound public health practice. The manner and extent to which the latter is true has been presented in an excellent manner by Mattison,[3] who describes and compares the model of a public health program as seen from the viewpoint of a politician in contrast with that of a health director and indicates points at which common interests and goals may come together. Attention should also be directed to a symposium, The Politics of Public Health, presented at the Eighty-sixth Annual Meeting of the American Public Health Association.[4] One of the participants (Richardson) stated that "Politics has a depth and complexity encountered in no other human pursuit. Einstein perceived this and succinctly summed it up when he was asked why it was that men who can develop wonder drugs and stamp out epidemics cannot understand politics. The wise old man answered, 'Politics is more difficult than medicine.' "

Public health work itself has certain characteristics that give rise to peculiar personnel problems in contrast to most businesses and industries. It is a curious mixture of public and social responsibility and service. It is notable in this respect that, despite what was said in the preceding paragraph, public health as a social movement has only recently been adopted by government, that much public health work is still carried on by private voluntary organizations, and that not infrequently the budgets of official health agencies are still augmented by funds from private sources. In a real sense it is still in the process of organizational development. In public health work the major expenditure is for personnel. A complex spectrum of ability and function is required that necessitates the activity of many different specialized types of personnel. In the same organization there may be physicians, engineers, sanitarians, chemists, nurses, bacteriologists, educators, social scientists, management specialists, and many others, each with particular pride and interest in his specialty.

Not only are the activities of many types but they are continually undergoing change, adaptation, and evolution. What is good and adequate practice today may be inadequate or outmoded tomorrow. Furthermore, we are dealing with an expanding field, one that began with the barest essentials of sanitation and expanded into the fields of preventive medicine and health promotion. In contrast to most other private and public businesses, there are relatively few activities in public health that are subject to formalization or formularization. In most instances the product to be sold tends to be intangible and the consumers are all the people with their varying types and degrees of need, pride, prejudice, reticence, and intelligence. Often the selling literally involves a change in the habits, de-

sires, and customs of people so that a successful approach in one instance, time, or location may fail in other circumstances.

Because of the relative newness of public health work and the great recent demand for services, additional difficulties have arisen, many of them involving personnel. For a considerable period there were no special facilities for training individuals for this field. In the absence of trained specialists it was considered satisfactory to employ a wide variety of generally unqualified individuals, including retired or unsuccessful practicing physicians as well as political appointees. Related to this was the inability to attract and retain capable personnel because of insecurity of tenure, low salaries, and competition from other fields, and also because the profession of public health was not yet well enough known to be attractive. The problem was summed up by Rosenau,[5] who commented:

> The time has long since gone by when the physician can spend a few hours from his busy day to look after the duties of the health office. The situation demands the entire time and energy of those who consecrate their lives to the public welfare. In order to attract capable men to the new profession it is important that the health officer should have an assured tenure of office with adequate pay and freedom from politics.

To complete the circle, due to the previously mentioned inadequacies, there was a corresponding lack of established, well-organized agencies in which at least practical field training experience might be obtained.

As time went on, however, the public health profession undertook to solve these problems on many fronts. Through the efforts of those concerned with public health work as a career there occurred a fairly rapid maturing of the profession, which resulted in widespread public and professional acceptance, accumulation of sound experience, and the application of more scientific procedures. Gradually medical schools began to include preventive medicine and public health in their curricula. The recency of this, however, is emphasized by a prophecy by Rosenau[5] in an article written in 1915. "The modern practitioner of medicine is fast adding prevention as one of the tools of his equipment.

The future student of medicine will make a study of health and how to maintain it, as well as a study of disease and how to cure it."

The fact is, however, that even to this day it is a rare medical school that does even a reasonably competent job in this respect. Medical curricula are still almost completely illness oriented, and most medical schools and teaching hospitals are more interested in clinical departments that bring in sick patients, most of whom someone or some agency pays for, than in a department that strives to prevent illness and promote positive health. A significant trend for the better should be noted, however. An increasing number of medical schools are discovering that patients originate from someplace—the community with all of its complexities—and that the genesis of most illness, hence the more complete handling of the case, is to be found in the community and not merely within the walls of the hospital or the physician's office. As a result experimentation is occurring in a number of the more progressive centers of medical education in the teaching of comprehensive medicine, community medicine, or social medicine.

Because of the rapidly evolving scope of public health, medical training alone was soon recognized to be inadequate preparation for a health officer as well as not serving the needs of the nonmedical personnel in public health work. In pleading for specialized training and degrees for public health workers, Rosenau[5] said:

Public health work is becoming, in fact, has already become, a separate profession. It has split off from medicine just as medicine long ago split off from the priesthood. Public health service, as a career, must be an end in itself. It is often difficult and sometimes impossible to bend the physician into a health officer. The ordinary medical training does not qualify a person to be a health officer.

In 1912 there was established at Massachusetts Institute of Technology in cooperation with Harvard University a program of basic training in the biologic sciences similar to the first 2 years of medical school, followed by courses in public health science instead of the usual clinical courses pursued by medical students. In 1914 a conference of leaders of education, medicine, and public health called by the General Education Board recommended that public health schools of high standards be established as separate entities affiliated with universities and their schools of medicine. The first distinct school of this type was established in 1916 at the University of Pennsylvania; however, this school is no longer in existence. As time passed, additional schools were established.

But an additional complication had arisen. Due to the acceptance of the value of public health programs and the resulting demand for personnel, a large number of educational institutions of all grades of quality began to grant degrees in public health, more often than not on the basis of grossly inadequate training. By 1939 a total of 45 schools and universities were listed as granting 18 different kinds of degrees in public health.[6] The situation became so undesirable and confusing that finally in 1941 there was established an Association of Schools of Public Health consisting of schools later accredited by a system developed by the American Public Health Association.[7,8] As a result there are at the present time 17 schools accredited for the granting of acceptable professional degrees in this field. These are the University of California at Berkeley, University of California at Los Angeles, Columbia University, Harvard University, the University of Hawaii, Johns Hopkins University, Loma Linda (Cal.) University, University of Michigan, University of Minnesota, University of Montreal, University of North Carolina, University of Oklahoma, University of Pittsburgh, University of Puerto Rico, University of Toronto, Tulane University, and Yale University.* Several other educational institutions are also contemplating the establishment of schools of public health. In Latin America a similar Association of Schools of Public Health was formed at a conference of deans in Mexico in 1959. As yet no accrediting system has been established, but biennial meetings

---

*For a detailed discussion, see *The School of Public Health: Past, Present, Future.*[9]

which have been held since with the assistance of The Pan American Health Organization have gone far to enhance professional education in public health in Central and South America.[10-13]

In order to establish criteria for the accreditation of schools it was logically necessary to first determine qualifications and standards for prospective personnel of public health agencies. In other words, what was the final product of the schools to be? Efforts toward this end were begun in the late 1930's by the Committee on Professional Education of the American Public Health Association, with the result that educational qualifications have been established for the majority of the various kinds of professional personnel that might be employed by an official or nonofficial public health agency.[14]

Although each specialty is of necessity dealt with separately, those usually considered to represent the basic personnel of a health department, i.e., health officers, public health engineers, and public health nurses, have certain requisites in common. These may be summarized as follows:

1. Graduation from an approved professional school (medicine, nursing, etc.)
2. An academic year in a school of public health or, in the case of nurses, a school approved by the National League for Nursing, leading to a degree
3. A period of practical supervised experience in a health department
4. The customary desirable personal qualifications

It was soon realized that just as an internship was necessary to round out the academic training of the medical graduate, so a period of practical field training should supplement study at a school of public health. Therefore a special Subcommittee on Field Training analyzed the types of field training desirable for public health personnel, dividing them into the following five categories[15]:

1. Observation—duration: 1 day to 1 week. The individual takes no direct part in the activities of the health department. It is best suited for a well-trained, experienced person who simply desires to learn of new procedures or to discuss new policy.
2. Orientation—duration: 1 to 2 months. This is training to prepare an individual for a specific position in a specific place. It is intended to familiarize a skilled person with the particular problems, laws, codes, customs, and procedures of that area or state in which he is about to work.
3. Field Experience—duration: 3 to 6 months. This training is supplementary to a theoretical, academic training in public health. It is comparable to an internship which follows medical training. The training areas should be carefully selected and require teaching personnel, in addition to standard personnel.
4. Apprenticeship—duration: 3 to 12 months. This training is given before the candidate has had his academic year of work at a school of public health. It has special advantages in the selection and training of medical health officers. The individual is employed as an apprentice by the health department, and if he likes the work and proves to be capable he is then given a period of academic training by the state and returns to his official sponsor at the completion of the theoretical work.
5. In-service Training—This is simply a continuous educational program for all types of personnel in the health department, in order to keep them abreast of the times. It is a special function of the local health department, with aid from the state health department.

The next step taken was the development of accredited field-training areas to supplement the academic training received in a school of public health. This began in 1950 and has been carried forward under the tripartite egis of the Committee on Professional Education of the American Public Health Association, the Council on Medical Education and Hospitals of the American Medical Association, and the American Board of Preventive Medicine and Public Health.[16] By now about one half of the states and through them a number of localities have programs approved for residency training.[17] The program is analogous to the approving of hospitals for internships and residencies. Still another step was the establishment in 1949 of the specialty board, the American Board of Preventive Medicine and Public Health, by the Council on Medical Education and Hospitals of the American Medical Association assisted by the American Public Health Association in order "1. To encourage the study, improve the practice, elevate the standards, and advance the cause of preventive medicine and public health [and] 2. To grant and issue to physicians duly licensed by law to practice medicine, certificates of special knowledge in preventive medicine and public health."[18]

In addition to these activities that relate only to physicians, several other professional disciplines engaged in public health work, notably environmental health and public health nursing, have also developed programs for approved field training and accreditation.

Further trends toward the solution of personnel problems in public health are the increasing adoption of merit systems, in which the American Public Health Association, the United States Public Health Service, and the Children's Bureau have taken leading roles,[19,20] and the gradual improvement of salaries resulting from a number of circumstances, including personnel demand in relation to supply, improved training, and recognition of the value of public health work. In relation to the health manpower shortage and training needs has been the important recognition that the problems are of national scope rather than simply state or local. An increasing number of fellowships for professional public health training have been made available to the states through federal grants; and in 1958 Congress passed the first bill to subsidize accredited schools of public health to a modest extent, partly on the basis of their representing regional training centers for the nation. Since that time several national conferences on health manpower and public health training have been held, leading to increased federal efforts to improve the situation.[21]

The need for these steps was indicated by the fact that, as recent as 1951, while the majority of physicians employed in public health agencies had attended various short courses and institutes on specialized subjects, only about one third had formal training leading to a degree in public health. About 36% of staff nurses employed in state and local health agencies had 1 year or more of study in public health or public health nursing. Of sanitation officers, ap-

proximately one third had no public health training.[22] This situation has improved somewhat since then, but there are still significant numbers of individuals in all categories working in public health with inadequate specialized training backgrounds. An analysis of educational requirements of local health officers has shown that by law or regulation only 26 states specifically require training in public health. In 19 others it is a commonly accepted practice, while 2 states by regulation say it is not necessary and 1 state actually prohibits the requirement.[23]

Because of the persistence of the health manpower shortage combined with the rapid development of new knowledge and techniques, the field of public health has been experimenting with a number of additional approaches. Among these have been not only programs for updating existing personnel[24] and many programs for the training of volunteer and ancillary workers but also more recently special programs to take advantage of the special cultural knowledge and abilities of individuals recruited directly from socioeconomically depressed neighborhoods.[25]

The generally accepted minimum staffing requirements for proper basic health services are as follows:

One public health physician for every 50,000 persons (or one for every local health unit, whichever is less)

One public health nurse for every 5,000 persons if bedside nursing is not included; otherwise, one per 2,500 persons

One supervising nurse for each 6 to 8 staff nurses

One sanitary engineer or sanitarian for every 15,000 persons

One clerk for every 15,000 persons

One of the most complete analyses of the quantitative needs for public health personnel was that presented by the Emerson report a quarter century ago.[26] While now obviously out of date, it does give perspective to the problem. It indicated that in 1942 there were 40,782 persons employed in providing local public health services under the auspices of the local, state, or federal governments. One fourth were part-time workers, three quarters of which were health officers and clinic physicians. It was estimated that at least 23,000 additional trained individuals were needed to provide the minimal public health services on the local level alone. Greatest needs were for public health nurses, dentists and dental hygienists, health educators, and environmental workers.

The past quarter of a century has seen slow improvement. By the end of 1949 the number of full-time personnel employed by full-time official local health agencies totaled 33,555. Fewer than half of the local units had sufficient physicians to meet minimum requirements. Approximately one fourth of all units reported no physicians employed on a full-time basis. Shortages were still much more pronounced for nurses than for any other types of personnel. Only 6.5% of local health units had enough nurses to meet the minimum standard. With regard to environmental health personnel, i.e., sanitary engineers, sanitarians, and veterinarians, nearly 63% of cities but only about 31% of counties met minimum standards. About 50% of units had adequate clerical and office staffs. According to accepted requirements, there were needed an additional 1,223 physicians, 11,826 nurses, 1,982 environmental health personnel, and 1,587 clerks.[27]

For other specialties, approximately 20% of budgeted positions for health educators, public health dentists, and medical social workers were vacant at that time. For nutritionists the figure was 16%, for laboratory workers about 10%, for veterinarians 10%, and for statisticians and analysts 15%.[28]

By 1965 the situation appeared on the surface to have improved somewhat with a total of 51,632 full-time workers of different categories reported employed by local health departments. This represented a 50% increase since 1949. Gains, however, have been uneven. Thus full-time public health physicians increased only from 1,609 in 1949 to 1,668 in 1965, and laboratory personnel from 1,391 in 1949 to 1,546 in 1965. The greatest gains made over this period were in environmental health personnel (from 6,531 to 10,369), in medical and psychiatric social workers (from 111 to 688), and in public health nurses (from 11,251 to 16,058). Despite this, when the increase in population during the 16 years is taken into consideration, it is found that, with the exception of social workers and dentists, no net gains were achieved and some significant decreases in relative numbers had occurred.[29] In order to evaluate the situation adequately one must also consider the significant increase in general earning power and the standard of living with a resultant greatly increased expectancy and demand for public health services on the local and especially urban level. It is interesting but not surprising to note that, although in absolute numbers the need is greatest in the larger, more populated communities, the proportionate need is greatest in the smaller, less populated areas. Undoubtedly this is attributable to the many attractions of work and life in urban and suburban as against essentially rural or small-town circumstances.

In summary it might be stated that the consensus at the present time is that the two intimately related factors that contribute the most to retarding the development and expansion of public health work are (1) inadequate competitive salaries and (2) inadequate personnel, both quantitatively and qualitatively.[30]

PERSONNEL MANAGEMENT

It has been stated that one of the health administrator's chief responsibilities is the direction and supervision of the function and activity of the other members of the health department staff. This is important in any organization, but its relative importance is perhaps accentuated in public health practice because to an unusual degree the personnel is literally the health department, and, furthermore, the successful function and behavior of the members of the health department's staff determine in the last analysis the acceptance and success of the organization's work. This is true because acceptance and success depend on the reaction of the public and it is through personal contacts of the department's staff with the public that the health program operates.

In view of this, it is tragic to see how frequently health officers ignore the personnel aspects of their programs. Too often the health officer looks upon himself as the source of medical knowledge and activity in the department, having essentially a nominal appointment as the representative head of the agency, perhaps by virtue of age, length of education, or community prestige. Common as this attitude may be, it is certainly not good practice and is naive from the viewpoint of legal and executive responsibility. The capable administrator, in public health work as elsewhere, must assume an active interest and responsibility for every phase of personnel management, from recruitment and employment to dismissal if necessary.

RECRUITMENT AND EMPLOYMENT

Merit systems

Recent years have seen the development and wide acceptance of the merit system principle for the purpose of recruiting and selecting capable individuals to fill specific positions in the civil service. It is curious to find occasionally among administrators of public health programs a certain amount of conflicting resentment toward the civil service or merit system idea and at the same time complaint against political patronage pressure as a handicap to efficient service. This dissatisfaction may perhaps be attributed to three things: lack of understanding by the executive of the essential purposes and potentialities of the merit system; the unfortunate fact that some civil service agencies still think of their original "fight the spoilsman" slogan and consider themselves more as policemen than as program facilitators; and lag in the development of new personnel techniques to aid effective administration. Despite these attitudes and difficulties, it is obvious that merit systems are here to stay and generally speaking have already resulted in considerable improvements in public service.

By now the majority of governmental employees in the United States serve under merit systems and each year sees more

added to the list. White[31] has pointed out that:

> . . . the basic conditions of government are such that the eventual triumph of the merit system seems inevitable. The ever-increasing technological aspects of governmental operations; the greatly intensified social responsibility of government, making the risk of administrative failure equivalent to the risk of social catastrophe; the emerging professional point of view in many branches of administration; and the expansion of civil service unions intent on protecting their own interests by the steady application of the merit system, these and other circumstances forecast the certain destruction of patronage in due course of time.

Civil service systems and merit systems have had a long and slow history, and only recently has there occurred accelerated adoption of the idea. Although the first but unsuccessful measures were taken by the national government as early as 1853, it was not until the assassination of President Garfield in 1881 by a disappointed office seeker that increasing sentiment was crystalized. As a result Congress reluctantly approved the Pendleton Act, which serves as the basis of civil service regulations in effect today. Originally the Pendleton Act included only about 14,000 federal positions, chiefly those in the postal and customs services. Successive presidential orders have increased the number of federal employees under the merit system to over 2 million, representing 86% of the total. Of particular effect has been the Ramspeck Act of 1940, which gave the President wide authority to extend the scope of the civil service act and the classification act. The first state civil service law was passed by New York in 1883. Two years later Massachusetts followed suit. Twenty years passed before any other states took action (Illinois and Wisconsin in 1905). More widespread adoption continued slowly until the late 1930's. By 1937 only 10 states had adopted merit system legislation. When many states finally introduced the principle, it was due largely to pressure from federal agencies rather than to an appreciation on the part of the states themselves of the value of civil service or merit systems.

Concerning public health agencies, with but rare exceptions states establishing civil service or merit systems did so because of restrictions in the federal laws and regulations governing financial payments to the states for the much needed grants-in-aid programs of the United States Public Health Service and the Children's Bureau under the Social Security Act. The effect of the federal requirements is dramatically indicated by the fact that in 1940 alone, the year following their adoption, 12 states established merit systems affecting public health personnel! The purpose and method were described as follows[32]:

> In the interests of promoting and maintaining sound personnel policies, Federal administrative agencies are authorized to examine civil service or merit systems of states and territories receiving "grants-in-aid" funds. Such systems when submitted by the state and territories are considered by Federal agencies under two headings and approval or disapproval is given either or both of these. The parts thus examined are: (1) the basic or rule, (2) the classification and compensation plan. The score by 1945 for 51 states and territories with the United States Public Health Service is:

	Reviewed	Approved
Law or rule	50	45
Classification and compensation plans	46	20

By now less than 10% of local public health workers are not included in some type of merit system.

The terms "civil service system" and "merit system" are often used interchangeably as if they were synonymous. There is a difference, although the distinction is slight from a practical standpoint. Both are nothing more or less than organized methods of selecting and advancing employees on the basis of their qualifications in relation to the aptitudes required by a particular job, together with relatively assured permanency of tenure, prescribed personnel benefits, and equal pay for equal work. If the plan exists by virtue of a statute, it is usually referred to as a civil service system. If it originates from an administrative ruling, it is called a merit system. A merit system therefore might be considered a civil service system without benefit of legislation. However, as this newer term gained in popularity and generic use, it appeared also in legislated plans so that one cannot automatically infer the structure from the name. Neither term has yet been supplanted by the preference of personnel administrators to speak of public personnel programs in which the merit principle is assumed.

In order to accomplish the purposes outlined a number of prerequisites are indicated. In a civil service system the first essential is the necessary enabling legislation accompanied by adequate appropriation for the satisfactory operation of the program. The legislation should provide the necessary authority to the civil service agency so that its activities may not be circumvented or ignored. If a number of agencies are involved, of which the health department is only one, provision should be made for uniform policies and procedures inasmuch as possible. The law itself should give attention to the removal of the system from the influences of local politics. This is desirably accomplished by providing for a separate personnel agency administered by a career executive under a nonpartisan advisory, regulatory, and appellate commission whose members serve for overlapping terms.

Of more recent origin is the trend toward professional personnel divisions within large functional agencies such as health departments of states or large cities. This unit reports to the agency administrator, assisting him in carrying out his personnel responsibilities, and provides liaison with the civil service agency. In order to provide for the selection and promotion of employees on the basis of their qualifications or merit a civil service agency is faced with the preliminary problem of position analysis and classification. This is further necessary in order to make possible the desired uniformity of policy previously mentioned and in order to prevent a number of individuals doing essentially the same type and amount of work from getting widely varying compensation. Needless to say, position analysis and classification and the resulting qualifications for prospective personnel should be carried out jointly by the administration of the functional agencies and the civil service agency, or a personnel department under the latter's control, with an attitude of helpfulness. It should be revised periodically to reflect changes occurring in the content of positions.[33]

Once position classifications and personnel qualifications have been established, the next step is to provide for the recruitment and examination of applicants. In the field of public health more recruiting activities are carried on by the public health agency itself than by the civil service agency since in most instances the health officer is in a better position to know the type of individual he wants and where he might look for him and candidates usually do not abound. Examination may consist of one or all of the various approaches, including substantiated records of training and experience, written examinations largely for the purpose of determining technical knowledge, and personal interviews chiefly to get an insight into the personality of the applicant. Since achievement of a high grade is not invariably indicative of desirable personnel and since, as will be discussed, an important phase of operation is the interplay between the personalities of the executive officer and his subordinate personnel, it is only reasonable to allow the executive officer a choice among the top two or three candidates who were successful in the examination.

When circumstances result in a surplus of desirable applicants, it becomes an added function of the civil service agency to maintain a register of qualified personnel. Where retirement plans have been put into operation, responsibility for them has often been given to the civil service agency. In addition they frequently serve as places of appeal and review in instances involving disciplinary measures, dismissal, or overt employer-employee conflicts.

Compensation, tenure, and promotion

As previously stated, one of the essential purposes of a compensation plan based on position classification is equal pay for equal work. In the absence of such a plan the weak executive tends to be unconcerned or ineffective in obtaining increases for his personnel in general. At the other extreme is the executive with a strong and aggressive personality who may tend to secure increases for favorite employees without consideration of the absolute or comparative value of their services. Compensation in such instances may then depend largely on political influence, friendships, favoritism, and nepotism. Needless to say, the morale of the employees of either of these types of administrators rapidly degenerates.

The position in an organization having been classified and a general policy of compensation having been decided upon, the next step is the allocation of pay rates to the various position class titles. Usually this is done by establishing a range from the minimum rate to be paid to new employees up to a maximum that may be paid to anyone in the particular position class. In setting this salary scale consideration should be given to numerous factors, among which are payment for comparable work elsewhere in the same locality, cost of living, wage trends, the financial condition of the community and agency, legal restrictions that may exist, and recognition of union rates. In many professional health classes the national mobility and recruitment of personnel cause salaries for comparable work in agencies across the country to become a significant factor. Once set, salary scales should be reviewed regularly to maintain currency.

It is usually desirable that the minimum rate of a position class should not be less than the maximum rate of a lower class. Between the minimum and maximum there should be one or more intermediate steps. A usual compensation policy is to start the new employee at the minimum of the range, granting the first increase at the end of an introductory or probationary period, followed by further increases annually thereafter until the maximum salary for the particular position class has been reached. It should be clearly understood, however, that compensation advancement is not automatic but only follows demonstrated and continued proficiency. Whenever possible the decision concerning an increase should be made by more than one person. For example, in larger organizations the decision might involve the combined judgments of the executive health officer, the immediate supervisor of the employee in question, and the personnel officer.

Of considerable assistance in making decisions concerning compensation increases is the use of efficiency and service ratings. It is recommended that the administrator periodically and systematically survey or study the efficiency of his employees and that the results be made part of a permanent personal history file of each employee. Inasmuch as possible the evaluations should be based on factual data, measurable performance, and work records rather than on purely personal judgments, although the latter should be included as auxiliary information. An important personnel function of the administrator therefore is an attempt to develop practical and equitable standards of measurement or evaluation. There should also be included in the employee's personal history file memoranda concerning specific and noticeable changes in behavior, attitude, or efficiency. Contrary to all too frequent practice, these memoranda should relate to changes for the better as well as for the worse. Furthermore they too should consist of statements of fact rather than mere supervisory deductions, impressions, or opinions, which not infrequently are biased.

The factors involved in determining tenure and promotion are essentially the same as those that determine the granting of step increases in compensation. It is customary and proper that an employee expect to hold a position so long as he adequately fulfills its purpose and so long as his behavior is not detrimental to the interests of other employees or of the organization.

Vacancies in the organization may be filled in essentially two ways: promotion of an employee already working in the organization or employment of someone new from outside. If the position is other than the lowest in the scale and if it is filled by promotion from within, the executive is faced with the possibility of having to carry out promotions all down the line, involving considerable reshuffling, readjustment, and retraining.

While on the surface this may appear to have the disadvantage of upsetting the work of the organization to a considerable extent, it also has definite advantages. First, if it is wished that employees approach their work from the point of view of possible careers in public service, promotion from within can be considered a fundamental premise and is conducive to desirable organizational morale and loyalty. It also develops a staff with wider interests and abilities than is otherwise possible. Furthermore, to follow a policy of filling upper positions from outside discourages the really capable individuals from remaining in the organization, with the result that over a period of time there is built up a residue of predominantly disappointed, disillusioned, and mediocre employees. Once this occurs the responsible executive, or one so unfortunate as subsequently to take his place, finds himself with no choice but to go outside for capable personnel. Finally, if there is any reason for employees to suspect that an outsider has been brought in because of personal or partisan favoritism, a disastrous lowering of morale is sure to follow.

It must be realized of course that some positions must be filled from the outside, especially during a period of organizational growth or when there is no one within the agency truly capable of filling the vacancy. Occasional problems of intra-agency frictions, favoritism, and cliques may be effectively solved only by the reallocation of certain of the present employees and the introduction of one or several new employees. In general, perhaps the best course to follow is in the middle, filling positions from within as much as possible but always keeping in mind the basic interests and purposes of the organization. Accordingly, many capable administrators follow a policy of occasionally introducing a few new, particularly well-qualified leaders in key positions made available by retirement of older employees or by their reassignment to other duties, in conjunction with the development as rapidly and as extensively as possible of a group of promising younger employees well trained from within.

Some ill-advised executives avoid the advancement of younger capable employees either from fear of their possibly presenting eventual competition to themselves or from fear of losing them to another agency. Such an attitude is of course absurd since the truly capable administrator need have no fears of competition from loyal staff members, and should his capable assistants advance into other fields or agencies, that might be considered a measure of the successful nature of the administrator's policies and leadership. In fact the wise executive should derive considerable satisfaction from seeing individuals trained by him go out and spread his philosophy and viewpoint much farther than he could ever hope to do by himself.

THE EXECUTIVE AND HIS PERSONNEL

Administrative management is essentially a question of the organization of manpower, materials, resources, and strategy for the accomplishment of a desired goal. This is impossible unless the administrator has successfully organized himself so as to intelligently understand the causes of the problems he meets in his day-to-day work and the remedies for their adequate solution. It requires therefore an intimate knowledge and understanding of a great many factors, including people as well as materials, plus a great deal of curiosity, imagination, determination, integrative ability, and good judgment. In a field such as public health there also is required a greater than usual social consciousness and understanding. Accordingly, the work of the public health administrator becomes much more than a matter of writing rules and regulations, issuing orders, or establishing clinics. In effect it involves the power and ability to influence if not to determine the happiness, welfare, and even the lives of a large number of people, beginning with the staff of the agency and extending out to include every member of the public. This is statesmanship in the correct sense of the word in that the executive health officer, in keeping with executives of other fields, plays an active and significant role in shaping the future not only of his organization but also of a community and of a society as a whole. This represents a truly great responsibility.

In order to be successful the executive officer must be well balanced. He should possess the type of personality that marks him naturally for a position of leadership and inspires the confidence of others because of a mature interest in them rather than using them for his own selfish purposes. He should demonstrate a constant sense of fairness, giving his employees the assurance that their individual and collective welfare and interests are safe in his hands and that they will not be subjected to the undesirable influences of prejudice, favoritism, or arbitrariness. The most effective administrator is one who is not specialized in any particular field, which would make him a technician and would result almost certainly in an unbalanced program. He should, however, gain enough knowledge and understanding of the various technical phases and activities of the organization to enable him to coordinate them intelligently and assist administratively in their development.

It therefore follows that the administrative health officer, like executives in other fields, must establish his goals, make plans for their attainment, create a sound organization providing for practical levels of authority and coordination, recruit and manage good personnel, delegate responsibility and its concomitant authority, establish whatever rules and regulations are needed for smooth operation, develop a sound financial policy and an efficient work plan, provide continued leadership, education, and inspiration, maintain good morale, secure cooperation, and keep the plans and programs of the organization constantly in tune with the social forces on which depends its success and survival. To accomplish all this he needs personal characteristics such as those summarized by Dimock[34]:

> The successful executive, therefore, is he who commands the best balance of physique, mentality, personality, technical equipment, philosophical insight, knowledge of human behavior, social adaptability, judgment, ability to understand and to get along with people, and a sense of social purpose and direction.

This sounds as if some type of superman is required. However, this does not necessarily follow since, stripped to the essentials, what is required is a determination to carry out a certain few proved administrative principles, e.g., that authority should equal responsibility or that functions should be defined, plus a genuine liking and understanding of human nature. The administrator's function is to maintain a sense of goals, strategy, and timing and to supply specific encouragement, instruction, and pressure at the right point and time. The executive is most effective when, having delegated as much detail as possible to his subordinates and their having contributed everything of which they are capable, he provides the extra 5% of knowledge and leadership with which to turn out a completed and workmanlike job.

The executive health officer should always bear in mind that he is placed in a managerial position for a social purpose and not because of any personal interest in him or his welfare. He is employed for more than routine management and housekeeping. He is expected also to be a tactician and social philospher, using his wits, his ability as a leader, and his understanding of social forces to improve the state of society. Since society and the forces influencing it constantly fluctuate, he never operates in a fixed environment. He must constantly adapt himself, his program, and his organization to these environmental changes and further must try to influence the environment in any way that might seem indicated for the accomplishment of the ultimate purpose of the program.

With this in mind, there should be mentioned a not unfamiliar type of administrator commonly referred to as a promotor, who, although possessing great imagination, enthusiasm, and salesmanship, lacks the ability or momentum to follow through. He finds it difficult to sustain an interest in any one thing for long, dislikes routine, and is constantly searching for new worlds to conquer. Accordingly, his interest and energy jump unpredictably from one thing to another, with the result that his personnel never knows in what direction they are going next or what their relative positions will be. Particular subordinates may receive concentrated attention and support one day, only to be ignored and forgotten the next. That this is conducive neither to a sound balanced program nor to high morale is obvious.

There are others, however, who achieve a balance between promotional ability and executive leadership. They, while never satisfied with the status quo, realize nevertheless that "the show must go on," that all parts of the program must be continuously sustained. Possessing strong imagination, they are ever on the alert to new problems and methods of attack, carrying a promotional activity to the point where it has been established and accepted and may be turned over to a capable subordinate for its complete development, without at any time unbalancing or confusing the program as a whole. This is the difference between the will-o'-the-wisp promoter and the executive with promotional ability.

While the latter type of leadership is desirable in every organization at all times, it is of particular importance in the initiation and development of a new enterprise. Such circumstances require an unusual amount of imagination, courage, exploration, self-confidence, and planning ability, plus a sense of good timing and an ability to combine what is in the process of creation with what already has been brought into existence. In this regard it should again be realized that public health work, being a rapidly expanding field, requires that to be effective, the executive health officer constantly face the problem of initiation and promotion of new programs.

It is therefore clear that the health executive of a functioning agency must be three things: a trouble shooter constantly expecting the unexpected and always ready to deal with crises, a supervisor delegating everything he can to those working under him, and a promoter of new programs to increase the usefulness and effectiveness of his organization. As pointed out by Dimock,[34] this order is reversed in the formative stages of a new organization. Many executives successfully carry out one or two of these, but the test of a truly competent administrator is if all three can be accomplished.

It may be appropriate to give some consideration to what makes an effective chief executive officer. Perhaps the most comprehensive general statement that could be made is that the characteristics of a good administrative officer are in many ways similar to those required for good parenthood. A primary function of the executive health officer is to provide leadership. His usual problem is how to lead his organization in the face of the limitations and obstacles found in most situations. There is no standard answer to the question. Solution depends to a considerable degree upon the individual and his personality rather than upon his technical knowledge. This explains why capable technicians are often unhappy failures when placed in administrative position. The answer to the question varies by place and time. The problems encountered in a new organization are quite different from those of an old established agency. It should also be recognized that different organizations have different backgrounds of development that condition the rate and manner in which they move. Executive manner and action are certain of course to differ under emergency conditions, in contrast with normal circumstances.

Perhaps the most important philosophy for the executive to adopt is that the end results are the products of the organization, not those of any one individual, even himself. In the long run any effect he has is due to his influence and not to his command. Whether or not he wants to, he must rely upon his subordinate staff in order to accomplish the purposes of the agency. Even if this were not true, the executive should not attempt to take over the tasks of those on lower levels. To do so invariably confuses and antagonizes the personnel in general and the division and bureau heads in particular. The executive health officer's position is that of a catalyst dealing with people, assimilating their ideas, evaluating them, and determining lines of action and seeing that action is taken. He should do everything possible to conserve his time and energy for these higher level administrative functions by adopting the policy of Andrew Carnegie, who never did anything he could hire someone else to do for him. The executive health officer should approach his position with a long-range view, recognizing that most administrative changes and advances take a long time. This means that he must balance his type or method of action to fit particular situations, slackening the line at this point and at this time and reeling in or striking out at other places and at other times.

A popular picture exists of an executive austerely established behind a shiny desk in a comfortable office, granting a series of interviews to a parade of subordinates and others who appeal for advice and guidance. This presents a poor picture of administrative practice. As in any other field, the chief executive in public health is neither the ultimate fountainhead of all knowledge nor physically capable of personally directing the activities of a large number of individuals. The numbers of those within his agency with whom he has intimate working relationships should be limited, otherwise he misses the forest for the trees. This is not meant to imply that the executive should confine his contacts or relationships to those who voluntarily come to him; rather he should actively seek out those who need his help and who can be of assistance to him.

Delegation

An organization functions most effectively when a capable executive officer, rather than attempting to control and supervise intimately each of the various activities that make up the total program, is able to delegate control and supervision to responsible subordinates. This is unquestionably the most important single factor in successful administrative practice. The executive has to decide what part of his responsibilities and authority he will entrust to those immediately below him and what he will withhold for himself. Each of these key subordinate executives should be allowed to choose those who will work under him or he cannot fairly be held responsible for results. The subordinate executives in turn delegate to those next in rank such parts of their own specified responsibilities as they may choose, and so on down the line. As Dimock[34] has described it, the executive in effect says to his department heads, "You know our objective. You know the plans. You know the policy. Now the job is to see that this part of the work is done. I am holding you responsible for it. It is up to you to get results."

This type of leadership almost certainly pays dividends since it gives competent individuals pride in their work and encourages initiative, self-confidence, and ability. The opposite and usually unsuccessful approach is that of the executive who insists that all actions and decision originate with him, and that everything go in or out over his desk. This inevitably causes division heads either to leave the organization for more reasonable and stimulating fields or to lose interest and initiative, thereby becoming intimidated "yes men" of little real value to the organization. The latter, while they may appear to be obedient, gravitate into a sullen rut, secretly delighting in the event of administrative errors. Equally inevitable in such cases is the puzzlement of the executive over the apparent lack of cooperation, understanding, and support from his subordinates.

It is not to be inferred that the job of the executive is merely to find capable subordinates, to delegate authority to them, and then to sit back in ease and watch the wheels go round. The real test of sound leadership involves the ability, after delegating authority, to step in unobtrusively at appropriate times to give suggestions or directions on the basis of greater knowledge and a more complete understanding of overall strategy. Pfiffner[35] has listed certain rules and prerequisites for the successful delegation of authority and responsibility. The first, most important, and most frequently overlooked of these is simply that the executive must honestly want to delegate. If responsibility is to be delegated, subordinates must be carefully chosen and must be capable of bearing responsibility. Their responsibility must be defined for them and they must be trained to carry it. Furthermore, if responsibility is delegated, there must also be delegated with it the appropriate type and amount of authority. Failure to do so is the second most common error. If subordinates are good enough to employ in the first place and to assume responsibility, they are good enough to trust.

Delegation has been referred to as fundamentally necessary for successful administrative management. In fact administration might with considerable truth be defined as getting things done through others. In present-day public health organizations as well as in other organizations it is impossible for one person to do the whole job. The head of an organization should not try to handle all of the details himself; it is a physical and mental impossibility and it is not expected. Decisions should be made at the lowest possible point in the organization's line of command. Were this not true, there would be little use or justification for creating an organization in the first place. The wise executive will employ as subordinates individuals who are more capable than he is in each of the various functions of the organization and will let them take care of the details. Far from indicating weakness, it is a sign of a good administrator for subordinates to be called upon to present detailed information to outsiders as well as to the executive himself. Furthermore to do so boosts the ego, job interest, and loyalty of the subordinate.

Probably the average executive does not adequately understand the basic principles involved in delegation. Not uncommon is the pitiful spectacle of an executive who, feeling that only he can do each job correctly, is trying to face all points of the compass at once and has become a slave to nonadministrative minutiae with which others are better fitted to cope. He lets the job run him instead of the preferred and intended reverse. Meanwhile his subordinates must helplessly stand by, losing interest and initiative, merely nodding assent to the wishes and actions of their superior.

On the other hand, there are the many executives who, apparently lacking the courage of their convictions, delegate responsibilities to a greater or lesser extent but avoid establishment of clear-cut lines of command and neglect to invest the employee with the corresponding authority needed for adequately meeting the added responsibility. They thereby tend to expect more from their subordinates than they have a right to, expressing great surprise and disappointment when their subordinates appear not to stand up fully to their responsibilities. They appear not to realize that a subordinate under such circumstances, in addition to feeling a lack of recognition and trust, is in great danger of being left out on a limb, caught between an employer who demands that he carry out a delegated responsibility and other employees who understandably question his right to make requests or issue orders.

Failure to delegate therefore has many undesirable consequences. First, and probably of least importance, is that the executive tends to drive himself toward a physical or mental breakdown, following never ceasing high-pressure workdays coping with annoying details and sleepless nights fed by bulging briefcases. Inevitably the organization suffers because the executive himself is the chief bottleneck and the work is incompletely and inefficiently done. The agency loses the benefit of whatever abilities exist in the rest of the personnel, capable potential employees shy away from the uninspiring environment, and those within the organization soon ask themselves either, "Why stay?" or "What's the use of working or trying?"

All who have studied the problem agree that in practically all instances of "one-man shows" with the absence of delegation the essential difficulty is one of psychologic inadequacy on the part of the executive. This masquerades in many forms: conceit, boorishness, false pride, false interest, fussy perfectionism, or obvious lack of self-confidence. As Dimock[34] has said:

> Show me the man who does not delegate and it will frequently be found that he is a bundle of fears and misgivings. He is afraid to make mistakes. He is afraid that he will be tricked or embarrassed. He is afraid that others would not do it his way.

This gives a sadly accurate word picture of more than one executive officer in the field of public health.

Certain few essentials are necessary for successful and effective delegation. The first requisite is that the executive must truly and consciously want to do it. It is never a subconscious action. The executive must look upon his function as essentially that of a coordinator of the activities of many others, each of whom has been entrusted with specific responsibilities and authority. He must consider his position akin to that of the conductor of a symphony orchestra through whose coordinating activity inspiring music results where there might otherwise be cacophony.

The organization must be set up with clear-cut and well-understood lines or channels. In delegating, these lines must be respected, never making one person responsible for a job only to give the job or the authority for it to someone else. Perhaps the most important consideration involved is the realization that delegation properly involves a multiple action. The key setting off the chain reaction is the necessity of delegating work load or function. This infers a delegation of responsibility. In turn, to make the fulfillment of the responsibility possible, delegation of an appropriate additional amount of authority is necessary. In some instances a change in the title or rank of the employee is indicated as part of the delegation of authority in order to implement it.

In discussing the relationship between delegated responsibility and authority most writers speak in terms of equality. Actually what is called for is an even more delicate adjustment. The good executive has a real interest in the development of his subordinates as well as in getting the work done. Accordingly, he will grant to the responsible subordinate the amount of authority required by the responsibilities plus just enough in addition to allow expanded opportunity for experience and improvement without risking marked difficulty and a sense of failure.

It must always be understood that delegation is in effect a loan that is never permanent and that it can be recalled at any time. Delegation is most effective in an atmosphere of mutual understanding and respect. The executive has the right to expect that his trust will not be abused. He should, however, be constantly alert to the possibility that his trust as manifest by delegation might not be justified. Unfortunately he will occasionally find this to be the case. Such instances are not always easy to handle, as Dimock[34] has emphasized:

The worst kind of a person to deal with in any organization is the slippery evasive individual who gives the appearance of a good fellow and a square shooter, who pays a sort of obsequious deference to the wishes of his superior, but who goes contrary to known policies and abuses his authority to the extent where it cannot help but be noticed, but not quite to the point where the official is justified in chopping off his head. It is this kind of person more than any other who gives the executive pause when it comes to delegation, and who is most likely to damage the morale of the organization as a whole. The egoist is soon discovered and can be eliminated. The man with an inferiority complex can be built up and restored to normalcy. The devious person is the hardest to handle on all scores, but especially in any situation requiring a delegation of authority.

Another important aspect is the power relationships of the head of an organization. The successful leadership of an organization involves a constant struggle with those in other organizations or groups who also possess power. The executive health officer must recognize this and be ever ready and able to engage in a struggle for proper power. This is vital if his organization is to survive and if he is not to betray it, its employees, and those it serves. He should not allow himself to be deluded or deterred in this by false modesty, weakness, or complaisance. Of course a struggle for power should never be simply for the accumulation of power for its own sake or for self-aggrandizement but should be engaged in in order to assure that no important or essential part of the organization and its program will be lacking or misplaced.

A most succinct summary of the approach to such situations has been given by Upson[36]:

As an executive, you must expect some people to disagree with you—some who are smarter than you are and honestly object to both your methods and objectives; some who are less smart than you are and out of that inadequacy damn what you are doing in an effort to make themselves appear big; some, who dislike or misunderstand your motives and who will fight everything you try to do simply because you are doing it. Of these groups, respect the first, ignore the second, and fight the third—and fight them without compromise, winner take all.

Morale and discipline

In every organization some rules or regulations will be necessary, but if they are to be effective they must be few, simple, readily understood, and inflexible. Items that may be effectively included are limited largely to such matters as the hours of work, the length of the lunch period, the handling of certain records and correspondence, holidays and leaves. The administrator's real difficulties begin at the point where objective inflexibility ends. He cannot hope to constantly police the work and behavior of all of his subordinates and even if he could, it would preclude the possibility of good leadership. The best he can hope for, and what is probably most desirable in the long run, is to develop inasmuch as possible an almost subconscious self-discipline within the group itself so that improper behavior of a particular employee is considered by his fellows as an infraction against their self-developed and self-enforced code of working ethics.

The executive and his supervisors should always bear in mind that although most people are quite willing to be subordinate to good leadership they are not willing to be subservient. Even though the person in authority may have the legal or financial power to demand obedience, the subordinate similarily has the power to refuse to obey or, what is more practical from his standpoint, the power to circumvent orders while appearing to obey.

Individuals in an organization may often with relative ease find it possible to chronically arrive late and leave early or to spend considerable time visiting with fellow workers. If promptness and attention to work has over a period of time become part of the organization's code of working ethics, in most instances the administrator will find it unnecessary to deal with the individual situation himself. The other employees by virtue of their own interest in the matter will handle it for him. They will take the attitude that the individual is trying to get away with something that is contrary to the best interests and welfare of the group. If, on the other hand, there is a tradition of slipshod management and administration, the affairs of the organization will tend to assume the atmosphere of a routinized semi-social event to the detriment of the program and the morale of all concerned.

The question of attendance control is only one example of a great many problems of administrative management for which there is more than one answer. Depending on the type of activity in which the organization is engaged, attempts to obtain strict adherence to the scheduled hours of work may be a deterrent to wholehearted cooperation and high personnel morale. This probably applies to most phases of public health work, where a reasonable degree of latitude allowed by a good leader will in most instances result in greater loyalty to and interest in the work than would otherwise be attained. An organization is recalled where unusually high morale, evidenced by interest, willing overtime, and loyalty, was definitely jeopardized by the installation of a time clock for the professional personnel by an overenthusiastic efficiency expert from the mayor's office.

In terms of what has been said therefore the goal for which the good administrator will aim is a cooperative team, which is probably most successfully achieved by the development of a logical organizational structure with well-defined and understood lines of authority and responsibility and a well-established tradition of good self-discipline. Good personnel management depends partly on sound organization and partly on sound individual guidance, correction, reward, and punishment. It has been said that the administrator must understand people and be a leader. There are two kinds of leadership, the first demonstrated by a person with superior ability whom people gladly follow, the second consisting of mere possession of authority. Authority in itself is of limited value. It is well to remember the adage, "You can lead a horse to water but you can't make him drink."

The wise executive will understand the difference between a well-balanced person and one who is emotionally disturbed, and he will be conscious of the gap that may exist between ability and achievement. He will recognize that these characteristics apply to himself as well as to his subordinates. He will realize that an emotionally immature person will tend to measure accomplishments against those of more gifted or more fortunate people or against some un-

reasonable standard he has set for himself. Such a person remedies failure by daydreaming, rebellion, self-pity, bullying, bragging, or even by deliberate failure, a form of overcompensation. The well-balanced person, on the other hand, will measure his accomplishments against his honestly recognized aptitudes and share of luck. His aim is to seek a cause worth serving, one for which he has an aptitude and in which he can find mental and emotional satisfaction. In dealing with personnel therefore the executive should be aware of the various types of behavior defenses that may arise from a feeling of failure or dissatisfaction. These are of many types: "If I give in, you won't need to hurt me." "If I am humorous, you won't think to hurt me." "If I flatter you, you will be deterred from hurting me." "If I am sick and unfortunate, you will be ashamed to hurt me." "If you love me, you won't want to hurt me." "If I hurt you first, you won't be able to hurt me."

This leads to the question of discipline. As White[31] has indicated:

In a healthy organization the staff possesses a high morale which relegates discipline of any type to a position of secondary importance. For most persons the attitude and morale of the group are a sufficient guide to conduct; and where effective leadership and good supervision exist, problems of discipline largely disappear. The basic attack on disciplinary problems is therefore an indirect one, rather than the search for new forms of action or the imposition of heavier penalties.

Practically every instance requiring discipline comes after a failure of some kind on the part of management. This applies even to cases of "born troublemakers" since an effective personnel program would preclude their employment in the first place. It should always be realized that a disciplinary act deals with much more than the immediate present and the individual directly involved. The case at hand merely concentrates in the present the results of the past and possible consequences of the future. Futhermore, literally every other member of the organization is alert and watching for the outcome because the solution will show him what to expect under similar circumstances. Magoun[37] has illustrated this point with the story of the office boy who was disciplined for absenting himself from work to attend a family funeral after having been refused by the boss, who suspected that he went to a World Series baseball game. Needless to say, such an employer would never be forgiven by those working under him for his bad judgment and ill-considered disciplinary action.

While avoidance of conditions requiring discipline is much better than successful discipline, failure to discipline when it is indicated is demoralizing to the group. There are a number of behavior patterns that require action of some sort on the part of the administrator or supervisor. Among these are inattention to duty, including chronic tardiness, laziness, carelessness, breakage or loss of property, inefficiency, insubordination in the form of violation of an order, regulation, or law, or disloyalty to the organization. Certain personal behavior such as continued and overt intoxication, immorality and lack of integrity manifest by violation of a recognized code of ethics, soliciting, accepting a bribe, or deliberately neglecting to enforce a law also requires action.[38]

A poor executive, in approaching disciplinary problems of this sort, will tend to rely merely on his power to coerce and command. In so doing he is actually attempting to reassure himself for his own feeling of inadequacy and weakness, refusing to recognize that perhaps he and his lack of leadership had something to do with the development of the problem at hand. The capable executive, on the other hand, sees unbalanced behavior as a symptom of wrong conditions either in the way the employee has been handled or in some external situation such as the work, social, community, or home environment. He will recognize the importance of the employee's stage of emotional development and even consider the possible influence of frustrations and insecurities of earlier origin along with those developed in the recent past.

In dealing with an upset employee one should ask himself a number of questions of a psychologic nature. What accounts for the emotional insecurity that resulted in the employee's decision to press the rebellion, to sidestep the basic difficulty, instead of consciously and honestly recognizing his feelings and responding to them in an intelligent manner? What opportunity can be given him to gain self-assurance so the solution will be permanent rather than temporary?

Some may consider an approach such as this as being unwarranted, patronizing, and out of place in business, industry, or public service. It might be pointed out, however, that considerable attention is paid to inanimate machinery and, if something goes wrong in its mechanism, we go to great lengths to discover the seat of the trouble rather than to discard the whole machine or to rely on makeshift repairs. It is high time that we realize that the animate mechanism, the human employee, merits this and much more attention and consideration.

The actual approach to a disciplinary action should never be casual or momentary. A series of steps should be taken. The executive officer should first study himself to discover and eliminate personal bias as well as to discover any personal responsibility for the situation. He should make a many-sided approach to the problem, looking at it through the eyes of the employee himself, his family, his fellow employees, and his immediate supervisor. The entire situation should be investigated, giving consideration to the condition of work at the time, the employee's past record, the morale and behavior of the employees as a group, the type and degree of infraction, the organization's tradition in such cases, and any outside conditions that may have influenced the employee. An attempt should be made to discover whether the failure was due to misunderstanding, an emotional upset, lack of experience, some irregularity in working conditions, or poor leadership. Throughout the whole process, the executive should look upon his function as that of a counselor rather than that of a judge and should be alert to opportunities to solve the problem from the point of view of the welfare of the organization while enabling the employee to save face.

Magoun,[39] in teaching human engineering at Massachusetts Institute of Technology, used the case analysis method to considerable advantage. The approach to disciplinary situations that he suggested is outlined in some detail because of its value as an exercise in the solution of personnel problems.

Prepare

I. Study the situation until you feel completely clear as to
   A. How your habits and emotions color what you see in it
   B. How the other people concerned are affected by it
   C. All the significant facts
   D. Exactly what the problem is that requires solution (problems in human relations are almost never what they seem to be on the surface)
II. Write down the essential facts of the problem
   A. Be sure to avoid any interpreting and include only accurate concise statements of fact
   B. Be sure to include material other people recognize as facts, even though you may not
III. Write down the emotions involved in the problem
   A. What desires created the situation?
   B. What desires are maintaining the situation?
   C. What long and short term goals are desired by you and others and why?
IV. Check by making believe you are each person involved, and see whether you have made a valid presentation of his facts, problems, and desires from his point of view

Analyze

I. Separate the fundamental from the trivial (beware that your emotions do not fool you in this)
II. What are the key logs in the jam?
   A. Make a careful and exhaustive analysis of each person's acts and reactions, step by step. Begin by finding out first, in detail, all the consequences each person's attitude has for him and what satisfactions it fulfills. Then be sure to get to the bottom of what actually happened, and work out an exact explanation of why. Does it make psychologic sense? Common sense?
III. Write all of this out in its proper relationship
   A. So that you can see the problem as a whole
   B. So that you can see where the situation is going and how fast
IV. Write out in significant detail the requirements for a total solution
   A. What are the things it must accomplish—can accomplish? Why is any given goal desirable? Why are there only certain ways of achieving it?
   B. Check for the immediate and total satisfaction of each person involved
   C. Note conflicting desires that must be harmonized by a successful solution
V. Contrive a total solution
   A. Write out every possible alternative showing how you derived it, and choose the best one (usually the simplest) that offers the interweaving of interests.

Handle

I. Once the goal has been determined, the means become the most important thing; now that you have decided what to do, plan to do it
   A. With a minimum of self-assertion or disturbance to habit patterns
   B. With careful consideration of time, place, and individuals
   C. With reference to the various possibilities that may arise
II. Write out your plan concretely, accurately, and in detail
III. Rehearse your plan as one would familiarize himself with a detailed map
   A. Go through it step by step, with the help of someone else, looking for flaws in your plan, flaws in

your attitude, ways of bettering your presentation in terms of the individual involved and places where you might meet failures due to the unexpected

IV. Wait for the appropriate time and conditions. Then try out your plan

  A. Be thoroughly sincere and keep voice, eyes, posture emotionally calm

  B. Begin by getting the facts understood

  C. Present your case in terms of his intelligence, viewpoint, and emotional responses

  D. Listen to his case so that you can express it to him better than he did to you; then he knows you understand it; you may also catch any new evidence that you overlooked

  E. Together come to a decision based on the facts

Evaluate

  I. Review the entire case

  II. Write out its lessons

    A. What almost failed and why?

    B. What almost succeeded and why?

    C. What did you do for yourself and others?

    D. What did you do to yourself and others?

The types of disciplinary action that may be taken in specific situations can be divided into several categories. First, there is what might be termed the indirect or informal approach. Here there is no specific or explicit reference made to dissatisfaction, and reliance is placed on inference by the employee as a result of a change in attitude in the executive officer or supervisor. There may be developed, for instance, a more or less obvious chilling of the atmosphere, closer supervision of work, a failure to invite the employee to confer or consult with reference to relevant matters, a rejection of proposals, or a reduction in estimates. The employee might further experience some loss of privileges, a curtailing of authority and responsibility, or actual reassignment to less desirable work. The assumption of this approach is that the employee will be intelligent enough to "get the point" and without further action spontaneously undertake a program of self-improvement.

A more explicit approach may be the application of what are sometimes referred to as direct or formal penalties of the first degree. Usually these are imposed and enforced by the head of an office or division on his own responsibility and without review. They may take the form of formal notice and warning, reprimand, delay in salary increment, loss of seniority, or requirement of overtime. The use of the last two disciplinary actions is somewhat open to question. The employee may with considerable justification and support object to unpaid overtime as a means of getting some work done for nothing. With regard to seniority, the supervisor or administrator may find himself involved in a controversy, very often with the employee and the civil service agency on one side and himself on the other, since for some reason it is not rare to find civil service agencies considering as one of their functions the protection of the misunderstood employee from an overbearing or malevolent supervisor or administrator.

The transfer of an employee might be considered a penalty of the first degree and in many instances solves the difficulty to everyone's satisfaction. Not infrequently the problem employee may cease to be a problem if he is reassigned to work under another supervisor, put in a new social or physical environment, or assigned a different type of work. This is understandable, considering that personnel problems involve much more than the employee, i.e., fellow employees, the physical environment, the supervisor, the type of work, etc. The surly and careless file clerk may turn out to be an excellent receptionist. The inefficient and unproductive field nurse may develop into an exceptional clinic assistant. Although often very effective, there is one objection to this approach: it encourages some supervisors and executives to feel justified in dodging personnel problems, to the development of which they have often contributed, simply by transferring them to others. Much more than a transfer is needed in every instance—a complete study of the circumstances of the problem is indicated.

If more drastic disciplinary action is indicated, what have been referred to as penalties of the second degree may be applied. They usually require the action of the head of the department or organization itself, and sometimes the employee has the right to appeal to a board, a civil service commission, or occasionally to a court. The first penalty in this category is temporary suspension. It is questionable if this is ever sound or justified. The fact that the employee is subjected to enforced although temporary absence from work and therefore loss of salary inevitably results in his return to work in a more disgruntled, defensive, and vengeful frame of mind than when he left.

The same objection may be raised to the use of demotion as a penalty. Occasionally, however, if the employee has great intrinsic desirability for the organization, a temporary demotion, with the clear understanding that reinstatement will readily follow demonstration of good intentions, may be indicated. One might well raise the question, however, whether some of the less drastic methods of approach would not be equally or more effective in such instances.

Dismissal or removal for cause is of course the extreme and final measure. A word of caution is indicated here, and applies to all types of disciplinary action. When it first appears that an employee may be a problem, a detailed documentary record should be made of pertinent instances and facts for possible reference and use in the event that subsequent disciplinary action may be appealed. It is a good policy to keep the employee in the case informed at every step concerning his status rather than to subject him, as too often happens, to a sudden release of pent-up managerial objections. This always should be and can be done with an atmosphere of counseling, which shows a genuine concern for the employee's welfare as well as for that of the organization. True, this often takes much time, but in the long run it pays great dividends in the maintenance of high morale. In the past and to a considerable degree in

the present the attitude of executives toward dismissal has been that it represents merely a disagreeable experience for the employer involving simply the summary discharge of the employee. If dismissal is necessary, the employee should be made to realize that it is in his best interest as well as the organization's and, in effect, presents an opportunity for his rehabilitation elsewhere.

One final word of caution: Under no circumstances should a worker be subjected to any active form of disciplinary action in the presence of his fellow employees. While some of them may appear to enjoy it, they will all resent it.

CONDITIONS OF WORK
Job appeal
A high level of employee morale has been referred to repeatedly as a prime essential for the satisfactory and efficient operation of a public health program. Good morale is difficult if not impossible to define. Perhaps, like health, the best way to recognize it is when it is not present. If the state of mind and the working relationships of a group of people are satisfactory, one seldom if ever finds himself even thinking about the problems involved in the development and maintenance of good morale. In contrast one becomes acutely aware of the problem if things are not what they should be.

The nature of high morale might be better understood by some of its symptoms, such as a pride of the employees in being identified with the organization and their pleasure in working for it. There are health departments, unfortunately, the employees of which look upon their activity as merely a means of earning a wage or salary. On the other hand, health organizations exist in which everyone, including the office boy, the elevator operator, and the lowest clerical worker on the staff, feels that the organization is his health department and that he is contributing something essential to its activity; he thereby derives considerable happiness and satisfaction from his daily work.

Although morale is determined by a great many factors, unquestionably the most important is the quality of leadership of the "line officers," i.e., the immediate supervisors of the workers, and the amount of inspiration and job interest they can impart to the personnel. The concept that once prevailed with regard to subordinates was, "If you don't like the orders or the work, you can quit or be fired." The complete futility of this approach is exemplified by the attempts of the Nazi conquerors to force the people of the countries they overran into productive labor. The whole world knows the devastating and significant effects of the slowdowns to which these conquered workers resorted.

Now, instead of trying to prod or drive the employee into doing work, the approach is based on good leadership, example, and respect, job and employee analysis, and employee training. From this is seen the great importance of the specific job in relation to the specific worker. Very often both an employee and a job are individually desirable and important but simply may not mix. As previously mentioned, an unsatisfactory file clerk may on reassignment turn out to be an excellent receptionist. Very few situations in life work only in one direction. If an employee is expected to give his best effort to his job, the job should be expected to give him something in return. The activity must appear to be something more than busy work or dull routine. The worker must have the opportunity to realize its significance and its contribution to the attainment of the total goal.

An excellent example of this was found in the attitudes of the large number of clerical workers who were engaged by state health departments during World War II to handle the routine paper work of the Emergency Maternity and Infant Care Program for the wives and infants of servicemen. Unfortunately most state health departments simply employed clerks, assigned them to tables and desks, distributed pens or rubber stamps, and subjected the clerks to a continuous rapid flow of inanimate sheets of paper. This gave them no real understanding of the significance of the program and the vital part they were playing in it. It was not surprising that these organizations ex-

perienced considerable difficulty, not merely in obtaining personnel but also in holding them. In fact in many instances personnel turnover was truly appalling and seriously hampered the effectiveness of this important program. In a few states, however, some consideration was given to the worker, his intelligence, and the possible monotony of the job and the relation of it to the employee's morale. It was refreshing to visit these few state health agencies and to notice the alert and satisfied expressions on the faces of the workers. In discussing the work with them, the same interpretations were repeatedly encountered. They were not working with pieces of paper and rubber stamps; they were making it possible for a large number of women and children to obtain necessary medical attention. They looked upon the beneficiaries involved as "their mothers and their babies" and thereby received considerable satisfaction from the work they were doing in helping them. As might be expected, while these latter organizations had the same difficulty in obtaining new personnel, having done so they kept them, and in a highly satisfactory state of morale.

The administrator's responsibility for seeing that his staff is well informed of the agency's current goals, its progress toward them, and the importance of every job in their achievement is too often overlooked or is exercised casually. While free communication may be conducted best on an informal personal basis, there must be planning to assure that it does occur. In large agencies use of mass communication techniques is often a necessary and desirable supplement to building a staff that knows what is going on and feels that it is part of the organization.

Dimock,[34] in the course of management studies, asked a number of businessmen for their views concerning factors that determined employees' activities. In other words, for what reason do men and women put forth their best efforts? The replies received were so consistent that he felt justified in suggesting the incentive scale shown in Fig. 13-1. Up to a point, the chief incentive is increased income in order to give a sense of

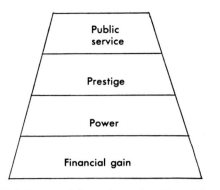

Fig. 13-1. Personnel incentive scale. (From Dimock, M. E.: The executive in action, New York, 1945, Harper & Brothers.)

security. At some point there is superimposed upon this financial urge a desire for power and position, an opportunity to determine policy and to make one's own work. This in turn is eventually replaced by a desire for recognition and prestige, and eventually when these three urges or appetites are appeased, there is added a spirit of altruism and a desire for public service. Dimock concludes that the latter is the ultimate and most rewarding of all incentives.

The question of job appeal might be summarized therefore as including serious consideration of two factors: the assignment of the right employee to the right job, and the provision to the worker of an opportunity to realize and understand the significance of the work he is being called upon to do and to obtain a fair measure of personal reward and satisfaction.

Certain physical factors should not be overlooked in considering job appeal. It is a definite responsibility of administrators and supervisors to be constantly alert to needs and methods for the improvement of the physical environment in which their personnel must work. It has often been said, and with considerable justification, that health departments traditionally are relegated to the least desirable rooms in the basement of a city hall, county courthouse, or a state capitol building, preferably as close as possible to the public comfort station. Unquestionably there have been many instances of progressive public health personnel leaving positions because of an undesirable working environment. A health officer should always attempt to make his department an outstanding physical example of the cause for which it works. It is illogical to expect the public to respond to the educational efforts or even to the statutory measures of an organization that tolerates itself being housed in quarters that exemplify all the circumstances it criticizes and condemns.

A satisfactory working environment is in reality a sign of administrative efficiency. It has been shown repeatedly by industrial and other studies that the improvement of lighting, ventilation, and attractiveness is invariably followed by a significant increase in work output, a decrease in physiologic fatigue, and greatly improved employee satisfaction and morale. Unquestionably public health officials in the past have been guilty of unwarranted complaisance and timidity in competing with other public officers for desirable quarters and in the promotion of attractive and efficient health centers. The health officer should realize that few things are truer than "Do not ask and you shall not receive."

Overtime

In every organization work during time other than the regular working hours is occasionally necessary. Emergencies and pressure periods are certain to occur, especially in a field such as public health. It is reasonable to expect the personnel to have sufficient interest in the program of their organization to do their part willingly in meeting emergency situations, and if the personnel relationships are satisfactory, no difficulty or opposition will be encountered. However, the amount of overtime work should be kept at a minimum and should be engaged in only after careful study and with adequate reason.

Continued or repeated overtime is administratively unjustifiable. A habit of overtime indicates either inefficient work methods or personnel, either of which signifies inefficient administrative management. It is patently unfair to expect effective work and satisfactory function during the regular workday when the employees have been mentally and physically fatigued by chronic overtime requirements. When overtime is necessary, provision should always be made for compensation either in time off or in additional pay at the rate of time and one half. Whenever possible, the latter method should be followed. Generally speaking, to allow addition of accumulated overtime to the annual vacation is undesirable since it encourages deliberately sought for overtime and may result in considerable personnel depletion for part of the year.

Leaves

Annual vacation leave with full pay of the personnel should always be planned for and encouraged. This bears many advantages for the organization as well as for the employee himself. The physical and psychologic need for weekend rest and for an annual vacation has been well established by social custom and proved by scientific investigation. An organization should have a definite policy concerning vacations. Usually an employee is not entitled to vacation until he has rendered at least 6 months of service. Many organizations, however, allow 1 day of cumulative vacation time per month of service, which is due the employee regardless of the date of his employment. It is most common at this stage of our social and economic progress to allow for an annual vacation period of 2 weeks. This applies particularly to office and other nonprofessional personnel. Scientific, professional, and educational workers often are allowed longer vacations, perhaps in consideration of their greater period of training or in relation to the vacation time of their professional brethren engaged in teaching. Justification of this distinction is somewhat vague and untenable; undoubtedly the ideal would be an annual leave of about 1 month for all.

It is decidedly undesirable to allow employees to work for additional pay instead of taking their vacation since this defeats the purposes of the vacation idea and usually results in employee regret and inefficiency. Similarly it is unwise to allow the addition of unused sick leave to vacation time since this defeats the purpose of sick

leave. If a holiday occurs during the vacation period of an employee, it is only fair to allow him an extra day off. However, the additional day off usually should be taken at a later date and not added to the vacation period since this tends to cause difficulty in scheduling the vacations of the other employees.

Provision for sick leave should be considered a protection or insurance against a time of potential future need and not simply an added benefit to which the employee is entitled whether or not he becomes ill. In an increasing number of public agencies it is supplemented by various forms of disability and hospitalization insurance. Policies with regard to sick leave vary considerably. In smaller organizations there are often no specific provisions made, illness among the personnel being dealt with on an individual basis as it occurs. In other organizations, especially in larger agencies, a specific number of days per year is allowed for sick leave.

This frequently gives rise to several difficulties. Some workers look upon the total number of sick leave days as their inevitable due whether or not they become ill. If no administrative controls are applied, there may develop considerable abuse of sick leave privileges, causing resentment by conscientious employees and an undesirable state of morale in general. Some organizations attempt to solve this by requiring a visit by a city physician or a report from a private attending physician. However, this is an administrative and personal nuisance, necessitates added expense, and develops a not unjustified feeling of resentment among employees that they are not being trusted. It has been suggested by some that the solution is to make sick leave cumulative. This encourages employees to regard it as a saving or an investment and is a sound policy considering the occasional but inevitable occurrence of prolonged and catastrophic illness.

Of course the ideal approach to the problem is one that is aimed at the reduction of the need for absence due to illness. This is desirable from the point of view of both the organization and the employee. A number of simple principles are involved. The first is provision for preemployment physical examinations and periodic reexamination. Although essentially most benefit accrues to the employee, the fact that an organization requires these examinations makes it duty bound to bear whatever cost is involved.

Those returning to work following a period of illness should undergo careful examination, both from the point of view of protecting the other employees and of preventing premature return to work followed by a more serious and prolonged breakdown. If necessary, provision should be made for the follow-up and correction of physical defects, and employees with physical handicaps should be assigned to work with this in mind and supervised with particular care. The importance of a desirable working environment was previously referred to in relation to morale. This factor is of significance also in the prevention of illness and accidents. Many studies have demonstrated significant reductions in illnesses and accidents following improvement of the physical circumstances in which people must work. In-service training will be discussed in the next section, but here might be emphasized the importance of including education in personal health and safety practices.

Provision should be made for certain other types of leave. If an employee is asked to serve as a witness or as a member of a jury, it represents a civic responsibility concerning which he has no choice. It is therefore only right that the meeting of this responsibility be made possible. Of similar nature are leaves for military purposes. In no sense should absence from work for these reasons handicap the employee's reinstatement or his opportunities for advancement.

A number of strictly personal matters that require consideration are perhaps best dealt with on an individual basis. If illness or death occurs in the family of an employee or if it is necessary for him to move during a working day, it is justifiable to grant a reasonable time away from work. Not infrequently employees request the privilege of extended leave without pay. If a sound reason exists, it is usually well to grant the request. However, it is administratively unwise to allow repeated or extended leaves without pay for personal activities that are strictly matters of choice, such as extra vacations, fishing trips, and the like. It is recommended that this be avoided as much as possible since it serves to interrupt and confuse the work of the organization and since some other employees and possibly the public are apt to misunderstand the situation and consider it evidence of favoritism.

Certain types of personnel, particularly those who are members of professions, are entitled to leaves within reasonable limits for the purpose of educational and professional improvement. Everything possible should be done not merely to allow this but to encourage their attending and taking an active part in the meetings of the professional societies and associations to which they do or should belong. Here again there is a reasonable extent to which time away from the job should be allowed to any one person. There are occasional individuals who tend to be professional conventioneers and who unless restrained will spend the majority of their time attending meetings and conventions away from the job for which they are presumably employed. Not only does the work of the organization suffer but the other employees are thereby prevented from obtaining their fair share of this privilege.

In-service training

The process of learning should stop only with the last breath of life. The knowledge and ability that the public health worker brings to his job in the first instance should represent at most only the beginning of an ever growing fund of ability upon which he may base professional action. An organization that does not aid and abet continued improvement of its employees is remiss in its responsibilities and in the long run handicaps itself. There are many ways of accomplishing the desired purpose, all of which may be included in the term "in-service training." As one writer[40] has put it: "In-service training is a big thing, in-service training is many little things." The purposes of an in-service training program have been well summarized by Palmer[41] as follows:

1. To make up for deficiencies in technical and scientific information required for the job generally.
2. To enlarge the outlook and understanding on the specific job.
3. To acquaint the staff with the fundamentals of personal and public relationships in order to encourage smoother functioning of the day-to-day job.
4. To keep the staff abreast of newer technical, procedural, and administrative developments as derived from experience in other jurisdictions.

A good program will follow many different approaches and most desirably will involve in one way or another all of the personnel from the administrator himself to the custodian. The methods used may consist of a formal orientation course or a field orientation in a well-organized health department. Of importance are conferences, both individual and group, institutes, staff meetings, and refresher courses. There is a growing feeling of a need for a more intensive practical experience comparable to an internship. Often visits to other health departments are worth while in order to acquaint the personnel with problems and procedures in other areas. As mentioned previously, attendance at business and professional meetings and conferences should be encouraged. If an employee has enough interest and ambition to cause him to attend a school while continuing to work, particular consideration during the period of time involved is often justified. A policy of granting full-time leaves for professional education is a highly desirable adjunct to the effective development of a staff in a career service. An in-service training program is as important and as possible in a small organization as in a large one and in a rural area as well as in a city with many facilities available. Successful and worthwhile programs have been carried out on all levels of government. Special mention is merited of the work of the Joint Committee on Executive Development. This committee, sponsored by the Health Officers

Section of the American Public Health Association and the Association of Management in Public Health and assisted by the Training Branch of the Public Health Service, has planned and conducted over the past decade a series of excellent in-service training programs in the various administrative, management, and planning aspects of public health. The programs, in the form of seminars lasting from 3 to 5 days, have been presented in various parts of the nation, usually under the local sponsorship of a state or local health department or a school of public health.

Retirement

Retirement systems have become increasingly important in public health recruitment. Security is a basic desire, especially in one's later years. Even though retirement systems have multiplied in recent decades, they are still not available to about one third of local employees. A good retirement system does at least three things. It aids in organizational efficiency by making it possible to replace older personnel with younger people who possess more recent training and greater physical ability. A good retirement system does justice to all existing or prospective employees. Furthermore a retirement system aids in the solution of one of the greatest social problems that exists, that of the dependency of the aged. Finally, from the individual's point of view, a sound system coupled with preretirement counseling represents good gerontologic practice by making possible a gradual tapering off of activities as physical stamina decreases.

If a retirement system exists, it is fundamental that payments be adequate, for if they are too small, there will develop a tendency to refuse the pension and to remain on the job at a salary for as long as possible, thereby defeating the purposes of the plan. For the same reason and in order to conduct the retirement system on a sound insurance basis it is equally fundamental that participation in the plan be compulsory.

There are two principal types of retirement plans. The first is a simple cash disbursement plan that consists essentially of including an item in each budget to provide for pension payments. In this system total payments are small at first when few are entitled to benefits. As time passes, however, and more employees become older and eligible it becomes necessary to budget and therefore to tax for greater and greater amounts, resulting in a large proportion of the budget being for the payment of pensions rather than for actual services. Repeatedly organizations that have used this plan have become insolvent and in many instances have had to decrease or completely stop pension payments to which they had committed themselves and to which they had led their employees to look forward.

The second and more sound approach is through the use of an actuarial plan. Here future retirement objectives are calculated and planned for in advance for each employee. Such a program begins with larger payments than does the cash disbursement plan, but it builds up a reserve, the compound interest from which considerably lightens and in some instances completely absorbs the immediate financial burden.

The retirement plan may consist of contributions from employees alone, from the organization or government alone, or from the employees and the organization or government jointly. Typically, Social Security retirement benefits are part of the plan. The last is probably the best method since it gives both the employee and the organization an interest and a stake in the solution of the problem. For the employee it represents enforced savings with interest, plus reward for continued good service. For management it represents an orderly and socially responsible system for extending security to the current employee and separating the superannuated employee. If an employee leaves the organization before becoming eligible for pension payments, he should have the right to receive the total of whatever contributions he has made to the plan, plus whatever interest has accrued to that total. Under such circumstances, however, he should not expect to receive any of the contributions made by the organization or government since that too defeats the purpose for which the plan has been established.

The fact that public health personnel tend to move from job to job and from one state to another in improving themselves and advancing themselves professionally indicates the desirability of some type of interagency and interstate reciprocation with regard to retirement plans. No one would question the desirability of workers in a field like public health obtaining many and varied experiences. Rigidly provincial retirement plans already are acting as a deterrent to this. P.L. 89-749, the Comprehensive Health Planning Act of 1965, took an initial step to provide some latitude. However, this still remains one of the most critical and difficult personnel problems in the field of public health.

REFERENCES

1. Parran, T.: Public health schools and the nation's health. Dedicatory address, School of Public Health, University of Michigan, Sept. 19, 1944 (official publicaton).
2. Bailey, S. K.: Ethics and the public service, Public Adm. Rev. 24:234, Dec. 1964.
3. Mattison, B. F.: Political implications in good public health administration, Amer. J. Public Health 55:183, Feb. 1965.
4. Tucker, R. R., Richardson, E. L., Lifson, S. S., and Aronson, J. B.: The politics of public health—a symposium, Amer. J. Public Health 49:301, Mar. 1959.
5. Rosenau, M. J.: Courses and degrees in public health work, J.A.M.A. 64:794, Mar. 6, 1915.
6. Committee on Professional Education of the American Public Health Association: Public health degrees and certificates granted in the United States and Canada during the academic year 1939-40, Amer. J. Public Health 30:1456, Dec. 1940.
7. Editorial: Accreditation of schools of public health, Amer. J. Public Health 35:953, Sept. 1945.
8. Criteria and guidelines for accrediting schools of public health, Amer. J. Public Health 56:1308, Aug. 1966.
9. The school of public health: past, present, future, Public Health Rep. 78:867, Oct. 1963.
10. Conferencia sobre escuelas de salud publica, Bol. Ofic. Sanit. Panamer. 48:4, Apr. 1960.
11. Conference on schools of public health, Mexico, Amer. J. Public Health 50:1039, July 1960.
12. Recommended norms, schools of public health in Latin America, Washington, 1965, Pan American Health Organization.
13. Directory of schools of public Health in the Americas, Washington, 1966, Pan American Health Organization.
14. Committee on Professional Education of the

American Public Health Association: Individual reports, Amer. J. Public Health

15. Proposed report on field training of public health personnel, Amer. J. Public Health **37:** 709, June 1947; **45:**1351, Oct. 1955.

16. Editorial: Field training for public health personnel, Amer. J. Public Health **36:**178, Feb. 1946.

17. Guide for residencies in public health, Amer. J. Public Health **48:**1407, Oct. 1958.

18. The American Board of Preventive Medicine and Public Health Inc., Amer. J. Public Health **39:**425, Mar. 1949; **49:**561, Apr. 1959.

19. Burney, L. E., and Hemphill, F. M.: Merit system in public health, Amer. J. Public Health **34:**1173, Nov. 1944.

20. Mountin, J. W., Cheney, B. A., and Simpson, D. F.: Merit system administration in official health agencies, Amer. J. Public Health **37:**23, Jan. 1947.

21. Peterson, P. Q., Murray, L. J., Crabtree, J. A., and Amos, F. B.: The 1963 national conference on public health training, Amer. J. Public Health **54:**1049, July 1964.

22. Flook, E.: Public health service, personal communication, 1955.

23. State laws governing local health departments, Washington, 1953, Public Health Service Pub. No. 299.

24. Weiss, R. L., et al.: Retreading public health workers through training, Amer. J. Public Health **55:**242, Feb. 1965.

25. Bellin, L. E., Killeen, M., and Mazeika, J. J.: Preparing public health subprofessionals recruited from the poverty group, lessons from an OEO work-study program, Amer. J. Public Health **57:**242, Feb. 1967.

26. Emerson, H.: Local health units for the nation, New York, 1945, Commonwealth Fund.

27. Report of local public health resources, 1951, Washington, 1953, Public Health Service Pub. No. 278.

28. Building America's health. Report of the President's Commission on the Health Needs of the Nation, Washington, 1952, Vol. 3.

29. Health resources statistics, 1965, Washington, 1967, Public Health Service Pub. No. 1509.

30. Health manpower—Report of National Commission on Community Health Services, Washington, 1967, Public Affairs Press.

31. White, L. D.: Introduction to the study of public administration, New York, 1955, The Macmillan Co.

32. Mountin, J. W.: On making public health positions more attractive, Amer. J. Public Health, **35:**1150, Nov. 1945.

33. Donovan, J. J.: Career service classification, Amer. J. Public Health **51:**591, Apr. 1961.

34. Dimock, M. E.: The executive in action, New York, 1945, Harper & Brothers.

35. Pfiffner, J. McD.: Public administration, New York, 1946, The Ronald Press Co.

36. Upson, L. D.: Letters on public administration from a dean to his graduates, Detroit, 1947 (privately printed by the author).

37. Magoun, F. A.: New phases in personnel training, Public Health Nurs. **38:**592, 1946.

38. Allen, F. E.: Remedies against dishonest or inefficient public servants, Annals **169:**172, 1933.

39. Magoun, F. A.: Personal communication, 1948.

40. Underwood, F. J.: Inservice training in a state department of health, Amer. J. Public Health **36:**352, Apr. 1946.

41. Palmer, G. T. Quoted in Bearg, P. A., and Stockle, R.: Inservice training in a rural health department, Amer. J. Public Health **36:**1304, Nov. 1946.

Chapter 14

Planning and evaluation

INTRODUCTION

During most of public health history, programs and activities have been developed in a generally unplanned manner. Several phases may be identified. In the earliest phase much of the effort proceeded on the basis of crises—an epidemic, a flagrantly unsalubrious situation, or a natural disaster. The carry-over of this approach is still observable to an unfortunately common extent. Next, due to the efforts of the American Public Health Association's Committees on Administrative Practice and Evaluation coupled with the development and increasing sophistication of professional public health training, increasing numbers of health officers began to give serious attention to better planning. To no small degree this depended upon their personal interests and former experience, but gradually their staffs and even members of the community began to be involved. This led in recent years to the development of special short training courses, sometimes in schools of public health and sometimes within operating agencies, on the planning and evaluative aspects of public health. In this regard particular mention should be made of the numerous excellent seminars sponsored by the Joint Committee on Executive Development of the Association of Management in Public Health and the Health Officer's Section of the American Public Health Association as well as by the Communicable Disease Center of the Public Health Service.

As funds became more plentiful for pub-lic health work, as the perimeters of the field were extended by legislation, as public demands and expectancy for service increased, and as government and management in general became more sophisticated, health agencies became more visible and began to be held more accountable for their stewardship. This of course brought about a greater consciousness of the importance of more careful planning and programming. Two recent events have served to crystalize this trend and have caused more interest and activity in health planning on the part of a wide variety of individuals and organizations during the past 2 or 3 years than at any time in the past quarter century. The first of these was the development and refinement of certain planning techniques designated as PPBS (Planning-Programming-Budgeting-Systems) by the Department of Defense. The success of this prompted the President in August 1965 to direct his Cabinet members to apply the approach to the activities of the departments and agencies under their direction. The second event was the enactment by Congress in 1966 of P.L. 89-749, The Comprehensive Health Planning and Public Health Services Amendments. The significance of this act is threefold in that (1) it moves federal health assistance away from categorical grants toward block grants in order to make possible greater state and local program determination, (2) it encourages and requires more deliberate and hopefully more efficient program planning, and (3) it recognizes the breadth of social concerns and potential involvement by requiring the establishment of state (and local or regional) planning commissions broadly representative of various professions, agencies, institutions, and citizen groups.

These trends are certain to generate problems for the professional public health administrator, and the procedures proposed are not without their limitations. Gorham,[1] who had much to do with their development in the Department of Defense and who subsequently moved to the Department of Health, Education, and Welfare for the same purpose, has commented on the limitations of planning techniques. "Anyone in government knows that most decisions on spending emerge from a political process and are most heavily influenced by value judgments and the pressures brought to bear by a wide range of interested parties." He points out that the leaders of government may have preferences about programs, unrelated to costs, benefits, or efficiency. One may be interested in a particular program because its beneficiaries are numerous or politically powerful or vocal. Another may have experienced a heart attack or have a crippled child and therefore tend to favor programs aimed at these conditions. A program conducted as part of Social Security benefits financed from a payroll tax may be favored over another perhaps more important program that would necessitate increased tax revenues. Hilleboe and Schaefer[2] also indicate the problems imposed by inadequate data, insufficient attainable resources, the current rapidity of scientific and technologic changes, and the scattered responsibility and authority in health matters. Nevertheless, as Gorham[1] concludes, while ". . . the tools of analysis are still fairly primitive—we are learning as we go along—and the best they can now do is to clarify some of the consequences of choices. . . . But the very process of analysis is valuable in itself, for it forces people to think about the objectives of Government programs and how they can be measured. It forces people to think in an explicit way. It is an important tool in the fight against creeping incrementalism—'ten percent to those with the most bureaucratic or political muscle, five percent to all others.' "

With reference to the comprehensive and total community approach to planning, this too has its inherent problems. Public health workers, prideful of their educations, experiences, and professionalism, cannot be expected to be entirely pleased with situations in which their ideas, proposals, or decisions are subjected to the scrutiny and even veto of "the uninformed," be they from the governmental or community agencies or from the public at large. However, "the increased community involved, always sought but seldom attained, will more than make up, in the long run, for the transient confusion or the few moments lost while these new elements become familiar with the facts and figures and gear themselves to the mechanics and procedures essential to sound program planning. Given the motivation and a blueprint, the effective delivery of the requisite health services will not be far behind."[3] This viewpoint is emphasized more strongly by the National Commission on Community Health Services.[4]

The nature of today's society and the complexities of health and other community services require a broad approach to planning and action which can be fitted to each particular community situation, yet is in harmony with broader trends and is capable of further development and change. The Commission believes that planning is an action process and is basic to development and maintenance of quality community health services. Action-planning for health should be communitywide in area, continuous in nature, comprehensive in scope, all-inclusive in design, coordinative in function, and adequately staffed.

The responsible participation and involvement of all sectors of the community, coordination of efforts, and development of cooperative working arrangements are fundamental to effective action-planning. Health service objectives can be met through processes which provide opportunity for citizens to work together to understand, identify, and resolve problems, to set intermediate and long-range goals, and to act to achieve the goals.

The readiness and ability of communities to respond to health needs and problems are dependent, in large part, on the presence of effective mechanisms for planning.

In a pluralistic society wise and acceptable decisions and policies can be made less and less by the single channel approach.

This is why interorganizational and community planning approaches and the systems analysis devices are becoming ever more important. Already, for example, a number of state governments specify that certain policies, such as those relating to water use and conservation, be made by a cabinet rather than by a single departmental director or board. In other words it is becoming increasingly important to find the multiple interfaces among organizations, programs, and groups that have some commonality of interest, concern, responsibility, or action.

OBJECTIVES OF HEALTH PLANNING

In recognition of the growing importance of improved planning by health agencies the Program Area Committee on Medical Care Administration and Public Health Administration of the American Public Health Association addressed itself during recent years to the development of a formal statement on the subject.[5] The statement as adopted presents the following useful list of the purposes or objectives of careful health planning:

1. Improve organizational patterns for health services.
2. Speed development of needed new health services, strengthen existing services, and improve utilizations.
3. Discourage programs not needed in the community.
4. Improve the quality of health care through better coordination.
5. Eliminate duplication of health services among official and voluntary agencies at all levels.
6. Reduce fragmentation of health services at the state and community levels.
7. Help to achieve better geographical distribution of health services, with optimum utilization.
8. Establish priorities among new health programs and services, develop better balance among health programs, and provide services more responsive to the special health needs of the area.
9. Foster better use of scarce health manpower and more effective development of training resources.
10. Identify health needs and problems and help to set realistic goals, keeping expected changes in the area's characteristics in mind.
11. Spur faster application of new health knowledge.
12. Encourage closer relationships among health services, research, and training.
13. Help to integrate health needs into physical, economic, and other areas of planning for community development.

Particular attention should be directed to the last of these objectives since it is so often overlooked or ignored. Earlier, public health administration was defined as "the planned and organized social application of the knowledge and techniques of various and varying disciplines to the biological, physiological and sociological advantage of man." In this definition emphasis is placed not only upon the importance of planning but also upon planning within the total social context. In other words it is important at the outset to regard planning in the field of public health as only one facet of total social and economic planning.[6] This was stressed also by Seipp[7] in a discussion of health planning and economic development:

While program planning continues to be of major importance to health workers in the developing countries, there has emerged today an essentially new emphasis to plan for health as part of the totality of developmental effort. In this context, health measures are evaluated in terms of their significance for the process of development as a whole. The essential planning problem is to maximize the contribution forthcoming from the provision of health services to the total nation-building efforts of society. Planning within the health sector thus is undertaken in the terms of the larger framework of national developmental planning. . . . Health, it is obvious, cannot be overlooked as an end in itself. At the same time, the improvement of the health of a population represents an essential means or instrument for the developing society to attain its social and economic goals. It is when health measures are assessed from this instrumental point of view that they can be recognized as productive in character. They represent a necessary element in the total process of development, facilitating the attainment of the general goals of a society.

The World Health Organization understandably has also addressed itself to this aspect of planning of public health services and urges more attention to it by economists, political leaders, and health workers.[8]

At one time I was called upon to advise a developing nation whose economy was based primarily upon mining under exceedingly poor conditions. At the time the government was also encouraging the settlement of potentially good agricultural areas. After careful study, the primary recommendations were for the establishment of a strong occupational health program and an intensive antituberculosis program based essentially upon almost universal ambulatory prophylactic and therapeutic drug administration to miners and their families, among whom the incidence of tuberculosis was tremendous. The intent was obvious—to shore up the immediate economic producers upon whom the nation depended almost entirely at the moment. Next, emphasis was placed upon malaria eradication and the establishment of effective health posts along the routes of forest clearance and settlement. The intent here was to protect the health of the new group of producers upon whom the nation would depend more as time passed. It was felt that other activities could and indeed would have to wait their turn. A number of subsidiary recommendations might be of interest— (1) a thorough hydrographic survey of the rivers to determine appropriate sites for dams; this would assure a constant supply not only of water but also of electricity important to community development, education, food preservation, etc.; (2) the construction of refrigeration plants for the preservation of meat and other foods; cattle raising had already begun to prosper, and meat spoilage was becoming a problem; (3) the construction of some chicken-packing plants; this was aimed particularly at providing a year-round source of low-cost poultry protein in a protein-deficient society; (4) a celotex factory adjacent to one of the large sawmills that had already been constructed to process lumber for export; housing had already become a severe problem to the solution of which inexpensive celotex could contribute; (5) the pavement of certain feeder roads in the area being settled; this would make the settlements more accessible year round for health, educational, and other purposes. These and some other recommendations for planning may appear remote from health interests, but in each case they would eventually contribute in some way and to some extent to the attainment of good health.

By like token each of the health measures recommended very clearly would contribute to the social and economic development of the area.

TERMINOLOGY IN PROGRAM PLANNING

Already a considerable number of source and reference materials have developed on the subject of planning.[2,9] Terminology in this relatively new field has already become somewhat confusing. A variety of names, achronymic or otherwise, have been invented and applied to the analytic methods involved by various writers, teachers, and practitioners. Among those encountered are program development, program planning, program analysis, decision trees, program cost accounting, cost-benefit analysis, operations research, systems analysis, PPBS (Planning-Programming-Budgeting-Systems), PERT (Program Evaluation and Review Technique), and ASTRA (Automatic Scheduling with Time Integrated Resource Allocation). Many of these names and methods are synonymous, some represent parts of others, and many overlap. The more encompassing are PPBS, operations research, and systems analysis. Essentially these are synonymous and are concerned with the complete spectrum, from fact-finding, problem definition, goal setting, programming, controls and evaluation with proper feed-ins and feedbacks of information, resources, and results to subsidiary or final outputs or solutions. An example of this systems approach is shown in Fig. 14-1, which represents the elements of a research procedure and the ways they may be systematically interrelated.

PPBS (Planning-Programming-Budgeting Systems). PPBS is a procedure intended to make possible the better allocation of resources among alternate ways to attain a desired objective. "Its essence is the development and presentation of information as to the full implications, the costs and benefits, of the major alternative courses of action relevant to major resources allocation decisions. . . . Such problems as budget and implementation, manpower selection, the assessment of the work efficiency of operating units and cost control of current opera-

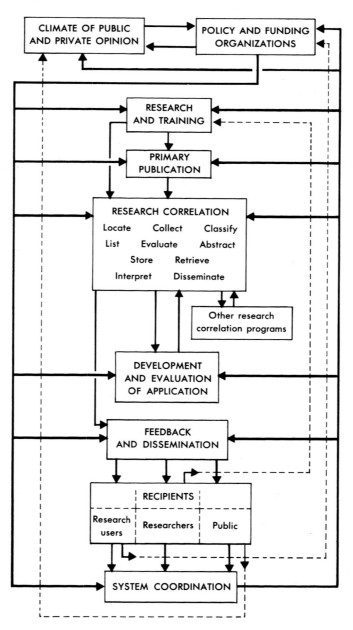

Fig. 14-1. Example of systems approach—the research context. Boxes represent activities; solid lines, flow of information, influence, or funds; dotted lines, feedback. (From Blumenthal, M.: Traffic accident prevention as a system component, Public Health Rep. **81:**569, June 1966.)

tions are generally considered to be outside the purview of PPBS. Cost accounting and non-fiscal performance reporting systems are very important in providing basic data required for PPBS analyses (as well as for fiscal accounting and management control purposes). However, such systems are usually considered complementary to PPBS rather than directly part of it. . . . The main contribution of PPBS lies in the planning process, i.e., the process of making program policy decisions that lead to a specific budget and specific multi-year plans."[10]

Operations research. Operations research originated from the efforts of scientists of many disciplines to solve military operations problems during World War II.[11] It is a term applied to "research into some or all aspects of conducting or operating a system, a business, or a service, while treating the system as a living organism in its proper environment . . ." According to Andersen,[12] its major phases are as follows:

1. Formulating the problem, including definition of the objectives.
2. Collection of data relevant to the problem.
3. Analysis of data to produce a hypothesis and a mathematical model to represent the system under study.
4. Deriving solutions from the model.
5. Choosing the optimal solution and forecasting results.
6. Testing the optimal combination of interventions, with controls built into the system to keep continuous check on the hypotheses.
7. Recommending implementation of the solution, including the control system.

Systems analysis. Systems analysis is primarily focussed upon the first phases or parts of PPBS or operations research procedure; i.e., ". . . the interpretation of broad objectives and guidelines, and the structuring of information in such a way that the decision maker can see and evaluate the options available to him. . . . The realistic goal of systems analysis is the improvement of the decision-making process, not the creation of a mechanism that automatically produces ideal decisions."[10] Hopefully the method provides the decision maker with more accurate or dependable information with reference to the cost and value of po-

tential programs. The process involves the following steps:

1. Definition of the problem
2. Projection of determinants of the problem
3. Generation of alternative approaches to solving the problem
4. Evolution of the cost-effectiveness of the alternatives
5. Interpretation of the qualitative results

PERT (Program Evaluation and Review Technique). PERT is adapted from the work-flow studies long used in industrial management. Proceeding on the basis that the relations within the planning process are dynamic, it provides a graphic detailed representation of the components of a program. "It is most useful when planning the implementation phase of a program. Essentially, it is a method of mapping future activities so that anyone can visualize the total plans of action for a program."[13] However, it is useful in planning only objective-oriented programs with specific measurable end results. The characteristics of the technique are as follows[14]:

1. A work breakdown structure, beginning with a final objective subdivided into a series of smaller subobjectives.
2. A network including all activities and events necessary to reach each subobjective. Activity is an effort required to move from one event to another. An activity may also indicate simply a connection or interrelationship between two events which does not require any effort. In the latter instance, estimated time for the activity would be zero. Specific and definable program accomplishments that do not require time or resources are events.
3. Identification of time estimates for various activities as well as the total process, including a critical path. The longest path, in terms of time, through the network from the beginning to the ending event is the critical path.
4. A method of network analysis that provides continuous evaluation of program status and identification of problem areas so that preventive action can be taken. The network is a diagram of activities and events necessary to reach a program objective. It shows sequences of accomplishment, interrelationships, and dependencies. Analysis of the network by the administrator at any stage of the program permits him to determine whether anticipated progress is being made and if not, specifically where the bottleneck is occurring.

APPROACHES TO PLANNING

With this general background, what types of problems and factors must be considered when we attempt to develop programs for the achievement of public health purposes and goals? Generally they appear to fall into three categories:

Plan—including programming, control, and evaluation

Money—including its acquisition, management, and accountability

People—including recruitment, training, organization, and management as well as relationships with other parts of the government and with the public in general

For our purposes it should be pointed out that, although planning appears to be only one of the three considerations, everything in each of the other two factors is in fact involved in program planning. In other words a plan is incomplete if it does not include consideration both of what resources exist and how best to use them and also of what methods of evaluating results it is hoped will be obtained. It might also be worth indicating that the plans of an organization, to the extent that they exist, are usually illustrated in a general sense by (1) the organization chart, (2) the staffing pattern, and (3) the budget.

In modern public health administration it is becoming evermore necessary to develop and use effective and objective approaches to program planning, establishment of program priorities, program control, and program evaluation. This is important in order to know (1) What are the goals and standards? (2) What should be done? (3) What is being done? (4) What does it cost? (5) Is it being done efficiently and effectively? (6) Is it worth doing?

Goals and standards

One of our most serious limitations in the past and one of the chief reasons why we have often found ourselves ineffective and in difficulty is that we often have not defined our goals and standards in sufficient detail, with adequate enough precision, and with consideration of all the community's interests or needs.

The determination of goals and standards depends upon a number of factors, each of whose relative significance varies through time. The initial approach is to find out what the government and the people that it represents had in mind as their purpose in establishing and continuing the health agency. This is important, regardless of the amount of agreement with that purpose. To ignore it may doom one's best intentions and efforts to failure. A more familiar approach to the determination of goals and standards is the collecting and analyzing of statistics, reports of births, illnesses, and deaths, or the conducting of special surveys and studies. Information from such sources, if properly obtained and logically analyzed, points to problems that suggest desirable goals to be attained or desirable standards to be established, achieved, and maintained. Obviously the problems indicated by such data should be studied in relative terms, i.e., in relation to other times, in relation to other places, and in relation to each other.

Priorities

The relation of possible goals to each other is of particular interest and concern to public health administration because it necessitates the development of some means of determining the relative importance of various health problems and hence various public health activities. In other words it involves the establishment of *priorities* in relation to goals. At any given moment or place there are many different public health problems, always many more than can be attacked adequately with available resources. Some problems obviously must take precedence over others. As previously indicated, it is unfortunately frequent that the decision is made on the basis of whim, on some personal interest of the public health administrator, or in deference to particular political or public pressure groups rather than as a result of careful study and analysis.

How may this important early step in program planning be approached? There are certain fundamental factors that should be considered in program priority determination. For example, a problem that affects a large number of people ordinarily should take precedence over one that affects relatively few, but not if the former is the common cold and the latter is endemic smallpox. A disease that kills or disables should take precedence over one that does not, but only if an effective method of scientific attack is at hand. There are many such factors that should be taken into consideration: existence of scientific knowledge and techniques, economics, cultural acceptability, availability of suitable personnel, and propriety and legality of the contemplated action, to mention only a few. In addition, as Nathan[15] has pointed out, one should consider pressures and interests of special and local groups, expressed views of the chief executive, editorials in the local newspapers, official policy expressed by the legislature, opportunism when funds are made available with regard to a particular problem, sudden advances in knowledge or techniques, and the need for research and demonstration. Further exploration, experimentation, and trial are needed in this field.

A somewhat detailed and complicated approach is one first developed as an administrative aid in connection with the International Technical Assistance Programs of the United States Government. It has subsequently been refined for provocative, experimental, and in-service training purposes.[16] It is presented here for the possible interest it may have. Actually the process of its development by the staff of an agency, rather than its end product, is perhaps its most valuable characteristic. The first step is for the key professional and management personnel to meet together and to list every conceivable type of activity and program that is being engaged in, might be instituted, or has ever been requested. The number of items may easily number in the hundreds. Following this listing down one axis, across the other axis is listed every conceivable factor that might be considered in judging whether or not a particular activity or program should or could be engaged in at the moment or in the near future. Then there is discussion of each possible activity or program in terms of these many factors, resulting in a rating of each from 0 to 4+. By this means it becomes possible to consider existing or potential activities or programs from a broad overall objective yet relative point of view. From the concensus that develops the results usually fall into three broad priority categories:

1. For activities or programs that are consistently rated 3+ or 4+ for every qualifying factor the conclusion is that under all circumstances these particular activities should be carried out.

2. Of secondary importance are certain activities or programs that ordinarily might not merit attention without special precise explanation and justification because of reservations with regard to one or several of the qualifying criteria.

3. In the third category are certain activities or programs that are not justified and should not or cannot be engaged in. It is recognized, however, that in unusual instances certain non-health considerations might result in a decision to engage in one of these activities.

Repeated trial of this procedure appears to indicate the existence of a dynamic formula consisting of four components as follows:

Component A = Size of problem $\left.\begin{array}{l}\end{array}\right\}$ Public
Component B = Seriousness of problem health
Component C = Effectiveness need
Component D = PEARL

The formula then appears as:

$$\text{Basic priority rating (BPR)} = \frac{(A + B)C}{3}$$

$$\text{Overall priority rating (OPR)} = \frac{(A + B)C}{3} \times D$$

The range of scores for each of the four components is decided upon as follows:

$$A = 0 \text{ to } 10$$
$$B = 0 \text{ to } 20$$
$$C = 0 \text{ to } 10$$
$$D = 0 \text{ or } 1$$

The maximum obtainable product of the four components (A,B,C, and D) is therefore 300. By an arbitrary division of this maximum product by 3, the maximum score becomes 100. Every computed rating will then be in the range 0 to 100.

It now becomes necessary to consider certain fundamental qualifying factors. These are shown as PEARL, the meaning of which is explained later.

As in the case of many evaluative procedures, a large so-called subjective element enters into this exercise. The choice and definition of the components in the formula and the relative weights assigned to them are based upon group concensus. Application of the formula in the rating of programs and activities involves the judgments of individual raters. However, some scientific control may be achieved by the use of a representative sample of qualified raters, a precise definition of terms, the delineating of exact rating procedures, the utilization of statistical data to guide ratings when feasible, and a statistical averaging of scores derived by raters working independently. However, some further detail on the components of the formula is necessary.

Component A—size of problem. For purposes of assignment of priorities, size of problem is defined as the *total number of persons having the problem or being directly affected by the problem expressed in rates per 100,000 population.* Qualifying within this population are those persons who may reasonably be expected to receive services if the services were available. Not qualifying within this population are those persons who have the problem or are directly affected by it but for whom public health services are inappropriate.

Since there are many problems that will be defined in terms of comparatively small demographic groups, it was arbitrarily decided that size of problem be scored according to the following scale:

Units per 100,000 population (component A)	Score
50,000 or more	10
5,000 to 49,999	8
500 to 4,999	6
50 to 499	4
5 to 49	2
0.5 to 4.9	0

Thus if a problem is defined in terms of the population of a large city, it is obvious that the following scale would result and apply:

Population in city (component A)	Score
1,000,000 or more	10
100,000 to 999,999	8
10,000 to 99,999	6
1,000 to 9,999	4
100 to 999	2
Less than 100	0

Component B—seriousness of problem. Seriousness of problem is defined in terms of four factors: urgency, severity, economic loss, and involvement of people. The component "seriousness" is assigned a range of 0 to 20 in the formula. Each factor of seriousness is assigned a range of 0 to 10. Thus it is possible to obtain the maximum score of 20 for seriousness even though only two factors contribute to it. However, if all four factors rate 10, the maximum for all four would still be limited to 20.

Factors comprising seriousness	Range of score
Urgency	0 to 10
Public concern	
Public health concern	
Severity	0 to 10
Mortality	
Morbidity—degree and duration	
Disability—degree and duration	
Economic loss	0 to 10
To individuals	
To community	
Involvement of people	0 to 10
Potential—number of persons who may acquire problem or be affected by existing problem, and relative degree of involvement	
Indirect—number of persons affected socially, economically, psychologically, etc., and relative degree of involvement	

Component C—effectiveness. Effectiveness is yet to be studied comprehensively. It involves the difficult field of evaluation, for which valid measuring devices are largely yet to be developed. It is felt that this component should be assigned two values:

C_1 for the program or activity as it is now being carried out

C_2 for the program or activity as carried out optimally

Component D—PEARL. PEARL consists of a group of factors not directly related to the actual need or effectiveness but which determine whether a particular program or activity can be carried out at a specific time.

> P = Propriety
> E = Economics
> A = Acceptability
> R = Resources
> L = Legality

Each of these qualifying factors is given a value of 0 *or* 1, and since together they represent a product rather than a sum, if any one of them is rated 0, it not only gives PEARL a total rating of 0 but also makes the OPR score 0. Therefore, although the BPR might be high, the proposed activity or program is impossible or impractical at the moment, and certain intermediate steps are indicated.

Program inventory and performance reporting

The question, What is being done? is not so simple as it sounds. It is essentially a matter of *program inventory*. Fundamental to a useful program inventory is an adequate *performance reporting system* in which the various activities engaged in are reported in terms of the nature of the work performed. An important distinction must be made here. Whereas the more usual type of reporting is focussed upon personnel function, activities carried out, or services rendered (e.g., number of inspections made, laboratory specimens examined, or homes visited by public health nurses), to be of true value, performance reporting should be focussed upon a program purpose such as food establishments supervised or individuals immunized (in other words results actually achieved). This has been emphasized by Flook[17] in the following statement.

> There is a fine distinction between the traditional activity counts—enumerations of nursing and clinic visits for various purposes or of sanitary inspections of different types of establishments—and the kind of statistics which focuses attention on numbers of persons served and types and amount of service received. With the traditional counts, quantitative evidence is being accumulated to describe how each public health worker spends his time—how much effort is being expended for each separate program. With the latter type of statistics, information is being collected on the results of that effort.
>
> Measurement of results then, is the key to what we want to achieve with service statistics. The term service yield indices is an apt phrase. Just as a farmer finds it necessary, if he is to know whether he is operating at a gain or loss, to reckon the number of bushels of wheat or bales of cotton he gets per acre in return for the labor and expense of production, so the public health worker must calculate the service being rendered to the community in relation to the need for service.

Nathan[15] has commented on this important point from a slightly different viewpoint:

> There is not enough known about methodology to make such a broad, sweeping statement. Perhaps a case in point may help to illustrate: Let us consider inspection of pasteurizing plants. We know that certain communicable diseases may be transmitted through milk. We know that proper pasteurization of milk will establish a barrier preventing the transmission of the organisms causing these communicable diseases. We therefore require the pasteurization of milk and establish a procedure of inspection of pasteurizing plants. To assure proper pasteurization we say that a certain number and type of inspections are necessary. Is our goal in this instance the prevention of communicable diseases, the carrying out of a certain number and type of inspections, or is it to make sure that the pasteurizing plants adhere to standards?

Performance budgeting

The development and availability of a program inventory based upon valid performance reporting makes possible an approach to the fourth and fifth questions: What does it cost? Is it being done efficiently and effectively? This is the realm of performance budgeting, which is discussed in Chapter 15. As stated there in its simplest terms it is nothing more than the application of benefit-cost accounting to a performance report. It summarizes the program activities performed in terms of unit cost, telling the total cost of achieving immunization of an individual or the cost of obtaining compliance with a food ordinance. With this available for all parts of a program a further step becomes possible, the determination of the cost of total program in relation to what it achieves. One then has a true program budget that measures the total impact of a program in terms of its cost.

With this, in relation to the first question listed (What are the goals and standards?), it is then possible to answer the sixth and final question, Is it worth doing? At this point we have reached the area of evaluation.

EVALUATION

The subject of evaluation and the many ways in which it may be and has been approached are large, complex, and dynamic. The approaches have been summarized in an especially worthy manner by Hilleboe[18] in his address at the Second Annual Award Lecture on Public Health at the Fifty-Ninth Annual New York City Health Conference on June 12, 1963. The subject has also been dealt with extensively in the Proceedings of the First and Second National Conferences on Evaluation in Public Health.[19] There are certain subjective and philosophic determinations necessary before one proceeds to the details or mechanics of evaluation. Thus what is to be evaluated—services, activities, results, or qualifications? If performance or services are to be measured against certain standards, as they must be in the final analysis, how firm, objective, valid, or applicable are the standards? Who develops them and on what basis? If an activity or program is to be evaluated, for what purpose, toward what end is it to be evaluated? Earlier there was brief discussion of the importance of measuring end products or end results rather than motions by employees. At the same time it was emphasized that, cruel though it may seem to some, programs designed to benefit certain individuals or groups may be much more valuable in the long run than certain others. Sanders[20] emphasizes this further by saying, "To answer the question of what constitutes adequate health care for a community, we must be able to identify the contribution which that care makes, and the extent to which a reallocation of resources is required to maximize productive man-years per life. This should be the acid test in appraising the efficacy of health services, and in determining whether a community is making optimum outlays for health care. The goal is difficult of attainment, but the stakes are enormous for our nation and for mankind."

The meaning of evaluation is of great importance in relation to any efforts to achieve it. The American Public Health Association has defined evaluation as it relates to health as "the process of determining the value or amount of success in achieving a predetermined objective. It includes at least the following steps: formulation of the objective, identification of the proper criteria to be used in measuring success, determination and explanation of the degree of success, recommendations for further activity."[21] Although each of these steps is of obvious importance, particular attention is directed to the last, the feedback aspect of evaluation, the recommendations to be derived from the evaluation process that may serve to alter or improve the program or activity that has been evaluated. James[22] states this well in saying that evaluation "differs from research primarily in that it does not seek new knowledge, but attempts to mark progress toward a prestated objective. While research can end with the presentation of results, evaluation is viewed as part of a circular process. Its findings are reincorporated into the specific program from which they came."

It is also important to distinguish between evaluation and the mere development of indices of health or of health practice and the surveys necessary to obtain them. Indices and surveys of this type can be of great value in a number of ways—problem identification, need definition, public relations, and statistical comparison[23,24]—but they must not be confused with true evaluation. Brief descriptive reference has been made earlier in this chapter to PERT. This systematic approach to problem solving or goal achievement illustrates very well the most desirable and useful approach to evaluation. Here evaluation is very deliberately built into the planning process not only at the beginning but as one of the major phases or purposes of the planning process. Then in order to justify having done this the products or results of evaluation, i.e., the evaluative output, is fed back into the dynamic system as it proceeds.

Another interesting way of evaluation of health services has been developed by Greenberg,[25] who also emphasizes that evaluation is not an assessment of need or community diagnosis but a follow-up procedure to ascertain effectiveness or goal fulfillment among the recipients of service in a program. After considering the components of program input, e.g., organization, personnel, funds, data, etc., he visualizes evaluative output as follows:*

Immediate goals

Increase in knowledge; improved attitudes and practices

Reduced *d*isinterest; reduced *d*issatisfaction

Intermediate goals

More positive health; improved status

Reduced *d*iscomfort and *d*eprivation; reduced *d*isease

Long-range goals

Reduction in morbidity and mortality

Reduced *d*isability; reduced *d*eath

Other types of output may take the form of accompanying favorable effects in the community other than among recipients of service or of untoward side effects. Overall efficiency may then be expressed as

Output (in terms of goal fulfillment)
———————————————————————
Input (in terms of dollars, services, and/or personnel time)

Evaluation aids. The *Evaluation Schedule For Use in the Study and Appraisal of Community Health Programs,*[26] developed over many years by the American Public Health Association, deserves particular mention since it has provided an admirable, stimulating, and convenient tool for administrative control and coordination as well as for appraisal. Referring to this

*From Greenberg, B. G.: Personal communication from lecture material, University of North Carolina, 1967.

study, Pfiffner[27] makes the following statement:

Probably no administrative field has gone further than public health in developing criteria to judge the effectiveness of its work. Since public health administration in its present form is so young, this fact becomes especially significant. The standards and measurement referred to are the results of experiences growing out of a number of public health surveys covering a period of years. . . . The criteria are so objective that little is left to the opinion of the appraiser. . . . Indeed, it has been shown quite conclusively that there is a very direct relation between the amount that is spent for public health administration, score achieved, and the health of the community as shown by the mortality and morbidity rates.

Rating was based upon performance rather than results. In other words the schedule took cognizance of the administrative organization and facilities of the health administration rather than sickness and death statistics. It considered in separate detail the following 16 phases of the public health program:

1. Personnel, facilities, and services
2. Public health problems
3. Community health education and staff training
4. Communicable disease control
5. Tuberculosis control
6. Venereal disease control
7. Maternal health
8. Infant and preschool health
9. School health
10. Adult health
11. Accident prevention
12. Water supplies and excreta disposal
13. Food control
14. Milk control
15. Housing
16. Financial support for local health work

For a period the American Public Health Association also published a document entitled *Health Practice Indices,* which consisted of an extensive series of line charts relating to the particularly significant items in the *Evaluation Schedule.* Each chart presented the reported experience of several hundred investigators. It had value in allowing a health officer to insert the position of his community in each chart. Concurrently the Association published a summary scoring sheet that made it possible to obtain an overall view of the strengths, weaknesses, balance, and coordination of the program of a public health agency. Certain items were graphically emphasized, being considered of such great importance that a poor score for them outweighed any benefits that might result from other activities. Thus an approved water supply, a satisfactory sewage disposal system, and pasteurization of milk were considered fundamental to the health of a community regardless of whatever other accomplishments were achieved.

More recently the Association has developed *Guide to a Community Health Study*[28] for use by community organizations and agencies in studying and improving all aspects of their community's health structure and program, both official and nonofficial. Every public health worker should become thoroughly familiar with this valuable document.

The use of administrative control tools such as these is of great importance in measuring success and progress toward the goals and objectives that should always consciously exist. Generally speaking, once the administrator determines the needs, goals, obstacles, facilities, and abilities, failure to reach the goals can be due only to poor administration and inattention to duty.

This brief and general discussion of program planning and evaluation can have no better closing than a comment by the late James A. Crabtree[29] while Dean of the Graduate School of Public Health of the University of Pittsburgh:

Perhaps todays greatest challenge to public health administration is to advance and accelerate the pace of research aimed at the establishment and validation of a body of administrative theory applicable to its broader dimensioned problems and issues. To take the attitude . . . that administration is only an art and will never become a science is to say that every outcome of any administrative action is altogether unique, and therefore there can be no transferable knowledge or understanding of either the administrative process or the phenomena involved therein.

That administration can become a science rests on the assumption that regularities can be detected and identified in the phenomena involved in the administrative process and that there must be an orderly arrangement of the elements of the process itself. The administrative process basically is a systems process. . . . There is encouraging evidence today that public health is becoming alert to these possibilities.

REFERENCES

1. Gorham, W.: PPBS, its scope and limits, The Public Interest 8:4, Summer 1967.
2. Hilleboe, H., and Schaefer, M.: Papers and bibliography on community health planning, Albany, 1967, Williams Press.
3. Editorial: Planning for healthful communities, Amer. J. Public Health 56:1987, Dec. 1966.
4. National Commission on Community Health Services: Health is a community affair, Cambridge, 1966, Harvard University Press.
5. Guidelines for organizing state and area-wide community health planning, Amer. J. Public Health 56:2139, Dec. 1966.
6. Hanlon, J. J.: Can accounting sell health? In Economic benefits from public health services, Washington, 1964, Public Health Service Pub. No. 1178.
7. Seipp, C.: Health planning and economic development. Address given at the John Grant Memorial Session, Ninety-First Annual Meeting, American Public Health Association, Kansas City, Nov. 13, 1963.
8. Planning of public health services, WHO Techn. Rep. Ser. No. 215, 1961.
9. Anderman, R. C.: Bibliography on program planning, budgeting and evaluation in public health, Philadelphia, 1967, Fels Institute of Local and State Government (mimeographed).
10. Hatry, H. P. and Cotton, J. F.: Program planning for state, county and city, Washington, 1967, George Washington University Press.
11. Flagle, C. D.: Operational research in the health services, Ann. N. Y. Acad. Sci. 107:748, May 22, 1963.
12. Andersen, S.: Operations research in public health, Public Health Rep. 79:297, Apr. 1964.
13. Arnold, M. F., et al.: Health program implementation through PERT, San Francisco, 1966, Western Regional Office, American Public Health Association.
14. Merten, W.: PERT and planning for health programs, Public Health Rep. 81:449, May 1966.
15. Nathan, M. R.: Some steps in the process of program planning, Amer. J. Public Health 46:68, Jan. 1956.
16. Hanlon, J. J.: The design of public health programs for underdeveloped countries, Public Health Rep. 69:1028, Nov. 1954.
17. Flook, E.: The value of good service statistics in a modern health department, Public Health Rep. 68:811, Aug. 1953.
18. Hilleboe, H.: Improving performance in public health. Second Annual Award Lecture on Public Health presented at the Fifty-Ninth Annual New York City Health Conference, June 12, 1963 (mimeographed).
19. Proceedings of the First and Second National Conferences on Evaluation in Public Health, Ann Arbor, 1955 and 1960, University Publications Distribution Service (mimeographed).

20. Sanders, B. S.: Measuring community health levels, Amer. J. Public Health **54**:1063, July 1964.
21. Glossary of administrative terms in public health, Amer. J. Public Health **50**:225, Feb. 1960.
22. James, G.: Evaluation in public health practice, Amer. J. Public Health **52**:1145, July 1962.
23. Conceptual problems in developing an index of health, Washington, 1966, Public Health Service Pub. No. 17, Series 2.
24. Measurement of levels of health, WHO Techn. Rep. Ser. No. 137, 1957.
25. Greenberg, B. G.: Personal communication from lecture material, University of North Carolina, 1967.
26. American Public Health Association: Evaluation schedule for use in the study and appraisal of community health programs, (reprinted) New York, 1937, The Association.
27. Pfiffner, J. McD.: Public administration, New York, 1946, The Ronald Press Co.
28. American Public Health Association: Guide to a community health study, New York, 1961, The Association.
29. Crabtree, J. A.: Plans for tomorrow's needs in local public health administration, Amer. J. Public Health **53**:1175, Aug. 1963.

Chapter 15

Fiscal management

INTRODUCTION

Since public health activities are usually performed by governmental agencies, it necessarily follows that public revenues must furnish the most stable and largest part of the funds supporting them. This being the case, it is important that public health personnel and especially the administrators of official public health agencies constantly bear in mind that the handling and administration of these funds represent a public trust. It is obviously impossible to separate public health administration and public finance. Every act performed for the promotion of public health involves an expenditure of money, whether for supplies, transportation, or salaries of personnel. In fact the very nature and extensiveness of the public health program is determined in the final analysis by the amount of the funds available for its conduct. Accordingly, an understanding of the sound management of the public financial program forms one of the most important responsibilities in public health administration.

It is surprising to realize that until 1910 no executive budget existed on any level of government in the United States. Until that time operating bureaus and departments approached appropriating bodies individually and directly requested and received for the most part "omnibus" appropriations for support of their respective activities. The following item from the budget of the city of Chicago for 1909 may serve as an example of this highly undesirable procedure and make evident the opportunities for inefficient if not dishonest public administration under these circumstances.

For repairs and renewals of wagon and harness, replacement and keep of livestock, identification, police telegraph expenses, repairs and renewals of equipment, hospital services, printing and stationery, secret service, light and heat, 25 more horses for mounted police, and for repair of Hyde Park station; also other miscellaneous expenses . . . $205,000.

Since about 1910 the trend on all levels of government has been toward centralization of the responsibility for public financial management. In the larger units of government, i.e., federal, state, and large cities, separate fiscal departments have usually been established to meet the need. Thus there now exist the federal Bureau of Budget, many state departments of finance, and municipal comptroller offices. Within the large operating departments one frequently finds a central accounting office organized as a separate bureau or division, directed by a person specially trained and directly responsible to the executive head of the department. The trend in fact has been to go even further and attempt the coordination of the accounting functions with those of revenue administration, budgeting, purchasing, and in some instances even treasury management. White[1] accounts for this trend in terms of "loss of confidence in legislative bodies as agencies for fiscal management; realization of the desirability for fixing responsibility for the management of fiscal affairs; rapidly rising governmental expenditures and debts which emphasized the necessity for fiscal reform; and the studies of research bureaus, which made apparent the waste due to disorganized fiscal management and which offered promising, reasonable alternatives."

This trend toward centralizing fiscal activities in no way removes the need for interest and responsibility on the part of public health officers in these matters since of necessity part of the responsibility for fiscal matters must rest with the operating department as well as with extradepartmental budget officers, comptrollers, finance directors, and others. There is involved here a series of relationships that constitute one of the most important aspects of public health administration. In general the functions are divided in somewhat the following manner. The health administrator is responsible for estimating the needs of his organization, which the budget office has the right to review and modify. Expenditures are initiated by the health department but they may require approval by the central comptroller. The health department is responsible for the preparation of reports indicating and justifying expenditures to provide accountants and auditors from central fiscal offices with information necessary for their analyses. Within the functional health department responsibility for financial matters rests nominally with the administrative health officer. Usually he is the one authorized to incur expenditures, as indicated by his signature on payrolls, requisitions, and other financial documents. In large organizations this authority is sometimes delegated to division or bureau heads. The tendency has been to establish a fiscal officer under the health officer to assume immediate concern for the financial aspects of the operation of the department as a whole.

FISCAL POLICY MAKING

Before either the health officer or the various fiscal officers may function it is necessary that legal policies be established governing the operation of financial matters. Traditionally this responsibility for determining fiscal policies and objectives has rested with the legislative branch of government, which must provide the legal framework for the creation of a sound financial structure to implement the public health and other objectives that the legislature as representatives of the people outlines. Therefore, it is the legislative branch that must decide upon the general nature and extent of the public health services to be provided, appropriate whatever funds are necessary to meet their cost, and put into effect whatever revenue measures are necessary for financing the appropriations made. It must fix the authority and responsibility for the collection and expenditure of these revenues, establish the operating units, organize the machinery through which the operating units are financed, and account to the public for the revenue measures enacted, the expenditures incurred, and the services rendered. The progressive health administrator might well assume an honest responsibility for providing inasmuch as possible information and advice for the guidance of the legislators in the performance of these functions.

FINANCIAL OPERATIONS

Financial operations, the second phase of the public financial program, is concerned with implementation of the policies and plans of operation that have been outlined by the legislature. It includes revenue administration, treasury management, budgeting, accounting, and purchasing. The first two of these are seldom of direct concern to the health officer and are mentioned here merely in order that the public health worker will be acquainted with their general content. Revenue administration is concerned with the assessment, levying, and collection of taxes; the study of proposed tax measures; advice to the legislature, the executive head of the unit of government, and the budget officer on problems relating thereto; the preparation of revenue estimates and proposed revenue measures for the executive; and the maintenance of records and accounts of all revenue assessed, levied, adjusted, collected, and deposited with the treasury. Treasury management is concerned with the custody and disbursement of public money and the custody of whatever securities are held in trust by the governmental unit. The treasury accepts money and gives receipts, assures that a cash reserve is constantly maintained, and disburses money on the presentation of legally authorized warrants or disbursement orders.

Budgeting

Of direct concern to the health officer is the problem of budgeting. Since he is responsible for the public funds provided to him for the operation of his department, it is only reasonable and logical that he conduct some system of financial bookkeeping that will give a continuous, accurate, and verifiable account of his stewardship. A departmental budget provides such a system.

The question might be raised concerning the fact that frequently many of the funds that are made available, especially to local departments of health, come from sources outside the local governmental unit, some even from private sources. Among these are the increasing number of grants-in-aid from the state and federal governments, private foundations, and various voluntary health agencies. For administrative purposes all monies, regardless of their source, should appear in the budget and be placed in the custody of the state or local treasurer. This of course does not preclude their being credited to a health department account or fund in order to assure their being used only for the purposes for which they were granted.

A fund may be established by the legislative body of the government, by a contractual agreement, or by an executive order, and may be abolished only by the agency establishing it. The number of separate funds should be kept at a minimum since a multiplicity of them effectively hampers the development of broad, well-balanced programs. In general, funds may be considered in the following categories:

Expendable funds
General fund—this usually contains most of the available funds. It represents the unrestricted fund of the organization as far as budgeting and expenditure are concerned. It can be spent for any legal purpose for which the organization may wish to use it and may be drawn upon for the replenishment of other funds.

Special funds—these are restricted as to use since they are established for specific purposes. They cannot be transferred to other funds. Some originate by means of the government levying a special millage tax to pay for a particular function. This forms a kind of special appropriation and is usually not considered in the budget, thereby confusing budget planning. Special levies as a whole are undesirable. Much more preferable is a general levy adequate to cover all the needs of a government with the exception of sinking funds, the proceeds of which, however, should go into the general fund.

Sinking funds—these are a form of special expendable funds set aside for the redemption of bonds or other similar obligations. They are nontransferable.
Working capital funds
The purpose of these is for conducting the many organizational and institutional activities. They are usually replenished by means of transfers from other funds.
Endowment funds
The principal of these funds cannot be expended but the income accruing their investment may be spent for the purposes specified in the conditions of endowment.
Suspense funds
These are not funds in the true sense of the word. They consist of sums of money made available for special purposes, their distribution and use pending transferal to other funds.

The average person interprets the word budget as meaning a complicated scheme devised for the purpose of saving money, a scheme he wishes he had followed when the income tax form arrives. In one sense this interpretation is correct; in another it is not. Although it is true that a budget may help in saving and planning for future needs, that is not its primary purpose. To the contrary, in public service a budget is most concerned with the manner and rate at which available resources are to be expended. In brief, therefore, a budget may be defined as an administrative tool for the purpose of (1) estimating future needs and future resources and (2) the wise apportionment and systematic expenditure of the resources that are available during a given period of time.

The public health administrator should realize that the construction of a budget not only fulfills the demands of the agencies providing the funds but also may hold many advantages and uses for him in his management of the health department. It has a marked influence on the economical use of working resources since it is intended to make possible the maximum use of the facilities and current assets of the organization. It prevents waste and conserves resources by regulating expenditures for definite purposes and in accordance with appropriations established by the administrative head of the organization. A well-constructed budget places definitely, exactly where it belongs, the responsibility for each function of the organization. It makes for coordination by causing all individuals and departments of an organization to cooperate in attaining the goals fixed by the budget. A budget presents in cold figures the best judgment of the executive responsible for a definite organizational objective and thus guards against both undue pessimism, which leads to underactivity and poor work, or undue optimism, which leads to overexpansion. By indicating variance between estimates and actual results obtained it may serve as a danger signal for the administrator and thereby show when to proceed cautiously as well as when expansion may be safely undertaken. Similarly it is valuable in determining the relative effectiveness and cost of activities and procedures since it tests the ability of the organization to make things happen in accordance with a well-ordered plan. A very important benefit is that it compels the organization to study its market (the people) and its own methods and services, thus disclosing ways and means for strengthening and enlarging the organization. It provides the only means for predetermining when and to what extent financing will be necessary and serves as a guide to future needs, possibilities, and sources of revenue. Finally, organizations that develop and follow a well-ordered budget plan find greater favor from their administrative superiors or boards of directors, business associates, and potential sources of income.

Once the decision is made to use the budget idea, certain principles should be followed in order to assure its success and helpfulness. Perhaps most important, and so often overlooked, is confidence in the idea and willingness to cooperate with it. Nothing will ensure its failure more effectively than skepticism of its value, apprehension of the work involved, and a feeling that it is simply a red-tape requirement to which adherence after completion is not necessary. Related to this is the importance of enlisting the interest, aid, and cooperation of all subordinates in the preparation of and adherence to the estimates relating to their work. Estimates should be based on past performances and existing assets as well as upon plans for expansion and anticipated assets. The amount of estimates should be based upon the total probable assets available rather than upon that which is desired or ideal. All sources of income as well as all anticipated expenditures should be included in the budget, which should indicate clearly where the funds come from since this in itself has an educational value and paints the total financial picture. To indicate all sources of funds may also serve to cause awareness to future budgetary problems. This is always an important consideration in any future program planning. It follows that the interval over which a budget is to be effective should be restricted to a period for which dependable estimates of sources and expenditures may be prepared.

The mechanical procedures involved in setting up the budget should be kept as simple yet as useful as possible; this necessitates the attainment of a practical balance between the two. The items might best be classified primarily by units of organization, e.g., division of preventive medical services, division of environmental sanitation, bureau of vital statistics, etc. Such a classification requires a sound organization with well-defined lines of authority and responsibility. Beyond this, provision should be made for reasonable flexibility within the budget with a not too detailed breakdown of items. With regard to the relative advantages and disadvantages of a lump-sum budget as against a more detailed budget, it may be pointed out that, while the former provides more administrative leeway, the latter makes possible more effective control and planning and has an educational value entirely lacking in a lump-sum type of budget. For further breakdown, analysis by function or type of service is one of the most convenient and useful methods. This is particularly true in public health agencies since the units of organization (bureaus, divisions, etc.) are essentially functional, e.g., vital statistics, sanitation, health education, communicable disease control, etc.

Expenditures may be broken down to administrative advantage in terms, for example, of (1) operating expenses, i.e., salaries, travel, supplies, repairs, etc.; (2) capital costs;

GENERAL FUND— Health—General

Items numbered are the appropriations.
Items following in detail are explanatory of the appropriations—see city charter title VI, chap. 1, sec. 7.

	Account code		Items	Expended 1966-67	Budget allowance 1966-67		Adjusted allowance Dec. 31, 1966		Expended July 1, 1966 to Dec. 31, 1966	Requested 1967-68		Revision by the Mayor		Revision by the Council	
	Function	Object			No.	Amount	No.	Amount		No.	Amount	No.	Amount	No.	Amount
1	3010		ADMINISTRATION:												
2		111	Salaries	66,439.72	19	73,835.00	19	74,287.00	32,707.25	19	74,182.00				
3		301	Duplicating and Office Supplies	3,475.74		4,000.00		4,000.00	1,436.39		4,000.00				
4		302	Postage	10,000.00		9,000.00		9,000.00	4,200.00		10,000.00				
5		303	Reimbursement, Purchase, and Repairs of Badges	67.25		300.00		300.00	52.50		250.00				
6		405	Telephone and Telegraph Services	6,925.60		7,300.00		7,300.00	3,546.56		7,200.00				
7		414	Rental of Buildings and Space	23,500.00		23,500.00		23,500.00	11,750.00		25,000.00				
8															
9				110,408.31		117,935.00		118,387.00	53,692.70		120,632.00				
10	3020		Health education												
11		111	Salaries	24,416.59	15	43,861.00	15	44,163.00	12,631.96	15	44,724.00				
12		301	Purchases and Rental: Educational Films, Publications, and												
13			Displays	138.00		600.00		600.00	53.20		600.00				
14															
15				24,554.59		44,461.00		44,763.00	12,685.16		45,324.00				
16	3030		Vital statistics:												
17		111	Salaries	33,896.72	15	38,013.00	15	38,887.00	18,174.59	15	39,032.00				
18		113	Salaries—Issuing Birth Certificates	11,161.64		19,550.00		19,734.00	4,535.66		15,000.00				
19		301	Supplies	1,759.00		1,770.00		1,770.00	627.83		1,770.00				
20															
21				46,817.36		59,333.00		60,391.00	23,338.08		55,802.00				
22	3041		Sanitary engineering:												
23		111	Salaries	94,617.99	31	106,420.00	31	106,940.00	48,568.74	31	107,210.00				
24	3042		Sub-standard housing inspection:												
25		111	Salaries	39,509.83	18	53,605.00	18	53,927.00	19,563.22	18	54,397.00				
26		301	Supplies	90.79		200.00		200.00	17.27		200.00				
27															
28				39,600.62		53,805.00		54,127.00	19,580.49		54,597.00				
29	3043		Food inspection:												
30		111	Salaries	289,923.92	97	325,294.00	97	325,900.00	147,882.28	97	321,102.00				

Fig. 15-1. Example of budget form for a city health department, presenting data based on unit of organization and purpose.

GENERAL FUND—HEALTH—GENERAL

#	Function	Object	Items numbered are the appropriations. Items following in detail are explanatory of the appropriations—see city charter title VI, chap. I, sec. 7.	Budget allowance 1966-67 No.	Rates	Adjusted allowance Dec. 31, 1966 No.	Rates	Request for 1967-68 No.	Rates	Revision by the Mayor No.	Rates	Revision by the Council No.	Rates
1			Public Health Nurses	4	6,595 to 6,967			4	6,595 to 6,967				
2													
3				15		15		15					
4	3030	111	**Vital statistics:**										
5			Deputy Registrar of Vital Statistics	1	7,651 to 8,285			1	7,651 to 8,285				
6			Junior Statistician	1	6,657 to 7,095			1	6,657 to 7,095				
7			Technical Aid (General)	1	5,327 to 5,459			1	5,327 to 5,459				
8			Senior Clerk	1	6,525 to 6,936			1	6,525 to 6,936				
9			Intermediate Clerks	9	5,261 to 5,393			9	5,261 to 5,393				
10			Intermediate Typist	1	5,261 to 5,393			1	5,261 to 5,393				
11			Junior Stenographer	1	5,327 to 5,459			1	5,327 to 5,459				
12													
13				15		15		15					
14	3041	111	**Sanitary engineering:**										
15			Sanitary Engineer and Secretary	1	10,613 to 11,441			1	10,613 to 11,441				
16			Associate Sanitary Engineers	2	8,761 to 9,476			2	8,761 to 9,476				
17			Head Health Inspector	1	8,047 to 8,761			1	8,047 to 8,761				
18			Senior Assistant Sanitary Engineer		8,047 to 8,523	1	8,047 to 8,523	1	8,047 to 8,523				
19			Principal Health Inspectors	7	7,492 to 7,809	6	7,492 to 7,809	6	7,492 to 7,809				
20			Senior Health Inspectors	10	6,859 to 7,174			10	6,859 to 7,174				
21			Junior Health Inspectors	2	6,459 to 6,723			2	6,459 to 6,723				
22			Senior Sanitary Engineering Aid	1	7,095 to 7,571			1	7,095 to 7,571				
23			Junior Cartographic Draftsman	1	5,723 to 6,174			1	5,723 to 6,174				
24			Intermediate Clerks	4	5,261 to 5,393			4	5,261 to 5,393				
25			Junior Stenographer	1	5,327 to 5,459			1	5,327 to 5,459				
26			Junior Typist	1	4,752 to 4,980			1	4,752 to 4,980				
27													
28				31		31		31					

Fig. 15-2. Example of budget form for a city health department, presenting data based on unit of organization and function.

and (3) fixed charges, e.g., interest on bonds, etc. Figs. 15-1 and 15-2, which show portions of the budget of a large city health department, illustrate this.

In most instances it is desirable to include a contingent fund which, however, should be kept small (3 to 5%), a large contingent fund being indicative of poor planning and mangement. It should be used as sparingly as possible and should be applicable to all items in the budget with one exception, i.e., salaries should never, for any reason, be augmented from a contingent fund. A final requisite, and perhaps one of the most important, to a successful budget is placing the responsibility for its maintenance in the hands of one capable individual. Since a budget is essentially an estimate of future needs and activities, its construction should take into consideration the cost of operation on the present scale, including administrative, functional, and depreciative costs, the anticipated cost of operation of expanded activities, and the need for coordination of the existing and anticipated activities into one well-balanced whole so that the expenditures of money, time, and effort for the various activities will be in a proper and balanced relationship to one another.

Concerning the detailed steps involved in drafting the budget, no single method or technique exists that will satisfactorily fit all situations. It is strongly suggested that the newly appointed public health official assume as one of his earliest duties the acquiring of an intimate acquaintance not only with his own budget but also with the total budget of the governmental unit with which he is identified and the budgetary methods and forms being used. However, since the budgets of all governmental agencies have the same general purpose, certain similarities exist in their form. Geiger[2] summarized these well-accepted basic principles as including the following eight factors:

1. Expenditures of a preceding period equal in time to that for which the budget is being prepared. The period should be closed, so that actual expenditures as they occurred are stated in this column.
2. Budget of the present period. These figures can include only the budget as it was set up, since expenses thereon are still being incurred while a budget for the future is being prepared.
3. Changes in the present budget period. These figures should include any significant changes in the present budget that have occurred or that may be anticipated, such as changes in salaries or in departmental organization, which will have the effect of modifying the present budget. This column thus has the effect of bringing the present budget up-to-date.
4. Expenditures of the present period, given as actual expenditures to the time the next budget is being made, and as estimates of the expenditures to the end of the present period. The actual expenditures and estimates are totaled.
5. Object of expenditure. This column designates each item for which expenditures have been made or are requested. This should include the salary group, classed as permanent, as temporary, or as services secured on a contract basis. Other groups will include materials and supplies, fixed charges, foodstuffs, equipment, and any other divisions of expenditures.

   The remaining columns refer to estimates and requests for future activities, for which the preceding columns have provided a basis.
6. Budget request for the next period. Each item should be arranged in such a manner that comparison with the present budget will be as simple as possible.
7. Comparison between the present and anticipated budgets. Since comparison of present and requested budgets (items 2 and 6) is crucial in the consideration of new budgets, this column should indicate all items for which an increased expenditure is desired, items which are not changed from the present budget, and items which are dropped or in which a decrease in allotment of funds is desired.
8. The adopted budget. At least one column will be necessary for the budget adopted. As many additional columns should be provided as may be demanded in accordance with the number of official approvals required. This greatly facilitates the recording of recommendations by different officials empowered to approve one or all phases of the budget previous to its final adoption.

The preferred steps that lead toward the development of a final budget for a public agency are usually as follows. The date on which the department must submit its budget request to the bureau of the budget or budget officer is usually fixed by custom in relation to the fiscal year. With this date as an anchor point, about 2 months prior to this time the department director should send out to the director of each division or other unit of organization in the department a memorandum concerned with the approaching budget exercise. It should include a calendar of events or deadlines that indicates what steps are to be completed as of certain dates. It should also direct each division director to develop the budget request for his division preferably in consultation with his chief program aides. Any general statements or special policies relating to the budget year under consideration should be included in the memorandum. All divisional budget requests should be submitted to the departmental director (or his departmental budget officer) by a specified date. The department director, preferably in company with his budget director and any other pertinent staff members, should then carefully review each divisional budget proposal, annotating items to be deleted, altered, or added. The departmental director should then schedule a series of departmental budget hearings to provide each divisional (or program) director an opportunity to explain or defend the proposals he has put forward. On the basis of these hearings the departmental director should then refine the budget further, add his own ideas and provisions for the needs of his office, and submit the final departmental budget proposal to the director of the bureau of the budget or the budget officer of the jurisdiction. This officer in turn should schedule a hearing at which the departmental director may defend or explain his budget. He should be allowed to be accompanied by whichever divisional or program directors and administrative staff he wishes. On the basis of this hearing the budget officer will readjust the departmental budget request and submit it to the chief of government (e.g., the mayor or governor) and the comptroller. They in turn review the proposed departmental budget as readjusted by the budget officer. The departmental director is again scheduled for a budget review session, this time with the chief of government and his comptroller, who subsequently accept the proposed budget or revise it according to

their views. It is then sent to the legislative branch of government (the city council or the state legislature), where still again the departmental director has an opportunity to defend it or to express his needs in relation to whatever might have been eliminated by the budget officer or the chief of government and his comptroller. The legislature then takes it under advisement in relation to the budget requests of all parts of the government, fiscal resources, and their own interests. The result is the final approved budget.

Increasingly another step is being added to the process. It takes the form of an interim or preliminary budget hearing much earlier in the year at which department heads have an opportunity to discuss their existing and anticipated needs with the budget officer and sometimes with other officials. This has the advantage of giving everyone a preview of what in general to expect during the actual subsequent budget exercise.

In counties without a chief executive or comptroller the procedure varies. Preferably it involves hearings before the county budget officer, the county board of auditors, and the county ways and means or finance committee. The latter might be regarded as the counterpart of the legislature or city council, and the board of auditors the counterpart of the chief of government and his comptroller.

In the construction as well as in the operation of his budget the health officer should make it a practice to maintain contact with the budget director and the finance or ways and means committee of his government. He should keep them constantly informed and call upon them for advice, causing them to realize that the financial problems are theirs as well as his. This may present a delicate problem in personal relationships but usually results in benefits that are well worth the effort.

There may be a tendency for some health officers to take the attitude that it is necessary to work on the budget only as budget time approaches. To so restrict one's use of this valuable administrative tool eliminates most of the possible benefits that might be forthcoming from its existence. The wise administrator works closely and constantly with his budget the year round and on a long-term basis, using it as one method of continuously feeling the pulse of his organization. Trial balances should be run as often as is indicated. He should regard the budget as inviolate and as one of his most important administrative tools. He should adhere to its contents as strictly as possible, deviating from it only as a means of last resort. A certain amount of transferring of funds is inevitable but should be kept to a minimum since it is a sign of poor management and again defeats the purpose for which the budget was originally brought into existence.

If an emergency or other situation that requires an unexpected and unpredictable expenditure of funds should arise, the health officer should feel free to appeal to the appropriating body for an emergency appropriation rather than attempt to meet the situation by transference of monies that have been set aside for other predictable expenditures. It is believed that in most situations, if an honest and understandable explanation of the need is given, an additional allotment will be forthcoming. In this connection it might be well to point out here that a good administrator will not attempt to use emergency situations as leverage to increase his general budget or to make up deficiences arising out of poor management.

In the process of obtaining the appropriations requested in his budget the health officer should not assume the entire burden himself but should share it with others in the community such as his health council and other groups of interested and influential citizens. By convincing them of the need for the services for which the money is requested, the health officer may increase the forcefulness of his requests and arguments manyfold with greater assurance of the appropriation being granted.

The efficient health officer will be constantly alert to discover new ways in which to use the budget. He may use it to demonstrate the public health activity in his own area or to show what is being done else-where in comparable situations. The use to which the taxpayer's dollar is being put is always of public interest and can be used for very effective publicity and educational purposes. A budget may be used as the starting point for requests for state and federal grants-in-aid for the health program and also furnishes a fundamental source of information for self-evaluation and appraisal. It may furnish the key to the determination of the efficiency of various public health procedures and show the way to the achievement of better results per dollar of tax money spent.

It has been pointed out that the budget should be based not on a series of guesses but rather upon estimates arrived at inasmuch as possible from the past experience of the organization. It is obvious therefore that to be satisfactory the budget should result from a careful analysis of accounting data, including actual previous experiences and current cost and price trends. Most states provide for the installation and maintenance of a system of uniform accounting by local governments and often provide further for periodic audits by a central state fiscal authority. However, legal provision does not necessarily imply action, and effective enforcement of these provisions appears to be the exception rather than the rule. The lack of an efficient system of accounting makes sound budgetary methods impossible and often results in expenditures that comply with only the barest minimum requirements that may be specified in the law.

Accounting

A sound system of accounting serves many purposes. It provides a financial record of the activities of an agency, reveals its financial condition at all times, provides very necessary data upon which the departmental administrator may base plans for future action, gives substantive protection in case of question, and provides the fundamental starting point for audits. White[1] states this as follows:

From the point of view of the department head or the chief executive early and accurate accounting reports are necessary in order to direct the course of the work and future expenditures. They also provide the essential record to demonstrate the appropriate and legal use of funds, making certain that each subdivision of an organization is actually using money for the purposes for which it was appropriated. The accounts and supporting financial documents provide the evidence on the basis of which each spending officer justifies his expenditures, either to the finance director or to the auditor. While the accounting system is thus essential as a means of preventing the wrongful uses of funds, it also underlies all other types of executive control of fiscal operations. It is the basis on which executives act to prevent deficits as well as the documentary foundation for questioning the care and wisdom with which the funds have been used.

Health departments should maintain at least the following basic accounting records: (1) general ledger and (2) complete and detailed record of receipts and expenditures. The general ledger, illustrated by Fig. 15-3, is the record of the various accounts or controls pertaining to assets, liabilities, and types of revenues and expenses of the health department. Posting to these

accounts or controls are made from the books of original entry, namely the cash receipts and expenditure record (see Fig. 15-4) and the book of transfer vouchers (Fig. 15-5). All departmental receipts and warrants, including their amounts, should be recorded in the combination cash receipts and expenditure record in their respective numerical order and classified as to source and type of expenditure. Receipts should be posted in the treasurer account-deposits column and classified under the miscellaneous accounts-credit column (see Fig. 15-4). Similarly the amount of each warrant should be recorded in the column entitled treasurer account-amount of warrants and classified in further columns according to the monies used and type of expenditure. The code number of the general ledger control account should be used to designate proper postings to the general ledger. Great care should be given to using

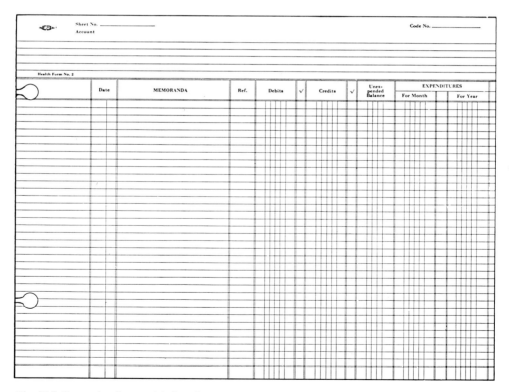

Fig. 15-3. Example of general ledger form.

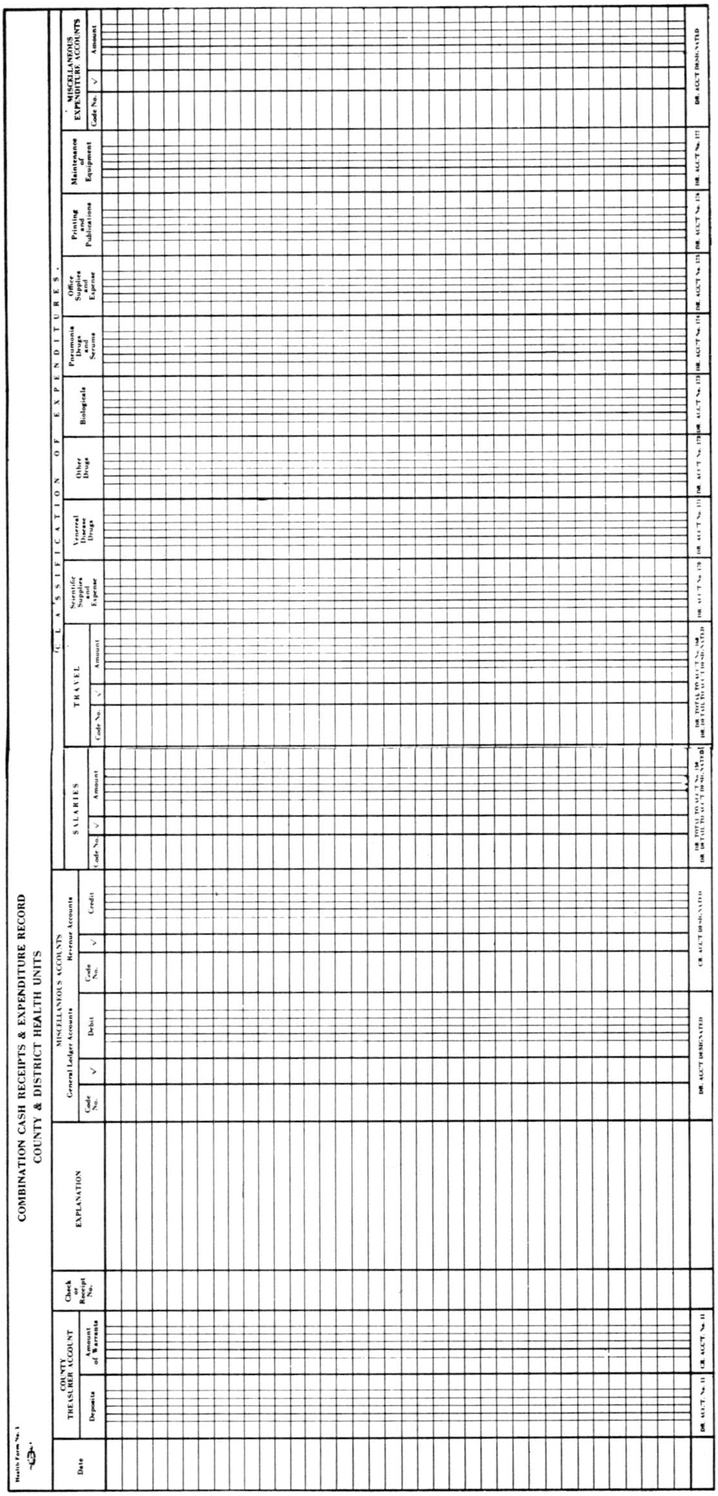

Fig. 15-4. Example of combination cash receipts and expenditure form.

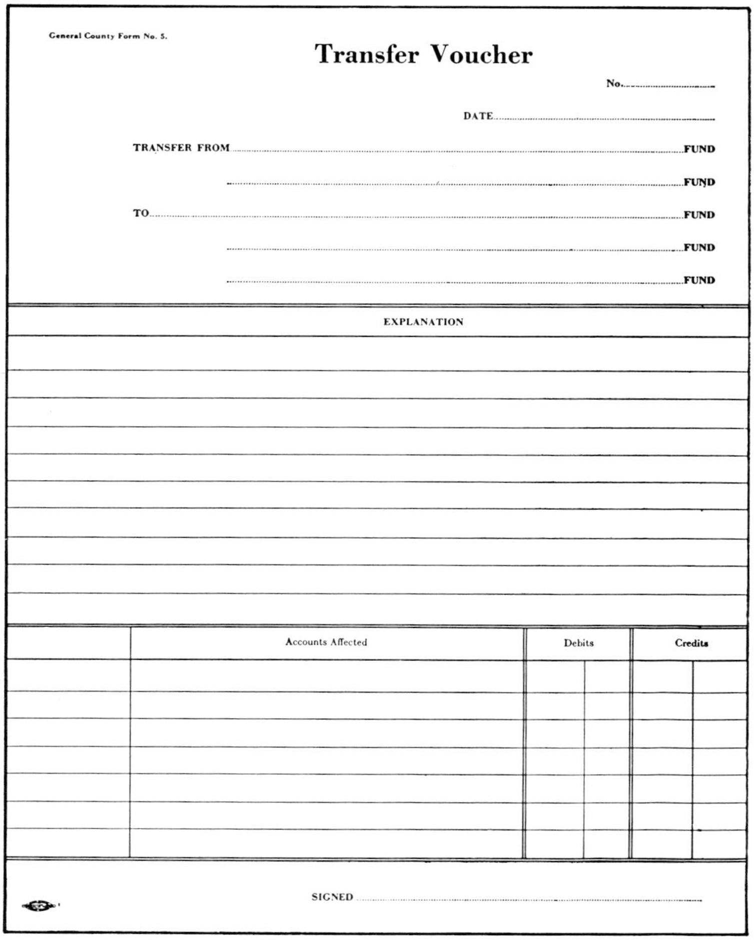

General County Form No. 5.

Transfer Voucher

No.........................

DATE.........................

TRANSFER FROM.........................FUND

.........................FUND

TO.........................FUND

.........................FUND

.........................FUND

EXPLANATION

	Accounts Affected	Debits	Credits

SIGNED.........................

Fig. 15-5. Example of transfer voucher form.

the proper code number as this governs the final classification of expenditures.

During the course of recording and posting items to the general ledger controls and accounts, numerous errors will arise that if left unchanged will not reflect a true statement of revenues and expenditures. For this reason the record of transfer vouchers is used to correct erroneous postings to accounts and to adjust and close out revenue and expense accounts at the close of each year's business. For future audit and reference purposes, full explanation for each transfer should be recorded in the space provided.

An important accounting procedure increasingly used by public health and other agencies is encumbrance control. This is designed to ensure adequate funds for future payment of obligations made in the present. The Emergency Maternity and Infant Care Program which operated during World War II provides a convenient example. Lump-sum allotments were made to the states each month on the basis of the estimated number of births that would occur during the following month. In order to forestall the great possibility of committing itself to future payments in excess of the sums allotted to it for the purpose, each

Table 15-1. Maternity and infant care encumbrance control record*

Date	Description	Transactions: Increase—Decrease			Totals to date		Balances		
		Allotment	Expenditures	Purchase orders (Requisitions)	Total allotment	Total expenditures	Unexpended balance	Accounts payable	Unencumbered balance
2/ 8/45	(1) Medical	$24			$ 74				$74
2/ 8/45	(2) Hospital	50			84				84
2/18/45	(3) Hospital	10			84				24
2/22/45	(4) Hospital		$60		84	$ 60			
2/23/45	(5) Medical		24		84	84			
5/ 8/45	(6) Medical	24							
5/ 8/45	(7) Hospital	50			158	84			74
5/26/45	(8) Medical to adjust	−24							
5/26/45	(9) Medical	36			170	84			86
6/ 3/45	(10) Medical		36		170	120			50
6/ 3/45	(11) Hospital to cancel	−50							

*Explanation: Child becomes ill and mother applies to participating physician for care. Physician decides hospital care needed, so sends in applications for medical and hospital care. These are both authorized and funds encumbered (1) and (2). (Maximum of $24 for first medical authorization and 10 days at $5 per day for hospitalization.) Two additional hospital days are needed, so reauthorization for them is made and $10 additional encumbered (3). After hospital service rendered, the hospital submits a bill for $60 (4) for which a check is made and sent. The physician, having completed care, submits a bill for $24 (5) for which a check is made and sent.

Several months later the child again becomes ill and the standard amount of funds for hospital and medical care are encumbered as before (6) and (7). The physician requests further authorization to provide for a minor operative procedure for which funds are then encumbered by canceling out the previous medical authorization (8) and encumbering the new amount necessary (9). The physician subsequently submits his bill which is paid (10) and notifies that the care was rendered at the patient's home so the allotment for hospitalization is canceled (11), bringing the unencumbered balance to zero.

state was encouraged to set up an encumbrance control procedure that simply deducted on paper from the total funds made available the amount of money that eventually would be required for payment of physicians and hospitals. It was somewhat as if payment were being made before the services were actually rendered rather than on their completion some months in the future. In this way the state could ascertain at any time the total amount of nonobligated funds available with which to provide care for additional individuals. In addition it provided a basis on which to apply in advance for deficiency allotments.

The program involved various types of services, e.g., obstetric, medical, surgical, hospital, and nursing. With cases of uncomplicated pregnancy and delivery the procedure was relatively simple; a standard fee was agreed upon by the medical profession and each state health department. Similarly per diem bed costs were determined and agreed upon for the participating hospitals. When a private physician notified the health department that he was assuming the care of a woman who was expected to de-

liver normally, say, 6 months hence, it was a simple matter to immediately set aside or encumber a sum of money sufficient to cover the physician's standard fee and the anticipated hospital bill. The latter could be rather accurately estimated as the product of the hospital's per diem bed cost times the average number of days that patients in the locality or state stayed in the hospital following delivery.

The procedure for encumbrance control becomes slightly more complicated when dealing with a service that is not as predictable as to time and cost as a normal pregnancy. Success depends on standardized fees and costs for services and materials. Insofar as possible, estimates of the probable extent of the services needed should be based on averages for the particular condition and/or type of patient in the particular area, and large sums should not be encumbered over long projected periods for the care of patients the cost of which is impossible to estimate with reasonable accuracy. An example of the manner in which a case of illness in an infant would be satisfactorily handled is given in Table 15-1.

Table 15-2. Record of encumbrances and unobligated balance for maternity care

Date	Authorization numbers	Amount encumbered	Amount paid	Adjustment	Unencumbered balance
6/30/43	(Received from U. S. Treasury $50,000)				
7/ 1/43	1–50	$ 3,750			$46,250
7/ 2/43	51–125	5,200			41,050
7/ 3/43	126–300	12,200			28,850
7/31/43	301–499	14,000			14,850
Total for July		$35,150			
8/ 1/43	(Received from U. S. Treasury $35,000)				$49,850
8/ 5/43	500–650	$13,000	$ 2,500	$ 500*	37,350
8/10/43	651–675	1,750	5,000	200	35,800
8/20/43	676–801	5,715	5,000	250	30,335
8/31/43	801–950	14,235	7,500	50	16,150
Total for August		$34,700	$20,000	$1,000	

*The first entry in this column ($500) is based on the assumption that authorizations totaling $3,000, issued early in July, were paid on August 5 in the amount of $2,500, or $500 less than the amount encumbered. This amount is therefore released for the commitment and added to the unencumbered balance in the last column.

The Children's Bureau, which was responsible to Congress for the program, naturally did not wish large unused and unencumbered sums accumulating in the individual states. On the other hand, it wanted to give assurance to each state that sufficient funds would be available at all times for payment of statements received. The states therefore maintained a summary record of encumbrances and unobligated balance such as that presented in Table 15-2. In addition to using it for their own guidance the states submitted their totals each month to the Children's Bureau to serve in determining the amount of money that should be sent to each state for the forthcoming month from the United States Treasury.

Performance budgeting

In Chapter 14, which deals with program planning, brief mention was made of cost-benefit analysis leading to the development of a program performance budget. Performance budgeting has been well described by Klepak[3] in his discussion of its application to public health. In effect it summarizes the program activities performed in terms of unit cost. Thus performance budgeting tells what it costs to immunize the individual against a specific disease or to supervise the average food-handling establishment. When such detailed cost analysis or inventory is available for all components or functions in a program, the determination of the cost of the total program becomes possible. One then has a true program performance budget that provides a measure of the total impact of a program in terms of its cost.

The advantages of a program inventory and the resultant performance budget that it makes possible may be summarized as follows:

1. Provide effective tools in planning a well-balanced program
2. Assist in developing short- and long-range program objectives
3. Provide elements for the control of programs and their costs
4. Provide detailed information concerning work volume and unit costs
5. Provide a sound basis for comparing past, present, and future activities, programs, and performance
6. Aid greatly in supporting requests for funds on a demonstrable and realistic basis
7. Discourage "padding" of the budget by program directors
8. Aid in the sound expansion and contraction of program activities
9. Permit personnel to see relationships among activities and programs
10. Provide qualitative and quantitative measures of personnel and departmental efficiency

This is the theory. However, certain general precautions are necessary. The program inventory, the performance report, the performance budget, and the program budget are only administrative tools. They must be used properly as aids to administrative evaluation—not in place of it or as ends in themselves. The performance budget specifically must be regarded as a classification of proposed expenditures in terms of things to be done or accomplishments to be achieved rather than things to be bought. Furthermore, yardsticks of performance standards have not yet been developed in many important areas. Ideally there should be standard cost tables and quantitative measurement devices for every important element of the health program.

Performance budgets cannot be used in every organization and program. If activities are of a highly routinized and objective nature and large numbers of people and objects are involved, a performance budget can be an invaluable aid to an administrator in learning not only what may be accomplished but also how well it is accomplished. In smaller organizations, dealing with less tangible objectives as, for example, a small local health department concerned with total health conditions, there are better ways of determining efficiency and more simplified methods of expressing end products in budgetary terms. In such instances supervisory impressions, reporting, inspection, and other subjective approaches may be useful and dependable.

A basic problem is that by their very nature preventive medicine and public health deal with negatives—cases and epidemics of disease prevented, home or industrial accidents guarded against, disasters avoided, and the like. To attempt to measure the value and efficiency of the efforts applied to such ends is quite different from measuring the cost of gallons of water processed, miles of streets paved, or radios manufactured. To place a monetary value upon the prevention of an epidemic is largely conjectural. Public health programs are actually a form of investment. When one deals with investment as a primary consideration in the performance of a function, the ordinary accounting rules do not apply. In the final analysis the only rule that is possible is that of the net return, which is the net of the benefits over costs otherwise incurred.

Many examples might be cited to illustrate these reservations. A few may be worth noting. Public health is an organized endeavor involving constant dynamic change toward improvement of the social and environmental scene. The more effective and efficient its performance, the higher the relative unit costs tend to be. The elimination of each remaining case of tuberculosis is necessarily increasingly costly. As communicable diseases are conquered and the age distribution of the population shifts upward, there occurs a shift from low-cost mass communicable disease laboratory examinations to the more time-consuming, hence more expensive, laboratory examinations for the more individualized cases of chronic diseases. In this dynamism we also witness increasingly the sudden availability of newer, more effective, and often less expensive methods of diagnosis and treatment. Tuberculosis provides a good example. Within a few years it has become possible to treat patients effectively at a much lower cost and for a shorter period of time than before. The effect of such changes upon comparative performance budgeting systems is obvious. Then there is the example of two child-health clinics, in one of which each physician examines an average of 10 children per hour, in contrast with the other clinic, where each physician examines an average of 4 children per hour.

How does one properly evaluate the efficiency of these two clinics on the basis of costs per child examined? A final example relates to food sanitation where the obvious ultimate goal is a uniformly sanitary food service. If, as often suggested, function and efficiency were to be measured in terms of violations investigated and corrected, the best program would appear to be the least effective or efficient in terms of costs.

While the foregoing qualifications and examples are proper and valid, they do not, however, justify an attitude of defeat or an unwillingness to search for some useful measures of achievement and efficiency in public health practice. Within the inherent limitations it is felt that some practical measures exist. Perhaps the problem is not so much the discovery and development of such measures as is their interpretation and use. If these measures are considered only as stable as the activities and programs they measure and are subject to parallel change, then no serious difficulty should ensue. Any attempt therefore should be based upon the following premises:

1. All costs should be accumulated, if possible, to reflect major functional activities or programs. (Compromises are necessary because the broader the program category used, the more difficult it is to find a common performance unit to reflect the total activities of the program.)
2. Fixed costs should be separated from variable costs. (This is especially important when dealing with a declining problem and program with a declining work load situation, such as tuberculosis.)
3. Variable costs should be related to work load and accomplishments. (These costs, while not including all direct and indirect expenditures devoted to the achievement of a particular goal, do provide the best and perhaps only real reflection of operational efficiency.)
4. Cost standards thus established can be used to appraise program and activity performance.

5. Since by their nature public health activities involve for the most part interpersonal action, the costs of materials in most instances are considered to represent a relatively insignificant proportion of the total cost. In many instances therefore the cost of materials may be ignored. In certain other instances, e.g., laboratory work or immunizations, materials do add substantially to the total cost of the function or activity and should be included.

6. While attention should be focused primarily upon specific program areas, there is some value in attempting to develop cost centers in certain broad across-the-board service areas, e.g., laboratory work, public health nursing, and district health operations, in order to attempt to obtain some overall operational cost and efficiency figures.

The following are a few examples of the many cost centers which actually or theoretically may be measured. It must be recognized that the best of them are subject to many intrinsic and extrinsic influences over which a public health organization and its staff has limited or no control and that may cause considerable fluctuation.

Food protection.

$$\frac{\text{(a) Cost of manpower per year}}{\text{(b) No. of establishments supervised per year}}$$

$$= \text{Cost per establishment supervised}$$

Here the numerator (a) should include the total number of man-years of time devoted by inspectional staff to routine complaint, violation, and follow-up inspection of establishments in which food is received, stored, processed, sold, or served. It also includes the time devoted by clinicians, public health nurses, disease control investigators, and laboratory personnel involved in the examination and follow-up of present and prospective food-handlers to the point where they might be diagnosed as having some communicable disease, under which circumstances the problem becomes one of epidemiology. Since all these categories of personnel are generalized, it is

necessary for each staff member to record the number of hours devoted each workday to travel, inspection, office and clinical work relating to the foregoing purpose. The total man-years that results is multiplied by the average actual salary of currently employed personnel to obtain the numerator. The denominator (b) is the total number of separate establishments in which food is received, stored, processed, sold, or served with which the division of environmental health of a community health organization has direct or indirect contact in relation to supervision, inspection reports, complaints, violations, or follow-up.

Epidemiology. A number of cost centers are possible in this area. The first example relates to the general efficiency of the overall program as follows:

$$\frac{\text{(a) Cost of manpower and materials per year}}{\text{(b) No. of cases, contacts, and suspects investigated per year}}$$

$$= \text{Cost per individual investigation}$$

This is a very general index that interprets investigation in its broadest sense to include routine and special case finding based upon x-ray examinations, blood tests, and clinical or laboratory examinations in health centers, central diagnostic units, mobile diagnostic units, street-corner campaigns, etc. It also refers to both endemic and epidemic situations. The justification for so doing is based on the premise that in the final analysis most of the time of an epidemiologic staff is devoted to investigation of cases, contacts, and suspects toward the end of getting them under treatment. In order to be valid, however, (a) must exclude the time of physicians, nurses, and clerical personnel who work in relation to treatment. Also it must include the value of the man-years of time devoted by generalized public health nurses and by disease control investigators. This necessitates their keeping a daily log of the amount of their field, travel, and office time devoted to this purpose. The denominator (b) is the total number of individual cases, contacts to, or suspects of acute communicable diseases, venereal diseases, and tuberculosis that are investigated throughout the year by the community health organization.

An example of a cost center of a more specific nature is in relation to the cost of finding a new case of tuberculosis. The same procedure applies to a long series of disease-related activities. It must be recognized that the more successful the activity, the more the cost per case found will rise.

(a) Cost of manpower and materials per year
(b) No. of new cases of tuberculosis

= Cost per new case of tuberculosis found

The numerator (a) is based upon the man-years devoted by physicians, radiologists, x-ray technicians, clinic nurses, clinic clerks, field public health nurses, field disease control investigators, and clerical personnel to the discovery and investigation of new cases of tuberculosis and the placing of new patients under treatment. It is necessary for each worker to keep a daily log of the amount of time devoted to the clinical, travel, home visit, and office aspects of this activity, which multiplied by their respective salaries and totaled provides the cost of the manpower per year for this purpose. Added to this is the cost of expendable materials requisitioned and used by such personnel for this specific purpose. The sum of these two figures provides the cost of the activity. The denominator (b) is the number of new cases of tuberculosis diagnosed and brought under care during the year by staff of the community health organization. Not included in this sum are cases of tuberculosis diagnosed for the first time after death of an individual.

Maternal health.

(a) Cost of manpower in maternal health clinics per year
(b) No. of patient visits per year

= Cost per maternal patient visit

The numerator (a) is the number of man-years of each physician, nurse, and clerk working in relation to maternal health clinics, including field follow-up by public health nurses, times the sum of their salaries. The denominator (b) is the number of patient visits to maternal health clinics during the year.

Vital records.

(a) Cost of manpower per year
(b) No. of certified records processed per year

= Cost per certified record processed

The numerator (a) consists of the sum of the salaries of the individuals employed in the vital records office. The denominator (b) is the number of vital records for which certified copies are requested and delivered.

Laboratory.

(a) Cost of manpower and materials per year
(b) No. of laboratory examinations per year

= Cost per laboratory examination

The numerator (a) consists of the cost of all salaries in the public health laboratory plus the cost of all expendable materials requisitioned by the laboratory, including the value of all specimen kits distributed to physicians, hospitals, and others, and any postage or other transportation costs involved. The denominator (b) includes the total number of all laboratory examinations performed (not specimens received) during the year.

Public health nursing.

(a) Cost of PH nursing time for each type of program per year
(b) No. of nursing visits for each type of program per year

= Cost per visit

This example provides a series of figures, one for each type of program, e.g., tuberculosis, maternal health, child health, etc. The numerator (a) is based upon the total number of man-hours devoted by members of the field public health nursing staff to various types of programs. This necessitates each field nurse's keeping a detailed record of her time and activities throughout each day, which separated into program categories and each multiplied by her individual salary provides the value of her time devoted to each program. This sum combined with similar data from all other field nurses provides the cost of the field nursing component of each major program. The denominator (b) is the number of nursing visits for each type of broad program area per year.

Air-pollution control.

$$\frac{\text{(a) Cost of manpower per year}}{\text{1}} \div \text{(b) Amount of air pollution}$$

$$= \text{Efficiency quotient of program}$$

This represents a more difficult type of activity to measure. Air pollution is obviously less tangible than a person immunized or a visit made. Here, the numerator (a) includes the total man-years of time devoted by field, environmental health laboratory, and central office staffs to routine, complaint, violation, and follow-up inspection of residential, industrial, and dump sites that may or actually contribute to controllable contamination of the atmosphere. Some of these individuals devote all of their time and others devote part of their time to this purpose. It is necessary for each of them to keep records of this time to be accumulated and translated into man-years or fractions thereof which, when applied to their respective salaries and totaled, provides the total cost of personnel time devoted to this activity. The reciprocal (b) is of the amount of air pollution. The reciprocal is used since otherwise the more effective the program, the higher the apparent cost would be to the limit of infinity. Air pollution can be measured by instrumental determination of the total amount of suspended particular air pollutants (in milligrams per cubic yard) times an appropriate standard number such as 1,000. A reading may be made once each month and the 12 readings averaged.

It is recognized that this quotient is not a cost figure. However, it is desirable to begin exploring the development of the true indicators of program usefulness and efficiency. It must be recognized that this efficiency figure is subject to alteration by nonprogram factors such as meteorologic changes, fires, emergencies, and especially by an increase in industry or in the use of motor vehicles.

Purchasing

Related to accounting or expenditure control is the obtaining of materials and supplies involved in the operation of public agencies. Until relatively recently the pattern followed was largely the provision to each individual operating department of lump sums of money for operation or maintenance. There existed also a general feeling that purchases and contracts should be distributed as widely as possible throughout the various business concerns existing in the area served, apparently with the end in view of obtaining their goodwill and support of the government and its program. Why this was felt necessary is somewhat difficult to understand since business and industry has always followed a more progressive and efficient course.

The recent trend therefore has been toward the development of central public purchasing agencies with the authority to purchase or to formulate regulations governing the purchase of all materials, equipment, supplies, and contractual services for all of the public agencies in the particular unit of government. As this approach developed, in order to promote their effectiveness public purchasing agencies have generally been given the authority to inspect all goods delivered, to test samples submitted with bids or deliveries, to transfer or dispose of any materials, supplies, and equipment from operating agencies, and to maintain a central warehouse. Centralized purchasing has many advantages, including lower unit costs, better delivery service, reduction of overhead costs, standardization of products and of purchasing and expenditure documents, more efficient accounting control over expenditure, and simplification of the ordering, delivery, and storage problems of both vendors and operating agencies.

Complaints are frequently raised against central purchasing agencies, usually to the effect that they hamper the activity of the functional department by causing delays, red tape, and the acceptance of substitute or unsatisfactory materials. The subject of most controversy is whether or not the purchasing agent should have the right to modify the requisition sent to him, to substitute for a specified material or brand, or to refuse to place an order for materials requested by a functional agency. The statutes of some states specifically allow this right, some imply it, others deny it, and worst of all in a number of states the issue is entirely ignored. It is felt that most or all of these objections may be easily avoided, provided the purchasing agency, on the one hand, constantly considers that its existence is justified only in terms of the auxiliary service it finds possible to render to the functional agency and if the latter, on the other hand, takes pains to make clear to the purchasing agency its exact needs and the reasons for them. The problem therefore is essentially one of proper interagency relationships and understanding.

While a system of continuous expenditure control assures the efficiency of operation and expenditure, only an audit following the completion of the budget period can determine their legality. Therefore it is necessary in the public interest that there be some method of assuring not only that the public money is being legally spent but that the public is receiving reasonable value for it. The auditor is in effect an arm of the public's legislature, which not only has established a public program but has provided appropriation for its fulfillment. A system of postauditing involves the examination and appraisal of accounts, records, and statements as well as accounting and operating procedures. It provides the legislature with information and analyses arrived at independently of those who are directly responsible for expenditures and operations. It provides data for reviewing past and for planning future budgets, revenue and expenditure programs, and for drafting needed additional legislation. The personnel of the functional units subject to postauditing should in addition look upon it as a protection to them and a means of providing for official and public recognition to their honest and efficient fulfillment of the duties and responsibilities entrusted to them.

FISCAL RESPONSIBILITY

The placement of fiscal responsibility in any political subdivision may vary from place to place. However, the principle exists and must be maintained that a public health officer must always be in the position of knowing the current status of his budget appropriation limitations.

In large cities where there tends to exist highly centralized financial operations with fiscal controls established therein and where an "executive type" rather than a "legislative type" of budget is effective, it is especially important that the health officer establish a firm fiscal basis upon which he may successfully operate. A brief review of the successive steps involved in such a community that adopts this newer concept of fiscal control is presented for those who may be confronted with such an operation.

In a certain year the voters of a particular city adopted a home rule charter that had recently been authorized by the government of the state. The new charter, among other benefits, established new fiscal policies for governmental operation in the fields of budgeting, accounting practices, collection of taxes and other revenue, and the related responsibilities thereto.

The mayor of the city was made responsible primarily for the efficient fiscal operations of the various governmental functions, and through his finance director, the city's principal finance officer, was charged with the responsibility of submitting to the city council the budget requests of the various governmental units.

The city council's authority in the field of finance was restricted in the charter in favor of wider authority to be exercised by the mayor. The council retained the right to adopt the annual operating budget and the capital budget, to levy the taxes necessary for the support of the government, and to authorize debt, contingent upon the approval of the voters. Under these circumstances the council was bound by the mayor's estimate of receipts and was guided in the determination of its budget appropriations by consideration of the line type budget, with detailed justifications thereof, which was submitted to the council by the mayor. This budget was presented on an "object detail class" basis. All the positions to be financed were segregated on a budget schedule, with separate schedules for personnel, contractual services, materials and supplies, equipment (detailed), and such other additional classes as the mayor recommended in his proposed annual operating budget ordinance. All budget appropriations were made in lump-sum amounts and according to the foregoing classes of expenditure for each office, department, board, or commission.

This approach to budgeting produces the executive type budget rather than the legislative type budget and gives the administrative officials of government more flexibility within broad limitations but does not destroy the possibility of close administrative supervision and control. Thus the responsibility for fiscal direction and control is placed more firmly on the executive rather than on the legislative branch of the government. The city council is required by law to adopt the annual operating budget ordinance for the next fiscal year at least 30 days before the commencement of that year.

Upon receipt of the approved budget, the director of finance, with the approval of the mayor, sets up allotment accounts by departments on an expenditure class basis. Personnel appropriations may be established on a quarterly allotment pattern, and materials, supplies, and equipment on an annual basis. In the larger departments allotment accounts are set up on a departmental functional basis, with subaccount allotments for detailed object classes exceeding $20,000, for closer appropriation controls.

The multiplicity and volume of fiscal transactions handled in a centralized fiscal office of a large city necessitate the utilization of mechanized facilities. Since the director of finance is the chief fiscal officer of the city, all budget, fiscal, and accounting practices are centrally controlled in his office. There are released from the offices of the director of finance all of the official financial statements of the city. For day-to-day operations the fiscal office of each department receives from the director of finance a daily statement that reflects the current status of each of their allotment accounts. Each transaction listed on his daily statement is documented by a copy of the voucher related thereto. These statements, however, do not include all of the encumbrances that may be involved in proposed commitments that have not reached the stage of machine recording. Therefore for this and other reasons there still remains the need of a departmental fiscal office. This need is apparent when the following are considered:

1. Most of the initial action in all fiscal transactions originates in the operating department.

2. The original departmental budgetary appropriation request is prepared in each operating department.

3. The various types of requisitions covering departmental needs are processed from each department.

4. Appropriation accounts authorized for the general fund, capital fund, and special funds must be maintained at the department level in order that the health officer may direct and plan his program during the course of the year from the unencumbered balances. Therefore the departmental accounts must include those planned and proposed commitments that have not as yet currently reached the stage of machine recording.

5. Although payrolls may be prepared by mechanized methods in the finance department, the initial official time record of personnel work must originate and be prepared at the operational level.

6. Costing for evaluation of programs and activities is also essentially the responsibility of the departmental fiscal office.

In the capital fund area the principles of responsibilities are practially the same as those applicable in the general or operating fund field. However, the details of handling are somewhat different. For example, a city council may adopt each year a 6-year capital program, wherein is listed each project to be financed during these periods, showing the amount proposed to be spent for each of the 6 future years covered. The council then would also adopt a capital fund budget for the forthcoming year where the amounts authorized to be spent therein are recorded projectwise.

In the preparation of the capital program and capital budget it is probable that the director of finance and a city planning commission, if one existed, would work jointly with the approval of the mayor to furnish the city council with a budget document that would best reflect the needs of the community with regard to the various proposed capital improvements. However, the initial budget requests would originate in the fiscal office of the operational departments.

It is evident from the foregoing that the health officer, in order to plan his health programs efficiently, to utilize the health dollar to the best advantage, and to remain within his budget limitations, must assure himself that he has prepared his budget properly, that its terms are applied correctly, and that shifts in programs are adjusted as the funds permit. In order to do this he must familiarize himself with the principles of the local fiscal requirements and must obtain the best fiscal advice and aid available.

REFERENCES

1. White, L. D.: Introduction to the study of public administration, New York, 1955, The Macmillan Co.
2. Geiger, J.: Health officers' manual, Philadelphia, 1939, W. B. Saunders Co.
3. Klepak, D.: Performance budgeting for the health department, Public Health Rep. **71:**868, Sept. 1956.

Chapter 16

Public relations

PURPOSES AND OBJECTIVES

Ours is a society of increasing complexity and sophistication. One of the requirements of both private and public organizations in such a society is a concern for customer or patron understanding and attitude, commonly referred to as public relations. The term is admittedly general and vague; it is used to describe a variety of techniques, practices, and activities, some good, some bad, designed to win the goodwill and cooperation of people individually and collectively. These activities are never an end in themselves; rather they are important merely to the extent that they enable employees to fulfill adequately their intended responsibilities to the satisfaction and understanding of all concerned. The field of public relations is not only difficult to define but also presents a problem when one merely attempts to list or describe the various factors that contribute to it. All too often are seen instances in which executives point with pride and satisfaction to their publicity programs and refer to them as public relations programs. While press releases, public addresses, and the like are of great importance in their place, public relations encompasses far more. It includes every conceivable factor and circumstance that may influence people's attitude toward the organization, its goals, its activities, and its personnel. Most important it includes the many seemingly incidental and casual relationships between the organization, its personnel, and those who are served. In this sense public relations may be looked upon to a considerable degree as the summation of personal relations.

Another misconception with regard to the purpose of public relations activities is that they are developed for the purpose of having a reserve of support and defense when the going gets rough. While a really good public relations program will go far in accomplishing this purpose, it is an incidental or secondary effect; the primary purpose is to make the road as smooth and effective as possible in the first place. As one writer[1] has described it: "Public relations is not an ambulance parked at the bottom of a precipice. Rather, it is a fence built at the top."

Although the public relations problem of a public health department is essentially the same as that of any other type of enterprise, certain differences in the reasons for the existence and manner of operation of the organization make good public relations peculiarly important. A health department is a tax-supported public agency that belongs to the people it serves. Its existence in a democracy depends in the final analysis upon their wish to maintain it. In the long run this wish can be sustained only by public understanding and satisfaction. Such reactions naturally give rise to pride of ownership, which in turn enhances cooperation and support. It might be pointed out further that modern thinking in public health is along the lines of doing things with people, not for them or to them. "With" is an interesting word which, when applied jointly to a health agency and the people it serves, implies everything that contributes to good public relations.

GENERAL CONSIDERATIONS

Fundamental to a successful program of public relations is the desire to sell the organization and its program, not the individual. It is true that the public is interested in personalities and figureheads, but it soon tires or becomes suspicious of too frequent references to a particular public employee, even though he be the health officer. Perhaps the most important public relations consideration for the health officer is not to regard the health program as a one-man show but to share credit as well as responsibility. When this policy is followed, the individual is automatically benefited. Thus when Dr. Enion Williams, the eminent health commissioner of Virginia, was asked to account for his long tenure of office, he replied, "I have never tried to sell the people of Virginia on the name Williams, but I have sold them on the Virginia State Department of Health."

What has been said is not meant to imply that the health officer does not have a most important personal part to play in the public relations program of his organization. After all, he is the responsible leader. It is his job to ascertain that desirable relationships are formed and maintained. Beyond planning and directing the program he must cultivate certain relationships that he alone is in a position to do and is expected to carry out. He makes these contacts with other governmental officials, prominent citizens, and various important key people including representatives of the communications field in the interests of the program for which he is responsible.

This leads to a second basic consideration. Good public relations, particularly those of large organizations, seldom if ever come about spontaneously. Sometimes they may appear to, but to be effective a public relations program must be carefully and conscientiously planned and constantly watched. To do this requires initially a clearly determined overall policy of the organization and its attitude toward the public in relation to the purposes and aims of the agency. Cognizance of all potential contacts must be taken and insofar as possible arrangements made for their occurrence in the most mutually satisfactory manner. Provision must be made for employee training in good public relations, followed by checks and evaluations of the success of this aspect of the life of the agency.

With regard to the first of the two words in the term "public relations," it must be fully appreciated that there is no such thing as "one" or "the" *public*. In even the most primitive societies more than one public exists. Usually there are many, each with its particular interests, needs, and demands. The population of the typical community is subdivided into a large number of groups or publics on the basis of many characteristics, e.g., religion, economic status, education, race, nationality, age, sex, and occupation, to mention but a few. The public relations program must be broken down into a similar number of subprograms. No single approach will bring success because it will touch only one or at best a few of the publics. The program must be designed as a jigsaw puzzle that eventually succeeds in reaching in one way or another all of the publics involved.

Attention should be drawn to several other general considerations. The first of these is the often overlooked fact that public relations is a two-way process. It involves a flow of information, reactions, and understanding, not only from the agency to the public but also in the reverse direction. Accordingly, it is important that the health agency devise and use some method of periodic determination of needs, wishes, understanding, and motivational inclinations of the public. Overlooked with equal frequency is the part played by the many informal as well as formal contacts between public employees and the citizenry. A health department may have the support of the press, the professions, and the business groups, and may be doing a scientifically splendid job, but all this may be negated in the mind of the citizen if he is slighted, dealt with flippantly and rudely, or in any other way made to feel dissatisfied.

One final consideration, which is related to the next discussion, is an appreciation of the competition for the attention of the public. In our modern society the senses of the average citizen are bombarded constantly throughout his waking hours by a barrage of publicity, propaganda, advertising, and promotional and educational forces. Some of them are subtle, while others resort practically to brute force. The public health worker must recognize all this as competition and must devise and employ techniques that will meet it on its own ground and obtain a fair share of public attention. In this very real struggle for public attention and support the public health agency is handicapped by certain obstacles that act as deterrents to desirable public relations. Some of them relate either to the nature of the product (health) or to the means of providing for it (a public agency). Others stem from outdated, impractical, and supercilious approaches.

OBSTACLES TO GOOD PUBLIC RELATIONS

It must be frankly recognized that people are seldom interested in public health in the general sense. Individuals are concerned with their own personal health or with that of the members of their families. By and large they are willing to pay attention to some of the larger community aspects of health only insofar as they may readily appreciate its effect upon them. Even then they may weigh the possible benefits against certain other considerations such as personal freedom of action or business advantage. In other words, strange as it may seem to those imbued with the "public health spirit," public health is not necessarily a natural or spontaneous concern, interest, or wish of all people. It is in fact more than a little distressing to find that an appreciable percentage of the population is quite ignorant of the existence of the field and not particularly interested in enlightenment.

Another obstacle is related to the fact that activities engaged in for the protection and promotion of health require employees with a scientific, technical, or professional background. Their training and experience usually emphasizes the scientific and technical aspects of the problems and their solutions and ignores more often than not the human factors involved. Thus it is easy for public health workers to be so intent upon their activities, programs, or goals that they

lose sight of the personal and human aspects of the work. This professionalism may sometimes give rise to feelings of discomfort, awe, and even resentment on the part of the members of the public in their contacts with the personnel of the health department. If this occurs, it is of course a deterrent to good public relations and understanding.

Particular difficulties arise from the fact that public health programs are in large part activities of official governmental agencies and therefore subject to all of the attitudes that the public and community groups tend to have toward government. Unfortunately public employment has been held in low esteem by many in the United States, although some improvement has been noticed in recent years. All too often the public servant, professional or otherwise, has been regarded as someone incapable of successfully engaging in private business or professional practice and interested only in a political sinecure. This is due partly to the traditional American admiration of rugged individualistic business and industry and partly to occasionally unsatisfactory if not unsavory governmental operations. In addition, it must be recognized and accepted that a public agency must function much more in a glass case than does a private agency in which for some reason citizens tend not to feel a vested interest and demand accountability. Business and the private professions have always regarded government as a natural enemy that always seeks to control or to take over. Under these circumstances the opposition to the development and expansion of public programs is not surprising.

Related to this and accentuated by traditionally low salaries in governmental service is the not infrequent inferiority complex that has developed in many public employees. An unfortunate method of compensation for this is the occasional exercise of injudicious authority based upon public position. This, when resorted to, only aggravates the situation.

It is not difficult to understand how many citizens may misinterpret planned public relations activities of public agencies as representing propaganda for the purpose of self-aggrandizement at public expense to assure reappointment or continued employment. For this as well as other reasons the public has been loath to provide funds for public relations purposes, thereby often making it necessary for the public agency to resort to subterfuge in order to accomplish this important purpose.

Finally, it should be recognized that a great many citizen contacts with the health department are unwilling contacts whereby the individual is called upon to do something not to his liking, e.g., to obtain a permit. From the point of view of development of desirable public attitudes, the health department finds itself with two strikes against it from the onset. This makes it all the more necessary that the personnel of the health department take full advantage of every possible opportunity for the development and maintenance of good public relations.

METHODS IN PUBLIC RELATIONS

Since in every community there are many publics and since societies have become so complex, it necessarily follows that there are many different approaches to the development of improved public understanding and support.

Personal contacts

This is mentioned first, not only because of its importance but also because it is so often overlooked or neglected. A health department exists to serve the public, and most of its work involves contact between its staff and the individuals who comprise the public. It naturally follows that these contacts should be of a desirable nature. If a contact or association of a citizen with the personnel of the agency is unsatisfactory and leaves an unpleasant memory, the contact is a failure despite whatever service is rendered in the process. In addition to this, if the attitudes of the employees toward the public health organization, its policies, and its management are unsatisfactory, they are certain to influence the nature of the employees' contacts with the public, and this in turn will adversely affect the community's attitude toward the department.

On-the-job personal characteristics of health department employees that influence the reactions and attitudes of the public they meet may be considered under the categories of appearance, behavior, and capability.

Appearance. Most large private organizations have found it desirable to impose certain requirements concerning dress and other aspects of personal appearance upon their employees. To do so is not without risk since requirements of this nature, if unexplained, misunderstood, or too strict, are apt to lead to considerable intra-agency friction and personnel dissatisfaction. Most employees, however, if worthy of employment in the first place, can be made to realize the purpose and desirability of their requirements.

The average person on entering a business office, especially if the office is tax supported, does not react favorably to flashy clothes or an excess of jewelry, cosmetics, or perfume. Male employees should avoid sports clothes and dazzling neckties in favor of more dignified or professional dress. Women should be similarly conservative, tending toward suits and tailored clothes. The use of cosmetics, jewelry, and perfume occupy a very real place in our culture and are by no means to be denied. However, in a business environment their use should be judicious and in good taste. Under all circumstances the personnel should be neat and clean, there never being any excuse for appearance to the contrary. That this is possible is given testimony by the level of neatness and cleanliness maintained by many industrial workers and gasoline-station attendants.

No discussion of clothing can be concluded without reference to the question of uniforms. The problem arises especially in connection with one large group of employees, public health nurses. It is possible to set forth many arguments pro and con the wearing of uniforms. The chief advantages relate to ease of identification and recognition of professional standing. Many feel that the public expects to find nurses in some type of uniform, lacking which they may be less acceptable. It is further felt desirable by many that a corps of readily identified uniformed workers provides visual evidence of the importance and activity of the health department. In this sense the argument rests upon the promotion of public relations. Some also claim that the wearing of identical uniforms by a group of employees promotes an esprit de corps. The opposing view points to the frequent drabness of public health nurses' uniforms. This is not necessarily a valid complaint in view of the very attractive yet dignified uniforms designed for airline stewardesses and many nursing agencies. With reference to identification, some call attention to the resentment felt by many citizens when their neighbors see the "city nurse" knock at the door. Added to this, they claim, is the embarrassment of both the citizen and the nurse caused by the frequent identification of a public health field visit with venereal disease or some other problem of similarly unpleasant connotation. I do not feel it within my province to render a judgment in the matter. Rather this is a question that requires separate answers by each individual health department and its community.

Behavior. While the first impression in a personal contact is a visual one depending upon appearance, the subsequent and most telling impressions are of an even more direct and personal nature. Much depends upon the manner in which employees approach individual citizens or patrons in the office or in the field. Everyone has at some time found it necessary to visit offices where, after a seemingly needless wait, he has been called upon with bluntness, curtness, and occasional rudeness to state his business. In such instances the visitor is made to feel that he is an outsider, an intruder, an interruption, a nuisance to be disposed of as quickly as possible. In contrast are offices equally if not more busy where the approach is friendly, as one human being to another, where any delays are courteously and regretfully explained, and where the visitor is made to feel at home, expected, and wanted.

In their contacts with the public there are certain principles or rules that public health workers would do well to follow.

The key to the situation is to look upon those contacted as the real and only reason for the job and for the department. Each contact should be regarded as a contest rather than a boring routine, the goal being to win the other person over to your side, your point of view, your program. In order to accomplish this the public health worker must first attempt to put himself in the position of the caller, remembering that in most instances that person would much rather be doing something else. The measure of success is for the visitor to depart with no regrets. At best the circumstances of the contact will be strange to him, therefore the employee should make every effort to call forth associations that are familiar and pleasant. Explanations should be in simple terms, and strange and technical terminology should be avoided. "Vaccination," "immunization," and "shots" are examples of complicated and rather frightening words, whereas "protection" bears a connotation of something positive and desirable. A woman would much prefer to be spoken of as an "expectant mother" rather than as a "prenatal." All of us resent being referred to as cases, subjects, or numbers; we are human beings and are worthy of address as such.

Every organization of whatever size should make provision for some type of information desk. In a small organization such as the typical rural county health department this desk will not be difficult to find. In larger agencies that occupy many rooms on several floors the information desk should be placed as close to the main entrance as possible. The person in charge should be selected with care; she should appear approachable, friendly, and desirous of being of assistance to all types of persons. Her manner, while dignified, should be somewhat informal, and it is perhaps preferable that she be allowed somewhat more leeway in the matter of dress than the rest of the personnel. In order to fulfill her purpose it is of course necessary that an individual in this position possess an encyclopedic knowledge of the organization and its program, the building in which it is housed, and also of related organizations in the community. Placed near the information desk should be an easily read and interpretable directory that indicates the location of each of the functional units in the organization and lists the names of unit directors and of any other persons frequently sought.

Next in line of travel is the office receptionist, who to a considerable degree conditions the attitude of the caller toward the organization. This position is usually filled by a woman who also serves in a secretarial capacity. She should have an air of alertness and industry backed up by competence. The position is not necessarily an easy one since the occupant may often find herself in the middle between the person for whom she works and the visitor. By no means are all visitors important, and the receptionist has the responsibility of husbanding the limited time of the executive. On the other hand, each visitor naturally considers himself and the reason for his call of importance, otherwise he would not have taken the trouble to come to the office. The receptionist therefore must have as an outstanding qualification a sound understanding of human nature and the ability whenever necessary to turn some visitors away in such a manner as to preserve their pride and dignity and make them feel satisfied at least in some degree. Whether or not the receptionist attempts to forestall or divert the visitor, she may by her manner convey the impression that the appearance of the visitor was the most important event during the day and that any delay or refusal is extremely regretful to her, her employer, and to the organization.

When a visitor approaches, the receptionist should greet him pleasantly, arise if circumstances allow and warrant, and ask in a pleasant tone of voice, "May I help you?" When a request to see the executive is stated, the receptionist should counter with, "May I ask who is calling?" whereupon, unless impossible, she should immediately take steps to notify her superior. Should it be necessary to turn away truly important persons or individuals whom the receptionist feels her superior would want to see, she should if possible arrange or at

least suggest a subsequent appointment. If the visitor is to be seen, she should usher him into the presence of the executive, announce his name, and if necessary the organization he represents. If the visitor has given her a calling card, she should place it before her superior.

An annoying problem is posed by the visitor who never knows when to leave. The time of most professional workers and executives is limited and frequently they are tempted to terminate a call impatiently or brusquely. This is apt to be misunderstood and resented by the visitor, even though he may have inconsiderately usurped more than a fair share of time. It is possible to circumvent such occurrences either by means of a prearranged signal to the receptionist-secretary or by routine interruption on her part after a reasonable interval to remind the executive of another appointment. This allows the executive to terminate the contact regretfully and gracefully.

A common cause of ill feeling towards public officials and agencies is the manner in which visitors, clients, or patrons are frequently shunted from one place to another, no one taking the trouble to ascertain exactly what they want or assuring that they get it by the shortest possible route. This type of runaround or buck-passing has proved costly to many organizations in terms of public relations. Accordingly, the person at the information desk and the receptionist and secretaries in the organization have the important responsibility of adequate referral. Moreover, whenever indicated they should take the trouble to follow up referrals in order to assure the satisfaction of the caller. Usually a caller has several reasons for contacting the agency, but in each instance there is one predominate reason for the visit having been made. Under no circumstances should the visitor be allowed to depart with the feeling that absolutely nothing was done with regard to that particular reason.

Some organizations have found it possible to improve their public relations by coordinating certain services and activities and by centralizing the location of places to which the public must come. A good example of this is in connection with building permits. Ordinarily a citizen who wishes to construct or alter a building finds it necessary to make the rounds of the building department, water department, fire department, health department, and possibly others in addition to the city clerk in order to obtain approval of all parts of the building permit. Some communities out of consideration for the taxpayer have brought together into one office, at adjacent desks, representatives of each of the branches of government involved so that all requirements may be fulfilled in one place and in a single visit.

Many health departments have effectively built up an extensive backlog of ill feeling through their public counters. This problem was magnified during the war years as a result of the tremendous demand for birth certificates as a prerequisite to work permits. The same applies to demands in relation to marriage and burial permits as well as to foreign travel. Admittedly the extent to which health department offices have been deluged with often hurried requests has not been conducive to good temper and patience. Nevertheless, by attempting to be overly efficient by the use of impersonal mass production methods, health departments have sometimes irritated large numbers of individuals. Some of the difficulty can be attributed to personnel shortages and inadequate funds. Over and above this, however, is the ill-advised policy followed by many organizations of placing at public counters employees who do not seem to fit in anywhere else. It is strange that positions that involve the most frequent contacts with the public so often are used as reservoirs or wastebaskets for employee misfits. Examples of improper behavior at information desks and public counters are not difficult to find. I once had the misfortune of inheriting a county health department officer manager who seemed to resent the appearance of anyone and who all but physically drove out anyone who dared enter. She was promptly relieved of her duties. Another well-remembered instance concerns the front information desk of the health department of a large city which was staffed by two formerly profes-

sional employees who had become too addicted to alcohol to render professional service. In still another agency the office of statistics and records was considered more or less a place of retirement wherein the older, worn-out employees found it definitely not to their liking to have to get out of their chairs to serve applicants for copies of vital records. The organization was widely known for its outstanding achievements. Nevertheless, within its community it was evaluated by many citizens in terms of the poor, ingracious service at the counter of the office of statistics and records.

Every public agency including the health department is the recipient of many complaints. From the point of view of public relations one of the worst things that can happen is for the public to feel that it is wasted effort to call any dissatisfaction or shortcoming to the attention of the organization. Errors of omission and commission are certain to occur to some degree, particularly in an agency that must deal with large numbers of people and problems. A forward-looking organization should welcome complaints from those whom it is supposed to serve since this is one way to evaluate and improve the program. Furthermore, to give the citizen the feeling that his complaint or criticism was justly and fairly received, considered, and investigated is one of the best ways of making him a community salesman for the department. Certain steps should be followed in handling complaints. The first is to assure the individual that the organization is willing and in fact anxious to hear what he has to say. Related to this is the important necessity of allowing the complainant to tell his complete story in his own words and as he sees it without excuses or alibis on the part of the listener. The next step is to check at once if possible whatever records exist that might substantiate, explain, or disprove the complaint; e.g. a complaint against the health department for failure to deliver a copy of a birth certificate sometimes may be resolved by immediately checking to see if the birth was registered in the first place. Following this there should be made a clear and understandable explanation of whatever contributory factors or circumstances relate to the situation and its solution. One failing of many health departments that conscientiously investigate complaints and make necessary corrections is to neglect making known what it has done, even to the complainant. People want to know what happened.

Field contacts made by representatives of the health department are subject to the same public relations influences as those that occur in the office. There should be evident a desire to help rather than to enforce or compel. The same care should be taken to make proper and effective referrals and to secure necessary follow-up. These are the things that decide the difference between cooperation and resistance or at best passive acquiescence. In addition there are certain public relations circumstances peculiar to field visits. Relatively few health departments have made any effort to give advance notice by mail or telephone of intended field visits by members of their staffs. Some may object to the procedure on the basis of cost or the possibility that some persons may attempt to forestall or avoid the contact. Against the first of these objections is the fact that notification by mail or telephone costs only a few cents, in contrast with an average cost of several dollars for a field visit. One of the most difficult administrative problems of a health agency is the reduction of unprofitable and costly field visits caused either by the patron not being at home or having moved elsewhere. Many fruitless visits may be avoided by a program of advance notice, and a considerable saving will result. As an example, an important aspect of the disease prevention program of the Detroit Department of Health has been educational home visits of public health nurses to parents of infants between 6 months and 1 year of age. A study of a sample of 14,028 nurses' visits showed that almost 30% were wasted. In 2,568 instances, or 18.3%, the family was not at home when the nurse arrived. In 1,511 instances, or 10.8%, the nurse found that the family had moved and could not be located. The procedure was instituted of preceding the first public health nursing

visit by a letter that explained the reason for the forthcoming visit and asked for confirmation of address and whether or not the child had already been immunized against certain diseases. By this means, not only was the percentage of "not home" visits reduced to 8.7%, but in addition 33.8% of the families who ordinarily would have been "unable to locate" were located by means of the mail-forwarding procedures of the postal department. Without presenting financial figures it is obvious that the procedure not only paid for itself but also resulted in a significant saving. In addition to the saving were the educational value of the letter and the preparation it gave for the nurse's subsequent entry into the home. In other words it was of good public relations value.

The validity of the objection to previsit contacting or notification that some people may be forewarned and thereby forestall or avoid the visit depends of course on the type and content of the correspondence or telephone conversation. If properly planned and conducted, it may in itself be of educational and public relations value and make the subsequent visit more acceptable and fruitful. Furthermore, it may be pointed out that citizens, particularly housewives and mothers, are frequently annoyed by nurses and other health department employees arriving when they are in the middle of their housework or caring for a child. A stated wish to avoid doing so is apt to bring about a more receptive feeling toward the health department.

Attention must be given by the health department to the frequency and multiplicity of calls. Even the most cooperative citizen becomes understandably and rightfully annoyed when health department employees arrive too often or more than one at a time. This indicates the desirability of some form of field activity coordinating device, something too frequently overlooked in health department practice. One manner in which some form of control may be exercised is by means of a central file in which are kept all records pertaining to each person, family, household, or premise. The checking out of a folder from the file indicates that some employee is presently engaged in some activity relating to the person or household.

One final remark concerning field visits has to do with the desirability whenever possible of following up the visit with some other type of contact to promote good continuing public relations. One suggestion is that each visitor, whether nurse, sanitarian, or other professional person, ask before leaving if there is anything pertaining to health or sanitation about which the householder would like further information, to be provided by a mailed brochure or a visit by some other employee of the health department.

Capability. A third characteristic of health department employees that influences the attitudes of the public is the extent to which they are able to demonstrate their knowledge and ability in the solution of problems with which they are faced. Little need be said with regard to this obvious requirement. Capable service breeds respect on the part of the public and their elected representatives. Continued capable professional service is the most potent safeguard against political interference. When it becomes obvious both to the public and to elected officials that here is a necessary and vital technical and professional job that requires trained and capable professional personnel, that personnel is most apt to be left alone to function.

Private life

In a certain sense public employees, particularly those in executive positions, have no private lives. Not only are they under constant scrutiny during working hours but also at all other times. Their behavior is always associated with their public positions, the citizenry always asking themselves, "Is this the kind of person I want as a health officer or public health nurse or sanitarian?" Often the public applies standards to public officials it is unwilling to apply to itself. The citizenry further tends to consider public officials and employees on call and personally accountable 24 hours of every day. "Isn't that what we taxpayers are paying them for?" This perhaps applies particularly to public health workers since

the nature of their responsibility implies a round-the-clock vigilance. With reference to personal habits and behavior, if the public employee feels that he must drink or engage in extrafamilial activities not generally accepted by society, he owes it to the organization for which he works to avoid open scandal. As Pfiffner[2] has stated, large numbers of influential citizens do not approve of the new freedom as to liquor and domestic relations. On the other hand, there are ways to do things without necessarily soliciting the attention of those who disapprove. To say this is not to suggest hypocrisy and subterfuge but simply to point out that it is the better part of discretion to avoid attracting public attention in such matters.

Public employees as social human beings have many off-the-job contacts with fellow citizens. These may occur in the home neighborhood, in churches, clubs, lodges, and many other occasions for social intercourse. In all such circumstances the health department worker should speak and behave in terms of the best possible representation of himself, his family, and his organization. In addition to strictly social contacts an important phase of off-the-job public relations is the participation of the health department worker in various civic and professional group activities. The health officer had best be an active member of the local and state medical societies. Similarly the other professional personnel should be active in their respective professional societies. Of a somewhat similar nature is the participation of public health personnel in chambers of commerce, councils of social agencies, service clubs, and the like. The individual employee must always realize that others may evaluate his organization through him. In relation to this subject, it is inadvisable for a public health worker to develop a reputation as a perennial joiner, handshaker, or backslapper. Membership in organizations should be judiciously and carefully decided. More than one prominent public servant has been embarrassed by association with politically or socially unsavory organizations. In most communities there exists one or two outstanding groups or organizations that are the most influential and professionally valuable. They do not always appear to be so on the surface. In one city it may be a women's club, in another an athletic club, and in a third it may be a voluntary tuberculosis and health association around which cluster the most prominent and influential citizens. The health officer and his co-workers would do well to evaluate the organizations in their community and ascertain if possible health department representation in each of the most significant groups.

Before leaving the subject of behavior in private life, some comment should be made concerning gifts or gratuities. A large segment of the public takes it for granted that public service is characterized by a strong inclination toward graft and corruption. Almost every health department employee in a position of any degree of authority is certain at one time or another to become aware of this. Restaurant owners will suggest free meals, and gifts of liquor, cigars, and other things will be offered. Such forms of apparent friendliness always carry some implication of future reciprocity. It is doubtful that any citizen likes a public servant so much that he will freely press him with gifts. Once an employee falls into this trap it is most difficult to escape. Few such gifts are worth the psychologic quandary that usually results. The best and only policy for the public health or other public worker to follow is consistent refusal accompanied by a pleasant explanation that the gift is not expected by the worker or allowed by the position.

Professional contacts

Telephone etiquette. Each day about 300 million telephone conversations are held in the United States. Most of these are in relation to business and public affairs. The possibility that both friends and enemies may be made over the telephone is often overlooked, many people apparently feeling that the absence of physical and visual contact allows a certain amount of leeway in behavior. It is an interesting psychologic fact that everyone engaged in a telephone conversation consciously or subconsciously visualizes the person with whom he is speaking. Employees therefore should approach telephone contacts in the same manner as all other types of contact. The rule suggested by telephone companies themselves is to "phone as you would be phoned to." The goal should be to make these contacts brief, friendly, and fruitful. Persons calling the organization should never be left holding a silent phone for any length of time. If a protracted delay is anticipated, the caller should be so notified and asked if he wishes to be called back later. Particularly annoying is the practice of having phone connections completed by one's secretary, who must then ask the person called to hold the line while the one placing the call is located. In other words, if you place a call, be immediately available when the connection is made.

In any type of contact the first words are of great importance in conditioning the tone of the entire relationship. This is particularly true of telephone contacts since the relationship is entirely auditory. When a call is received, the person called should identify the organization and perhaps himself in a pleasant and friendly tone of voice: "Jones County Health Department, Mr. Smith speaking." Or if a receptionist or information clerk answers, "Jones County Health Department, may I help you?" If the person placing the call neglects to state his name, it is proper to ask "May I ask who is calling?" rather than "Who are you?" or "What do you want?" No offense will be taken at the former statement, while the latter tend to make the backs of most people stiffen.

If the department is large enough to justify a private switchboard, the operators should be chosen with great care as in the case of information desk attendants. They must be quick and accurate, with a pleasant and even disposition, and have a complete knowledge of the organization and its personnel. All of these characteristics are necessary. I recall a delightful lady who operated the switchboard of a large health department with the greatest efficiency. She was always cheerful and had an uncanny knowledge of where everyone was and what they were doing. Her attitude had much to do with the development of public good-will for the department.

If an employee or a division is called by mistake, the courteous and wise thing to do is to assist the caller in making contact with the right person or the one who can best help him. Thus: "That problem is handled by the nursing division. If you wish, I will have your call transferred." If it is uncertain which unit or agency is indicated, the employee, in the interests of good public relations, should say: "I am sorry, but that is not handled by this division. I'll be happy to try to find out whom you should speak with and ask him to call you."

Courtesy demands that the person placing a call identify himself as soon as a connection is made. This should be immediately followed by a statement of the reason for the call, e.g., "This is Dr. James of the Jones County Health Department. May I speak with Mr. Smith?" The business at hand should then be discussed as briefly as possible, giving the other person a chance to express his opinion, and then the call should be terminated.

Correspondence. A significant proportion of the contacts of an organization occurs by means of correspondence. It is often overlooked that a piece of written or printed material may be as personal as an expression on a face or an inflection in a voice. Since friends and enemies may be made by a piece of paper, it is advisable that special attention be given to this important form of social and business intercourse. It is desirable therefore, that a health department establish a favorable organizational tone in its written contacts with the public rather than to leave the matter entirely to chance. There are several ways in which this may be accomplished. The organization should have a written standard practice with regard to incoming and outgoing correspondence with which all employees should become familiar. It should give consideration to matters of routing and handling of mail, restrictions concerning who in the organization should write what letters, priorities in answering, and even matters of phraseology. An important phase of correspondence control is to include instructions relating to it

in preservice and in-service training programs.

Insofar as possible letters should be personalized since the average recipient enjoys seeing his name in print. Certain words should be avoided as much as possible. Among these are "I," "we," "order," "must," and similar words implying egocentricity, compulsion, or command. By like token, "you," "your convenience," "your cooperation," and similar words and phrases should be stressed. The use of standardized, impersonal, printed form letters should be avoided. When there is indication for their use, e.g., when large numbers of persons must be contacted for the same reason, it is still possible to personalize the written contact. This may be accomplished by means of electric typewriters that operate automatically in a manner similar to a player piano. A master roll or tape is made that provides for the automatic typing of the routine parts of the letter. The machine stops automatically when certain personal items in the letter are reached so that names, birthdates, "he" or "she," "him" or "her" may be typed by hand or by means of a coordinated punched card. Thus it is possible to write a letter that is both standardized and personalized.

Studies have indicated a significantly greater response to this type of written approach which, while slightly higher in cost per letter, is well worth the difference in terms of results.

Employee training

It has been indicated that good public relations do not just happen. They result only from a planned program of employee training and example. It does little good for a few at the top to formulate techniques and programs to promote good feeling on the part of the public if the rank and file of the employees of the organization are not involved. If they are not provided with opportunity to develop feelings of pride and loyalty toward the organization, if they are kept in the dark with regard to the program and its progress, if they are not taken into at least the general confidence of the organization concerning plans and aims for the future, and if they are not impressed with and shown the importance of each of their contacts with the public, the organization cannot hope to achieve an atmosphere, employee borne, that speaks for good public relations.

Some industrial concerns have found it much to their advantage to pursue a consistent employee training program for public relations. One of the most outstanding of these is the program of the Bell Telephone Company, which is well worth a few sentences of description. Before they report for work, all persons employed receive a manual by mail entitled *You are the Company*. On reporting for work the new employee is assigned to a school for an induction course that has three phases. First, the employee is told about the electrical and communications industry as a whole. Then he is told about the company for which he is going to work. Finally, he is told about the department in which he is going to work and the job he is going to do and its relation to the company, the industry, and society. Following this he begins training to enable him to master all the technical details of his specific work. Finally, he is rated periodically by his instructors and office managers at the end of the first, third, sixth, and twelfth month. It is of interest that one phase of the customer interview rating procedure used by Bell Telephone Company is controlled by the employee himself. He records transactions and listens to the playback, comparing them with standard records. He may stop or start or discard records, depending only upon his wish. After he has listened to a recorded transaction, he is allowed to dispose of the record.

Programs and techniques such as these are well worth trial and development by public health agencies. Certainly every health department employee should be made to feel that he is taking part in much more than a means to a personal livelihood. If he feels this, and it can result only from planning and encouragement from the top of the organization, his contacts with the public are certain to be more satisfactory.

Quarters and equipment

As the appearance of the health department employees is important, so too is the appearance of their quarters and equipment. One of the most unfortunate characteristics of official health agencies is that they are so often forced to be satisfied with physical facilities left over after the needs and wishes of the other branches of government have been satisfied. For many years the physical appearance of many health departments was the antithesis of what they attempted to preach and, even more serious, of what they demanded of others. Under the circumstances there is little wonder that many people do not take too seriously the proposals of health departments. To require that others be what one is not oneself is hardly conducive to good public relations.

Fortunately the situation has been undergoing considerable improvement. Many local health departments have moved into quarters similar to those occupied by business organizations. An increasing number are housed in buildings designed especially as health centers. This trend has been significantly aided by the Hill-Burton Act and more recently by the Hill-Harris Act, which provide matching federal funds for this purpose. In addition to going far to provide health departments with community dignity and respect, these trends have the added value of removing the public health agency from physical connection and therefore association with the centers of partisan politics and all they represent in the public's mind.

A few specific details are worthy of mention in connection with the reactions of the public. Health in the public's mind is intimately associated with cleanliness. This being the case, the premises of the health department, of all agencies, should be clean and bright. Soap and paint alone considerably improve even the oldest quarters. If there is any question, attention is directed to the remarkable change that has taken place in the appearance of gasoline stations, earth-moving equipment, heavy-duty trucks, and the like during the past decade. If they can look neat, so too can a health department. If at all possible, dark woodwork and dark heavy furnishings should be avoided. The present trend in office architecture is away from a multitude of stuffy poorly lighted cubicles toward the open-office type of layout. An increasing number of private agencies even place important executives in large open areas, set apart perhaps by a railing. It is thought that this general plan is conducive both to better personnel morale and efficiency and to better public relations since the visitor receives a strong impression of serious business activity.

As few movable items as possible should be kept on the top of desks. In fact it is stated with good reason that only papers and other items in immediate use should be visible at any given time. In this regard a modern filing system contributes importantly to the general air of neatness and lack of confusion as well as to efficiency. It should always be remembered, however, that files are business tools, and not completely enclosed wastebaskets simply for the purpose of getting things out of sight.

AVENUES OF PUBLICITY

In any society in which they are available the formal channels of community communication play a very important role in public relations. Predominant among these communication channels are the press, radio, and television.

The press

One of the most important phases of public relations deals with how to obtain and retain the cooperation of those who command the channels to community public opinion. Outstanding among these are the representatives of the press. There are in the United States over 2,000 daily and 10,000 weekly newspapers that blanket the population. Rare indeed are individuals who do not have some contact with the product of the press. An ever present problem facing the health officer is how to reconcile his interests and those of the newspaper published in his jurisdiction. As one authority[3] has pictured it, the ideal situation would be one in which the press and the institutions in the community would have similar noble interests and in which the press could fulfill all the varying demands of all the community's institutions. No such situation exists, however, for there are no perfect newspapers with perfect pub-

lishers, editors, and reporters, and there are no perfect directors of community institutions. It is from these imperfections and also from healthy, honest differences of opinion regarding the nature of community institutions and their proper place that problems in press relations arise. It must be realized that publishing a newspaper is a big business and that each paper has a policy regarding what it considers to be news and what it will publish. That policy, while colored somewhat by altruism, idealism, and civic interest, in most instances is determined primarily by what the publisher thinks the public wants to read, which will therefore sell more newspapers and thereby attract more advertising. The average newspaper will be inclined to print material relating to health and to the health department only if it feels that it is in and of the public interest.

It must also be remembered that the press is traditionally a critic of government and its agencies. Fortunately in most instances this critical attitude is potential since the press generally offers strong support to what it considers a good government or a good health department. Nevertheless, because it regards a government, a public health department, or any other public agency as potentially inadequate and their personnel as potentially self-seeking, the press is constantly alert, acting as the guardian of the public interest.

Each newspaper has it own style that has been developed over a period of time. It has been developed for the purpose of reader appeal. In order to accomplish its purpose the newspaper must write in a manner simple and interesting enough to appeal to the largest possible number of the people. This means that technical and scientific information must be translated into simple language than can be understood by the average or subaverage person. General, tedious, verbose statements must give way to sharp, precise, concise, and specific information readily applicable to the reader. It is true that sometimes emphases are changed and important points missed, but by and large the press has proved itself amazingly competent in getting rather complex ideas across to the average citizen.

A particular newspaper style is not something that the health department employee can expect to master overnight.

Because of this and in the interests of good press relations it is best that the public health worker respect the newspaper man as a specialist in his field. Therefore it is worth while to consider the following suggestions from an experienced newspaperman to public officials.[4] These suggestions resulted from years of practical experience and contact with public agencies.

1. If I were a city official, I would have a clearly defined and systematic policy in all press relations. I would either supervise execution of such policies myself or have a responsible person, preferably with a knowledge of news and reporting techniques, do so under my direction. I would not deny reporters access to department heads but I would consult with the latter from time to time on matters of policy in regard to their own press relations.

2. I would, after this policy is clearly understood, arrange conferences with the publishers and city editors of each of the local newspapers. I would ask their advice on how to clear the news for their convenience, and how to make that news accurately reflect the best values in public administration. I would discuss the result of these conferences with the reporter on my beat and get his reaction to them. He is my daily contact; I would never make him feel I was "going over his head."

3. I would arrange a convenient, regular "press conference" time to see all newspapermen, although I would never deny any one of them admittance at any time.

4. I would develop my own "nose for news." If I found it necessary to make off-the-record statements, I would be sure the reporter understood at the outset that I was talking off-the-record. I would be free and helpful to reporters in their news-gathering jobs and answer all questions I thought fair and proper. If I could not answer a question, I would, if possible, explain why. If a reporter were after a story which would be detrimental to good government if announced prematurely, I would tell him all the facts on that story, appealing to his sense of fair play in holding it. However, I would promise his paper an equal "news break" when that story was ready.

5. I would see that news breaks were distributed as evenly as possible between the morning and evening papers. If I talked to competitive reporters individually I would be careful to give each exactly the same story.

6. I would not exaggerate the occasional petty criticisms that newspapers print so long as my general press relations were good.

7. If a "news leak" occurred and the report, because of inadequate information, was misinterpreted, I would call in newsmen and explain the proper interpretation to them.

8. I would ask editors to give me a fair chance to answer critical "letters-to-the-editor" in the same column printing such letters.

9. I would insist that all municipal and departmental reports designed for public reading be written in terms understandable to the layman, with the qualities of clarity, simplicity, and directness, and with a format that would make people, including newspapermen, want to read them.

10. On major public reports I would make the matter available to reporters from time to time before the report itself is actually published, if that is possible. These releases would be carefully timed. I would point out to the reporter the significance of more complicated passages in these reports and interpret them so he could write accurate and intelligent stories. I would also point out to him the infinite possibilities in various departments for news features and special Sunday articles. I would help him to get pictures for such articles.

11. I would prepare releases or formal written statements only on those stories of important policy where misconceptions or misquotes might result. Newspapers generally prefer to do their own local stories in their own way, and if I have the right to contact with them I can explain any story clearly.

12. I would look upon newspaper people as intelligent men engaged in a reputable work, and I would instruct all department heads and employees to treat them with respect and courtesy.

13. Finally, I would make the newspaper an effective instrument in accounting to the public for my stewardship, and I would keep in mind the significant motto of a great newspaper chain: "Give light and the people will find their way."

A number of additional hints may be made with regard to relationships with the press. Occasionally public health workers, particularly some health officers, have a tendency to irritate if not insult reporters and editors by adopting a superior professional air. Overly impressed by their own apparent importance, their attitude is one of suspicious condescension. Much more is to be gained by accepting the newspaperman as an equal. The public health director can often profit from the advice and criticism of the reporters assigned to his beat. They and their editors can often give invaluable advice regarding public feeling, anticipated reactions, and timing of reports and announcements. It is much better to follow their opinions in these matters than to demand arbitrarily that a certain item appear on the front page of this evening's paper.

Articles should emphasize problems, programs, and the organization, not the individual. Both the press and the public soon tire of the health worker who appears to want his name in every issue of every paper. Share the credit; stress the organization. In submitting copy the customs and requirements of the trade should be followed. Material should be typed double-spaced on one side of the paper only, with extra space at the top of the first page for placement of a headline. Let the reporter reword, revise, and cut the material and write his own headline. These are his professional prerogatives that allow for individuality and pride in his work. The best safeguard against errors in reporting and headlining is to state and emphasize clearly the basic idea to be communicated. Advance copies of announcements, speeches, or articles are always appreciated by busy reporters and editors. They should not be expected, however, to use all material submitted. After all the newspaper is theirs, and so should be the choice of material.

Persons writing copy should guard against verbosity. We each tend to feel that what interests us must naturally interest everyone and that every word we take the trouble to write is worth everyone's time. Newspaper writing and for that matter newspaper reading are specialized forms of writing and reading. News items must be presented "in a nutshell," for that is the form in which the newspaper reader wants them. Feature articles are seldom read in toto. Brevity and conciseness therefore are the characteristics to be sought. A page and a half, double-spaced, is a moderately long story; two typewritten pages are too long for most purposes; three and a half pages make a whole column and except in most unusual circumstances are an imposition upon any editor.

Care must be given to impartiality in the handing out of newsworthy stories. Papers and editors are in competition with each other and naturally resent signs of favoritism. One of the first things a public health worker should do on beginning work in a new community is to make a complete list of all papers published in the area. Those most apt to be overlooked are the county papers in contrast with those published in the county seat, weeklies as against dailies, and foreign-language papers. The latter are of particular importance in many metropolitan cities that contain large numbers of non-English-speaking residents.

A final suggestion to be made in the interest of improved press and therefore public relations is that consideration occasionally be given to inviting reporters and editors to "come and see." If an opportunity is provided for them to visit the various activities of the health department and to take part in field trips and other in-service training activities, benefits will be reflected in better appreciation and reporting.

Audiovisual methods

No one medium of publicity can be used to the exclusion of all others. While the press is unquestionably of great importance, it is often credited with more power and influence by the general public and many organizations than most editors and reporters would privately give it. As some newspapermen have pointed out, if the press does appear to have more power and influence than any other community institution, it is probably because the other channels of publicity and public education have been neglected. One probable reason for this neglect is that these other approaches are not as easy to use as is the press. They are more expensive, require more specialized skills and equipment within the health department, and are more time consuming because they require planning, rehearsing, or construction. Yet it must be realized that the press is applicable only to certain problems and even then only serves one phase of the total publicity. The same of course is true of all avenues of approach to the public. Thus an important program may be announced through the press, on the radio, on posters, or in organized meetings. The actual launching of the program may be accomplished by exhibits, leaflets, demonstrations, and personal visits. Finally, there must be publicity follow-up, presenting the progress and results of the program.

Among the audiovisual approaches to the public, radio and television are perhaps the most important. Most stations feel some responsibility for public welfare and improvement. In order to meet this responsibility they follow the policy of setting aside a portion of their air time for public service programs, among which may be some dealing with public health and the health department. There are certain reservations with regard to the value of such programs. In the first place the time periods that radio and television stations donate are most apt to have low listener ratings. This is understandable since after all the stations are in a costly business and naturally reserve their most valuable time for the profitable commercially sponsored programs, particularly broadcasts over nationwide hookups. Another handicap is that the writing and presentation of satisfactory programs is a highly technical and fairly expensive job and not one for amateurs. There is a tendency on the part of many professional people, including those engaged in public health work, to feel that everyone is ready and willing to listen to them. They overlook the fact that radio and television developed primarily as entertainment media and that the busy housewife or the tired workingman is not particularly interested in avidly following the serious opinions of a public health worker presented more often than not as a monotonous monologue. To insist and persist in the presentation of such performances is poor public relations to say the least. The average member of the listening public, if he happens to hear the program at all, is most apt to turn the program off. In order to do even that involves interruption and physical effort that the average listener is apt to resent.*

Despite this, radio and television may oc-

*For one interesting analysis, see *Radio Listening Habits of Mothers Who Attend Well Baby Clinics* by Murray and Turner.[5]

cupy real places in the educational and public relations programs of the health department. In order to do so, careful planning and judicious use are required. The very fact that it is primarily a means of entertainment may be used to advantage. Many people simply turn a good program on and leave it on, tolerating short commercial or spot announcements with the knowledge that in a few minutes another entertaining program will be forthcoming. It is suggested therefore that more consideration be given to the use of spot announcements by health departments.

Beyond these short attention-getting auditory contacts that are essentially of a sensitizing nature, health departments may find value in certain types of longer programs of 15 or 30 minutes' duration. They should not, however, take the form of talks or addresses. Instead the patterns long since proven of value in other fields should be adapted. Certain types of audiences are attracted by quiz programs, others by round-table or town-hall types of discussion. For many listeners the drama has great appeal. In any case the total program should be planned and written by professional producers and writers and if possible presented by professional actors. The period of the novelty of television is past. The role it will play eventually in social and cultural life is not yet fully determined. Already, however, it has brought about very real changes, some desirable and others not desirable, in family life. Indications are that it will become a significant means of public education as well as entertainment. In fact it may eventually replace in large measure not only radio and motion pictures but also to some degree the newspapers. Many health departments in urban centers are using it as an effective means of health education of the public.

Other media of public relations as well as educational value are exhibits, public talks, and such miscellaneous approaches as billboards, filmstrips, streetcar and bus advertisements, throwaways, "comic" books, and paid advertising. Each of these may be made to serve particular purposes and to reach certain groups. No one of them is an end in itself but must be a part of and tied in with a larger overall program. If poorly done, they do much more harm than good and should therefore be carefully planned and evaluated.

Many public health officials attach considerable importance to their annual reports as implements for the development and maintenance of good public relations. Annual reports may be made to serve this useful purpose, but there is cause for serious doubt that they actually do in most instances. It is the uncomfortable truth that, from the viewpoints of both content and format, most health departments' annual reports make very poor reading. Financed usually by inadequate funds, they are often poorly printed on cheap paper and consist largely of a series of disconnected reports from each of the functional units of the organization and are illustrated merely by uninteresting columns of statistics plus perhaps the photographs of the members of the board.

An interesting and pertinent analysis of municipal public reports was made by the editors of *Public Management* in 1938[6]. Their criticisms, which deserve serious consideration by public health workers, may be summarized as follows:

1. Complete failure to make any kind of report
2. Extensive use of uninterpreted statistics
3. Use of graphs and statistics that may be falsely interpreted
4. Use of superfluous statistics unrelated to any purpose or accomplishment
5. Poor makeup, arrangement, paper, type, and printing, and poor or no illustrations
6. Lengthy financial statements of interest only to a few individuals
7. Disconnected combining of a collection of unrelated divisional or departmental reports rather than the synthesis of one general overall report.

The distribution of annual reports presents a problem in itself. The typical situation is one in which a few thousand are printed and copies sent to the members of the board of health, city councilmen or county supervisors, prominent citizens, representatives of voluntary health and social agencies, and fellow public health workers elsewhere in the country. In many instances a sizable proportion of the edition rests in a storeroom to await some future housecleaning. The point of significance is that rarely is a copy seen by the average citizen. This gives rise to the question whether or not the annual report should be regarded at all as an education tool or a public relations technique. There appears to be a growing opinion in public health circles that the essential purposes and objectives of an annual report should be redefined. This opinion is given substance by the trend toward fulfilling legal requirements by submitting typewritten or mimeographed descriptive and statistical reports to city or county officials, conserving other efforts and funds for attractive picture-magazine types of publications designed specifically for wide public appeal and distribution.

COMMUNITY GROUPS

Most citizens of civilized society live two lives—one as individuals, the other as members of groups. Aristotle had this in mind when he observed that the man who can live without society is either a beast or a god. Furthermore, even among primitive people a single group seldom if ever satisfies. Thus there may be found the family group, the clan or tribal group, the secret male societies, the religious groups, to mention but a few. This is the basis for the statement that there is no such thing as one public but that every community consists of many publics, each with its own characteristics. These community groups or publics manifest themselves in most instances in some form of organization. Advantage may be and should be taken by public health officials of the existence of these organizations since they serve the triple functions of channels, audiences, and sounding boards. It therefore is important for those in responsible public health positions to establish and maintain close and friendly relationships with those in command of these valuable channels. Such relationship is dependent upon three things: mutual interest, mutual understanding, and mutual respect.

It should be realized that public health agencies do not operate in a vacuum. Problems of public health are related to many other community problems. In other words many other individuals in the community have public health as a subsidiary professional or occupational interest. The personnel of official public health agencies therefore should be constantly on the lookout for other community programs, agencies, organizations, or groups to which public health interest can be related. There should be a deliberate effort to make public health problems their problems.

While no single approach is universally applicable, there are a few planned or formal steps that may be taken to achieve greater success. It is suggested that there be compiled a list of all groups or organizations known to exist in the community. This list in many cases will be lengthy and may include some listings that will never be of value. Nevertheless it is well to have the information ready at hand in case it is needed. A few of the many categories of groups and organizations under which listings should be made are political, religious, racial, nationality, educational, professional, occupational, social, financial, and fraternal.

There are certain characteristics of organized community groups that must be kept in mind. It should be remembered that each is usually built around some special interests. Therefore if the list that is suggested takes the form of a private file, notations may well be made of any pertinent items of information relating to leadership, influence, age and social representation, chief and subsidiary interests, prejudices, and the like. This specialization referred to influences the fraction of the population that is attracted to membership in each organization. Yet, membership not infrequently overlaps several groups. Thus the same individuals may be found in the Eagles fraternal society who are also members of various labor unions. The Parent-Teachers Association may often have many members in common with the League of Women Voters and the Association of University Women. Because of this, if a group cannot be reached through one organiza-

tion, they may often be approached through one or two others. Significantly, members of city councils, state legislatures, or county boards may frequently be contacted under desirable circumstances through service clubs and other community organizations.

It should also be realized that the majority of service, social, and business clubs and organizations represent the more favored in the community. As a result they may be excellent for prestige and influencing public opinion but poor for obtaining direct results. This brings us to the most difficult aspect of the problem. Despite what was said concerning man's need for society, it is a curious fact that a large proportion of the population of any community does not appear to belong to any organized community group. Several studies have been made of the subject. One of the most complete was conducted in Springfield, Mass., in the mid-1940's. It was found that in that community almost two thirds of the population appeared on the surface to belong to no organized group, including churches and labor groups. It is certain that the proportion is subject to considerable variation and it is probable that two thirds is unusually high. Nevertheless it is of significance that those in the community who are in greatest need are usually those not included in an organized group. In other words the people who do not come to meetings or participate are the very ones who need the help.

In planning a program or activity the public health worker should be systematic in his analysis of the community groups and organizations that may be involved. It is suggested that the following lists be made:

1. A list of the problems of the community and of the health department
2. A list of each group of the population affected by each problem
3. A list of all individuals, groups, agencies, and organizations that also may be concerned with or interested in each problem and that therefore may be considered a potential source of help
4. From the foregoing, a list of methods or channels of attack

A program for the control of venereal diseases may serve as an example. The first three lists might appear in summary somewhat as follows:

Problems of the community and the health department

Incidence	Rehabilitation
Case finding	Education
Control of infectious individuals	Etc.
Treatment	

Groups affected

Young adults	Infants
Low-income groups	Prostitutes
Newlyweds	Etc.

Groups, individuals, agencies, and organizations concerned

Health department	Industry
Private physicians	Family and other social
Private laboratories	service agencies
Hospitals	Welfare agencies
Pharmacists	Recreation agencies
Police	Housing agencies
Schools	Etc.
Churches	

In view of the foregoing, it is possible to classify community groups and organizations according to their representation and potential use. The following is one such suggested classification that may be of value in planning and conducting the public relations and education programs of health departments.

   I. Top level (for prestige, political, professional, and financial support)
>   Governmental officials—elected and employed
>   Medical and other professions
>   Business and industry
>   Influential citizens

  II. Middle level (for influencing opinions of large key citizen groups)
>   PTA
>   A.A.U.W.
>   Labor unions
>   Grange, etc.

 III. Lower level (for neighborhood or individual contacts)
>   Local churches
>   Athletic clubs
>   Fraternal organizations
>   Veterans organizations
>   Block clubs
>   "Grass roots" clubs, etc.

 IV. Schools (too often overlooked as important to public relations program)

Several of the categories are worthy of special mention. The health officer has an important public relations job with regard to elected governmental officers and to his fellow public officials. Above all he must impress the elected representatives of the people with his practicality. In order to do this he must have some understanding of the total problem of civic government and management with which these representatives are faced. This may be exemplified in a negative sense by occasional county health officers who have read in a book that a health department budget should be of a certain magnitude. Lacking an appreciation of the limited tax resources of county governments and of the existence of outside potential sources of funds, they may make a request to their county supervisors for a local budgetary appropriation equivalent to most of the county income. From then on the members of the county government will look upon the health officer as ignorant of the facts of life.

In Chapter 25 the relationship between the medical profession and the health department with regard to medical care is discussed. It may be well to point out here that the achievement and maintenance of good relationships with this particularly important group depends upon observance of a number of considerations. Private physicians and the professions and institutions related to them have the same ultimate objective as public health agencies—that of raising the level of health of the people. Often attention must be called to this fact. Few things will contribute as much to obtaining the support of the medical profession as competent performance on the part of the health officer and his staff. In the past health departments have not always enjoyed good standing with the medical profession because members of their staffs have not been competently trained. This situation is undergoing rapid change. It is important that the health officer keep the medical group informed with regard to new programs that the health department is planning or is ready to inaugurate. If a physician in practice hears for the first time from some other source that the health department is going to do something, he will very probably react critically. If, on the other hand, he and his fellow practitioners have been taken into the confidence of the health officer, if his advice and opinions have been solicited, and best of all if he has been involved in the planning, he will most likely be cooperative.

As mentioned earlier, the health officer should preferably be a member of the local medical society and if possible an active member of its public health committee. He should if possible serve as secretary or some other officer of the organization. Adequate medical representation on boards of health and advisory committees is naturally important. Wherever possible and convenient, meetings of the medical society should be held occasionally in the health department quarters. If the department sponsors clinics, an attempt should be made to have the medical work performed by private physicians on a part-time or hourly fee basis. In that way, especially if the work is rotated among all the practitioners, they will become more familiar with the purposes and programs of the health department and will feel a personal interest and involvement in it. Finally, when the health officer and his department receive credit or praise, e.g., in the form of an award for service, the praise and credit should be freely shared with the medical profession as well as any other groups in the community that may have played a contributing role.

Before leaving the subject of public relations, reference should be made to public opinion polls. Frequently it is desirable to determine the attitude of the public toward particular problems and activities. This is practically a virgin field of public relations activity as far as public health agencies are concerned and one which should bear many fruits if properly utilized. It would seem possible for health departments through the efforts of their staffs to develop modest but effective sampling systems for this purpose. In addition to aiding in the planning of programs in a manner to which the public is receptive, the technique would undoubtedly cause many citizens to feel that the health department is truly concerned with their opinions and interests.*

There is one final method of positive publicity and public relations that is readily at hand yet usually overlooked—the employees of the public health agency itself. If each employee is kept currently informed about problems, programs, activities, and goals, and is actively encouraged to served as a purveyor of information, a very significant proportion of the public may be reached both directly and indirectly. Consider, for example, a city of 1 million persons. Its public health department may have a total of 400 employees. It is certainly not unreasonable to expect that each one has a circle of relatives and close friends totaling an average of about 25 persons. For the entire group this means about 10,000 persons, or 1% of the population, within easy potential reach. A rather good lawn would result from such a seeding! This emphasizes again the intimate interrelationship of the various aspects of public health administration, in this case, the relationship between personnel development and public relations.

---

*For examples of the application of this technique to public health, see *The Modern Public Opinion Poll* by Guernsey[7] and *Public Opinion Measurement as an Instrument in Public Health Practice* by Calver and Otis.[8]

REFERENCES

1. Harral, S.: Winning community confidence through public relations, Education **61**:168, Nov. 1940.
2. Pfiffner, J. McD.: Public administration, New York, 1946, The Ronald Press Co.
3. Maurer, W. H.: Public relations and the press. Talk presented at an in-service training course on public relations, School of Public Health, University of Michigan, Oct. 8, 1945.
4. Hazelrigg, H.: A newspaper man looks at city hall, Public Manage. **20**:67, Mar. 1938.
5. Murray, M. L., and Turner, C. E.: Radio listening habits of mothers who attend well baby clinics, Amer. J. Public Health **33**:952, Aug. 1943.
6. Editorial: Seven more sins, Public Manage. **20**:33, Feb. 1938.
7. Guernsey, P. D.: The modern public opinion poll, Amer. J. Public Health **32**:973, Sept. 1942.
8. Calver, H. N., and Otis, T. W., Jr.: Public opinion measurement as an instrument in public health practice, Amer. J. Public Health **37**:426, Apr. 1947.

Part IV

Substance of
public health

Although the chapters of this section are devoted essentially to a consideration of the activities commonly pursued by public health agencies, an appreciation by the reader of the point of view from which they are discussed is requested. A deliberate and not necessarily easy attempt has been made to avoid descriptive details of program content and technical procedures. These change too rapidly and relate more to practice and techniques than to administration. Each of the several fields generally discussed has merited numerous textbooks that provide much more adequately than is possible here the various program details and procedures. The intention here has been therefore to limit discussion as much as possible to some of the administrative considerations involved in each of the various components of the public health program. The presentation is necessarily incomplete, which in a sense is perhaps desirable if it serves to provoke discussion or even disagreement.

Viewed as a whole, public health activities now appear to fall into three broad categories or groups: (1) those concerned with the protection and care of the individual, (2) those that focus particularly upon factors in the environment that may be inimical to man, and (3) the variety of services provided by a variety of disciplines or professions in support of the first two categories.

Chapter 17

Control
of
communicable diseases*

Since this book deals primarily with the administrative phases of public health and since there are many excellent texts on the clinical aspects of the various communicable diseases, this chapter will present only certain broad aspects of the subject, particularly those concerned with administrative control measures. Some may question the need to devote much attention to the communicable diseases in view of the dramatic reduction of their incidence in many parts of the world. It is a false hope that man will ever be free from the threat of bacterial or viral infection—new or old. Complacency will lead with certainty to recrudescence of problems. At hand are examples of the resurgence of the venereal diseases and the slowing of the rate of decline of tuberculosis. Not without great significance is the compression of travel time combined with the massive movements of people for business, vacation, and military reasons. I have before me a current news report of the first instance in 42 years of a case of bubonic plague in the United States. Also before me is a departmental report noting epidemiologic surveillance visits made in Detroit during 1 week to a new case and a new carrier of typhoid fever, to an individual who has had contact with leprosy, to several persons from areas with cholera and smallpox, and to a number of returned servicemen who have acquired malaria.

It is assumed that the public health student or worker will be taking or will have taken courses in communicable diseases and epidemiology that present the details. Accordingly, the following should in no sense be considered a short course in itself or a substitute for more detailed study but should be regarded merely as a general introduction to certain aspects of the subject.

BIOLOGIC SIGNIFICANCE OF INFECTION

At first glance it may seem extraneous to discuss the essential meaning of infection. However, although we may be members of advanced societies, we are nevertheless influenced to a surprising degree by many elemental emotions and superstitions. We may strive to convince ourselves and others that we are different from the other creatures of the earth. Insofar as possible we consciously or subconsciously attempt to avoid recognition of the fact that we share with all living things certain fundamental needs, desires, and drives, i.e., the need for food and shelter, the desire for personal survival, and the drive for perpetuation of our kind.

Any approach to the communicable diseases and their control should be based upon a frank recognition and understand-

*For an excellent background discussion of this subject, see *The History of American Epidemiology* by Top et al.[1]

ing of these ecologic facts. It must be realized that the microorganisms that cause disease in man have no innate malevolence toward him, but in their struggle for survival and perpetuation have found in his body a convenient stepping-stone and have adapted their biology accordingly. By like token it may be said that man himself, probably more than any other species, has contrived in his adaptation to take advantage of many other living creatures, extending in kind from the myriad of microorganisms that exist in his intestinal tract and assist him in his digestive process to the fish, fowl, and cattle that give him sustenance and the beasts that bear his burdens.

By far the most desirable situation for a microorganism is one in which it lives in nonfatal harmony with the other creatures upon or within which it exists. For a microorganism to so evolve that its multiplication results in the demise of its host represents perhaps the ultimate in biologic failure; by killing its host, it kills itself. The anthrax bacillus, for example, depending upon multiplication in the bloodstream of its human host, completely defeats its purpose when it kills its host and thereby traps itself within the dead body, whence only with great difficulty it can be transmitted to others. If for the purpose of discussion we were to assume the tuberculosis organism to be endowed with some form of intelligence, it might be said that the more astute of its kind would be content with produc-

ing only moderate degrees of tuberculosis. By allowing its host to continue unsuspectingly his customary life, the organism assures itself not only of continued existence but also of ample opportunity for further transfer and perpetuation. In a biologic sense the more virulent and more toxic strains that kill and kill quickly also represent impatient and overambitious biologic failures.

GENERAL REQUISITES FOR MICROORGANIC SURVIVAL

In order for a microorganism that has involved itself in a biologic relationship with man to survive successfully a certain chain of circumstances or events must be followed (Fig. 17-1). As long as a parasitic microorganism is entirely confined within its definitive host it can in no way offer an immediate threat to other potential hosts. Many examples of this may be cited. Except for certain stages of the disease it causes, the spirochete of syphilis is completely contained within the body of its host, who, although actually infected, cannot transmit the disease. Similar to this in the field of protozoology is the malarial parasite, which except for relatively short intervals is nontransmissible.

The necessity for the parasite to leave the host implies a mode of exit. This is not as simple as it sounds since each parasitic microorganism has adaptively restricted itself to a few paths and often one particular

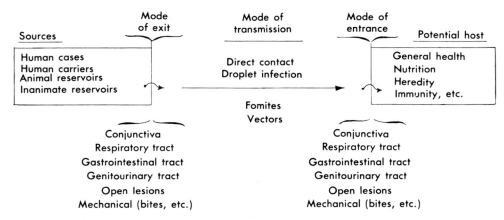

Fig. 17-1. Sequence of events in transmission of diseases.

path. Thus the parasite of malaria is restricted to egress through the skin of its host and even then only at certain phases of its life cycle. Except for biologic accidents the spirochete of syphilis, because of overspecialization that has resulted in marked frailty, must rely upon exit through the sexual organs of humans, which in the process of their use provide the spirochete with the maximum protection against its most lethal natural hazard, i.e., drying. A great many parasitic species have so adapted themselves that the nose and throat offer the most expeditious exit. Still others rely essentially upon the discharges of the gastrointestinal tract. If in some way the typhoid bacillus were suddenly to decide upon the skin or genitalia as a means of exit, it would in all probability cease to be a threat to man. All external parts of the human body, including of course the openings of the respiratory, genitourinary, and gastrointestinal tracts, serve as sites of exit for various microorganisms that affect man. Obviously the more limited the means of egress, the greater the opportunity for successful control, at least in a theoretical sense.

The picture becomes greatly complicated, however, by certain other biologic and cultural aspects of human existence. Thus, although for all practical purposes the spirochete of syphilis has restricted itself to a single mode of exit, successful control or elimination of the disease is more easily proposed than accomplished. In theory syphilis could be completely eradicated by prohibiting all human sexual intercourse. Such a prohibition, however, even if tolerated, would in turn eliminate man himself. This being impractical, it therefore becomes necessary to find some other approach to the problem. Theoretically typhoid fever and many related diseases could be eradicated by complete control over the defecatory functions and habits of man. This function, however, is essential to continued human existence, and the regulation of it is no mean task considering its involvement in various superstitions, social attitudes, and agricultural economies. Therefore it must be borne in mind continually

that the theoretically ideal or obvious approach to the control of a communicable disease is not necessarily practical or successful. The indirect attack is often the most fruitful. Furthermore in many instances the greatest handicaps to control are factors relating to man himself rather than to the pathogen.

On gaining exit the parasitic organism must find some means of transportation to the body of a new potential host. Here again, depending upon the biologic characteristics of the particular pathogenic organism, the method of this transfer is limited to a certain one or few ways. Some organisms, e.g., the syphilis spirochete, require very direct and intimate conditions of transfer. Certain others, of which those causing malaria and yellow fever are examples, must rely for transfer not only on another living thing such as a mosquito but even only on certain species of that insect. Many organisms, however, have made themselves more adaptable and have allowed for relatively prolonged existence outside the human host and for transfer in any one of a number of ways. The typhoid bacillus can be cited as an example.

Even when the proximity of a potential host is gained, successful transfer of infection does not necessarily follow. The pathogen must now find a biologically suitable mode of entrance. The limitations surrounding this requirement are similar to those that relate to the mode of exit. To be successful the choice must conform with the adaptive processes through which the organisms, both parasite and man, have gone. Generally speaking, but by no means exclusively, the mode of entrance is the same as the mode of exit, e.g., the diphtheria organism leaves and enters through the nasopharynx, the tuberculosis organism through the respiratory tract, the typhoid organism through the gastrointestinal tract, and the malarial organism through the pierced skin.

Finally, a number of factors come into play in deciding whether or not the parasite that has gained entrance is going to be successful in remaining and thriving. Among the most important of these may be mentioned the general state of health and nutrition of the host, the presence or absence of immune bodies, and the virulence and toxicity of the parasite. Because of the future need of the parasite to continue still further beyond the present host, consideration must be given to some other characteristics of the host. For example, the typhoid organism is most successful if it achieves infection of a food-handler or of someone who is indiscriminate in his defecatory habits. Its chances of future success are considerably limited when it finds itself within a business or professional person who works and lives according to a social pattern that

provides obstacles to further transfer. Gonococcal infection of the eyes of a newborn child does not nearly parallel the degree of success from the point of view of the gonococcus that is represented in the infection of a prostitute. In the first instance the organism has been sidetracked. Likewise infection of an individual about to move to a mosquito-free area is largely wasted effort on the part of the malarial organism.

Each one of the steps mentioned represents a necessary link in the chain of disease perpetuation. By like token each represents a point at which control measures

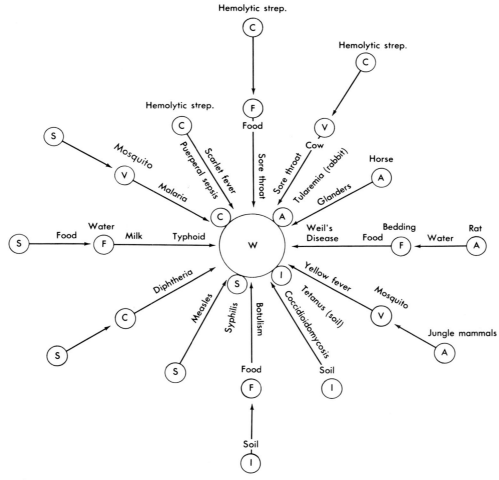

Fig. 17-2. Modes of spread of communicable disease. Symbols: *W*, Well human; *S*, sick infected human; *C*, well infected human (carrier); *F*, inanimate transmitter (fomite); *V*, animate transmitter (vector); *A*, animate reservoir; *I*, inanimate reservoir.

may be applied. The chain is only as strong as its weakest link, and the successful severance of any one link will go far in controlling and in some instances completely eradicating particular diseases.

This concept may be approached in still another way. In Fig. 17-2 the well person, represented by [W], is the center of potential attack by many types of organisms in many different ways. He finds in his environment a number of factors that threaten him: [S] clinically ill and infected humans; [C] apparently well but infected human carriers; [F] inanimate transmitters of disease (fomites); [V] animate transmitters (vectors); [A] animate nonhuman reservoirs of disease in the form of lower animals; and [I] inanimate reservoirs of disease, e.g., soil.

The well person may receive infection by means of many combinations of these factors, depending upon his biologically adapted habits and activities, those of other humans, and those of vectors, animal reservoirs, and the pathogens. In certain instances, as in the case of the venereal diseases, direct and intimate contact must take place between the well and the infected human. This is indicated diagrammatically as [S] [W]. In certain other instances the well person may be infected across a certain distance by droplets from an infected human in a nonintimate relationship, [S]⟶ [W]. Measles and smallpox present examples of this. With some diseases an apparently healthy human carrier may be interposed, as in the circumstance of a clinically ill diphtheria patient passing the organism to another human who remains apparently well but in turn transmits the organism to another well person who then becomes clinically ill, [S]⟶ [C]⟶ [W]. The intervening factor in some diseases, e.g., typhoid, may take the form of inanimate transmitters, often referred to as fomites. Thus the typhoid patient or carrier may transmit the disease indirectly to a well person by means of food, milk, or water, [S]⟶ [F]⟶ [W]. With diseases such as malaria and the rickettsial diseases the intervening factor may take the form of a mosquito, tick, louse, or other biting insect. The pattern here is [S]⟶ [V]⟶ [W]. Healthy individuals may sometimes be infected as a result of intimate contact with healthy carriers, [C] [W]. An example of this is found in the transfer of hemolytic streptococci from the hands of an accoucheur to the tissues of a woman in labor, thereby resulting in puerperal sepsis. Certain pathogenic organisms may be transferred over a distance from healthy human carriers to the well person, [C]⟶ [W]. Here again may be mentioned hemolytic streptococci, now causing scarlet fever in the recipient. Furthermore, many organisms, of which the hemolytic streptococcus is again an example, may be transferred first from a carrier to an inanimate fomite such as food, thence to the new human host according to the pattern [C]⟶ [F]⟶ [W]; if the organism is the hemolytic streptococcus, it may perhaps result in a case of septic sore throat. On the other hand, the healthy human carrier may infect an animate transmitter such as a cow, which develops mastitis and thereby infects its milk, causing septic sore throat in a new human host; the resulting pattern is [C]⟶ [V]⟶ [F]⟶ [W].

Animate but nonhuman reservoirs of disease may threaten the well person in a number of ways quite similar to the foregoing. Again instances exist in which intimate contact is necessary between the animate reservoir and the potential human host. Thus the handling of the carcass of an infected rabbit may result in the transfer of tularemia to man, [A] [W]. Bites from rabid animals and bites resulting in rat-bite fever are further examples in this category. Some animal diseases, e.g., glanders in horses, may be transmitted over a distance in a manner similar to measles, with the pattern [A]⟶ [W]. Other animal diseases may be passed on to human hosts by means of inanimate intermediaries, or fomites, [A]⟶ [F]⟶ [W]. Here might be mentioned the contamination by rats of bedding or food from which the human host becomes infected with the leptospira causing infectious jaundice. Some diseases which primarily affect lower animals but with which humans may be infected may require an intermediate vector, usually in the form of a biting insect. An important example is jungle yellow fever, transferred by mosquitoes from small jungle mammals to man. Here the pattern is [A]⟶ [V]⟶ [W]. Finally, even man's inanimate environment may be a source of infection, either by direct contact as in the case of tetanus acquired from the soil, [I] [W], or over a distance as may possibly be the case in transmission of coccidioidomycosis [I]⟶ [W].

The foregoing scheme by no means presents an all-inclusive picture. Some diseases of man, particularly those caused by protozoa and helminthes, involve far more complicated patterns of transmission. The large fish tapeworm *Diphyllobothrium latum*, for example, infects man according to the following scheme:

dog	water	crustacean	fish	human
[A] ⟶	[I] ⟶	[A] ⟶	[A] ⟶	[W]

Of a similar magnitude is the pattern of schistosome infection:

sick human	water	snail	water	human
[S] ⟶	[I] ⟶	[A] ⟶	[I] ⟶	[W]

A still more complicated cycle is that of the sheep liver fluke:

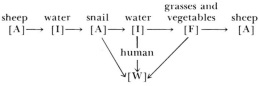

For purposes of further discussion, however, it is probably best to ignore these more complicated methods of infection and to limit consideration to the simple circumstances shown in Fig. 17-2. It is observed that the ultimate sources of infection in the diagram occur at the periphery and that, if it is found possible to place a block between any given peripheral source and the central potential host, infection cannot take place. Considering the problem from the standpoint of total diseases, it might be said that the central potential host would be completely safeguarded from all diseases if a cordon could be thrown around him at

any point between him and all of the various peripheral sources of infection. Careful consideration of the diagram indicates the possibility of a series of concentric cordons, the most central of which would bar all infections and the more peripheral affecting the more complicated types of infection patterns.

Theoretically speaking, the more links there are in a chain of infection, the more difficult it is for the organism to survive. Each link presents another place where something may go wrong. From the point of view of humanly conceived control measures each additional link provides another point of attack where obstacles to disease transmission may be interposed. Because of this, syphilis, with the simple [S] [W] pattern involving only the spirochete and man, is proportionately more difficult to control than malaria. In the latter instance control measures may be applied singly or jointly to any of a number of factors: the plasmodium (by treating or isolating infected persons), the adult mosquito, breeding places, the mosquito larvae, or the potential hosts.

By the same token it is equally true that the greater the number of ways an organism may be transmitted, the greater are its chances of survival. When a pathogenic organism is restricted completely to one particular path, e.g., the malarial parasite, the problem of control, once the basic facts about the disease are discovered, is theoretically simplified. Contrast with this the hemolytic streptococcus which, as shown in Fig. 17-2, may be transmitted by direct or indirect contact with either a sick infected human or a carrier or through a wide variety of fomites and vectors acting as intermediaries. An organism that could so adapt itself as to be transmissible by any or all of the paths indicated would present a dire threat indeed. Probably the best example of this is the *Pasteurella pestis,* which can spread by intimate contact, by droplet infection, by innumerable fomites, and by a number of animal vectors. It is not without significance that this particular organism came closer to eradicating the human race than any other known factor in human history.

In view of the foregoing the details of the control of specific communicable diseases must take into consideration the biologic characteristics of the pathogenic organism, of the potential host, and of any vectors or animal reservoirs that might be involved. In order to acquire essential knowledge concerning the disease and to apply that knowledge effectively attention must be given both to the adaptive habits of the organisms and to the social and cultural habits of the hosts.

GENERAL PRINCIPLES OF THE CONTROL OF COMMUNICABLE DISEASES

Control measures may be aimed at any factor or at any link involved in the chain of transmission, i.e., the organism, its present host, its vectors, its reservoirs, or the potential host himself. The following is a general classification of these measures.

Prevention of spread

Measures aimed at the organism. The ultimate point of attack here is the pathogenic organism itself. Since the goal is the destruction of the living cause of disease, any measures that could be devised to strike directly at it would be of great value. This is unfortunately difficult since pathogenic organisms by their very nature seldom exist in the free state. It is interesting that some of the earliest attempts by primitive people to combat communicable diseases were along these lines, taking the form of the generation of noise and smoke, the latter subsequently dignified by the term "fumigation." These methods were intended originally to drive away the evil gods of disease and were later continued against miasms. Although current scientific knowledge makes their use ridiculous, it may be pointed out that as recently as the beginning of the twentieth century pitch barrels were burned and cannons were fired in New Orleans as a means of combating yellow fever. Our ties with the past are further demonstrated by the continued sale of materials for fumigation and the wearing of asafetida bags in some areas of the world. A somewhat direct approach of attacking the organism is found in the treatment of persons who are infected. The community

as well as the personal benefit that results from so doing has justified even in the minds of those with narrow horizons the treatment under public health auspices of individuals infected with syphilis, tuberculosis, and certain other diseases.

Measures aimed at sources of infection. Sources of infection may be eradicated, their communicability may be reduced, or they may be rendered noninfectious by treatment.

Eradication of sources. When the source of infection is a known accessible animal reservoir, its elimination provides an effective means of eradication of the disease. Many instances of this method of attack in modern public health practice may be mentioned. Bovine tuberclosis has been practically eradicated in the United States by the destruction of infected cattle. However, this would be very difficult or impossible in a Hindu society for cultural reasons. Psittacosis may be eradicated by the elimination of infected parrots and other psittacine birds. Plague, typhus fever, leptospirosis, anthrax, tularemia, and a number of other diseases may be controlled by a similar attack against their animal reservoirs. Theoretically this approach could be applied effectively to diseases peculiar to man by the eradication of persons found to be infected. In a sense this was done at least partially during medieval times with regard to lepers, the deliberate neglect of whom was tantamount to elimination. A more conscious and direct use of this method was made occasionally in recent times by the leaders of the Nazi regime. A more humane and scientific adaptation of the method is seen in the surgical removal of a chronically infected part of the human body. Thus cholecystectomy has been used in an attempt to cure chronic typhoid carriers, and tonsillectomies have frequently been performed on chronic carriers of diphtheria and streptococci. Even these techniques, however, have become less justified with the introduction of antibiotics.

Reduction of communicability of sources of infection. The eradication of the sources of infections is often not necessary for the control of the infections they contain.

When dealing with diseases in human beings, the most practical primary point of attack sometimes takes the form of reducing the communicability of those infected. This may be accomplished by a combination of two control measures: (1) limitation of their movement, and (2) treatment of their infection. Limitation of human activity for public health purposes takes the form of isolation of those known to be infected and quarantine of those known or suspected to have been exposed to the risk of infection. Customarily the free movement of known infected individuals is restricted until clinical observation and/or laboratory tests indicate the absence of infectiousness. Quarantine for a disease usually has been extended over a time interval equal to the usual maximum incubation period of the disease.

These techniques, although of long historical standing, have never been too popular. First, it is human to resist and to circumvent restriction of personal action. Second, the measures are usually economically costly both to those restricted and to those enforcing the restriction. Beyond these objections are some more scientific reasons for their limited value. There are many unreported, hidden, or undected cases of most if not all communicable diseases. The ineffectiveness of isolation and quarantine for the control of measles is evidence of this. Of even greater significance is the large number of apparently healthy carriers of some diseases who effectively spread pathogenic organisms. For this reason isolation of a diagnosed case of poliomyelitis and its contacts is futile. Furthermore, the majority of acute communicable diseases are most infectious during their early stages before diagnosis is made or confirmed. Nevertheless, when rigidly applied under certain circumstances and to certain diseases such as smallpox and bubonic plague, isolation and quarantine may constitute effective means of control. This is particularly true in insular health programs. An interesting example of this is found in the rabies control program of England.

In order to be segregated and subsequently rendered noncommunicable, diseased individuals first must be discovered. Fundamental to this is a system for the reporting of cases of communicable diseases both by physicians in the area and by health authorities in other localities to which infected individuals may immigrate. Other sources of information are hospital records, requests for biologics, death certificates, and burial permits. The value of a report of a case of communicable disease is not in the counting of a "vital fact" or merely in the control of the patient but in the lead it gives in finding sources and contacts. This implies engaging in what some have termed "shoeleather epidemiology." A routine procedure must operate to determine and locate for subsequent examination the suspected individuals who constitute the group in which active infection of either recent or earlier origin is most apt to exist.

Human sources of infection may also be discovered by means of various screening and diagnostic procedures, e.g., tuberculin tests and chest x-ray examinations for tuberculosis, stool examinations for typhoid fever and other intestinal infections, nose and throat cultures for diphtheria, and vaginal and urethral smears for gonorrhea. Such tests are most useful when applied on a selective basis at certain times to certain groups of high average incidence and risk of infection.

Treatment of sources of infection. To find a source of infection is in itself of little value. Prompt treatment is indicated in order to render the patient noninfectious as well as to cure him. Thus treatment of individuals with communicable diseases is primarily for the protection of contacts and of the community and secondarily for the benefit of the patient. This has served in the past as justification for the establishment of publicly supported communicable disease treatment clinics and hospitals. In a few instances complete treatment or cure of the patient is not necessary in order to eliminate the threat to those about him. The syphilitic, for example, may be rendered noninfectious by prompt administration of therapeutic agents. Similarly many tuberculosis patients may be made noninfectious by means of collapsotherapy or drug therapy. It is important under such circumstances, however, that treatment be continued to ultimate success because the patient may relapse to a communicable stage. Furthermore, one must be concerned not only with the control of a disease from the standpoint of spread but also in terms of eliminating it as a cause of disability and premature death. In this sense public health is considered increasingly as a summation of personal health.

Measures aimed at transmitters of disease. Many communicable diseases require some kind of transmitting agent either in the form of an inanimate fomite or of a living vector. Not infrequently the most fruitful attack is one that is aimed at these transmitting agents. In fact some of the most spectacular examples of successful control have depended upon this approach. Truly remarkable results have followed programs of water purification, sanitary excreta disposal, food and dairy sanitation, and pasteurization. Success in these instances is greatly enhanced by the ability to apply effective control measures at central focal points such as water-treatment plants, pasteurization plants, canneries, bakeries, etc. It is worthy of particular mention that the healthfulness of our urbanized society and its economy depends in no small measure upon our penchant for convenient processed foods, the sanitary quality of which is controlled with relative ease.

Almost equally spectacular results are possible and in some instances have been achieved by the control or elimination of animate vectors of disease. Here the public health worker has the advantage of finding a chain of events with numerous links, each of which is subject to attack. For example, the control of mosquito-borne disease may be achieved in a number of ways: The adult mosquito may be destroyed by chemical or other means. Its breeding places may be eliminated by filling or impounding or made unsuitable by spraying with oils and other larvicides. The mosquito's effective biting contact may be eliminated by the use of screens, nets, mosquito bars, and repellents. Finally, persons with malaria may

be isolated from the mosquito, and healthy potential hosts may avoid the consequence of actual mosquito bites by routine chemoprophylaxis. Similar measures aimed at other vectors may take the form of delousing, cattle dipping, ship fumigation, rat proofing, proper garbage disposal, and the destruction of rats and biting flies. Measures relating to inanimate transmitters include the cooking of pork, the boiling of water or milk, the disinfection of typhoid stools, the burning of tuberculous sputum, and the ultraviolet disinfection of air.

Increasing the resistance of potential hosts

Maintenance of general health and nutrition. Although each communicable disease is attributable to a specific infectious agent, certain factors enter into the decision of whether or not the organism can thrive and cause disease once it gains entrance to the body of a potential host. The inverse relationship between general health and nutrition, on the one hand, and susceptibility to many infectious agents, on the other, is well established. Examples of this are found in connection with pneumonia, tuberculosis, some streptococcal diseases, and even some intestinal infections. A rather striking example is hookworm infection, in which spontaneous elimination of adult worms has been achieved merely by improving the diet of the host.

Production of passive immunity. If available, passive immunization is important when recent exposure of persons susceptible to diseases with short incubation periods is known to have occurred. Measures of this nature are exemplified by diphtheria and tetanus antitoxins. Still others are convalescent sera for the prevention of scarlet fever, measles, whooping cough, chickenpox, mumps, and some other diseases. Certain precautions must be observed in using passively immunizing products. Applicable to all of them is the need for prompt administration of large enough doses. In the case of antitoxin, particular care must be taken to avoid serum reactions by obtaining careful therapeutic histories and by testing for sensitivity to horse serum.

Production of active immunity. Where

available and popularly accepted, active immunization against communicable diseases offers the ideal control measure. It is in this area that spectacular successes comparable to those effected by sanitary engineering procedures are to be found. The widespread use of such simple measures as smallpox vaccination and diphtheria immunization has all but eradicated the threat of these two diseases in the United States and many other countries. Active immunization of a practical nature is also available against a number of other infectious diseases, including tetanus, pertussis, poliomyelitis, measles, mumps, influenza, cholera, typhoid fever, yellow fever, and spotted fever. Of more limited value and applicability are active immunizing measures against scarlet fever, meningococcic meningitis, and pneumococcal pneumonia.

Prevention of complications. A procedure similar to active immunization is the deliberate exposure of susceptible persons to measles, followed in 5 or 6 days by the administration of immune serum in an amount not sufficient to prevent the disease completely but enough to modify its clinical severity. In this way the patient obtains a lasting immunity by undergoing a controlled, greatly attenuated attack of the disease. The recent availability of an effective antimeasles vaccine, however, makes this procedure extraneous. For a somewhat different reason some advocate the deliberate exposure of female children to rubella (German measles) in order to preclude subsequent acquisition of the disease during the first trimester of pregnancy when certain malformations of the fetus may result.

Every communicable disease program must provide for the eventuality of dealing with incidences of communicable diseases, which occur in spite of preventive measures. Many large cities have met this problem by maintaining communicable disease hospitals wherein adequate isolation and treatment are concurrently effected. Smaller jurisdictions usually have not found this to be economically feasible and have provided treatment under the necessary isolation precautions either in a small general hospital or in the home of the patient. With the

dramatic decline in acute communicable diseases, the availability of antibiotics, and the perfection of isolation techniques special isolation hospitals have become less and less necessary.

ADMINISTRATIVE AIDS IN COMMUNICABLE DISEASE CONTROL

As with all other activities in public health work, certain administrative or management aids are necessary for the control of communicable diseases.

Legislation

A large part of public health law in the United States is concerned with the control of communicable diseases. The most important basis upon which rests the enactment and enforcement of public health law is the police power, which is considered in more detail in Chapter 9. For purposes of discussion it will suffice to remind the reader of the folly, even in a democracy, of allowing individuals complete freedom of action. In fact individual freedom in order truly to exist must be limited to the right to engage in all activities except those that may be detrimental to the common welfare. An individual infected with a disease transmissible to others must necessarily forfeit some of his personal freedom for the common good. It is the exercise of the police power over these restricted freedoms that endows the health officer with actually more power than any other individual or group in society. Only the health authority may summarily enter premises without a search warrant or deprive an individual of his personal freedom without a trial or even a subpoena. The necessity and legality for such action has fortunately been well established in the courts.

In order to make possible the administrative control of communicable diseases the states and the communities they contain have found it expedient and necessary to enact many types of legislation. The ultimate responsibility for the promulgation and enforcement of communicable disease laws, rules, and regulations rests with the state. All state and territorial health departments have this responsibility. In 15 states, however, power of enforcement is either not included in the regulatory authority or is limited to situations in which local action is inadequate. With regard to diseases of animals that are transmissible to man, the responsibility is shared with the department of agriculture in 25 states and with special commissions in 6 states. Other components of state government that are occasionally involved in communicable disease control include departments of welfare, social security, public assistance, education, and in two instances the state university. Where responsibility is thus divided, it is done in consideration for the particular portions of the general health program for which the respective departments are responsible. For example, in 5 states the department of education is responsible for the enforcement of the compulsory smallpox vaccination law, and in several states a department of public welfare or a state university has responsibilities concerning hospitalization of communicable disease patients.[2]

The problem of communicable disease is ever changing due to ecologic factors and to the application of newly acquired knowledge. It is important therefore that states revise their communicable disease codes periodically. Unfortunately many states and cities are long overdue in this important task. However, even many recent revisions are out of date because of the inclusion of antiquated and ineffective measures and requirements. In analyzing the undesirable features of communicable disease legislation, Emerson[3] has pointed to six characteristics in particular:

1. Lack of notification of some diseases for which modern standards of health service appear to demand notification
2. Placarding premises where cases of various communicable diseases are reported, under circumstances that make observance of isolation or quarantine neither likely nor helpful in preventing secondary or subsequent related cases in the home of the index case or elsewhere
3. Failure to verify the diagnosis of certain important diseases by an expert clinician, by laboratory test or by both
4. Requiring isolation periods for infected persons and quarantine periods for exposed susceptibles which are significantly inconsistent with the known periods of communicability and incubation of the particular disease

5. Failing to provide for a consecutive sanitary supervision of carriers from the time of the clinical course of the disease, or the first discovery of a carrier state, until it can be shown that these persons are no longer spreaders of infection
6. Use of fumigants for terminal disinfection in some diseases

Reporting

The most fundamental matter requiring legislation is concerned with the reporting to the official health agency of all cases of certain diseases listed in a communicable disease code. Acquisition of such information is necessary to any further steps the health authorities may wish to take in the control of those diseases. It provides the starting point for the application of isolation and quarantine measures and for all routine epidemiologic investigations. Although states vary somewhat in the particular diseases for which they require reports, the accompanying list (Table 17-1) is more or less typical.

In addition to those listed in Table 17-1, there are a number of other communicable diseases the reporting of which is not frequently required. Obligatory reporting of these diseases (Table 17-2) is not ordinarily considered justified by the benefits that may accrue from whatever steps the health authority may be in a position to take.

At the present time many states also include certain noncommunicable diseases in their lists of reportable conditions. Occupational diseases constitute the bulk of these, while some of the Southeastern states particularly include some of the avitaminoses, especially pellagra.

On the local level it is usually required that diseased individuals and carriers or suspected carriers of communicable diseases be reported to the local health officer, who acts as the agent of the state. In cities and counties without local health departments it is usually required that reports be made directly to the state health department. While "immediate" notification is ordinarily specified, in practically all cases this is interpreted to mean within 24 hours following diagnosis. Although in most instances it is the private physician who is in the position of having to make a report, a number

Table 17-1. Diseases usually considered reportable in the United States*

Anthrax	Psittacosis
Brucellosis	Rabies
Chancroid (soft chancre)	Relapsing fever
Cholera	Rickettsial fevers
†Conjunctivitis, acute infectious, in newborn infants, not including trachoma	†Ringworm of the scalp or body
†Dengue	†Salmonellosis
†Diarrhea of the newborn, epidemic	†Scabies
Diphtheria	Smallpox (variola)
Dysentery, bacillary (shigellosis)	†Staphylococcal infection
Encephalitis, arthropod-borne	Impetigo
Food poisoning (bacterial intoxications)	Pemphigus
Staphylomycosis	Surgical and nursery outbreaks
Botulism	Streptococcal infection, respiratory
Glanders	Scarlet fever
Gonorrhea	Streptococcal sore throat, streptococcal nasopharyngitis, streptococcal tonsillitis, septic sore throat
†Influenza	Streptococcal infection other than respiratory
†Keratoconjunctivitis, infectious	Erysipelas
Leprosy	Puerperal infection (puerperal septicemia)
Leptospirosis	Syphilis
Malaria	Tetanus
Measles (rubeola)	Trachoma
Meningococcic meningitis (cerebrospinal meningitis) and meningococcemia	Trichinosis
†Mononucleosis, infectious	Tuberculosis, pulmonary
Paratyphoid fever	Tuberculosis other than pulmonary
Pertussis (whooping cough)	Typhoid fever
Plague	Typhus fever
†Pneumococcal pneumonia	Yellow fever
Poliomyelitis	

*Adapted from American Public Health Association: Control of communicable diseases in man, ed. 10, New York, 1965, The Association.
†Epidemics only.

of other persons or institutions are usually specified in the laws, rules, and regulations as also having this responsibility. Generally included are physicians; dentists; directors of registered laboratories; veterinarians; parents and guardians; superintendents, principals, and teachers of all schools; nurses engaged in private duty and school, public health, or industrial work; pharmacists; keepers of hotels, lodging houses, motels, and trailer parks; superintendents of public or private hospitals, nursing homes, clinics, dispensaries, asylums, or jails; owners or managers of dairy farms or any place where dairy products are handled or offered for sale; and licensed embalmers when the death certificate certifies that the primary or contributory cause of death was one of the reportable diseases.

Reporting is effected locally in either one or a combination of two ways. Some jurisdictions require written reports on all reportable diseases; many others, however, make the much more reasonable compromise of accepting telephoned reports on all diseases and requiring written confirmation for only a few of the more serious diseases such as smallpox or typhoid fever. Written reports are usually in the form of printed postal cards that provide space for entry of the patient's name, address, age, color, sex, and disease, and the name and address of the person reporting.

Since the collection of data on the incidence of communicable diseases is a function of all state health departments, the regulations of every state provide for the transmission of information from the local health authorities or, in their absence, from physicians directly. About two thirds of the

Table 17-2. Diseases not ordinarily considered reportable in the United States

Actinomycosis	Hookworm disease (ancylostomiasis)
Amebiasis	Lymphogranuloma venereum (inguinale) and climatic bubo
Ascariasis	
Blastomycosis	Mumps (infectious parotitis)
Chickenpox	Pediculosis
Choriomeningitis	Pneumonia, bacterial, other than pneumococcal
Coccidioidomycosis (coccidioidal granuloma, valley fever)	Primary atypical pneumonia
	Rheumatic fever (acute rheumatic fever, acute rheumatism)
Common cold	
Filariasis (mumu)	Rubella
Granuloma inguinale	Schistosomiasis (bilharziasis)
Helminthiasis	Tularemia
Hepatitis	Vulvovaginitis in children
Histoplasmosis	Yaws (frambesia)

states collect weekly reports and only one-third require daily reports. Occasionally, states pay fees for reports of communicable diseases. In most instances this is in lieu of salary to part-time officials acting in the absence of a full-time health officer.

Despite the fact that failure to report a case of communicable disease usually implies liability to prosecution, it is common knowledge that reporting is far from complete. A health officer would be utterly lacking in wisdom if he were to attempt to obtain reports, particularly from private physicians, only on the strength of his legal prerogatives. A legal point and a demonstration of authority might be gained only at the expense of having made one or several lasting antagonists who henceforth might avoid cooperation with the general public health program.

Persistent tact, educational efforts, and good professional relationships are the keynotes to success. Certain generalizations may be arrived at in this regard. The more serious a disease, the more faithfully it is apt to be reported. Thus physicians seldom fail to report cases of smallpox; on the other hand, they might pay little attention to a requirement to report measles. Furthermore, it is not surprising that many physicians are negligent in reporting diseases when past experience indicates that little official action results. It is recommended therefore that requirements for reporting be limited to diseases that present a real social threat and about which some fruitful, official steps

may be taken or assistance might be given to the physician. Sometimes a public health agency requests information concerning minor diseases or those about which at present it can do little. In such instances it is advisable that the true reasons be presented frankly to those from whom the reports are requested rather than simply to notify them that as of a certain date a certain disease must be reported. The one approach invites cooperation based upon understanding, whereas the other suggests bureaucratic dictation.

The hesitancy of many physicians to report the names of patients suffering from certain socially stigmatized diseases such as syphilis is understandable. In many areas a practical compromise has been reached. In the long run, of course, public and professional education is the path to follow toward the attainment of a more mature attitude toward these as well as other diseases. Meanwhile it is possible to arrange for reports to list numbers rather than names, with the provision that an infectious patient who has become negligent in his treatment be subsequently reported to the health authorities by name and address in order that field follow-up may be carried out.

Isolation and quarantine

Until relatively recently legal authority was freely invoked to isolate diagnosed patients and to quarantine individuals who have had contact with any one of the many communicable diseases. Careful studies by a number of investigators, particularly Charles V. Chapin[4] in Providence, Peter Holst[5] in Norway, and Gordon and Badger[6] in Detroit, have brought out the limitations of these methods. The trend has been toward progressive shortening and individualization of the periods of restriction, using severity of infection, complications, age, and occupation of the patient as a guide. The decrease in the extent to which these restrictive measures are used has resulted not only in improved public relations but also in considerable financial savings, both to private citizens and to publicly supported hospitals and health departments.

Historically, isolation and quarantine have been associated with placarding, a procedure that is also becoming obsolete. The case against placarding was so well stated in *The Control of Communicable Diseases in Man,*[7] a report by the American Public Health Association, that it is included here as follows:

Placarding—This official procedure under local or State authority consists of posting a warning notice upon the door or entrance to living quarters of persons isolated because of communicable disease. The object of such placarding is primarily to keep unauthorized persons from entering upon the premises during the period of communicability of the isolated patient. Such placarding may incidentally protect the patient against additional or secondary infection which may be carried to him by visitors. Its use may have some educational value.

Placarding, however, does not aid significantly the efforts of a health department to control the acute communicable diseases ordinarily spread directly from person to person in the United States (chicken pox, mumps, pertussis, measles, diphtheria, scarlet fever, anterior poliomyelitis, meningococcus meningitis, pneumonia, tuberculosis, gonorrhea, syphilis) and consequently is not recommended for these diseases.

Placarding has definite disadvantages: it is difficult to enforce, it may be a deterrent to reporting, it is costly in transportation. The most serious objection is the loss of time of public health nurses and other public health department employees that should be devoted to practical instruction in the observance of isolation and concurrent disinfection at the bedside of patients suffering from the more serious of the communicable diseases.

The current policies of the health department of a large city illustrate the trend toward more reasonable control of communicable disease patients and contacts.

The requirements are summarized as follows:

Quarantine of contacts
Chickenpox—none
*Diphtheria—pending negative nose and throat cultures
*Poliomyelitis—none
*Scarlet fever—none
Measles—none
Pertussis—nonimmune children excluded from school and public gatherings for 14 days after last exposure
Smallpox—16 days after last exposure unless successfully vaccinated
Typhoid and paratyphoid—none; familial contacts should not act as food-handlers

Isolation of infected individuals
Until recovery—erysipelas, influenza, leprosy, meningococcus, meningitis, mumps, ophthalmia neonatorum (from other infants only), septic sore throat, typhus fever
For specific periods
Chickenpox—until skin entirely clear
Smallpox—until skin clear of crusts
Diphtheria—until two successive negative nose and throat cultures 24 hours apart, otherwise 14 days
Measles—7 days from rash minimum
Pertussis—3 weeks minimum
Poliomyelitis—7 days minimum from onset
Psittacosis—during acute clinical stage
Scarlet fever—7 days minimum in uncomplicated cases, otherwise until recovery
Typhoid and paratyphoid—until three consecutive negative stool cultures at least 24 hours apart
Excluded from school, public gatherings, or work until recovery—impetigo, epidemic keratoconjunctivitis, scabies, trachoma
Excluded from intimate contact—chancroid, gonorrhea, syphilis, granuloma inguinale, lymphogranuloma venereum
Not required but desirable—common cold, amebic dysentery, bacillary dysentery, pneumococcal pneumonia, primary atypical pneumonia, tuberculosis (preferably in hospital or sanatorium)
Separation from women in early pregnancy—rubella

Compulsory immunization

An important type of communicable disease legislation deals with immunization requirements. With the development of protective measures against specific major com-

---

*Wage earners are permitted to enter and leave premises provided they have no contact with the patient, with children, or with food intended for public consumption.

Table 17-3. Statutory prohibitions relative to vaccination*

State	Action prohibited or made unlawful
Arizona	Subjection of minor child to compulsory vaccination without parent's or guardian's consent
California	Adoption by school or local health authorities of any rule or regulation concerning vaccination
Minnesota	Rule of state board of health or of any public board or officer compelling vaccination of child or excluding, except during smallpox epidemics and when approved by local board of education, child from public schools because unvaccinated
North Dakota	Requirement of any form of vaccination or inoculation as a condition precedent to admission to any public or private school or college of any person or for exercise of any right performance of any duty or enjoyment of any privilege by any person
South Dakota	For any board, physician, or person to compel another by use of physical force, to submit to operation of vaccination with smallpox or other virus
Utah	For any board of health, board of education, or any other public board to compel by resolution, order, or proceedings of any kind the vaccination of any person of any age or to make vaccination a condition precedent to attendance to any public or private school, either as pupil or teacher
Washington	Requirement of child to submit to vaccination against parent's or guardian's will

*Adapted from Fowler, W.: Principal provisions of smallpox vaccination laws and regulations in the United States, Public Health Rep. **56**:188, Jan. 31, 1941.

municable diseases, it is natural that many persons in positions of authority have attempted to enforce their use by all people. Most notable in this regard is smallpox, a sufficiently serious disease for which a spectacularly easy, safe, and powerful preventive is available. Many countries have seen fit to require vaccination against smallpox by law. The pattern in the United States varies. By 1915, 15 states and territories* and the District of Columbia had laws that required vaccination as a prerequisite to school attendance. Twenty-one other† had laws or regulations that enabled local jurisdictions to enact compulsory vaccination regulations or to require vaccination under certain conditions, e.g., threatened epidemics, exposure to patients, or the existence of a case in a school or in the community. In striking contrast were several states that had certain statutory prohibitions concerning vaccination (Table 17-3). Some of these regulations have since changed.

*Arkansas, Kentucky, Maryland, Massachusetts, New Hampshire, New Mexico, New York, Pennsylvania, Rhode Island, South Carolina, Virginia, West Virginia, Hawaii, Puerto Rico, and the Virgin Islands.
†Alabama, Arizona, Colorado, Connecticut, Georgia, Iowa, Kansas, Louisiana, Maine, Michigan, Minnesota, Mississippi, Montana, New Jersey, North Carolina, Ohio, Oregon, Tennessee, Wisconsin, Wyoming, and Alaska.

Without question, where smallpox has occurred to a significant extent, compulsory vaccination brings about results, as illustrated in Fig. 17-3. The map shows that from 1936 to 1945 the incidence of smallpox was significantly lower in the states that had compulsory vaccination laws and higher in the states where compulsion was prohibited. Since that time the incidence of smallpox has undergone a marked reduction throughout the nation. In the process, those States that were negligent or those that opposed forthright action undoubtedly rode on the successes of the states and areas that undertook forceful epidemiologic action. Ordinarily, of course, acceptance of a procedure based upon understanding is the best long-term method.

Compulsory immunization laws are occasionally found in relation to several other diseases. A few states and a number of local communities have required immunization against diphtheria as a condition for admission to school. The inaptness of this is to be found in the study of the age distribution of diphtheria patients and deaths. Where laws of this nature exist, there is a known tendency on the part of parents to defer obtaining the protection until their children are ready to enter school. This practice overlooks the fact that the greatest threat

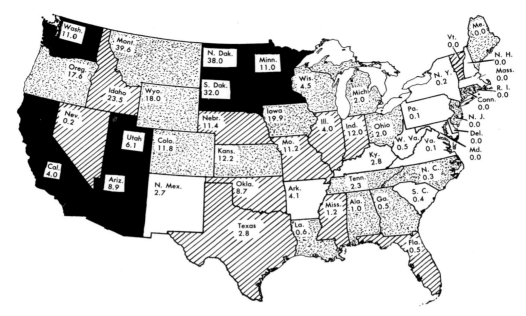

Fig. 17-3. Vaccination legislation and average annual smallpox incidence per 100,000 population, by states, 1936-1945. *White,* vaccination required for school; *stippled,* local option in face of threat; *diagonal lines,* no vaccination laws; *solid,* compulsory vaccination prohibited.

from the disease is during the preschool period from the first to the sixth birthday.

Arkansas, Mississippi, and New Mexico in the past have required immunization against typhoid fever for family contacts and known carriers, all food-handlers, and all susceptibles. While the development of immunity in such persons may assist in preventing them from acquiring clinical typhoid fever, it in no way assures their being noninfectious to others. Furthermore, in view of certain questions concerning the efficacy of typhoid vaccination and the current availability of a number of antibiotics that have considerable effect on typhoid and related organisms, the continuation of compulsory immunization in such circumstances seems inappropriate. More appropriately, certain countries require vaccination against yellow fever, and many nations insist upon valid evidence of vaccination against yellow fever, typhus fever, and plague as a condition of entry from areas affected by these diseases.

Related to the attempts to control communicable diseases in man is the legislative requirement in some jurisdictions that all dogs be actively immunized against rabies. Strangely, this sometimes calls forth greater public indignation and vituperation than do attempts to obtain immunization of children against various preventable diseases.

Compulsory examination

Another area in which legislative control of communicable diseases has been attempted involves the compulsory examination of certain people under certain circumstances. At the present time many states have laws that require examination of all applicants for marriage licenses. Unfortunately the premarital examination too often consists merely of the performance of a serologic test for syphilis and completely ignores other risks that one prospective mate may bring to the other. All but five states now have premarital examination laws. The majority of the states that have such laws requires that both the prospective bride and groom have a physical examination in addition to a serologic test for syphilis prior to issuance of a marriage license.[8,9]

Based upon the same general philosophy

as premarital examinations, legislation requiring prenatal examinations has been enacted by many states. Again the chief target is syphilis. At the present time all but eight states have enacted such laws. However, in two of these states prenatal tests for syphilis are recommended by statute or regulation. Prenatal health examination laws are confined to blood serologic tests for syphilis, with the responsibility placed upon the attendant of the pregnant woman. Exceptions to this are Georgia and North Carolina, where the pregnant woman also has the responsibility to request a test. One of the obvious difficulties is the time factor. Most state laws specify a serologic test during or within 15 days of the first examination. This of course is of limited value if the first visit is shortly before delivery. The remaining states' laws tend to be even more general.[9,10]

As a result of dramatic changes in the incidence, treatment, and control of the venereal diseases following the widespread use (and abuse) of antibiotics, the legal requirement of premarital and prenatal examination for these diseases became subject to question. Condit and Brewer,[11] for example, have pointed out that between 1949 and 1951 the 511,160 premarital examinations in California discovered only 1,079 cases of syphilis, of which only 162 were in the primary and secondary states, at a cost of $2,741 per new case found. Only 4.3% of all primary and secondary cases were discovered by this means. Hedrick and Silverman[12] have compared the experiences of the states that require premarital examinations with those that do not. They found that during the decade from 1945 to 1956 both groups enjoyed a dramatic 97% decline in infant deaths from syphilis and a 93% decline in primary and secondary syphilitic morbidity. They concluded that, since premarital blood tests had very little influence on syphilitic mortality and morbidity and were in addition very expensive to carry out, compulsory laws were no longer justified. However, there has been a resurgence of syphilis in recent years, partly as a result of changes in sexual mores and partly due to the appearance of more resistant strains of the spirochete. Thus an analysis of reports from 26 states in 1964 and 1965 indicated that about 1 out of every 85 prospective brides or grooms was suspected as having syphilis. Similarly, almost 1% of all pregnant women examined was suspected as having the disease.[13] In view of this, the continuance of premarital and prenatal testing appears wise.

A rather wide variety of laws and regulations exist through the country which require compulsory examination of various types of workers and groups in society. The most common and significant of these are persons known to have contact with individuals having communicable diseases. It is also common practice to require a medical examination as a condition for employment as a schoolteacher. It is not unusual, however, to find that no further periodic examinations are required after employment as a teacher is an accomplished fact.

Food-handlers have been singled out as a key group for which is required preemployment examination and periodic examinations and laboratory tests thereafter. It is unfortunate that more often than not the chief if not exclusive concern for the requirement of food-handler examination is a search for syphilis. Obviously this ignores the fact that it is highly unlikely that a food-handler will transmit the spirochete of syphilis while engaged in activities customarily related to food-handling. To examine these individuals for signs and symptoms of tuberculosis, the typhoid fever carrier state, and a few other pertinent conditions may well be warranted, but the singling out this occupational group with particular regard to the venereal diseases, however, does not appear to be justified.

Some states have enacted regulations that require the preemployment and periodic examination of workers in certain of the heavy industries, particularly those in which risk of silicosis or radium poisoning is known to exist. A few communities have adopted the policy of routinely examining all persons arrested for certain offenses, particularly prostitution, because those involved are considered to constitute key epidemiologic groups.

Compulsory treatment

The police power is sometimes resorted to in requiring treatment and if necessary enforced hospitalization of recalcitrant individuals infected with certain communicable diseases. Every large health department has found it necessary to resort to this undesirable and unpopular procedure occasionally with regard to cases of smallpox, typhoid fever, the venereal diseases, and even tuberculosis.[14] In a sense, to do so represents an admission of failure on the part of the educational and public health agencies of the community. However, a certain few adamantly unreasonable and uncooperative persons always exist and if necessary must be provided for by law.

Regulation of vehicles of disease transmission

Of tremendous public health importance are the regulations dealing with the many vehicles of disease transmission. There exists a formidable array of laws, regulations, and codes, unfortunately sometimes contradictory, concerned with the production, treatment, and distribution of milk, milk products, food, water, and drugs. Other factors that might be included deal with plumbing, sewage disposal, stream pollution, air pollution, and the care and transportation of the bodies of persons who have died from communicable diseases. No reasonable person would contest the wisdom of providing legislative regulation of these factors. The criticisms that may be raised against such laws, however, are based upon the wide variability of their provisions and their not infrequent contradictions and anachronisms.

Some mention should be made of the wisdom of placing too much reliance upon legislative action in the accomplishment of public health goals. It must always be remembered that it is natural for a free people to resent laws and restrictions and occasionally to regard them as challenges that provide an incentive for the popular game of circumvention. It should be realized further that the enactment of a law in no sense constitutes an accomplished end. Ill-conceived and poorly administered laws almost inevitably lead to undesirable and costly court actions that often end in dismissal for lack of evidence or the levying of a relatively small fine. Generally speaking, publicity attending such cases is not particularly desirable and often tends to crystalize hitherto unorganized opposition to the general public health program.

While it is always desirable to have a practical, scientifically correct, complete body of public health laws to fall back upon whenever necessary, it is equally wise to avoid insofar as possible the exercise of those laws. On the other hand, there is little sense in the enactment of laws and regulations in the absence of intent or ability to enforce them whenever truly necessary. For the greatest ultimate success, reliance should be placed upon intelligent cooperation by the public. This means that in the final analysis an effective program of community health education is the most fruitful approach to communicable disease control as it is to other public health problems. To tell an individual that he must not do a certain thing does nothing to make him a better person or citizen; this merely calls forth either dumb, unthinking acquiescence or sullen resentment. To educate him in an intelligent, cooperative manner, with regard to the undesirability of following a certain line of action, offers much more chance of success which, when it occurs, instills the idea not only in the individual but also in those about him and those who follow.

MATERIAL AIDS IN COMMUNICABLE DISEASE CONTROL

The provision or use of certain material aids has become standard practice in official public health agencies. Of primary importance among these are standardized forms furnished to private physicians on which they must report births, deaths, cases of communicable diseases, certain prophylactic treatments, and other significant information. The keynote for administrative success in designing such forms is simplicity and brevity. To require extensive written reports from busy medical practitioners, particularly if they have to pay the postage, is to invite failure. Such reports should be looked upon by public health agencies only as points of departure and should therefore be restricted to a minimum of requested information, e.g., identification and location of an individual affected, the condition with which he is affected, and possibly a few other items of basic information, depending upon the disease, service, and other circumstances. Prestamped or the more economical prepaid reply cards should be made freely available to all practicing physicians, along with simple instructions concerning their legal responsibilities. This is particularly important when physicians first enter practice in the locality and whenever responsibilities undergo a change.

An important adjunct to communicable disease control is the furnishing of biologic and certain other diagnostic, prophylactic, and therapeutic material and diagnostic laboratory service to physicians upon request and preferably free of charge. In addition the laboratory serves a fundamental function in the sanitary control of foods, milk, and many environmental factors that may influence the public health. This phase of the public health program is specifically considered in Chapter 31.

Consultation service

Consultation service in the diagnosis or control of communicable disease represents another type of material assistance often offered by public health agencies. All state health departments at the present time provide this service to local health departments, which in turn include it as a primary part of their service to local practicing physicians. There are two reasons for doing this: (1) the health department is responsible for the control of communicable diseases and (2) the health officer or his assistants usually see more cases of communicable diseases than does the average physician. Therefore they tend to have a more extensive diagnostic background in this field upon which to draw.

Graphic aids

Within the health department a number of material aids and techniques have been found useful for the efficient administrative control of communicable diseases. These fall into the two categories of graphic aids and registers. Perhaps the most common,

useful graphic aid is the spot map of cases as they occur in the area through time. Graphs showing the incidence of disease by day, week, month, or year are also frequently found useful. With certain diseases, particularly measles, incidence charts that include 5-year or 7-year moving medians for epidemic and nonepidemic years have been found to be particularly useful in estimating disease expectancy (Fig. 17-4). Every health jurisdiction and the statistical data relating to it should be fractionated to some degree in order to make more evident the predominant trends and problems. For this purpose health departments have relied particularly upon census tracts, voting areas, or sanitary districts for which basic population data may be conveniently available. A particularly interesting and useful adaptation of this is found in the so-called epidemiologic master chart, described in Chapter 30 and illustrated in Fig. 30-6. Rich and Terry[15] have suggested the use of the industrial type of control chart for epidemiologic purposes. It is only by the use of such tools that the public health worker can maintain a continuous and adequate grasp of the total disease situation and the factors relating to it.

Registers

The maintenance of case registers has proved to be of incalculable value in the operation of adequate programs for the control of many diseases. Most commonly used in connection with tuberculosis, registers have also been developed by some health departments for venereal diseases, some of the more important acute communicable diseases and their carriers, and occasionally for cancer, rheumatic fever, and other chronic diseases. To be of value the register should readily indicate by some combination of filing and tickler system the location of the patient or carrier, the stage of his condition, and the date of next indicated treatment or follow-up procedure.

ADMINISTRATIVE PROGRAMMING IN COMMUNICABLE DISEASE CONTROL

The official program for the control of communicable diseases should be based upon all the known epidemiologic facts and

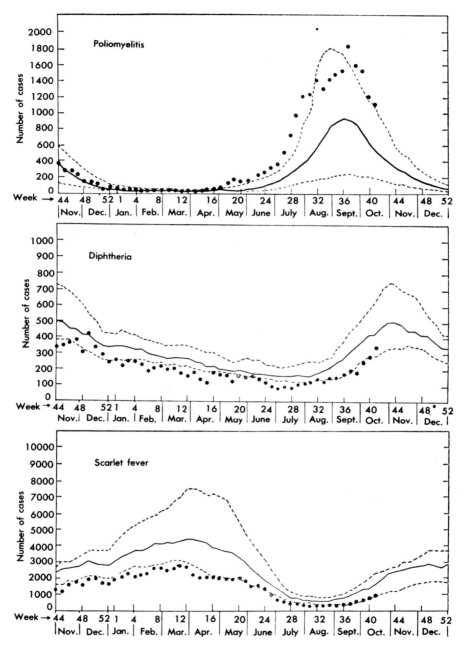

Fig. 17-4. Communicable disease charts. All reporting states, November 1947 through October 16, 1948. Upper and lower broken lines represent the highest and lowest figures recorded for the corresponding weeks in the 7 preceding years. Solid line is the median figure for the 7 preceding years. All three lines have been smoothed by a 3-week moving average. Dots represent numbers of cases reported for the weeks of 1948.

should be carefully and logically planned and balanced rather than allowed to pursue a hit-or-miss policy. The total program may be divided into routine control measures and those activities necessitated by emergency or epidemic situations. Much of the program may be routinized to a greater or lesser degree. In order to do so successfully it is necessary for the public health agency to obtain satisfactory answers to the following series of questions about each disease with which it is concerned:

1. What groups of the population are most apt to have or to acquire the infection?
2. Which of these groups is in the best position to expose others?
3. Where are they most conveniently and efficiently found?
4. What possible groups are most apt to be exposed?
5. When, where, how, and why are they subject to exposure?
6. What practical and economical control procedures and facilities are available?
7. What practical and economical control procedures and facilities are acceptable to the people involved?

For practical purposes the factor of timing is of paramount importance. Communicable diseases may be subdivided into those that vary in incidence by season and those that occur constantly, or endemically, throughout the year. Under usual circumstances a certain relatively constant incidence of new cases of tuberculosis and the venereal diseases may be expected. Programs aimed at combating them must therefore involve a constant hammering at the factors involved in their spread. Contrasted with these are the so-called acute communicable diseases of childhood that are subject to marked seasonal and in some instances annual fluctuation. A considerably simplified picture is presented in Fig. 17-5, which indicates the general seasonal prevalence of a number of these diseases as they have occurred in North America in the past. The incidences of a majority of the diseases usually increased during the spring months of the year. Whooping cough tended to lag a month or two behind the main group, while poliomyelitis was usually most prevalent in the fall and diphtheria occurred mostly in the winter months.

While it is desirable that children receive immunizing protection against various diseases routinely as they reach certain ages, it is obvious that any special immunization program that may be considered necessary should precede the period of expected high incidence. Accordingly, it would be more practical for health departments in the northern hemisphere to engage in a special whooping cough immunization program during February and March rather than to wait until August or September when the seasonal threat of that disease has passed. Similarly, antimeasles immunization is most practically provided during the late winter rather than in the summer or fall. Where

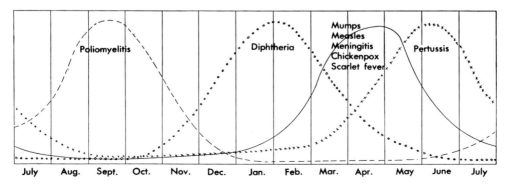

Fig. 17-5. Seasonal prevalence of acute communicable respiratory diseases.

the disease might occur, the promotion of a postgraduate institute in the management of poliomyelitis patients would probably be of greatest value in the late summer months rather than at any other time of the year.

Control programs should be similarly keyed with regard to age since particular diseases tend to affect certain age groups more than others (Fig. 17-6). A pertussis immunization program for entering school children would be of little avail since the period of greatest risk is during the first 2 years of life. Emphasis therefore should be placed upon the immunization against this disease during infancy. For similar reasons the diphtheria prevention program should stress immunization between the ninth and fifteenth months of life. The importance of this was clearly established many years ago by Godfrey,[16] who demonstrated that immunization of as high as 65% of entering schoolchildren against diphtheria was relatively ineffective in the community control of the disease, whereas immunization of as few as 35% of early preschool children would effectively prevent the disease from ever reaching epidemic proportions.

In this connection it is of interest to point out the statistical explanation for the lack of necessity, from a community's standpoint, of protecting every member of the community or even every susceptible member of the community. For the purpose of explanation it might be assumed that a given individual has an average epidemiologically effective rate of contact of two during the period he is infectious. That is, the average infectious person, while he is still able to circulate, may have contacts of an intimate enough nature to fulfill the biologic conditions necessary for the transmission of his infection to two susceptible persons. This of course varies with disease, location, culture, and many other factors. In a totally unprotected community therefore the original patient would give rise to two new patients, who in turn would produce a total of four, each of whom would infect two others to produce a total of eight. The picture therefore is one of geometric progression: 1-2-4-8-16-32-64-128, etc. (Fig. 17-7). If, on the other hand, merely one half of the susceptible individuals in the community are protected against the particular disease, the average rate of effective contact of patients with susceptible persons is reduced 50%. Each case therefore, on the basis of probability, will now give rise to only one new case, and everything but the main trunk of the tree of infection will have been pruned. The picture of transmission now becomes 1-1-1-1-1 (Fig. 17-8). While by chance an occasional case may give rise to two or more new cases, the chances are equally great that at some point the existing case will not have effective contact, and the chain of infection may die out completely.

The modern approach to tuberculosis

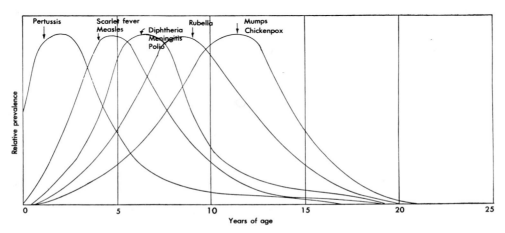

Fig. 17-6. Relative prevalence by age of acute communicable respiratory diseases.

provides an excellent illustration of administrative programming in the routine control and eradication of a communicable disease. Frost[17] stated the epidemiologic prognosis for this disease as follows:

We need not assume that tuberculosis is permanently and ineradicably engrafted upon our civilization. On the contrary, the evidence indicates that in this country the balance is already against the survival of the tubercle bacillus; and we may reasonably expect that the disease will eventually be eradicated. It is necessary only that the rate of transmission be held permanently below the level at which a given number of infection spreading cases succeed in establishing an equivalent number to

carry on the succession. If, in successive periods of time, the number of infectious hosts is continuously reduced, the end result of this diminishing ratio, if continued long enough, must be extermination of the tubercle bacillus.

However, there are many signs of impatience. A realization has come about that, although the biologic tide has turned in our favor, it is needlessly expensive and wasteful to be satisfied with the present rate of decline in the tuberculosis incidence and death rate. The question arises of how to accomplish the reduction most effectively and efficiently. Early case finding is ob-

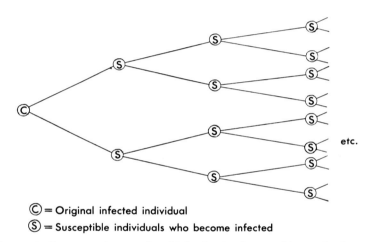

ⓒ = Original infected individual
Ⓢ = Susceptible individuals who become infected

Fig. 17-7. Geometrically progressive transfer of infection in absence of immunization.

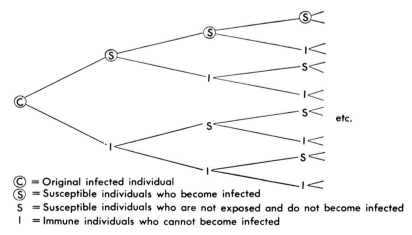

ⓒ = Original infected individual
Ⓢ = Susceptible individuals who become infected
S = Susceptible individuals who are not exposed and do not become infected
I = Immune individuals who cannot become infected

Fig. 17-8. Linear transfer of infection with 50% immunization.

Table 17-4. Summary of gastrointestinal diseases

	Typhoid fever	Paratyphoid	Bacillary dysentery	Amebic dysentery	Cholera	Brucellosis	Hookworm
Cause	*Salmonella typhosa*	*Salmonella* (several species)	*Shigella* (several species)	*Entamoeba histolytica*	*Vibrio comma*	*Brucella* (several species)	*Necator americanus*
Incubation period	3 to 38 days, usually 7 to 14 days	3 to 15 days, usually 4 to 10 days	2 to 7 days	2 days to several months, usually 3 to 4 weeks	1 to 5 days	6 to 30 days	None in true sense
Prevalence	Worldwide, warm seasons especially; affects mostly males and young adults		Tropics and subtropics, especially warm season; affects all ages and sexes		India and China	Mediterranean, U. S., Canada, Scandinavia; warm season	Limited to warm, moist sandy soil; affects white children especially

Period of communicability
Prodromes, illness, and convalescence until stools negative
Exception: Brucellosis, 20 to 300 days
Hookworm, While infected

Source
Feces and urine of cases and carriers
Exception: Brucellosis; milk, tissues, blood, and discharges of infected cows, swine, goats

Spread
Infected water, food, fomites, flies, direct contact
Exception: Brucellosis; milk and contact with tissues and discharges
Hookworm; contaminated soil. Neither man to man

Susceptibility
General susceptibility, decreasing with age
Exception: Brucellosis; most persons have some natural immunity

Immunity
Passive: None
Active: One attack gives long-lasting immunity to typhoid. Relative immunity in paratyphoid and bacillary dysentery. Short immunity with vaccines in typhoid and paratyphoid (about 2 years) and cholera (about 1 year)

Control measures
1. Early diagnosis and reporting of cases and carriers; laboratory tests
2. Isolation in all but hookworm, amebic dysentery, and brucellosis
3. Disinfection—concurrent—terminal in all but hookworm and brucellosis
4. Quarantine—cholera only (5 days)
5. Immunization (q.v.)
6. Source finding—cases and carriers, important in all
7. Water sanitation
8. Excreta sanitation
9. Food sanitation
10. Milk sanitation
11. Shellfish sanitation
12. Prevention of fly breeding
13. Carrier control
14. Education of patients and carriers

Table 17-5. Summary of acute respiratory diseases

	Diphtheria	Scarlet fever	Whooping cough	Measles	Smallpox	Chickenpox	Mumps	Meningitis	Poliomyelitis
Cause	Corynebacterium diphtheriae	Hemolytic streptococci	Haemophilus pertussis	Filtrable virus	Filtrable virus	Filtrable virus	Filtrable virus	Neisseria meningitidis	Filtrable virus
Incubation period	2 to 7 days	2 to 7 days	7 to 16 days	8 to 12 days	8 to 16 days	14 to 21 days	14 to 21 days	2 to 10 days	7 to 14 days
Period of communicability	Variable; usually under 2 weeks, seldom over 4	Variable; usually 3 weeks from onset until no discharges	Catarrhal stage (7 to 14 days) and 3 weeks of whoop	Catarrhal stage (4 days) and 5 days of rash	Catarrhal stage (2 to 4 days) to disappearance of lesions	Catarrhal stage (0 to 2 days) and during 6 to 10 days of lesions	Unknown; assumed while glands enlarged	From onset until 2 weeks after recovery	Unknown; assumed incubation period and first week of disease

Prevalence	Worldwide, but especially temperate zone—winter and spring except whooping cough (spring), polio (late summer), and diphtheria (fall and winter); affects children most; incidence usually less and older age group affected more in rural than urban
Source	Discharges from nose and throat of cases—occasionally other lesions in diphtheria, scarlet fever, and smallpox; carriers in diphtheria, scarlet fever, meningitis, and poliomyelitis
Spread	I° cases, II° fomites. Occasionally milk in diphtheria and scarlet fever (explosive epidemics); carriers in diphtheria, scarlet fever, meningitis, and poliomyelitis
Susceptibility	Everyone after 6 months of age not having active or acquired immunity. Exceptions: Scarlet fever varies geographically. Smallpox and whooping cough susceptible from birth. Some immunity probably acquired without disease by age and contact in all but smallpox and measles
Immunity Passive	Convalescent serum and gamma globulin give some protection for several weeks in all but smallpox. Whole adult blood in whooping cough, measles, mumps. Placental extract in measles. Antitoxin in diphtheria.
Active	An attack gives long-lasting immunity. Artificial immunity in smallpox, diphtheria, whooping cough, poliomyelitis, measles and mumps.
Control measures	1. Early diagnosis and reporting (laboratory in Diph., WC., Mening., Polio) 2. Isolation: Diph., SF., WC., SP. Of little value in the rest 3. Disinfection — Concurrent, Terminal 4. Quarantine like isolation 5. Immunization, q.v. 6. Source finding—D and SF (cases, carriers, milk); SP (cases). Of little value in the rest 7. Pasteurization of milk, especially in diphtheria and whooping cough 8. Prevention of overcrowding, especially in meningitis 9. Education

viously the key. By finding those who are already infected as early as possible, not only is it less expensive to restore them to health but the length of time during which they may infect others is significantly shortened. With the development of new and relatively inexpensive diagnostic tools such as the photofluorograph, the examination of large groups of people has become a practical technique. In addition there are now available drugs for more effective treatment and prophylaxis. It must be remembered that tuberculosis still requires a major part of state and local health expenditures. The economic savings alone, were the process of eradication adequately pursued, obviously would be enormous.

Tuberculosis is known to be a socially selective disease. The health department therefore must first familiarize itself with the extent and location of tuberculosis in its community. This involves a careful and fractionated analysis of all statistical and other sources of information, e.g., reports of cases, deaths, hospital admissions, etc. To

know that a community's tuberculosis death rate is 35 per 100,000 is not sufficient. Careful consideration must be given to the size and location of population groups in which the disease is apt to exist to an undue degree because of genetic, biologic, economic, or occupational influences. These are the groups among whom mass case finding techniques should be particularly stressed. Among the more important are (1) persons with suspicious pulmonary symptoms, (2) contacts to known cases of tuberculosis, (3) members of certain racial and nationality groups (e.g., Negroes, Amerinds, Scotch, Irish, Poles), (4) workers exposed to silica dust, (5) general clinic and hospital patients, (6) adolescents and young adults, (7) pregnant women, and (8) attendants of tuberculous patients. Several other groups should receive special attention by virtue of their occupational opportunity to infect others. Outstanding among these are schoolteachers and food-handlers.

Many of the groups mentioned are most conveniently and effectively reached for

STATE OF CALIFORNIA DEPARTMENT OF PUBLIC HEALTH

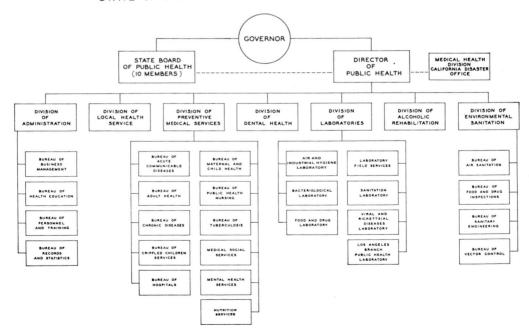

Fig. 17-9. Organizational plan of the California Department of Public Health.

diagnostic purposes through certain channels. Thus it is more efficient and fruitful to arrange for the mass examination of industrial workers at their place of work, schoolteachers and adolescents at their schools, and pregnant women and clinic and hospital patients at the time of their admission to service. Suspected cases and contacts of known cases require routine persistent field contacts by public health nurses.

While it is true that each of the communicable diseases is a biologic entity, certain similarities make it practical to group them into several categories for administrative and control purposes. Since control measures depend essentially upon modes of spread, this factor is also the most convenient for grouping diseases. Thus, while strictly speaking hookworm infection is not a gastrointestinal disease, the nature of the factors involved in its transmission justifies including it for administrative control purposes in that group of diseases.

The point of practical significance of course is that by grouping diseases in this manner many control measures may be applied to a group rather than to a single disease. This is illustrated by Tables 17-4 and 17-5, which summarize in a general manner the essential epidemiologic facts concerning acute respiratory diseases and gastrointestinal diseases. Similar groupings may be made for insect-borne diseases, chronic respiratory diseases, and genitoinfectious or venereal diseases. This concept is reflected organizationally in the frequent establishment, particularly in the health departments of states and large cities, of separate divisions or bureaus for venereal disease control, tuberculosis control, and occasionally in the past for certain of the gastrointestinal and insect-borne diseases. Present trends, however, are toward consolidation of all units into one major administrative division of communicable disease control or epidemiology, with bureaus for various subcategories, depending upon the relative magnitudes of problems. This trend is further manifest by the increasing number of organizations with a division of medical services, a bureau of which relates to disease control that may in turn be further subdivided. This is illustrated by a recent organizational plan of the California Department of Public Health (Fig. 17-9).

In addition to the more prosaic activities of the routine program of communicable disease control, public health organizations must be ever alert to the potentiality of circumstances that may be considered of an emergency or epidemic nature. The health department should be so organized that "without slipping a gear" it can marshal its resources and those of related agencies. An example of how this may be done is shown in the "responsibility schedule" shown on page 364. This represents one page of a complete responsibility breakdown of all of the components of the program of a large urban health department. It has been found useful to list points in the agency's effort in this form and to indicate exactly what part of the health agency is responsible for which activities, under what circumstances, and at what time.

Much has been said and written in an attempt to define the word "epidemic" in terms of the number of cases involved. At the present time this would seem to be similar to arguing over the number of angels on the head of a pin. From a practical standpoint, one might consider this to mean any communicable disease situation that calls for unusual or strenuous epidemiologic measures. The staff of a modern health department should become as concerned over a report of a single case of smallpox as it does with an outbreak of poliomyelitis or typhoid fever involving a score of persons. Both situations are unusual, present a serious threat to the community, and call for immediate action. Accordingly, a strong case could be made for avoiding the use of the word "epidemic" and substituting the term "communicable disease emergency."

On being confronted with evidence that indicates a possible emergency, the public health officer or epidemiologist must take a series of logical steps. Most obvious, although sometimes overlooked, he must first ascertain the true existence of an emergency. This involves careful consultation with those making the reports, followed by

RESPONSIBILITIES IN ACUTE COMMUNICABLE DISEASE CONTROL
Division with primary responsibility: Epidemiology

SCOPE AND PURPOSE

To control the incidence and transmission of acute communicable diseases.

COMPONENT PHASES

1. Acute infectious diseases
2. Parasitic infections
3. Food-borne outbreaks
4. Epidemic outbreaks of communicable diseases
5. Tropical and exotic infectious diseases

Typical activities

PRIMARY DIVISION

1. Furnishing consultation services to physicians requesting diagnostic help
2. Epidemiologic investigation and surveillance of diseases-medical
3. Food-borne disease investigation and control
4. Direction and control of follow-up procedures for the control of carriers
5. Validation of foreign travel immunization certificates
6. Professional direction of clinic for diagnosis and treatment of parasitic diseases
7. Detection and surveillance with epidemiologic services in occurrences of unusual, tropical, and exotic diseases
8. Direction of epidemiologic investigation and control of epidemic outbreaks of communicable diseases
9. Analysis of statistical reports
10. Research into cause and control of communicable disease

PARTICIPATING DIVISION

Public health nursing

1. Nursing services in clinics
2. Public health nursing services in the home for
   a. Nursing care when ordered
   b. Instruction and counseling for family health
   c. Referral to appropriate community agencies when indicated
   d. Epidemiologic investigation and follow-up in selected cases
   e. Consultation to other health and welfare agencies
   f. Interpretation of health department policies to families and social agencies

Laboratory

1. Providing laboratory tests to aid diagnosis and/or treatment including, but not limited to, the following:
   a. Enteric diseases
   b. Diseases of nose and throat
   c. Food poisoning outbreaks
   d. Hospital staph diseases

Environmental health

1. Food-borne disease investigation

Health education

1. Preparation and distribution of educational audiovisual materials
2. Preparation of educational-professional news releases
3. Promoting speaking engagements

confirmatory diagnosis in which the health officer or epidemiologist himself takes an active part. Diseases are poorly diagnosed or understood from behind a health department desk. The determination of the etiology of the disease is of obvious importance in deciding upon subsequent steps to take. Diagnostic assurance makes it possible to avoid some missteps and wasted effort and to decide what laboratory or other aids will be of assistance.

Once the nature of the condition is determined, the next step is to establish the fact of undue prevalence and incidence. False diagnoses due to either hysteria or faulty clinical judgment must be eliminated. By like token, missed cases must be found. These may be attributable again to faulty diagnosis or to unrecognized or un-diagnosed cases. Occasionally cases are missed, not because of lack of diagnosis but because they are deliberately concealed for misguided personal, social, or economic reasons. More than one vacation resort area, for example, has attempted to quash knowl-edge of the presence of disease. The occur-rence of typhoid fever in several places in the past has been ignored because of false pride in some new sanitary installation. These possibilities for missed cases there-fore make it necessary for the investigator to decide whether there is undue prevalence of recent origin or whether cases have been occurring for a considerable period of time and are just now being recognized. It is a common experience, for example, for the first one or two definitely diagnosed cases of poliomyelitis in a community to make the public and the private physicians particu-larly alert to the possibility of that disease in former as well as new patients.

Once the disease is diagnosed and a dis-tinct departure from normal prevalence has been noted, the next step in many situa-tions is to contact all persons involved, the public in general, and practicing physicians in particular in order to apprise them of the situation in a nonemotional manner and to solicit their assistance in whatever matter is indicated. This may take the form of public education to boil water or to avoid crowds, or of professional education in special diagnostic methods and tech-niques or in reporting.

Known patients should now be studied in relation to certain pertinent factors, in-cluding time, place, events, groups of the population affected, sex, race, age, and oc-cupation. Each of the patients or at least a representative sample of them, depending upon the disease and the size of the out-break, should be visited. A standardized epi-demiologic case card should be filled out for each patient. This has a twofold pur-pose: (1) to find the source and (2) to find contacts who may become future patients or in whom the development of the disease may be prevented. Out of a careful analysis of the epidemiologic case cards, it is hoped that some common denominator may be

discovered—a particular milk supply, social event, form of personal behavior, etc. If such a factor can be brought to light, it can then be made the subject of intense labora-tory or other study in order to confirm the suspicion of its causal nature, and appro-priate steps can be taken to prevent a re-currence of the emergency.

Anyone who has been engaged in such activities will agree that the foregoing para-graphs read much too easily. The investi-gation of a communicable disease emer-gency is no mean task. It involves intelli-gence, intuition, patience, and persistence. It is seldom a venture one can undertake alone. Reliable medical cooperation, lab-oratory assistance, and many other things are necessary for its successful comple-tion. When truly complete, however, an epidemiologic investigation is a work of art.

REFERENCES

1. Top, F., et al.: The history of American epi-demiology, St. Louis, 1952, The C. V. Mosby Co.
2. Christensen, A. W., Flook, E., and Druzina, G. B.: Distribution of health services in the struc-ture of state government, Washington, 1953, Public Health Service Pub. No. 184, part 3.
3. Emerson, H.: Uniformity in control of com-municable diseases, Amer. J. Public Health **32:**133, Feb. 1942.
4. Chapin, C. V.: Papers of Charles V. Chapin, M.D., New York, 1934, Commonwealth Fund.
5. Holst, P. M.: Concerning isolation in contagious disease, T. Norsk. Laegeforen. Nov. 9, 1933.
6. Gordon, J. E., and Badger, G. F.: The isolation time of scarlet fever, Amer. J. Public Health **24:**438, May 1934.
7. American Public Health Association: Control of communicable diseases in man, ed. 7, New York, 1949, The Association.
8. Shafer, J. K.: Premarital health examination legislation, Public Health Rep. **69:**487, May 1954.
9. Today's VD control program, New York, 1966, American Social Hygiene Association.
10. Halse, L. M., and Liberti, D. V.: Prenatal health examination legislation, Public Health Rep. **69:**105, Feb. 1954.
11. Condit, P. K., and Brewer, A. F.: Premarital ex-amination laws—are they worth while? Amer. J. Public Health **43:**880, July 1952.
12. Hedrick, A. W., and Silverman, C.: Should the premarital blood test be compulsory? Amer. J. Public Health **48:**125, Feb. 1958.
13. Resurgence of venereal disease, Bull. N. Y. Acad. Med. **40:**802, July 1964; **41:**820, July 1965.
14. Kupka, E., and King, M.: Enforced legal isola-

tion of tuberculosis patients, Public Health Rep. 69:351, Apr. 1954.

15. Rich, W. H., and Terry, M. C.: The industrial control chart applied to the study of epidemics, Public Health Rep. 61:1501, Oct. 1946.

16. Godfrey, E. S.: A study in the epidemiology of diphtheria in relation to the active immunization of certain age groups, Amer. J. Public Health 22:237, Feb. 1932.

17. Frost, W. H.: How much control of tuberculosis? Amer. J. Public Health 27:759, Aug. 1937.

Chapter 18

Maternal and
child
health activities*

INTRODUCTION

In a general sense the field of public health is concerned with the well-being of all people, regardless of age, sex, race, or other characteristics. Traditionally, however, there have been two groups to whom particular attention has been given: pregnant women and young children, particularly infants. There are sound reasons for this. Special attention to a pregnant woman brings double health benefits: first, to her as an adult member of society and, second, to the product of her pregnancy. Other reasons for placing special emphasis on the period of pregnancy are that this is a period of particular physical stress during which time the woman, who ordinarily may have no difficulties, may face the possibilities of unusual risk. Undesirable influences during the prenatal period may affect and even jeopardize the subsequent state of health of both the mother and the expected infant. Short of fatalities, these effects may take the form of health and economic disadvantages for the woman and child and even for the rest of the family if the mother's health is permanently impaired.

Remarkable progress has been made in many parts of the world in the saving of lives of expectant mothers and their infants. In the United States during the 50

*For a detailed discussion, see *A Bookshelf on Maternal and Child Health* by Schmidt and Valadian.[1]

years following World War I, maternal mortality declined about 95% and infant mortality about 75%. This may be attributed to many factors of which public health progress is only one. Hospital and medical standards have improved as have the national state of nutrition and the general standard of living. Also many new preventive and therapeutic agents have been introduced. Furthermore, while maternal and child health activities are usually given specific emphasis by public health organizations, every aspect of the public health program has had a marked effect upon the health and welfare of expectant mothers and particularly of infants and young children. In areas undeveloped in a sanitary sense the institution of an effective program of environmental sanitation involving the purification of water, the sanitation of milk and food, and the promotion of satisfactory facilities for the disposal of human wastes, will show its first effects in a reduction in infant morbidity and mortality. Vital statistics are involved in the maternal and child health program in various ways, especially by pinpointing specific problem areas. The public health laboratory is an essential tool, particularly in prenatal management where tests must be performed to indicate the presence of venereal diseases, the Rh reaction, eclamptic tendencies, diabetes, tuberculosis, and other ailments that considerably increase the risk incurred by

367

pregnancy and to determine appropriate medical management that must be followed. Throughout the entire antenatal, natal, and postnatal period there must be woven a strong thread of health education. The expectant mother must be constantly guarded against communicable diseases, particularly those of a streptococcal and influenzal nature, and early attempts must be made to protect the newborn child against gonorrheal ophthalmia, smallpox, whooping cough, diphtheria, measles, and other communicable infections. It is obvious, therefore, that the maternal and child health program cannot be considered by itself.

BACKGROUND OF MATERNAL AND CHILD HEALTH PROGRAMS

In the United States programs for the promotion of maternal and child health originated with the opening of the first milk station in 1893 in New York City. The original purpose of this and similar stations that subsequently were established was to combat the tremendous incidence of summer diarrhea in infants and children of the underprivileged by providing them with safe milk during the summer heat. In fact, the nature of this beginning had much to do with the ultimate development of municipal and state regulation of milk supplies. Observance of the benefits that resulted from this meager start led to the establishment of numerous infant welfare societies designed to bring medical and nursing knowledge and care to those in need. In 1908 the New York City Association for Improving the Condition of the Poor, in conjunction with the New York Outdoor Clinic, began to provide prenatal care for expectant mothers in the lower income groups. Simultaneously a Bureau of Child Hygiene was established in the New York City Health Department. These two moves were subsequently duplicated by many other communities throughout the nation. In 1912 the Children's Bureau was established under circumstances discussed in a previous chapter. Another development of significance at about that same time was the formation of the American Association for

the Study and Prevention of Infant Mortality. This was comprised of pediatricians, infant welfare nurses, who in a sense were the precursors of the present-day public health nurses, social workers, public health officials, and other interested persons, all of whom provided leadership in the rapidly expanding movement to protect the lives and health of mothers and children. This organization was the beginning of what in 1923 became the American Child Health Association, which provided most effective leadership until the time of its disbandment in 1935. The growing and widespread interest in the problem commanded national attention that resulted first in the passage of the Sheppard-Towner Act,[2] which functioned from 1922 to 1929, and later in the inclusion of broad national consideration of maternal and child health problems in the Social Security Act, which was approved in August 1935. These basic legislative acts which provided initial leadership and funds have had a marked and lasting effect upon the development of maternal and child health programs in state health departments and in local areas throughout the nation. Another occurrence of greater significance than was recognized by many at the time was the establishment during World War II of the Emergency Maternity and Infant Care Program. This program, designed to provide qualified obstetric care for the pregnant wives of servicemen as well as medical care for their infants, was administered by the Children's Bureau. This national program, by virtue of the necessity to establish basic standards for personnel, facilities, services, and fees in all areas that benefitted from the subsidies, had perhaps a greater effect upon the quality and quantity of care rendered to expectant mothers and their infants than any other factor up to that time. In addition, it provided some federal, state, and local health personnel with an opportunity to obtain experience in the administration of a medical care program. This experience proved to be of value to many subsequently.

The 1960's have witnessed the passage of some of the most significant federal and state legislation pertaining to health in the nation's entire history.* The Vaccination Assistance Act was passed in 1962. It made available almost $26 million to state and local health departments to conduct intensified immunization programs, especially among preschool children, against diphtheria, whooping cough, tetanus, and poliomyelitis. The act was extended in 1965 for another 3-year period, and measles was added to the list of diseases to be attacked. It also included measures designed to establish effective ongoing immunization programs.

In 1963, recognizing that about 3% of babies born are mentally retarded and that much of this problem is attributable to inadequate maternal and infant care, Congress passed the Maternal and Child Health and Mental Retardation Planning Amendments. This made possible the start of a 5-year, $265 million program to improve maternal and child health services, especially for high-risk prospective mothers who have or are likely to have conditions hazardous to themselves or to their infants during pregnancy. Particular emphasis is placed upon those who otherwise would not receive care because of low income or for other reasons beyond their control. The act also provides grants to states to plan comprehensive programs to combat mental retardation.

The year 1965 was a banner year; the nation through its Congress and the President entered into an unprecedented assault on its health problems.[4] More progressive health legislation was passed during that year than at any time previously. One indication is the fact that in the following year, 1966, the federal government expended through the Department of Health, Education, and Welfare about $3.1 billion for health purposes —a 50% increase in only 3 years.[5] The single most significant measure passed was the Social Security Amendments Act of 1965 (P. L. 89-97). It included a number of provisions designed to enhance the health and well-being of mothers and children. Not only did it extend the Maternity and In-

fancy Program which resulted from the 1963 legislation, but it also made it possible for state and local health departments to develop comprehensive health service programs, medical, dental and psychologic, for preschool and school children. Under the amendments the federal government through its Children's Bureau can provide up to 75% of the costs of projects to screen, diagnose, and treat children in low-income areas as well as carry out broad intensified child-health promotive and protective activities in the community. Funds for the program began with $15 million in 1966 and will increase to $50 million by 1970. The 1965 Social Security Amendments also extend and improve services to crippled children through case finding, diagnosis, and hospitalization with medical, surgical, and outpatient care. Provision is included for the training of more people who are needed to work with crippled children. Mention should also be made of legislation (P.L. 88-164, Title III, and P.L. 89-105) that provides support for research or demonstration projects relating to the education and training of youth handicapped by mental, physical, hearing, visual, or other defects.

Another event of considerable potential significance to maternal and child health was the passage of the Economic Opportunity Act of 1964 (P.L. 88-452). Through the provision relating to the Head Start Program medical and dental examinations and in some cases treatment and nutritional services may be provided to economically disadvantaged preschool children. Through its Community Action Program provisions numerous communities have added significantly to their services to the children of the poor, including in a number of instances the development of comprehensive medical or health centers. Similar provisions exist in relation to the Appalachia Regional Development Act (P.L. 89-4).

One other legislative action certainly destined to have far-reaching implications for maternal and child health as well as all other health activities was the passage of the Comprehensive Health Planning and Public Health Services Amendments Act of 1966 (P.L. 89-749). This act provides grants

---

*For a valuable reference volume on federal programs to further social and economic development, see *Catalog of Federal Assistance Programs.*[3]

to states to finance comprehensive planning in order to identify public health needs and to establish priorities for health services. The act also provides block grants in place of categoric grants to states to assist in the establishment and maintenance of comprehensive public health services, some of which may of course relate to or affect maternal and child health.

STATEMENT OF THE PROBLEM

Despite the significant advances in maternal and child health in the past few decades, there still is much room for improvement.

Maternal mortality

The unfinished business in maternal health becomes apparent even when the currently decreasing rates are compared with those of many economically less favored nations and especially when the rates are broken down geographically, economically, and by age, race, and other factors. During 1960, although the number of all maternal deaths per 10,000 live births was 3.7 and the rate for white women was 2.2, the risk for women of other races was 8.8

(Table 18-1). However, the proportionate decrease over the previous quarter century has been about the same for women of all races in the United States. It is important to note that 1960 was apparently a low point and that during the past several years maternal mortality rates have begun to increase in both white and nonwhite women.

These differences in the rates of maternal deaths by race are reflected partially in the variations observable among the states. Generally speaking, a line drawn along the 37th degree latitude, cutting across the northern boundaries of North Carolina, Tennessee, Arkansas, Oklahoma, New Mexico, and Arizona, divides the nation into a southern area with a high maternal mortality and a northern area of low to average rates. In 1960 maternal mortality ranged from 1.46 per 10,000 live births in Minnesota to a high of 8.60 per 10,000 live births in Mississippi.

There is no reason to believe that true racial or geographic differences should naturally exist. Analyses of economic status, standard of living, and availability and utilization of medical, nursing, and hospital fa-

Table 18-1. Maternal mortality, United States

Year	Total (per 10,000 live births)	White (per 10,000 live births)	Other (per 10,000 live births)
1930	67.3	60.9	117.4
1960	3.7	2.2	8.8
Percent of decrease	94.5	96.4	92.5
1962-1963		2.4	9.6

Table 18-2. Births by race, location, and type of attendant, United States and Mississippi, 1943 and 1960

Place, race, and year			Location Hospital %	Elsewhere %	Attendant Physician %	Other %
United States:	Total	1960	96.6	3.4	97.8	2.2
	White	1943	77.2	22.8	97.8	2.2
		1960	98.8	1.2	99.5	0.5
	Negro	1943	31.5	68.5	55.9	44.1
		1960	85.0	15.0	88.5	11.5
Mississippi		1943	26.6	73.4	42.8	57.2
		1960	72.7	27.3	76.0	24.0

cilities bring out striking parallels with the distribution of maternal mortality rates. If for purposes of comparison one goes back 25 years to 1943, a year for which much detailed data is readily available, in all of the southern tier of states referred to fewer than 60% of births occurred in a hospital, the figure in the case of Mississippi being as low as 26.6%. Similarly in each of these states many women were delivered by persons other than trained physicians, the extremes being Mississippi again with 42.8% and South Carolina with 36.3% (Table 18-2). When this is correlated with race, it is found that the majority of nonhospitalized and nonmedically attended deliveries in these states were those of Negro women. The overall figures for the nation in 1943 show that 97.8% of white women were delivered by physicians, 77.2% of them in hospitals, whereas 55.9% of Negro women were delivered by physicians, with only 31.5% of them in hospitals. In Mississippi over 80% of Negro women in labor had no medical attendance at all.

Since 1943 the circumstances of childbirth have improved considerably across the board, especially for those in the poorer areas and for nonwhite women. Thus in 1960 in Mississippi, although still with the poorest record, 73% of its women gave birth in hospitals. This represents a remarkable twofold improvement in less than two decades. Similarly the proportion of women in that state who were delivered by other than physicians was cut in half. By 1960 not only did practically all white births (98.8%) occur in hospitals, but even more significantly the proportion of Negro births in hospitals rose from 31.5% in 1943 to 85.0% in 1960 and medically attended Negro births rose from 55.9% to 88.5%. At the other extreme are North Dakota and the New England States, in which all but occasional births are medically attended and take place under hospital conditions.

Maternal mortality varies significantly with age. As illustrated in Table 18-3, it is lowest in all races in women under 20 years of age, after which it increases almost geometrically with each successive age span. Of considerable current importance is the fact that the rate of decline also varies with age. Among both white and nonwhite women the greatest gains have been made in the younger age groups. The discrepancy is most noticeable, however, with nonwhite women, among whom the rate of improvement in maternal mortality slows up significantly after 35 years of age.

With respect to time of occurrence most maternal deaths take place during or very soon after delivery or abortion. Thus a study in 1943, when the overall rate was 24.5 maternal deaths per 10,000 live births, showed that 65% occurred during or soon after delivery, 16% during or soon after abortion, 14% before delivery, and 4% related to ectopic pregnancies. About 90% of maternal deaths in 1943 were attributable to three categories of cause: infections, 36%; toxemias, 27%; and hemorrhage,

Table 18-3. Maternal mortality by age and race, United States, 1952-1953 and 1962-1963*

| Age period (years) | Deaths per 10,000 live births | | | | Percent decline 1962-1963 since 1952-1953 | |
| | White | | Nonwhite | | | |
	1952-1953	1962-1963	1952-1953	1962-1963	White	Nonwhite
All ages	4.6	2.4	17.7	9.6	48	46
Under 20	3.4	1.2	12.0	5.0	65	58
20-24	2.6	1.3	10.6	5.2	50	51
25-29	3.4	1.9	13.8	8.5	44	38
30-34	5.7	3.7	28.5	15.9	35	44
35-39	11.0	6.0	41.6	25.2	45	39
40-44	18.6	9.5	53.7	35.0	49	35

*From Statistical bulletin, Metropolitan Life Insurance Co., June 1965.

Table 18-4. Major causes of maternal mortality by race, United States, 1952-1953 and 1962-1963*

| Cause of death | Deaths per 10,000 live births | | | | Percent decline 1962-1963 since 1952-1953 | |
| | White | | Nonwhite | | White | Nonwhite |
	1952-1953	1962-1963	1952-1953	1962-1963		
All causes	4.6	2.4	17.7	9.6	48	46
Toxemias	1.4	0.4	6.5	1.9	71	71
Hemorrhage	0.9	0.4	2.8	1.7	56	39
Abortion	0.5	0.5	2.4	2.0	—	17
Sepsis	0.5	0.3	1.6	1.0	40	37
Ectopic pregnancy	0.2	0.1	1.7	0.9	50	47
Other complications	1.0	0.7	2.7	2.1	30	22

*From Statistical bulletin, Metropolitan Life Insurance Co., June 1965.

trauma, and shock, 28%. Since that time the greatest gains have been made against the risk of maternal death before and during delivery. The situation at the present time is shown in Table 18-4, which compares the major causes of maternal deaths in 1952-1953 with 10 years later, 1962-1963.

The decline in deaths from infection is undoubtedly associated with the recent advances made in chemotherapy, particularly in the development of antibiotics, the increased use of blood transfusions, the trend away from operative interference, and improved hospital standards. More frequent and better prenatal care with particular emphasis on diet and again the avoidance of operative delivery have undoubtedly played important roles in the great reduction of the death rate from toxemias of pregnancy. Significant inroads have been made against hemorrhage, trauma, and shock as causes of maternal mortality as a result of improved obstetrical management, fewer operative deliveries, and the more common use of transfusions of blood, blood plasma, and related products. It is to be noted that deaths from abortions remain about as important as before. A concerted attack must be launched against this needless killer of pregnant women. A major part is caused by illegal abortions carried out by unqualified individuals and women themselves often under extremely unsatisfactory and insanitary conditions. Fortunately this is increasingly recognized as an important social and public health problem,[6] and a number of states have revised their laws to liberalize the justifications for legal abortion, while a number of others are considering this move. The types of situations usually considered justifiable in the new state laws include rape, incest, risk to mental as well as physical health of the mother, eugenics, and exposure to certain viruses or drugs that tend to cause malformations.

Unquestionably, considerable further success is possible against deaths related to childbearing, especially in view of existing knowledge, obstetric techniques, and the existing remarkable pharmaceutic armamentarium. Faults of human motivation and behavior remain the single greatest deterrent.

Infant mortality

As would be expected, the factors involved in the problem of infant mortality and the improvements that have been made closely parallel the situations previously described for the mothers of the infants. Although there is cause for pride in the reduction that has been effected in the infant mortality rate, much remains to be accomplished. The situation has been depicted most vividly by comparison with war losses. "From Pearl Harbor to V-J Day 281,000 Americans were killed in action. During the same period 430,000 babies died in the United States before they were a year old— 3 babies dead for every 2 soldiers."[7] The nation still suffers a loss of about 85,000 infants each year. In 1966 this resulted in an infant mortality rate of 23.4 per 1,000 live births. During the first half of 1967 infant mortality dropped even more to 22.9, an all-time low for the United States. It is distressing to observe, however, that 17 other countries have lower infant mortality rates than the United States.[8] Of the possible causative factors studied, it appears that the most likely is the apparent higher proportion of low birth-weight infants in the United States, a problem which incidentally is increasing rather than improving.

Although the infant mortality rate has been steadily decreasing here as in the case of maternal mortality, internal disparities are to be noted: In 1963-1964, for example, the death rate for white infants was 21.9, while for other races it reached 41.3 per 1,000 live births. The rate of decline has been about the same, slightly above or below 60% for all races since 1960. It is noteworthy, however, that the rate of improvement in the infant mortality has not paralleled the improvement in maternal mortality. Thus between 1953 and 1963 the maternal mortality decreased 48% and 46% among white and nonwhite women, respectively; during the same period infant mortality declined only 11% and 5% among white and nonwhite infants, respectively. The geographic variation in infant mortality is approximately the counterpart of that observed with maternal deaths. Except for a few sparsely settled states for which the birth and infant mortality rates are of questionable statistical significance, the southern tier of economically ill-favored states again poses the greatest problem. In 1963-1964 infant mortality ranged from 19.3 in Utah and 20.2 in Massachusetts, on the one hand, to 32.1 in South Carolina and 40.4 in Mississippi, on the other. Again, as in the case of adult women, there is no evidence that the nonwhite infant is intrinsically less viable than infants born to white mothers. The same factors of lower standard of living, poor nutrition, and unavailability of professional services and hospital facilities play a predominant role.

In an evaluation of the problem, in order to formulate a sound program for control, a knowledge of the circumstances and causes of infant deaths is fundamental. A curve of infants deaths or death rates by age in hours, days, weeks, or months is characteristically a survivorship type of curve, asymptotic to both axes. It begins extremely high for the first few minutes, hours, and days of life and decreases sharply by the end of the first week. In 1960, for example, two thirds of infant deaths occurred during the first month of life and about one third during the first day. About 60% of neonatal deaths are due to prenatal or natal conditions or events, of which, as shown in Table 18-5, prematurity is by far the most important. The risk of death during the first month of life is almost thirty times as great for a prematurely born infant (2,500 grams or less) than for those who are of normal term (more than 2,500 grams). The problem of the premature and underweight infant, therefore, is of predominant and increasing concern. Interestingly there is excellent evidence that nonwhite premature and underweight infants have a significantly better survival rate than do white infants of the same condition.[9]

Deaths of premature infants have been reduced significantly during the past quarter century, particularly as a result of improved facilities and personnel for their prompt and adequate care. Pneumonia of the newborn used to be a much more important cause of neonatal death but has been reduced by improved nursery management and the use of antibiotics. Some inroads have been made in recent years not only against birth injuries but even against congenital malformations.

Table 18-5. Neonatal deaths by cause, United States, 1959

Cause	% of Deaths
Immaturity, unqualified	25
Postnatal asphyxia and atelectasis	24
Birth injuries	13
Congenital malformations	13
Ill-defined diseases peculiar to infancy, including nutritional problems	8
Pneumonia of the newborn	5
All other causes	12

Survival of the first few days or weeks of life does not mean that the health and life of the infant are no longer subject to risk. There are still many threats to his well-being, and there are necessary steps that must be taken in order to circumvent them. A list of the leading causes of infant deaths contains a number of factors that surprise many (Table 18-6).

Until only a few years ago infections and infectious diseases predominated. Now they are of secondary importance, with the exceptions of (1) pneumonia and influenza and (2) gastroenteritis. Even these have been markedly reduced in recent years—the first by better nutrition and antibiotics and the second by improved sanitation, nursery techniques, and chemotherapy. Of surprise to many and of much significance is the position of accidents in seventh place. Actually accidents represent the second leading cause of infant deaths after the first month of life is passed. Perhaps more interesting and surprising is the presence of heart disease and malignancies on a list of leading causes of infant death. Some success through survey is beginning to be achieved against congenital heart defects.

It appears obvious that the infant requires a spectrum of precautions and services to get him through his hazardous first

year: proper, adequate, and sanitary feeding; protection against infections and accidents; well-baby supervision, preferably by a family pediatrician, assisted if need be by a public health nurse; prompt correction of any defects that may exist; early diagnosis and treatment of any illnesses that may occur; and the provision of a satisfactory emotional environment. Failure to provide these needs invites more serious difficulties as well as personal and social loss later in life.

The preschool child

There are in the United States approximately 15 million children between the ages of 1 and 5 years, the period customarily referred to as the preschool age. When a child passes his first birthday, he enters a period of life that is most favorable from the standpoint of the risks of mortality. At the present time the risk of death between the first and the fifth birthday is only about 1 per 1,000 preschool children. This was by no means always the case; at the beginning of the century the death rate of this age group was about 20 per 1,000. It was this period of life that most benefited from many of the greatest triumphs of preventive medicine and public health. The decreases noted may be credited chiefly to the successful treatment and, what is of greater importance, to the prevention of the so-called acute communicable diseases of childhood. This is brought out forcefully by a comparison of the leading causes of death in this age group for 1900 as against 1965 (Table 18-7). In the earlier year, 1900, the preschool death rate from influenza and pneumonia was about 387 per 100,000 as compared with a rate of about 11 in 1965. At the beginning of the century diarrhea, enteritis, and dysentery were important causes of death, accounting for a combined death rate of about 330 per 100,000, compared with about 3 preschool deaths per 100,000 population in 1965. The decrease in deaths from diphtheria, measles, scarlet fever, and whooping cough have been equally dramatic. While deaths from motor vehicle accidents in this age group have necessarily gone up since 1900, it is interesting that accidents from other causes have

Table 18-6. Ten leading causes of infant death, United States, 1964

Rank	Cause	Deaths per 100,000 infants
1	Postnatal asphyxia and atelectasis	416.2
2	Immaturity, unqualified	396.6
3	Congenital malformations	352.5
4	Ill-defined diseases peculiar to early infancy, including nutritional maladjustment	265.4
5	Birth injuries	210.6
6	Pneumonia, except pneumonia of newborn	203.3
7	Accidents	84.6
8	Pneumonia of newborn	76.7
9	Gastritis, duodenitis, enteritis, and colitis, except diarrhea of newborn	50.3
10	Erythroblastosis	41.2

Table 18-7. Leading causes of death for children 1 to 4 years of age, United States, death registration area, 1900 and 1965

1900	Rates per 100,000 population	1965	Rates per 100,000 population
Influenza and pneumonia	386.6	Accidents	31.8
Diarrhea and enteritis	303.0	Pneumonia	11.1
Diphtheria	271.0	Congenital malformations	10.2
Tuberculosis (all forms)	101.8	Infective and parasitic diseases	5.8
Measles	87.6	Malignant neoplasms other than leukemia and aleukemia	4.4
Accidents (nonmotor vehicle)	75.3		
Scarlet fever	64.1	Leukemia and aleukemia	4.2
Whooping cough	60.0	Meningitis, except meningococcal and tuberculous	2.6
Dysentery	29.4		
Nephritis	19.5	Major cardiovascular and renal diseases	2.4
		Gastritis, duodenitis, enteritis, and colitis, except diarrhea of newborn	2.4
		Anemias	1.1
		Bronchitis	1.1

Table 18-8. Acute conditions, restricted activity days, and bed disability days by age, United States, July 1960—June 1961*

Age (years)	Acute conditions per 100 persons per year	Restricted activity days per 100 persons per year	Bed disability days per 100 persons per year	Bed disability days per acute condition per year
Under 5	373.4	1053.9	446.7	1.2
5–14	255.6	902.1	382.2	1.5
15–24	188.5	723.8	292.9	1.6
25–44	171.6	786.8	296.8	1.7
45–64	133.9	759.2	256.4	1.9
65+	119.0	1129.8	405.4	3.4
Total	201.9	856.9	332.3	1.6

*Health statistics, Series B–No. 34, Department of Health, Education, and Welfare, Public Health Service Pub. No. 584-B31, Jan. 1962.

decreased significantly. In fact, the 1900 rate was more than twice the current rate.

Of greater significance than the forces of mortality in the preschool ages is the fact that, although deaths are infrequent here, the age period is one of high morbidity. Thus the National Health Survey indicates an annual frequency rate of acute conditions for children during the first 5 years of life of 373 per 100,000. Similarly, restricted activity days and bed disability days are high during this period of life. Fortunately, as indicated in Table 18-8, not only is the recovery rate for preschool children high, but the duration of their illnesses is brief.

The preschool years represent a period of marked nutritional and emotional change for the child as well as one of increased effective contacts for the acquirement of communicable diseases and involvement in accidents. From the point of view of the public health approach, therefore, this stage of life is now one to which more attention must be given, not so much for the prevention of death as for the prevention of physical and mental illnesses and trauma that may handicap the future lives of those concerned. Since the individual in this age span is undergoing very rapid growth and development, what may often appear at the moment to be inconsequential influences of a nutritional, emotional, dental, or physical nature may have an ultimate cumulative effect far out of proportion to their initial appearance. The need, therefore, is for programs designed to minimize the daily impact of influences of this nature, programs for nutritional improvement, accident prevention, and continuous health and dental supervision, including, for example, the wider acceptance of techniques for the prevention of dental caries in the preschool child by the topical application of sodium fluoride. Mental illness is perhaps the greatest cause of disability in the adult population at the present time. It is in the preschool period of life where the seeds of much of this are sown. There is further indicated, therefore, a great need for the application of the principles of sound mental health and for the more widespread establishment and use of metal health and child guidance services.

APPROACH TO THE PROBLEM

Since so many factors can affect the well-being of mothers and children, programs related to them must be multifaceted.

General

In order to meet adequately the many problems presented in the field of maternal, infant, and child health, it is necessary for the official health agency of a community to carry out a well-conceived and interrelated series of activities, each of which looks forward to the subsequent periods of life. The objectives of all phases of the program should be both service and education. It must be realized, of course, that the health department alone cannot begin to render all of the service and education required. In fact, no other part of the health department program requires the cooperation of so many people and agencies in the community. In the final analysis, except in economically disadvantaged areas, most of the direct medical and dental service to mothers, infants, and children will be rendered by private physicians and dentists. Similarly the health department can probably never substitute for the health teaching of children in the home and in the classroom under the guidance of intelligent parents and

professionally trained teachers. No other phase of the public health program requires so many cooperative contacts with nonofficial nursing agencies and with the many social agencies that are found in the average community. Within the health department itself the cooperation of all the staff is necessary for success in this field. Everyone in the organization, including the vital statistics and engineering staffs as well as the nurses, contributes to the protection and improvement of the health and welfare of these population groups.

Beyond this, the active cooperation and assistance of many lay persons and groups in the community must be obtained. Few aspects of the public health program excite the active interest of the public as much as does the maternal and child health program. In addition to using lay advice and support by means of advisory committees, maternal health councils, or similar techniques, many health departments have found it possible to improve and expand their service programs considerably by using volunteer workers both in clinics and in the field.

One further general consideration deals with the necessity for conducting continuous research and surveys in order to keep the program in tune or in balance with the maternal and child health problem. This involves attacks from a number of angles. In areas with good reporting, morbidity and mortality data provide the most obvious source of guidance. In the United States a surprising amount of data is available through the publications of the Bureau of Census and the National Office of Vital Statistics as well as through analyses conducted by the states and communities themselves. Daily[10] has pointed out that, generally speaking, the statistical needs for maternal and child health programs can be divided into two categories: vital statistical data usually available in any state and supplemental statistical information that is usually necessary for the proper interpretation of the vital statistics. He lists the following vital statistics relating to maternity and infancy that are usually available for any state, county, or large city and that are a part of the basic information in planning any health service for mothers and infants:

1. Live births and stillbirths (number and rate)
   (a) Urban, rural
   (b) Resident and nonresident
   (c) In hospitals, in homes
   (d) Attended by physician, not attended by physician
   (e) Legitimate or illegitimate
   (f) Race
2. Maternal deaths (number and rate)
   (a) Urban, rural
   (b) Resident and nonresident
   (c) In hospitals, in homes
   (d) Attended by physician, not attended by physician
   (e) Causes
3. Neonatal deaths (infant deaths under 1 month of age) (number and rate)
   (a) Urban, rural
   (b) Resident and nonresident
   (c) In hospitals, in homes
   (d) Attended by physician, not attended by physician
   (e) Race
   (f) Causes of death
   (g) Age at time of death

This list must be supplemented by information relating to available medical and hospital facilities, the economic distribution of the population, the occupations of women in the childbearing ages, literacy, and many other socioeconomic factors. In addition, data must be sought with regard to the quality of care rendered and the complications of pregnancy and infancy that occur in the area under consideration. This will require the periodic or continuous analysis of hospital and medical records, an activity which is best performed for the health department by a committee of the medical and hospital groups in the community.

THE MATERNAL HEALTH PROGRAM

The natal process naturally divides itself into several rather definite phases, each of which presents certain problems and needs.

Preconceptional aspects

Contrary to the expectations of many, an adequate maternal health program should have its beginning long before the child is conceived and even before the expectant mother reaches physiologic maturity and marriage. The preconceptional aspects of the program involves a threefold approach

of education, medical service, and eugenics. Much education having a direct and significant influence upon future parenthood may be accomplished with the high school and even grade school girl and boy. Scientifically correct and socially acceptable facts may be presented to school children relating to many phases of social hygiene, including the anatomy and physiology of reproduction, the dangers of venereal diseases and abortion, the importance of medical supervision during pregnancy and infancy, and the responsibilities of parenthood. The staffs of health departments should cooperate actively with school and other groups engaged in such educational programs.

The health department is the chief agency for the promotion, implementation, and enforcement of legislation dealing with premarital and prenatal examination requirements of which serologic tests for syphilis and x-ray examination of the chest should be only a part.

The eugenic approach to maternity hygiene may be manifest by any one or a combination of three activities. The first of these is education, the basic principles of eugenics being an important and necessary part of any teaching program of sex education, social hygiene, or preparation for parenthood. Second, an increasing number of health departments sponsor programs on family planning often in cooperation with the Planned Parenthood Federation. These programs may provide contraceptive information and material and sometimes operate clinics for the remedying of sterility. Such programs are implemented in a number of ways: through supplementary service in maternal health clinics, through specifically established planned parenthood clinics, through the activities of the public health nurse in the home, or by means of referral to private physicians. A third manner in which the health department may be concerned with eugenics is where, as in a number of communities and states, commissions exist to pass upon the desirability of sterilization of certain defective individuals. In a number of such instances, the health officer is made a member of the commission.

Antepartum period

The antepartum period of pregnancy is most important. The objective is to get expectant mothers under early and continuous supervision of a qualified medical advisor. This objective should be supplemented by related activities including antepartum public health nursing service and instruction in the home; the provision of auxiliary facilities such as consultants, laboratory service, and nutritional aid; and an organized approach to special problems such as illegitimate pregnancy, abortion, care for women engaged in industry during pregnancy, and such technical problems as the management of Rh incompatibility.

So that as many expectant mothers as possible receive prenatal medical and nursing supervision, it is necessary to set up some form of administrative procedure to locate them as early in their pregnancies as possible. The need for and manner of doing this varies from one community to another, depending upon many social factors. The health department has at its disposal a number of sources of information. Knowledge of pregnancies may come to the health department staff through their personal observations during their daily rounds, by statements or suggestions from neighbors of expectant mothers, and from previous patients. Some health departments have found it worth while to maintain continuous contact with business establishments that sell layettes and other baby equipment. A highly desirable goal is for the private physicians practicing in the area to notify the health department of each new obstetric case. Part of the problem is already solved in that the patient is already under medical supervision. However, even here the health department may render service through public health nursing supervision and education wherever the medical attendant wishes and with follow-up of women who miss appointments.

Antenatal medical supervision may be rendered in one of three ways: by general practitioners, by obstetricians, or in prenatal clinics operated by the health department or other agencies. Considering the country as a whole, the first of these provides the largest part of the care, and the last the least. Great social and geographic variations exist. The majority of obstetric specialists practice in the large cities. Prenatal clinics are found serving primarily the lower economic groups in large urban centers and certain rural areas, particularly in the southern states. Most of the prenatal medical care rendered in rural areas is provided by general practitioners of medicine. It should be remembered, however, as previously pointed out, that although virtually all white women have some medical supervision during their pregnancies about 12% of Negro expectant mothers receive none.

Intrapartum period

Although the actual delivery of a pregnant woman would appear to be a matter of joint interest for the woman and her accoucheur, there are many places where the health department may enter into the intrapartum period. It has been pointed out in Chapter 9 that many health departments, primarily on the state level, have legal responsibility for the licensure, inspection, and regulation of maternity hospitals and nurseries. In many places public health agencies maintain active programs for the purpose of assuring hospitalization of selected obstetric cases and emergencies. Most states and cities where they exist have the legal responsibility for the regulation and control of midwives. Ordinarily this is accomplished by licensure, supervision, provision of some training, and examination. The ultimate goal in most instances, however, is the eventual elimination of this type of obstetric service in favor of medical supervision. A few health departments that serve areas with significant numbers of home confinements conduct programs designed for the improvement of this type of service. Some of the activities in this regard are the provision of sterilized obstetric packs and layettes, the preparation of the expectant mother for delivery in her home, and the provision of obstetric nursing assistance to the general practitioners who officiate at the deliveries. The purpose of the latter activity is threefold: service to the patient and the physician, education of the patient, and in some instances education of the physician.

Throughout the entire maternal health program, and particularly in its intrapartum phase, the intention of the public health agency must obviously be to support, assist, and promote the use of private physicians and not in any way to supplant them. Additional ways in which assistance is rendered are by provision of materials for ophthalmia prophylaxis, umbilical packages, birth registration materials, and in some instances loan of equipment for blood typing, transfusion, and other emergencies. Many health departments have been active in the development of standards for obstetric consultation and in some instances in the provision of the consultants themselves by direct employment or subsidization. A procedure of far-reaching consequence that has been promoted by many health departments in conjunction with their related medical societies is the formal review of all maternal deaths by a maternal and child health committee of the medical society. In many such instances the physician who attended the deceased mother must appear before the committee, outline his management of the case, and attempt to explain the reasons for its unfavorable outcome. This represents in effect a review of the attendant's work by a jury of his peers, and, where forthrightly carried out, it has undoubtedly encouraged more careful supervision and obstetric management of women in labor.

Postpartum period

As in the antepartum program, the first essential in the postpartum program is case finding. The location of women who have recently delivered is accomplished with relative ease. Where an efficient birth registration program is in effect, birth records provide a fruitful source of data. In addition to this is the arrangement achieved in some localities whereby hospitals routinely and promptly notify the health department of all deliveries that have occurred within their confines. In many instances the health department is notified when the patient is about to return home. Early notification is

most desirable, since it enables the public health nursing staff to make primary contact while the patient is still in the hospital, in order to facilitate her hospital discharge and reentrance into the home and to prepare her home to receive her. Unfortunately a great many postpartum public health nursing visits are first made after the mother and her new infant have been home for some weeks. By then much of the potential value is lost. It is when the woman first returns to the confusing cares of her home, with the added burden of a new infant, that she really needs and appreciates help. The value of meeting the mother and infant practically at the doorstep has been demonstrated by a number of health agencies, and the secret of its accomplishment is one of interagency cooperation and administrative timing. The problem of contacting women and infants after delivery has been greatly complicated during recent years by the current frequency of change of address and by the fact that many women come into cities for hospital delivery as a convenience but return to small communities or rural areas after discharge from the hospital. These factors have also caused much difficulty in the handling of premature and ill infants, especially those who are illegitimate.

The health department's postpartum program has two purposes: to provide whatever public health nursing service and education to the mother is indicated in each case and to accomplish a smooth and automatic carry-over to the infant health program. The The nurse often finds it possible to instruct the mother in proper infant care and formula preparation. She should make certain that the birth of the infant has been registered and that the mother and infant are both under medical supervision. She should maintain a watchful eye for the development of postpartum complications in the mother and of illness in the infant. Referrals should be made to appropriate agencies wherever medical, economic, or social problems are found to exist. Finally, the groundwork should be laid for the pediatric supervision of the infant, including all indicated protective treatments from either private physicians or health and well-baby conferences and clinics.

THE INFANT AND PRESCHOOL PROGRAM*

With regard to the neonatal program, early case finding is again a prerequisite and may be accomplished by means of (1) routine check of birth certificates, (2) notification from the accoucheur, the hospital, or the family itself, and (3) from the records of prenatal clinic attendance. Neonatal cases should be classified into priority groups, with premature infants at the top of the list, followed by those known to have been born with physical defects, and those who have become ill or injured during or following birth. Many health departments maintain a number of portable warm beds that may be loaned to parents of premature babies who have worked out arrangements, sometimes with other agencies, e.g., fire or police departments, for resuscitation services and for emergency transfer to hospitals. At least one large city has designed and provided electrically heated beds for prematures that may be fitted into taxicabs for the emergency handling of the premature infant.

For the usual infant and preschool child the health department's aim is one of supervision and education. As much as possible this aim is effected by reliance upon the many persons and agencies that exist as resources in the community. The most obvious and important of these are the private practitioner of medicine, the pediatrician, and the general practitioner. A large proportion of all well-child care is rendered by general practitioners. This occurs despite the fact that general practitioners tend to give less attention to health supervision as against therapy. Of general practitioner's visits to children (29% of his total practice), less than one in three visits are for health supervision. Thus while pediatricians see an average of nine children a day for health supervision, the general practitioner averages 1.3. Nevertheless it is the

general practitioners who provide most of the health supervision for the nation's children, for they outnumber pediatricians about twenty to one. Only about 1.5% of the total medical services to children is rendered in community health clinics. In view of these proportions it is all the more important for the health department to solicit the active and interested cooperation of the local medical society. One of the most effective steps in this regard is the promotion of an active participation in a medical society committee on maternal and child health by the health officer.

Within the health department the larger proportion of the visits and services of the public health nursing staff should be devoted to the infant and preschool program. The services are essentially educational in nature, the teaching being done wherever possible by demonstration. One of the primary objectives of the public health nurse in her visit to the home of an infant or preschool child is to assure continuous well-baby medical supervision, preferably by the family physician or pediatrician, and, failing that, in a well-baby conference conducted by the health department. Public health nursing visits on behalf of infants and preschool children should be made according to a set schedule that should be elastic enough, however, to allow for additional visits for special cases and emergencies. Generally speaking, at least two visits should be made during the first month of the infant's life. The first visit, as stated before, should be made within the first 48 hours following return to the home from the hospital or within the first 24 hours following delivery in the home. A third visit should be made as the child approaches 6 months of age, followed by another between the ninth and twelfth months. One of the primary purposes of the 6-month and 9-month visits is the promotion of the protective treatment of the baby against whooping cough, smallpox, diphtheria, tetanus, measles, and poliomyelitis. Chapter 29, which deals with vital statistics, includes a description of the manner in which this part of the program may be integrated with some other activities of the health depart-

---

*For a general overview, see *Standards of Child Health Care*.[11]

ment in order to achieve ultimately the desired result of a high level of community protection.

Despite the emphasis of the foregoing upon the well child, the infant and preschool program of the health department must take special cognizance of the sick and handicapped child population, seeking them out and referring them to the proper community or state facilities and agencies. It should be pointed out that in one half of the states services for crippled children are under the jurisdiction of the state health department. In the remaining states these services are usually found in departments of welfare; in six instances there are separate crippled children's commissions, in four states the program is conducted by the department of education, in two states by a branch of the state university, and in one state by a board of control.

Other activities that are gradually receiving increasing attention in infant and preschool health programs include the promotion of dental hygiene, nutrition, and mental hygiene.

REFERENCES

1. Schmidt, W. M., and Valadian, I.: A bookshelf on maternal and child health, Amer. J. Public Health 54:551, Apr. 1964.
2. Schlesinger, E. R.: The Sheppard-Towner era: a prototype case study in federal-state relationships, Amer. J. Public Health 57:1034, June 1967.
3. Office of Economic Opportunity: Catalog of federal assistance programs, Washington, 1967, U. S. Government Printing Office.
4. Forgotson, E. H.: 1965: The turning point in health law—1966: reflections, Amer. J. Public Health 57:934, June 1967.
5. A report to the people on health, Washington, 1967, Public Health Service (unnumbered publication).
6. Calderone, M. S.: Illegal abortion as a public health problem, Amer. J. Public Health 50:948, July 1960.
7. Committee for the Study of Child Health Services, The American Academy of Pediatrics: Child health services and pediatric education, New York, 1949, Commonwealth Fund.
8. International comparison of perinatal and infant mortality, Washington, 1967, Public Health Service Pub. No. 1000, series 3, no. 6.
9. Erhardt, C. L., et al.: Influence of weight and gestation on perinatal and neonatal mortality by ethnic group, Amer. J. Public Health 54:1841, Nov. 1964.
10. Daily, E. F.: Some statistical needs for proper administration of maternal and child health programs, Amer. J. Public Health 30:766, July 1940.
11. Standards of child health care, Evanston, 1967, The American Academy of Pediatrics.

Chapter 19

School health

THE SCHOOL CHILD

Following the preschool period, the child enters a world that involves more extensive contacts, a wider geographic range, an increasing number of personal and social conflicts, and many varied learning experiences. There are at the present time almost 40 million children in the age group between 5 and 15 years of age. The situation with regard to mortality and morbidity among school children is similar to that of preschool children. Again the death rates are low, having dropped from about 4 per 1,000 in 1900 to less than 1 per 1,000 at the present time. This reduction is largely attributable to success in prevention and treatment of acute communicable diseases of childhood (Table 19-1). In addition, the lowering of the threat of tuberculosis is noteworthy. At the beginning of this century over 36 school children per 100,000 died each year from this single cause. At the present time it is relatively inconsequential as a cause of death in this age group. Of further interest is the reduction in the number of deaths of school age children from diseases of the heart to approximately one tenth what they were in 1900.

As in the case of the preschool child, school children represent a group that, while subject to low death rates, experiences at the same time a high incidence of illness. To illustrate this, the number of acute conditions per year per 100 individuals in each age group is presented in Table 19-2.

As a result here again mortality data provide a poor measure of health problems and progress. Thus, while the death rate in this age group from heart disease, essentially rheumatic, was only 1.3 per 100,-

000 in 1960, it was estimated that almost 1% of the school population suffered from this disease, the crippling and life-shortening effects of which are delayed until later in life. Similarly, despite the great reduction in the tuberculosis death rate in this age period, it is undoubtedly here that a significant amount of infection with the tubercle bacillus takes place. Throughout this period of life the stresses of rapid growth remain evident and are emphasized both from a physical and mental standpoint by the sexual maturation of the individual in the later school years.

Two circumstances are of considerable importance to the community health program so far as the older school child is concerned: The first is that throughout this period the individual is preparing himself for living by learning. In addition, the often overlooked fact is that the older school child of today is the parent and citizen-voter of tomorrow. Both of these factors have a direct bearing upon the support and success of the public health program in any community. In other words this receptive impressionable period should be the most fruitful for the dissemination of health knowledge and for the establishment of understanding and support of community health measures.

SCHOOL AND COMMUNITY HEALTH

Between the fifth or sixth year and early adulthood children spend a large part of approximately one half the year in a school environment. During this important formative period the essential influences for physical and mental health and for education are shared by the home, the community,

Table 19-1. Leading causes of death for children 5 to 14 years of age, United States, death registration area, 1900 and 1965

1900	Rates per 100,000 population	1965	Rates per 100,000 population
Diphtheria	69.7	Accidents	18.7
Accidents, nonmotor-vehicle	38.3	Malignant neoplasms	6.5
Pneumonia and influenza	38.2	Congenital malformations	2.8
Tuberculosis	36.2	Influenza and pneumonia	2.1
Diseases of the heart	23.3	Cardiovascular and renal disease	2.1

Table 19-2. Acute conditions per year by age groups*

Age groups	Acute conditions per 100 people
All ages	201.9
Birth to 4 years	373.4
5 to 14 years	255.6
15 to 24 years	188.6
25 to 44 years	171.6
45 to 64 years	133.9
65 years and over	119.0

*Health of children of school age, Washington, 1964, Children's Bureau Pub. No. 427.

and the school. If the schools are to meet their responsibilities, it is necessary to formulate and to put into effect sound policies and programs for health protection and promotion during the hours of school experience.

The school is of particular importance for a number of reasons: In addition to its potential importance with regard to health instruction and the development of desirable habits it represents a gathering place for a population group that is particularly prone to many communicable diseases. School health must be thought of, therefore, as one part of the total community health pattern, concentrating its efforts upon the individual during a specific period of his existence. School health is actually the common concern of the school, the parent, and the community at all levels of government. The success and effectiveness of the program depends in large measure upon the common understanding on the part of each group and each individual involved as to (1) the precise scope of its sphere of action, (2) its role in the total community health picture, and (3) the need for consistent cooperation in its implementation. In other words at its best it must be a concerted attempt to put into practice for the school age child the thought embraced in the Children's Charter: "Every child has the right to be well-born and to attain the best possible quality of health of which it is capable."[1] All community health personnel need to pool their efforts in order to realize this obviously desirable goal to the greatest degree possible.

THE SCHOOL HEALTH PROGRAM

Because of the various influences and interrelationships as well as the dynamic nature of children and the health problems they may potentially develop, a program must be developed which focuses upon circumstances that may affect the health and well-being of the school child, that may derive from school personnel, and that may have their origin within the school and reach out to affect the home and the community or vice versa. With this purpose in mind the school health program has been defined as "the school procedures that contribute to the understanding, maintenance, and improvement of the health of pupils and school personnel, including health services, health education and healthful school living."[2] In other words we are concerned here with (1) the school environment, (2) the protection and promotion of health, including the handling of special problems of certain children, and (3) health instruction.

These three basic components of the school health program and the activities involved in each of them are presented in the accompanying table. Of necessity there is a certain amount of overlapping and interrelationship among these. This is desirable since each part of the program should be designed and used as much as possible to augment other parts. Thus certain aspects of the school environment or health appraisal activities should provide valuable firsthand health instructional material.

THE SCHOOL ENVIRONMENT

In relation to schools the term "environment" should be interpreted in its broadest sense. It should take cognizance not only of the immediate school premises but also of its surroundings and not only of its sanitation but also of its location and safety. In other words it should include consideration of every potential physical, mental, and moral hazard with which the child may come in contact in connection with his school experience. As stated by the National Committee on School Health Policies,[3] "The authority which requires pupils to attend school implies the responsibility to provide an environment as evocative as possible of growth, learning and health."

A discussion of the details of each of the many factors involved in the school environment is considered beyond the province of this book. Attention should be directed, however, to the general factors that call for supervision by public health and other au-

COMPONENTS OF THE SCHOOL HEALTH PROGRAM*

School environment	Health protection and promotion	Health instruction
Maintenance of a safe sanitary plant	Health appraisal	Planned, direct health teaching
Buildings	Periodic medical examination	Indirect health education
Grounds, playfields	Screening examinations	Assembly programs
Gymnasiums, swimming pools	Dental examination	Exhibits, etc.
Health service unit	Special examinations	Incidental health education
Seating, lighting, ventilation, heating, sanitation, drinking fountains	Referrals	Integrated health education
	Athletes	Correlated health education
	Follow-up procedures	Health units in other subject courses
Safety and accident prevention	Referrals	In-service health education
Protective equipment	Correction of remediable defects	School personnel
Fire drills	Care of exceptional children	Planning sessions
General safety	Prevention and control of disease	Workshops
Civilian defense and disaster	Planned emergency care	Conferences
Safety patrols, traffic safety	Illness	Courses
Transportation	Injury	Parent education
Driver education	Health counseling	Preparation of health curriculum guides
Administrator-teacher-pupil relationships	Health of school personnel	Utilization of resources
Recreation program	Cooperation with community agencies	Teaching aids
School luncheon	Official	Textbooks, supplementary books, periodicals
Custodial care	Voluntary	Community personnel
Healthful school day	Civic	Community facilities
Length	Parent	Museums
Class size	Program coordination	Libraries
Routine		Health centers
Grading and marking procedures		Cooperation with community health education efforts
Promotions		Official agencies
Classroom procedures		Voluntary agencies

*Adapted from Hanlon, J. J., and McHose, E.: Design for health—the teacher, the school, and the community, Philadelphia, 1963, Lea & Febiger.

thorities. Of primary importance is the location of the school. It should be chosen with a view to accessibility, salubrity, and adequacy. Proper choice of location will preclude the development of many sanitary problems. Attention should be given to drainage, shade and sunlight, freedom from industrial wastes, excessive noise, and excessive traffic. Provision should be made for adequate recreational space and for the possibility of future expansion. While the actual choice of location will not be a responsibility of the public health department, it should offer its consultative services to whatever agencies are involved.

The health department should play a role in the assurance of the proper construction and maintenance of the school. Conformance with accepted sanitary and safety standards should be assured by frequent inspection by representatives of the public health agency and by consultation with the school authorities. Consideration must be given to ventilation, lighting, heating, and acoustics; to adequacy and location of stairways and exits; to construction materials and methods from the viewpoints of sanitation and safety; and to the adequacy and design of toilet and handwashing facilities. Because of the numbers and characteristics of those involved, the water supplies and sewage disposal facilities serving schools are considered of a public nature. Even if they are part of larger municipal systems, facilities of this type merit particular scrutiny and supervision. In rural and developing suburban areas, the provision and maintenance of satisfactory water and sewage disposal facilities is particularly troublesome and requires especially persistent supervision by the health department.

Many schools, even in rural areas, provide lunchrooms and cafeterias that often have rather extensive facilities for the preparation and serving of foods. Such facilities should be under the constant surveillance of the sanitation staff of the health department in order to prevent their becoming a threat rather than a benefit to the children who use them.

Schools that contain gymnasiums, play areas, and swimming pools place an added supervisory responsibility upon the health department. Standards of construction and maintenance should be established by the health agency and enforced in cooperation with the school authorities. This becomes particularly important in view of the laudable trend toward making such facilities available to the entire community rather than to restrict their use to school children during school hours. Related to these facilities and to the school as a whole should be adequately equipped and adequately staffed health service rooms for the provision of first aid. This will be mentioned further in relation to health protection and promotion.

The most ideally located and constructed school can rapidly deteriorate and become a sanitary menace unless provision is made for its proper maintenance. As inferred above, many aspects of the physical school plant must be subject to frequent inspection. In addition, the health department staff, as a matter of policy, should annually conduct a complete and detailed survey of the sanitary conditions and facilities of each school, public or private, within its jurisdiction. Often this is best done during the summer months when some of the other community problems slacken and during which time whatever repairs as may be indicated may be made before the reopening of the schools in the fall. Written reports with recommendations for improvements should be submitted to the school principal and the superintendent of schools. Shortcomings should be discussed with them and all assistance possible given to remedy whatever defects are found. Subsequently follow-up inspections should be made to assure the correction of any undesirable conditions.

HEALTH PROTECTION AND PROMOTION

Present-day thinking indicates a social responsibility to prepare school children physically and psychologically as well as intellectually for adulthood. For many this means graduating them in better physical condition than when they entered school. In order to accomplish this purpose it is necessary to establish base lines by means of physical examination. At one time it was the custom to attempt to examine every school child every year. Eventually this was realized to be inefficient and pointless. This procedure had two undesirable features: So many children had to be examined each year that they usually received what amounted to a cursory scanning rather than ever getting a truly complete physical examination. Furthermore, so much attention was given to getting the children examined that it either became an end in itself or else left no time for the follow-up necessary to secure the correction of defects.[4,5]

Accordingly, a more reasonable approach has been developed and followed by more progressive communities whereby children are examined only three or four times during their entire school experience, for example, at entrance to grade school, the fourth grade, junior high school, and senior high school. Preferably a parent should be present at the examination of elementary school children for purposes of explanation and education. The examinations must be carefully conducted and complete examinations, regardless of the circumstances under which they are performed. By reducing the total amount of time spent on examinations more funds and personnel time and energy are left available for securing the correction of defects.

The arrangements whereby school children are examined varies. In some communities salaried school physicians do the work, whereas in others private physicians are employed on an hourly or daily basis. There may still occasionally be seen in large schools the grossly unsatisfactory system whereby one physician examines all throats, another all ears, another all chests, and so on without consideration of the total child.

A few large communities have followed the interesting policy of restricting the school medical work, particularly in relation to periodic examinations, to the younger and newer men just entering practice in the community. This is based upon the philosophy that everyone concerned benefits. The school and health departments get the examinations accomplished;

the new physicians not yet completely established benefit from the part-time salaries and from the experience and family contacts, and the children are given more thorough examinations because the new physicians have relatively more time, while the older busy practitioners are spared the necessity of using up their time in routine examination in which they often are not too interested. Finally, a learning situation is provided in which the younger physicians experience a satisfactory and helpful relationship with the health department which should bear sound fruits in terms of future professional relations.

Probably the most desirable system in the long run is one in which the health department and the schools educate and prompt parents to the maximum extent possible, to take their school children to their family physician, if they have one, for periodic physical examinations and other protective and promotive services as well as for their illnesses. Furthermore, when the school child becomes accustomed to going to his own physician for such services, the likelihood of his continuing to consult his private physician following his school years is considerably greater than if he had come to expect such services from a full-time school physician. Interesting and important variations exist as to the extent that this is possible.[6]

An important administrative technique which is of value as an adjunct to the periodic physical examination is the screening of pupils by their classroom teachers. The health department may cooperate by providing in-service training for teachers in order to acquaint them with the signs and symptoms of illnesses, particularly the communicable diseases. Without attempting to make diagnosticians out of them or to overburden them the teachers are encouraged to survey their pupils briefly each morning, referring any pupils with suspicious indications to the medical personnel available to the school. Comparative tests have demonstrated the ability of teachers to pick out sick or ailing children without reference to the exact cause.

The discovery of physical and mental defects or illnesses in school children in itself is of relatively little value. In fact, whatever value it has is contingent upon what is done with the information obtained. This means a successful follow-up program from the school and health department to the home, to the private physician or dentist, or to the social agency, whichever is needed for correction of the condition.

Another phase of the school health protection and promotion program deals with the control of communicable diseases. Of primary importance is the degree to which the parents of the community bring their children to school already protected against acute communicable diseases such as diphtheria, smallpox, whooping cough, measles, and poliomyelitis. Some school systems attempt to secure these protections by mandate. When this approach is followed, some parents tend to delay immunizations until the time of school entrance, which is too late for epidemiologic value. On the other hand, a high degree of community and school protection may be obtained by educational methods and it is foolish for a health department to make lasting enemies for its general program by stubbornly and needlessly insisting, on the basis of law or regulation, on the immunization of every last child. Too often some health or school officials have been so concerned with the achievement of high paper scores and ratings that they have overlooked much harm of a public relations nature that has been done in the process.

The screening of pupils by teachers has been discussed in relation to the periodic physical examination. When conducted routinely each morning, this becomes of some added value in the school's communicable disease control program and as an educational device. Children with suspicious signs and symptoms should be excluded from class and referred to the school medical service or to their private physician. It is desirable that there exist a policy of prompt notification of the health department. Similarly a release should be obtained from the health department or private physician before the child is readmitted to his classroom.

A question that inevitably arises in every community is whether or not schools should be in session during epidemic periods of communicable disease. In general the public tends to want the schools closed. However, when this is done, greater and more intimate contact between children usually follows since they tend to play in their neighborhoods and circulate among crowds rather than remain at home. Therefore, in communities with well-organized and efficient public health and school health services epidemics can best be controlled if the schools remain open and engage the children in controlled activities under intelligent and watchful surveillance.

In discussing the subject the National Committee on School Health policies suggested that the decision regarding the closing of schools when epidemics occur or threaten may be decided locally by answering the following two questions: (1) Are nurses and medical staffs so adequate and the teaching staff so alert that the inspection, observation, and supervision of students will keep sick students out of school? (2) If schools are closed, will students be kept at home and away from other students so that the closing of schools will not increase opportunities for contact with possible sources of infection?

As a general policy, when the first question can be answered affirmatively or when the second question is answered negatively, schools should be kept open in the face of an epidemic. This is most often the case in large public schools and in thickly settled communities. Schools should be closed when the first question is answered negatively or the second question affirmatively. In smaller communities with scattered homes, where chances for personal contact are limited, this is frequently the situation. In rural communities where pupils are transported in buses and close contact is unavoidable, it also may be advisable at times to close the schools.[7]

SPECIAL PROBLEMS

Of particular concern to the school health program are measures designed to meet the special needs of certain handicapped children. In every community there exist children whose needs for educational services must be met in conjunction with special care necessitated by physical or mental handicaps. Many localities follow a policy of complete segregation of these children, if not in special institutions, at least in separate classes for the blind, hard of hearing, crippled, pretubercular, or for those with cardiac ailments and epileptic tendencies. While such classes undoubtedly make possible much specialized care, they have the undesirable result of making the handicapped child feel still more apart and different from other children. This is not conducive to good mental hygiene and development or to complete rehabilitation. Most authorities consider that the best policy is to allow the handicapped to intermingle with other children in the same general classrooms and to provide special classes or rest periods if needed for them, depending upon their handicap. It is felt that this policy has a beneficial effect both upon the handicapped and their more fortunate classmates and results in all children considering each other as at least basically the same.

Programs of this nature may be criticized as being impractical, time consuming, and expensive. In many instances specially trained teachers are indicated. However, in terms of the most desirable end result such programs must be considered worth while. In any case time and money must be spent for the education and care of handicapped children and some specialized personnel will have to be employed. By careful curriculum and administrative planning and by using the specialized personnel partly as consultants and in-service trainers for the general teaching staff, possibly more can be accomplished than by any other approach to the problem.

HEALTH INSTRUCTION

Schools are primarily places where children go to learn for living. Most people consider health important for successful living. It logically follows, therefore, that school children should have presented to them in an understandable and interesting manner a considerable amount of informa-

tion dealing with the present and future health of themselves and their community. Customarily "health teaching" is a requisite in most school curricula. However, in a great many instances the job is poorly done. Too often "health classes" turn out to be physical training periods. With equal frequency the material is presented by unqualified and sometimes disinterested persons. On about the same level are the situations where didactically unsuited members of the health department staff or private physicians are asked to give "health talks" to the students. All of these are but poor substitutes for what is really needed. Empathy with students is a very important ingredient for success in this field.

Teaching is a profession in itself. Everyone is not fitted by temperament and training to teach. Certain skills, aptitudes, and training are necessary to accomplish a satisfactory result. Therefore, inasmuch as possible the teaching of health as well as of arithmetic and geography should be left to the trained classroom teacher who is already well acquainted with the pupils. The health department can be of greatest assistance to her by offering advice, consultative service, in-service training, and teaching materials and by aiding her in planning her health teaching program. This can best be done by a health educator or health counselor who may meet with the teachers collectively and individually to discuss goals and problems. Ever enlarging sources of visual aids are becoming available, and the health department, as one of its justifiable activities, should make them accessible to the schools of the community.

Wherever possible, health teaching should be related to other subjects or to other school activities. Civics, geography, and many other subjects offer opportunities for the incidental inclusion of health information. If a school lunch program exists, much education in food sanitation and nutrition may be associated with it. Many local health departments and school authorities have developed programs of field trips and special health study projects designed to demonstrate to school children community activities which have an influence upon the health and well-being of themselves and their families. When properly planned and carried out, these study programs can have a considerable educational impact. A few health departments have progressed further to the point of allowing high school students to take turns working at simple jobs in the health department offices or even clinics as volunteers or at a nominal temporary salary. This is a doubly worthwhile venture by virtue of its educational effect and because it is also a form of vocational guidance. To be of value, however, a judicious choice of jobs and constant supervision are necessary. Since, if properly planned and conducted, it represents a learning process under supervision, the granting of academic credit for the time spent is considered justified.

RESPONSIBILITY FOR THE SCHOOL HEALTH PROGRAM

A long-standing problem in public health administration but one that has been satisfactorily solved in many progressive communities is concerned with which agency in the community should be responsible for the school health program. Children are an important part of the total community. They can affect the health of the community, and the community in turn can affect them. It would appear obvious that to attempt to operate the school health program apart from the general community health program is inefficient, costly, and administratively unsound. An important factor is that in many communities, school systems were established earlier than public health agencies. In the absence of the latter it was natural and commendable for departments of education to attempt to provide for the health problems of the school child. However, the widespread development of sound community health programs tends to negate these excuses.

The Committee for the Study of Child Health Services of the American Academy of Pediatrics has found that 45% of school medical services are rendered by official education agencies, 41% by official health agencies, 11% by education and health agencies jointly, and 3% by other agencies. The pattern is by no means uniform. There was found to be a much greater tendency for education authorities to provide the service in metropolitan areas and for health agencies to be responsible in isolated counties.[8]

The advantages of operating the school health program as part of the community health program are many. Many more facilities, people, and sources of information are thereby readily available. Activities are more logical and fall more readily into their relative positions in the total picture of health. As just one example, consider the problem of securing the correction of physical defects. This is accomplished most effectively by qualified, generalized public health nurses who, rather than limit their interests and activities narrowly to the school situation, secure the correction of defects in school children as part of their general, family, and community public health nursing program. Such an approach cannot help broadening the understanding and increasing the capability and efficiency of the nurse, and what is said for her holds true for the other participants in the school health program. If adequate control and supervision of the school environment are outside the field of training of the medical, physical training, or custodial staffs of the schools, the well-organized local health department will have available the services and knowledge of a qualified engineer and sanitarian to perform this important function. The efficient health department will also have up-to-the-minute reports of illness in the community and can often prevent the infected child from reaching school in the first place. Furthermore, since the community health program operates the year around, the problem of lack of professional functions and activities during the summer months is obviated.

On the other hand, there are certain activities that are rightfully considered within the jurisdiction of the schools. The most important of these is the actual teaching of health, to which reference has already been made. This is best accomplished by the professionally trained classroom teacher who should feel free to call upon the official and nonofficial health agencies for assistance in planning and presentation. Many of the larger schools and departments of education employ a health coordinator to expedite these interagency relations and generally to plan and integrate the health instruction program. Beyond this all schools should have some system for providing first aid or emergency medical care or consultation. Many larger school systems employ full-time school physicians for this purpose, whereas many others rely upon one or a number of practicing physicians who agree to be on call as a public service or at a nominal fee. Even when the official health agency has general responsibility for the school health program, the employment of a school nurse by a large school or by a department of education is not unusual. In such instances her function, although subject to variation, usually includes responsibility for the first-aid or health room, care of minor injuries, referral to private physicians or school physicians, and consultant services to the teachers, the principal or superintendent, and the public health agency.

Under the circumstances, while it might be more advantageous to center responsibility for the school health program, reality will probably determine the situation. And the reality, as Wishik[9] points out, is that different patterns do exist, that they often have good bases, that they will continue to exist for a long time, and that the advantages of each type of administration need not necessarily be lost because of the existence of the other.

SCHOOL HEALTH COUNCILS

In dealing with most health problems of school children no single person or agency can bring about a complete solution. Fortunately interest in the health and well-being of school children is widespread. The primary responsibility, of course, rests with parents. In addition to them society as a whole and particularly private physicians, dentists, nurses, official and nonofficial health, social, and welfare agencies, and professional societies all have a rightful concern and responsibility. Here, therefore, intelligent and cooperative planning and teamwork are what spell success. Only thus

can balanced and effective programs of school health education, protection, and promotion be developed. School health policies must be formulated, therefore, in a manner that makes the maximum use of the resources of the community. This is best accomplished by means of school health councils. Every school and school system should have a health council or committee with representation from all groups concerned in school health. At the top level in the community, where general cooperative community relationships and policies are best developed, membership should include such persons as the superintendent of schools, the local health officer, the president of the parent-teacher association, a representative of the medical and dental societies, and whatever other individuals may be in key positions with relation to the health and well-being of the school child. The relationship of the central school health council to each of the individual school health councils or committees is best determined by experience in each community. In general it has been recommended that the central council guide and give leadership but leave each individual school health council with considerable authority.[3]

The health council or committee of each school need not follow any particular pattern. In a one-room rural school it might consist only of the teacher, an interested parent, and a public health nurse. In larger schools the numbers of those who may play an active role are many and varied and dependent upon local circumstances. The essentials are that they be representative of all in the community who are concerned and may be helpful and that they provide a simple, democratic, and orderly means of determining and implementing wise school health policies.

REFERENCES

1. The White House conference, New York, 1931, The Century Co.
2. Report of the Committee on Terminology in School Health Education, J. Amer. Ass. Health, Phys. Educ., and Recr. 22:14, Sept. 1951.
3. National Committee on School Health Policies, Health Education Council: Suggested school

health policies, ed. 2, New York, 1947, The Council.
4. Editorial: The annual school health examination—an archaic anomaly, Amer. J. Public Health 41:448, Apr. 1951.
5. Yankauer, A., et al.: A study of periodic school medical examinations, Amer. J. Public Health 45:71, Jan. 1955; 46:1553, Dec. 1956; 47:1421, Nov. 1957; 51:1532, Oct. 1961.
6. Cauffman, J. G., Petersen, E. L., and Emrick, J. A.: Medical care of school children: factors influencing outcome of referral from a school health program, Amer. J. Public Health 57:60, Jan. 1967.
7. American Academy of Pediatrics: School health policies, Pediatrics 24:4, Oct. 1959.
8. Committee for the Study of Child Health Services, American Academy of Pediatrics: Child health services and pediatric education, New York, 1949, Commonwealth Fund.
9. Wishik, S. M.: Administrative jurisdiction of the school health service, Amer. J. Public Health 41:819, July 1951.

Chapter 20

Adult health and chronic disease*

EMERGENCE OF THE PROBLEM

The form and substance of the practice of both medicine and public health have been undergoing considerable change during recent years. Not the least of the reasons for this is the spectacular shift that has occurred in the relative age distribution of the population. This shift may be attributed to three factors: (1) the decrease in immigration, (2) a decrease in the birthrate, and (3) an increase in the life expectancy and an accompanying rise in the average age at death. Of the three, the last has been of greatest significance and has been largely the result of prior activities in preventive medicine and public health. Up to the present time these activities have been designed of convenience or necessity to benefit primarily infants and children, with relatively little attention paid to those in the older age groups. That this has been true is not so surprising. In one sense it has been a case of first things first. In another sense it is characteristic of a growing nation that major attention be focused upon the younger age groups so necessary for the development of that kind of nation.

However, our population has matured as far as its age distribution is concerned. The extent to which this is true is shown in Fig. 20-1, which indicates the shift that has taken place in the age distribution of the population since the middle of the last century and the distribution anticipated by the end of the twentieth century. It will be

*For an excellent and convenient guide, see *Control of Chronic Diseases in Man.*[1]

noted that in 1860 only 13% of the population was 45 years of age or over, in contrast with an expected proportion of 40% by the year 2000. Similarly in 1860 51% of the population was under 20 years of age, in contrast with an anticipated 25% by the end of the twentieth century. Considering a shorter and more recent interval, in 1900 only 2.5 million persons or 4.1% of the population of the United States fell in the age group over 65 years. At the present time the corresponding figures are almost 20 million persons or about 9.4% of the total population.

When a population ages, many other changes necessarily occur. The relative need and demand for diapers and baby carriages necessarily decreases, whereas the need and demand for canes and wheelchairs increases. Similarly the need and demand for certain types of public health and medical care must be expected to change. With the increased control of acute communicable diseases the number of beds needed for patients being treated for these diseases has necessarily decreased. At the same time the need and demand for facilities for the care of chronic diseases and the aged have increased. By like token, private physicians and public health workers must expect to devote more and more attention to problems of a geriatric and gerontologic nature.

Although chronic and metabolic diseases are by no means restricted to the older age groups, the fact remains that it is that period of life in which they most commonly occur or become evident and cause disabil-

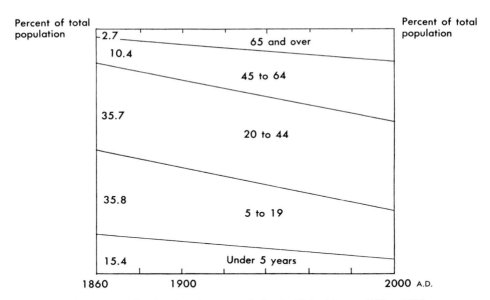

Percent of total population

Percent of total population

2.7 ── 65 and over

10.4

45 to 64

35.7

20 to 44

35.8

5 to 19

15.4　Under 5 years

1860　　1900　　2000 A.D.

Fig. 20-1. Change in age distribution of the population in United States, 1860 to 2000 A.D.

Table 20-1. Twelve leading causes of death, United States, 1900 and 1965

1900		*1965*	
Cause	*Death rate per 100,000 population*	*Cause*	*Death rate per 100,000 population*
Influenza and pneumonia	202.2	Diseases of heart	367.4
Tuberculosis	194.4	Malignant neoplasms	153.5
Diarrhea and enteritis	139.9	Cerebral hemorrhage	103.7
Diseases of heart	137.4	Accidents	55.7
Cerebral hemorrhage	106.9	Diseases of early infancy	28.6
Nephritis	88.7	Influenza and pneumonia	31.9
Accidents	72.3	General arteriosclerosis	19.7
Cancer	64.0	Diabetes mellitus	17.1
Diseases of early infancy	62.6	Other circulatory diseases	14.1
Diphtheria	40.3	Cirrhosis of liver	12.8
Simple meningitis	33.8	Suicide	11.1
Typhoid and paratyphoid	31.3	Congenital malformations	10.1
All causes	1719.1	All causes	943.2

ity and ultimate death. As a result of the population changes that have occurred many more persons are now surviving to ages that in our time are characterized by a high incidence of cardiovascular and renal diseases, cancer, diabetes mellitus, arthritis, rheumatism, gout, and the mental and physiologic changes associated with the climacteric. That this has occurred is em-phasized by a comparison of the leading causes of death in the United States in 1900 and in 1965 (Table 20-1).

The overall picture may be summarized by stating that, while at the beginning of the century 61% of deaths were caused by infectious and parasitic diseases and only 28% by degenerative diseases, the situation is now more than reversed, with over 80%

of deaths caused by degenerative diseases and only 1% by infectious or parasitic diseases.

EXTENT OF THE PROBLEM

It is difficult to determine accurately how many persons are affected at a particular time by the various chronic noncommunicable diseases. The insidious nature of most of these conditions results in delayed diagnosis which not infrequently is made first at the time of death.

However, interviews by the National Health Survey of a representative sample of families throughout the United States during the year ending June 30, 1958, indicated that approximately 70 million people or 41% of the population have one or more chronic conditions. Of these, 13.5 million were limited in the amount or type of their activity, whereas another 3.5 million

were unable to carry on their customary major activity. Thus it may be stated that 10% of the noninstitutionalized population has some degree of long-term limitation of activity due to chronic illness or impairment. The amount varies from about 1.5% among individuals 15 years of age to 55% among those 75 years and older (Table 20-2).

Beyond this, as might be expected, the frequency with which more than one chronic disabling condition exists increases with age. This is shown in Table 20-3. It is seen that among individuals 15 years of age or younger only 3.3% have more than one chronic condition. By contrast, 51% of persons 65 years of age or over have more than one chronic condition.

Only about 30% of those in the higher age group suffer 1 or more days per year from respiratory conditions. This is actu-

Table 20-2. Limitation of activity due to chronic conditions, percent of population by age, United States, July 1957—June 1958*

Age	All persons	Persons with no chronic condition (%)	Persons with one or more chronic conditions (%)			
			Total	With no limitation of activity	With partial limitation of activity	With major limitation of activity
All ages	100.0	58.6	41.4	31.3	8.0	2.1
Under 15 years	100.0	82.5	17.5	16.0	1.2	0.2
15 to 29 years	100.0	65.1	34.9	30.3	4.0	0.5
30 to 44 years	100.0	50.8	49.2	41.2	7.2	0.8
45 to 54 years	100.0	43.1	56.9	43.9	11.3	1.7
55 to 64 years	100.0	34.6	65.4	43.4	17.6	4.4
65 to 74 years	100.0	24.4	75.6	38.4	27.8	9.4
75 years and over	100.0	16.9	83.1	28.2	31.1	23.7

*Health statistics, limitation of activity and mobility, Public Health Service Bull. No. 584-B11, July 1958.

Table 20-3. Number of chronic conditions, percent of population by age, United States, July 1957—June 1958*

Age	Number of chronic conditions (%)				
	Total	None	One	Two	Three or more
All ages	100.0	58.6	23.0	10.0	8.4
Under 15 years	100.0	82.5	14.2	2.6	0.7
15 to 44 years	100.0	57.7	26.0	10.2	6.1
45 to 64 years	100.0	39.4	28.8	16.6	15.2
65 years and over	100.0	21.9	26.6	20.5	31.0

*Health statistics, limitation of activity and mobility, Public Health Service Bull. No. 584-B11, July 1958.

ally less than the incidence in the population as a whole. One quarter, however, have a degenerate disease, and about one eighth are ill from a digestive condition. About 6% suffer from a rheumatic or related condition, 3% from a chronic skin condition, and 2% from a nervous disease. More than 8% are incapacitated for a day or more because of accidental injuries. In addition, there is a considerable frequency of foot ailments and visual defects that limit ambulation and promote accidents, many hearing defects, and many dental problems that affect mastication and therefore diet and nutrition.

The prevalence of specific chronic diseases or impairments in the older component of the population is shown in Table 20-4. It is well to note that impairment of locomotion and limitation of relationship with the surrounding world (visual and hearing defects) are major handicaps which tend to be underrated by many, including health workers. Casual surveys under my direction have indicated that limitation of movement and of communication rank high among older people as most annoying and worrisome handicaps. This appears to hold true even when individuals are aware that they also have some more serious chronic

Table 20-4. Prevalence of chronic diseases and impairments, disabling and nondisabling, of persons 65 years and older*

Condition	Per 1,000 non-institutionalized persons
Arthritis and rheumatism	265.8
Deafness and other hearing impairments	171.8
Heart conditions	148.8
High blood pressure	129.1
Visual impairments	103.2
Hernia	54.6
Asthma, hay fever	53.6
Diabetes	40.4
Paralysis of major extremities and/or trunk	22.4
Peptic ulcer	22.3
Chronic bronchitis	18.9

*From Health statistics, Series C-4, National Health Survey, Public Health Service, Sept. 1960.

condition. Apparently many learn to live with the knowledge of the latter, whereas the less serious handicaps of locomotion and communication are constant limitations to daily living. With reference to the various chronic illnesses and impairments, it is of importance to note the consistent increases in the older age groups and the higher prevalence in most age groups for females in contrast with males. This is surprising, considering the significantly greater expectation of life for females. It could of course indicate a greater tendency on the part of women to be seen by diagnosticians.

There are estimated to be 5.5 million persons with chronic long-term disabilities serious enough to require some kind of care. Of these, 1.4 million are under 45 years, 1.8 million are between 45 and 64 years, and 2.1 million are 65 years of age or older. The respective prevalencies by age are 1.3% under 45 years, 5.8% between 45 and 64 years, and 17.1% over 65 years of age.[2]

CHRONIC DISEASES ARE INCREASING

There is no denying that many more people suffer from chronic diseases now than formerly. An important question, however, is whether the increase is real or apparent, absolute or relative. The use of crude morbidity and death rates in the evaluation of health problems is fraught with considerable danger. Unfortunately, because of the ease and convenience of their calculation and use, most of the information that is available to and discussed by the health professions as well as the public is of this nature. Since the older age groups in the population that are most prone to develop chronic ailments have increased, it would appear only natural that the crude morbidity and death rates from these causes should have increased. Thus the crude death rate for diseases of the heart increased from 137.4 in 1900 to 367.4 per 100,000 in 1965, and the rate from cancer during the same period increased from 64.0 to 153.5. These represent increases of about two and a half times for both diseases during the intervening 65 years. Quite a different picture is obtained, however, by a more careful analysis by means of age specific standardization of rates. In brief this procedure consists of the calculation of a series of death rates, one for each age group of the population, instead of a single crude rate for the entire population. These age specific death rates are then applied to the present population as it would appear if distributed by age in a manner similar to some standard or previous population such as that of 1900. Thus, when this procedure was applied to industrial policyholders of the Metropolitan Life Insurance Co., the surprising fact was brought out that during the third of a century between 1911 and 1945 the death rate standardized for color, age, and sex decreased 29% for diseases of the heart, arteries, and kidneys and increased only 8% for cancer. The observation was made that the slight increase recorded for cancer was rather less than might be expected from improvements in diagnosis.[3]

On the other hand, it has recently been pointed out that the population is not now aging as rapidly as before World War II and that the increase in chronic diseases cannot be linked as closely to increased age of the population as previously assumed.[4] Granted that older populations have more chronic diseases than do others, careful analysis indicates that there are not really enough of them proportionately to make the difference.

AGING VERSUS SENESCENCE

Information such as presented here is not meant to imply an inevitability of chronic illness and disability in the adult and aging population. Aging is not necessarily synonymous with chronic illness or senescence. This has been pointed out by many writers. Widmer,[5] having studied 100 persons past 90 years of age, summarized his conclusions in this forceful sentence: "The old people of sixty are all ill, the centenarians are healthy." He described his patients as taut, lean, and dry. None of them were invalid or bedridden, and all were rather young in appearance.

Rejoicing is heard on all sides for the consistent lengthening of the life span which has been the privilege of recent generations to experience. For many it would appear to represent a matter of scorekeeping in a contest with fate. If the increasing numbers of persons achieving advanced ages did so by being physically and mentally fit, there would be real reason to rejoice. The cruel fact remains that, despite any mathematic readjustments that may be made increasing numbers of individuals, not rates, are growing not only old but sick and senile as well. As Piersol[6] has opined, "Longevity marred by an accompaniment of a disabling disease and suffering has little to commend it; it is a distinct liability rather than an asset." He therefore considers that the most important responsibility of medicine and public health is prevention or delay of the development of the degenerative diseases in order that the potentialities of elderly persons may be more widely developed and utilized.

THE SOLUTION OF THE PROBLEM

Much attention is currently being given to steps that may be taken by the individual, the medical profession, and society in general to meet successfully the problems posed by the aging of the population and the accompanying increase in chronic diseases. The voluntary health agencies provided the first and continuing organized attack in the form of associations concerned with heart disease, cancer, arthritis, diabetes, and other chronic ailments.

A document entitled "Planning for the Chronically Ill," issued jointly in 1947 by the American Medical Association, the American Public Health Association, the American Hospital Association, and the American Public Welfare Association, contains this significant statement, "The basic approach to chronic disease must be preventive. Otherwise the problems created by chronic diseases will grow larger with time, and the hope of any substantial decline in their incidence and severity will be postponed for many years."[7] The ultimate hope is of course for prevention. With reference to chronic diseases prevention may be regarded in several ways. In general there are two kinds of prevention: (1) the total community approach as represented by the mass attack against certain public health problems and (2) the more individualized approach represented by the personal service rendered in the offices of private physicians or in a variety of public or private clinical settings. The total community approach is inapplicable to most problems of chronic disease and preventive geriatrics. The threats to the well-being of the older segments of the population or to any who may be subject to chronic illness cannot be avoided by the turning of a valve or the mass injection of an antigen. Necessarily, therefore, the predominant role must be played by physicians, assisted by a variety of other professionals and technicians, as well as by the increasing types of sophisticated devices for rapid and multiple screening and diagnostic tests. Geriatrics undoubtedly will pattern much of its thinking and development after the concepts and experiences of pediatrics. As a matter of fact, paradoxical as it may appear, pediatricians probably have been more conscious of the factors involved in aging than any other physicians.

The immediate problems that must be faced, however, are somewhat different. As pointed out by Stieglitz[8] in his discussion of the social urgency of research in aging, "Whereas the commoner diseases in youth have acute and florid onsets, obvious symptoms, and, being of infective origin, tend to be self-limited and self-immunizing, the disorders frequent in later years are characterized by insidious and asymptomatic onsets, slowly progressive course and endogenous, or at least nonspecific, etiology." Fundamental as it is to the solution of the problem of adult hygiene and chronic diseases, the personal approach of the private physician is not without its limitations and handicaps. Not the least of these are the expense and inadequacy of facilities for adequate early diagnosis and treatment. The inequalities in the distribution of members of the healing professions and of auxiliary aids such as hospitals is the subject of discussion in Chapter 25. Also discussed is the inability of a large proportion of the population to meet the mounting costs of medical care. The average elderly person can usually afford the fee for the first physician seen but in many instances finds it difficult to meet the costs of consulting physicians, diagnostic aids, hospitalization, and surgery. This problem was pointed up by President Johnson in a message to Congress: "One third of the aged who are forced to ask for old age assistance do so because of ill health, and one third of our public assistance funds going to older people is spent for medical care." The average annual income received by aged couples is half that of younger two-person families. For older persons living alone almost half receive a grossly inadequate $1,000 or less per year. The elderly, as James[9] states, have been pushed out of the mainstream of life ahead of their time. The percentage of older people in the labor force has declined by half since 1940. This necessarily makes more difficult the maintenance of proper health and nutrition and encourages a delay in prompt early diagnosis.

Prevention may be regarded in still another way. It includes measures that avert the occurrence of disease in the first instance and measures that halt or retard the progression of disease, which has been allowed to occur, into disability or death. These are referred to as primary and secondary prevention, respectively. While some might deny the possibility of prevention of chronic diseases, it is nevertheless possible to a significant although indirect extent. In fact, the Commission on Chronic Illness, which functioned between 1950 and 1956, listed more than 50 chronic diseases against which preventive action is possible.[10] The successful approach to the prevention and treatment of the communicable diseases of early life precludes the development of much tissue damage and foci of infection that, if permitted to occur, would be manifest later on as syphilitic or rheumatic hearts, nephritis, arthritis, or other chronic conditions. Careful obstetric management with the avoidance of cervical tears and the proper repair of those that occur is certain to prevent many future cervical carcinomas. The increasing precautions taken by industry for the protection of its workers not only prevent many disabling injuries but for some processes also remove potential hazards that might lead to bronchitis, silicosis, occupational cancers, and other chronic diseases. Breslow[11] emphasizes that better nutrition is a major immediate goal in the primary prevention of chronic disease. He points, on the one hand, to the common protein, vitamin C, and mineral deficiencies in the diets of many elderly persons and, on the other hand, to overweight as an increasingly important national health problem of the middle-aged. The latter, he indicates, accounts for a significant proportion of the unnecessary mortality from cardiovascular disease, diabetes, and other chronic diseases. These are but a few of the direct preventive measures that may be taken against chronic illness. The point to be realized is that the benefits should not be expected to become evident immediately any more than the effect of the injection of an antigen is expected to produce immediate and obvious immunity.

Secondary prevention, i.e., prevention of the progression of diseases that have already begun, is now possible with an increasing frequency. The keynote here, of course, is early diagnosis. This may be achieved in a number of ways. One is by intelligent and consistent self-observation and examination based upon sound personal health education. Self-palpation of the breasts, alertness to abnormal discharges, and other signs and symptoms are examples. Participation in screening programs as well as periodic complete medical examinations are other ways. Of great importance is the role of the personal physician, who should not be satisfied with treatment alone, much less treatment of only one complaint, but who should approach each patient as a total person with pathologic potentials as well as pathologic actualities. A serious handicap, of course, is the insidious nature of the development of the majority of chronic illnesses. Their onsets tend to be asymptomatic and they often progress slowly with

little or no pain or discomfort in the earlier stages. This encourages the person afflicted, even when he suspects the condition, to delay in seeking medical advice and care. One of the most fundamental handicaps, therefore, is the difficulty of getting persons to protect themselves, to obtain periodic medical examinations, and, if necessary, to obtain early and adequate treatment. Stieglitz[8] has aptly stated, "The privilege of longevity carries with it the obligation of personal effort toward health maintenance." This in consideration of the inherent frailties of human nature is the source of much of the problem. A number of psychologic blocks must be counteracted. The individual must overcome a considerable amount of inertia and do something that is not of immediate or apparent benefit, much less pleasure. For many a truly complete and adequate physical examination represents a decidedly unpleasant and embarrassing experience. Furthermore, it not infrequently requires time off from gainful work. Fear of a positive diagnosis serves as a deterrent for some, and others rebel at the thought of potential restrictions upon their personal habits and pleasures. The only weapon available against these deterrents is increased and persistent education. The ultimate goal should be the establishment of periodic medical examinations as part of the accepted process of living.

One effect of these psychologic and cultural blocks may well be the fact that the outlook for the reduction of deaths from chronic diseases in the United States and probably elsewhere is more favorable for females than for males. This has been pointed to by Bright[4] not only on the basis of the slight advantage that women have over men with respect to cardiovascular and renal diseases but also the trend of a declining cancer death rate among females, whereas the rate for males has been moving upward. These differences are observed in both the white and nonwhite races.

ROLE OF THE HEALTH DEPARTMENT

For a long period chronic diseases and adult health were not regarded by many as a concern of official public health agencies. Fortunately, this attitude has undergone considerable change. Interestingly it is often overlooked that the more commonly accepted public health activities may play a very important though indirect part in the eventual alleviation and prevention of many of the disease problems of advanced years. As pointed out previously, the reduction in morbidity from acute communicable diseases not only is important in the prevention of early death but also in the avoidance of infectious foci and structural changes that may give rise to chronic ailments that may impair or limit one's life. Maternal hygiene not only eases the burdens and immediate risks of motherhood but prevents the development of complications which formerly invalided many women in later life. Most of the benefits of services to children, such as well-child conferences and clinics, school health programs, and medical examinations for the correction of defects, are reaped in later life. Recognition should be given to the delayed benefits of the present extensive use of antibiotics, ataraxics, antihypertensives, and other drugs as well as to recent nutritional improvements.

Good nutrition of the expectant mother and the child is said to contribute more than anything to physiologic and mental health in later life. Davis,[12] for example, believes that "The involutional, biochemical processes which lead to senescence may be influenced by all factors that in any way modify cellular metabolism." He lists the following factors as important in determining the onset and relative severity of these changes: (1) heredity, (2) health and nutrition of the parents at conception, (3) health and nutrition of the mother during pregnancy and lactation, (4) any illnesses that the individual may have had at any time in his life, (5) quantity and quality of the nutrition at all periods of life and its relation to the individual needs, (6) environment of the individual during his past life, his occupation, habits, and manner of living, and (7) any gases, dust, or chemical compounds to which exposed and any drugs used at one time or another.

Official public health agencies should not be expected to assume the entire burden of the attack against the diseases of middle and older ages. As already indicated, the predominant role must be played by practitioners of medicine, and the place of the voluntary health and social agencies must likewise become increasingly important. The necessary combination to meet the need is a three cornered partnership made up of the medical profession, the social agencies, and the public health agencies working together toward the amelioration and solution of the problem. Such a partnership would not be new, having operated successfully for many years in other fields such as maternal and child health, tuberculosis, and venereal disease control. With the precedent well established it is logical to visualize, for example, the establishment of screening and diagnostic centers as well as home care programs financed wholly or in part by public funds, staffed by private physicians and consultants on any of the acceptable bases of payment, with the educational and promotional work carried on by the public and voluntary health agencies, and the necessary social service work performed by the appropriate agencies which exist for that purpose. The impetus and leadership, however, may well be furnished by the official public health agency, which may serve to stimulate, correlate, and integrate the contributions and activities of all concerned.[13]

DEVELOPMENT OF PUBLIC PROGRAMS

Chronic disease programs are being established at an increasing rate. Up to this time, however, the major focus of attention has been on cancer. This was the first of the chronic diseases to receive recognition in the official public health program. In this country Massachusetts merits priority for the provision in 1919 of funds for the establishment in its state health department of a program for the study of the prevalence, prevention, and control of cancer. As far as can be ascertained, Detroit was the first city to explore the problem, following a specific appropriation in 1928 to the health department for this purpose. The objectives of the program were: first, to get the factual information, i.e., the statistical background with regard to cancer in the community; second, to encourage physicians to diagnose and to treat cancer through the various channels of undergraduate and postgraduate medical education; third, to institute a service for early detection and the encouragement of treatment; fourth, to institute a follow-up system for cases that received surgical, radium, or x-ray treatment; and fifth, to educate the public in simple terms and with frank statements with regard to the existing knowledge concerning the early treatment of cancer.

Slow to develop, by 1950 every state had established a cancer program. Services are provided by 50 state health departments, 2 state cancer commissions (Arkansas and New Hampshire), most university medical centers, 9 departments of welfare, and 3 agencies of other types. A large share of the total statewide cancer programs is carried on with the assistance of the state chapters of the American Cancer Society, and state medical societies.[14] In most states the general ideals set forth by the National Advisory Cancer Council are more or less adequately approached. These include (1) statistical research to determine the nature and extent of the cancer problem of the state and to evaluate the results of activities, (2) educational activities for the public and all professional groups concerned in the detection, diagnosis, and treatment of cancer, (3) activities to provide adequate detection, diagnostic, and treatment facilities and services accessible to persons of all economic groups in all sections of the state, including facilities for care of the terminal case either at home or in an institution.

Progress has been much slower in relation to the other diseases and health problems of later life. A few states are beginning to turn their attention to some of the broader aspects of the situation. Here again Massachusetts has long been the leader, with Connecticut and New York not far behind. Already many public health programs include, in addition to the cytologic smear for detection of cancer, the clinitron for diabetes screening, the tonometer for

early glaucoma detection, and screening tests for various other chronic conditions. Significant also is the trend toward expanding programs for diagnosing tuberculosis into programs for diagnosing all chest disease, placing greater emphasis upon cardiac conditions, pulmonary carcinoma, and silicosis. The goal of such programs is the earliest possible diagnosis with referral to physicians and hospitals for prompt treatment.

Unfortunately, while a large number of local health departments now provide many *services* in relation to various chronic illnesses, few can be said to have yet developed what might genuinely be considered chronic disease *programs,* and surprisingly few have organizational units specifically concerned with chronic diseases.[15] This situation may very well stem from the categoric approach forced upon state and local health agencies by the various special legislative actions of Congress that have provided funds for the development and conduct of chronic disease services in a piecemeal and generally uncoordinated manner. It is to be hoped that this will be alleviated by the Comprehensive Health Planning and Public Health Services Amendments Act of 1965 (P.L. 89-749), which provides for block grants to states (and local agencies) in place of categoric grants.

CONTENT OF A CHRONIC DISEASE PROGRAM

Knott[16] has indicated five processes by which a community may establish and pursue a chronic disease program: (1) health maintenance, (2) prevention of disease or injury, (3) detection and treatment of illness in its earliest possible state when cure is often feasible, (4) limitation of disability to preserve the maximum normal function, and (5) restoration of the capacity for the highest level of independent activity of which the patient is capable. In other words, he emphasizes the critical need to regard chronic disease control in a broad comprehensive sense. For example or comparison he indicates that probably the nearest that public health and society have approached this goal is in the care of the individual during infancy and childhood. "Here," according to Knott, "to a greater extent than in any other stage of life, we more nearly practice—laymen and professional—the concept of total health care." Furthermore, "Examples of such health care during adult life are unfortunately few and far between. And even these seldom cover the entire life span of those individuals who are served." The development of a truly comprehensive and adequate program of chronic disease control requires very careful planning as a joint enterprise by a variety of disciplines. In this regard attention is directed to an excellent planning guide for the development of community chronic disease programs, recently produced by the Public Health Service.[17]

A complete program for chronic diseases should be based upon both primary and secondary preventive concepts and should include the following activities: (1) research, (2) case finding, (3) hospitalization and treatment, (4) follow-up, (5) rehabilitation, (6) education, and (7) custodial care.

Research

At the present time continued and expanding research is still a fundamental necessity. In addition to the obvious need for the study of the causes, diagnosis, and treatment of chronic diseases, research activities should include statistical studies of prevalence, incidence, and mortality in the various component groups of the population and administrative studies for the development of satisfactory and efficient methods of implementing a community program. The source of the greatest impetus in this regard are the National Institutes of Health. This does not preclude, however, an important role for state and local official and voluntary health agencies in research and demonstration.[18]

Case finding

Early diagnosis is a primary step in controlling any chronic disease regardless of whether it is communicable. For some diseases diagnosis is relatively simple and inexpensive, whereas for many others it is difficult, time consuming, and produces an economic burden of considerable magnitude. Several approaches are possible in order to overcome this aspect of the problem. Private physicians and hospitals might be called upon to render an increased amount of free or reduced-fee medical care. This, however, would be impractical and unfair to the medical profession and institutions as well as undesirable for the public. One compromise that has been arrived at and that has met with reasonable success is to provide periodic screening examinations of limited scope in the offices of private physicians with the patient paying the fee customarily charged for a general examination. If possible, medically indigent patients may be examined free or an agreement may be reached whereby the physician is paid out of public funds.

Up to the present this approach has been more or less limited to examination for signs of cancer. Studies have shown, for example, that more than 60% of cancer cases involve five readily accessible sites: the skin, lips, breasts, cervix, and rectum. These sites can be easily examined by any well-trained physician in his office without recourse to unusual equipment or procedures. The examination is so relatively simple, brief, and inexpensive that both the patient and the physician can afford its repetition every 6 months to a year. The only potential danger of this approach is that the patient, on receiving a negative report from this limited examination, may feel that he is free of all types of cancer and of all disease. It is of great importance, therefore, that these limitations be stressed to the public whenever such a program is put into effect.

Another approach has been the use of specialized cancer detection centers. Generally these have not been economical and efficient, and if the idea were extended to the establishment of similar special facilities for other chronic diseases, the cost would be prohibitive, and the program might well be very inefficient and ineffective in view of the total need. The approach therefore should be more general and concerned with broad aspects of the chronic disease diagnostic problem. Multiphasic screening programs have been developed as one attempt to meet the need. In these a variety of tests may be performed quickly and efficiently for large numbers of people. Carefully designed and conducted multiphasic screening tests would appear to provide the answer. At best they should be available on a continuous rather than on a one-shot basis.[19] Attention is also called to the use of the concept of prospective medicine, discussed briefly in Chapter 1, as a method of meeting the need.

Hospitalization and treatment

The majority of patients who are diagnosed as having a chronic disease are hospitalized for at least a period of several days or weeks in order for a complete decision as to diagnosis, therapy, and prognosis to be made. In addition, many hospital beds are needed for long-term care so that certain patients may receive the surgical, medical, and nursing treatment necessary to return them eventually to normal or near-normal existence. Here the problems of availability of sufficient hospital beds and the ability to pay for them appear. Private or public prepayment hospitalization insurance plans provide a possible solution to the problem of payment. Medicare and Medicaid, made possible by the Social Security Amendments of 1965, can be expected to have a significant impact on the payment aspect of the problem. There appears to be unanimous agreement concerning the need for large numbers of additional publicly supported hospital beds for chronic diseases. Some of these undoubtedly will have to be provided by additional appropriation and construction, such as are provided for by the Hill-Burton hospital survey and construction program.

The need for more beds for patients suffering from chronic diseases provides one answer, however, to a problem with which public health administrators have already begun to be concerned, i.e., the most efficient use of hospital beds formerly needed for acute communicable diseases and tuberculosis in the face of declining incidences and shortened hospital stays. It would appear logical that many of these beds might eventually be made available for the care of patients with chronic noncommunicable diseases. It is interesting that the first public hospital established for the care of cancer patients in Pondville, Mass., was a reconverted tuberculosis sanatorium.

Follow-up

The active follow-up of posthospitalized patients is an important and expanding part of the chronic disease program. Often the chronically ill and aged patient is happier and mentally better off in his own home with familiar surroundings and proximity of those he loves. It has been estimated that about 70% of such patients could be cared for satisfactorily in their own homes if adequate auxiliary services, such as visiting nurse, home health aid,[20] and housekeeper services,[21] were available and if the other members of the family were given some training. It is here that the public health nurse especially can make a significant contribution to the program for the care and education of the chronically ill and aged.[22] The needs and wishes have already been made evident by the public in terms of demands for this type of service. This constitutes a strong argument in favor of the more widespread and more effective joining of the forces of the official public health nursing services and the bedside nursing programs of the visiting nursing societies.

An early demonstration of the value of home nursing service in relation to chronic illness was provided by the home nursing service for policyholders of the Metropolitan Life Insurance Co. In 1925 nearly 50% of requests for service related to acute and communicable conditions, most of which occur in early life, and only about 5% for chronic diseases. Only 20 years later in 1945 the figures were reversed to 14% and 28%, respectively.[23] In addition to rendering direct services in the home the visiting nurse may be of assistance in returning the posthospitalized patient to the care of a private physician, providing him with information helpful in the handling of the case and assisting the patient in putting the physician's suggestions into effect. Patients may also be aided in the use of outpatient clinics and departments of general hospitals by patients residing in their own homes.

For those who no longer require the extensive medical services of a hospital but who are not yet ready to function on an independent basis the convalescent home provides an important bridge. Here, as is the case with nursing homes subsequently mentioned, the health department has an important role in establishing and enforcing standards and qualifications with reference to personnel, type and quality of care, and food quality and service as well as general sanitation and safety. Many health departments have the responsibility of licensing these institutions.

Rehabilitation

A program of rehabilitation for chronically ill and disabled patients should be carried on concurrently with other activities. The need for this is indicated from two points of view. The most obvious is assistance to enable patients to become partially self-supporting or at least to take care of their own personal needs and to be less of a burden to their relatives and friends. Many patients may be returned to their previous occupations although often on a reduced work-time schedule. Others may be guided into new endeavors more suitable to their present capabilities. Further mention will be made of this in the discussion of the role that industry may play in the adult health program (see subsequent section and Chapter 28).

Too frequently overlooked is the need for rehabilitation in the mental health sense. Not uncommon is the woman who, having undergone a breast amputation or a hysterectomy, is returned to her home and family with no psychiatric preparation and who spends the remaining years of her life feeling incomplete, half a woman, and perhaps unwanted. The same applies, although in a somewhat different sense, to the man who is summarily directed to give up his daily work, his sports, and his other activities that made life worth living because of a stroke or a cardiac ailment. The tremendous need for activity in this area represents as yet a vast virgin territory and provides an area of great potential service by public health nurses as well as medical and social service advisors.

Education

The need for public education with regard to the chronic illnesses of later life is very great. On first consideration it appears incomprehensible that large numbers of the population of the United States are so utterly lacking in knowledge and have so many misconceptions and superstitions regarding chronic ailments. Related to this is the substantial number of people who allow themselves to fall prey to all sorts of quacks and charlatans when afflicted with a chronic disease. However, when the fundamental forces which motivate human thought and behavior are considered, the result is not so surprising. Up to the present this challenge has been met almost singlehandedly by the various voluntary agencies, and as a result it is they who deserve the major credit for the contemporary interest and progress that is taking place in this field. In the final analysis it may well be that increased public education in these matters would represent the single most important service that may be rendered by public health agencies in company with the schools.

Custodial care

The final phase of any program designed to serve those who suffer from chronic diseases is the provision of custodial care. The extent of the need for this type of care is the best measure of the degree of defeat or failure of the total program. A certain number of patients require custodial care of long duration because of indigency and lack of family or because of progressive incurability of their illness. What is needed here is not so much medical and hospital treatment as mothering and the alleviation of pain and discomfort during the remaining period of life. At present relatively few facilities for this type of care are maintained at public expense. Dependence must be placed also upon facilities established and operated by religious and fraternal organizations or conducted as proprietary profit-making institutions—some excellent but others abominable. As indicated earlier in relation to convalescent homes, the adequate supervision of these institutions certainly is a justifiable public health function. With the inception of Medicare and Medicaid, the state health departments are being given the responsibility for the supervision of the sanitation and general operation of these institutions.

THE ROLE OF INDUSTRY

Industrial establishments are key spots of great potential advantage to any program of adult health and chronic disease service and control. They may be regarded as places where, because large numbers of adults are concentrated, they may be conveniently and efficiently reached and served in the same way that schools represent focal points for much of the public health programs designed for children. This is particularly significant when it is realized that chronic illnesses are particularly prevalent among wage earners in the lower and middle income groups (Table 20-5).

Progressive industrial concerns now realize that the promotion of the health and education of workers represents a sound investment. There are many ways in which industry may play an important role. An increasing number of businesses and industries are establishing policies which require preemployment and periodic medical examinations of workers. Considering the many persons involved, this serves as a fruitful means of diagnosing chronic illnesses in their early stages and makes a large part of the population aware of the need for constant self-surveillance. Many industries conduct praiseworthy programs of health education for their workers. Reference has already been made to the potential preventive value of the removal of industrial hazards. Hospital and medical care insurance is frequently an employment benefit and one increasingly demanded in union contract negotiations. Rehabilitation programs work to the advantage of business and industry. World War II brought about a belated realization that there exists in the population a large pool of industrial manpower in the form of persons only partially handicapped by chronic disease and disabilities. In the face of serious shortages of manpower the contributions of such persons to the national war effort was by no means insignificant and has been said by some to have turned the scale on the production front. As a result many industries have continued their wartime policy of job placement of partially handicapped workers on the basis of aptitude tests and a careful study of their physical capabilities. This is the best possible type of rehabilitation, physical, mental, moral and economic, and it should be done by more employers.

Table 20-5. Work-loss days from selected chronic conditions by family income, United States, July 1959—June 1960*

	Work-loss days (in thousands)		Work-loss days per 1,000 employed persons per year	
	Family income			
Selected chronic conditions	Under $4,000	Over $4,000	Under $4,000	Over $4,000
Heart conditions	6,247	7,821	318.4	184.8
High blood pressure	3,905	3,423	199.0	80.9
Varicose veins	950	1,023	48.4	24.2
Hemorrhoids	2,092	3,355	106.6	79.3
Chronic bronchitis	1,732	1,609	88.3	38.0
Peptic ulcer	4,759	4,412	242.5	104.3
Skin conditions	1,275	1,997	65.0	47.2
Diabetes	1,153	1,026	58.8	24.2
Fracture and dislocation residuals	1,739	1,419	88.6	33.5
Arthritis and rheumatism	9,014	2,220	459.4	52.5
Other diseases of muscles and joints	5,360	2,441	273.2	57.7

*Health statistics, currently employed persons, illness and work-loss days, Public Health Service Bull. No. 584-C7, Apr. 1962.

A very important contribution that may be made by industry is the development of more reasonable and individualized retirement procedures. The picture is all too familiar of an individual's having to accept retirement at a certain age on the basis of chronology rather than physiology, with the result that the enforced idleness and apparent lack of purpose limit the remaining years of life. Actually we are much less similar at the age of 65 than we are at birth. Productive potentials are subject to great individual variation until the end of life. Most men are not promoted to positions of great responsibility and opportunity until about the age of 50 years. This being true, it is important to find means to help the older individual keep physically and mentally fit and then to allow him to use his fitness and ability. It would appear, therefore, to be highly inefficient as well as illogical and cruel to attempt to place all persons in exactly the same retirement mold.

RECENT EVENTS ON THE NATIONAL LEVEL

Uncoordinated as the total picture has been up to the present, it now appears to be coming into focus. Not many years ago chronic illness and problems of adult health were subjects which tended to be underemphasized in public health as well as in other circles. The situation has rapidly changed during recent years, with the role of leadership being assumed more and more by agencies on the national level, perhaps most notably epitomized by the National Institutes of Health and the various chronic disease program units of the Public Health Service. One may also point to a number of important national meetings and conferences since the 1947 National Conferences for Planning for the Chronically Ill, which involved the American Hospital Association, the American Medical Association, the American Public Welfare Association, and the American Public Health Association.[7] Particular attention is directed to the National Health Forum on Chronic Disease in 1956[24] and the work of the Commission on Chronic Illness, a national voluntary group that carried out studies in the United States between 1945 and 1956. The Com-

mission has produced four extremely useful volumes on various aspects of the problem based upon its extensive deliberations.[25]

Finally, attention must be directed to the flood of recent national legislative proposals that relate to a long list of chronic ailments and disabilities including cancer, heart disease, arthritis and rheumatism, mental diseases, dental diseases, addictions, multiple sclerosis, cerebral palsy, birth defects, epilepsy, poliomyelitis, blindness, leprosy, and venereal diseases. Many of those have been enacted into law and have resulted in the establishment of a number of National Institutes of Health as well as in the promotion of many state and local chronic disease activities by means of grants-in-aid and consultation. Several recent acts of Congress deserve particular mention as major steps toward the more effective solution of the chronic disease problem. The first is the so-called Partners for Health Act or more correctly the Comprehensive Health Planning and Public Health Services Amendments Act (P.L. 89-749). Whereas this law applies far beyond chronic disease considerations, as indicated earlier, it should greatly assist and encourage state and local health agencies to develop broad gauged and properly balanced chronic disease control programs. In addition, because of the provisions that require the establishment of state and local or regional planning agencies and advisory committees with representation from official and nonofficial agencies as well as representatives of the public, voluntary health agencies and official health departments should be expected to work more closely and effectively together than previously. The Social Security Amendments of 1965 (P.L. 89-97) have also been referred to. This significant breakthrough assures payment for needed medical, hospital, and related services not only for the older component of the population by means of Medicare or Title XVIII but also for many young as well as older persons financially incapable of meeting medical expenses through Medicaid, Title XIX, or Grants to the States for Medical Assistance Programs. Obviously these provisions should encourage and make possible earlier diagnosis and secondary preventive treatment of many cases of chronic illness.

Another recent national legislative act of great and specific consequence for chronic disease control was the Heart Disease, Cancer, and Stroke Amendments Act (P.L. 89-239). This act grew out of the report of the President's Commission on Heart Disease, Cancer, and Stroke,[26] which recommended a series of regional medical complexes that would bring quality care direct to the patient with relation to these three diseases, which account for 7 out of every 10 deaths in the United States. However, the law as passed provided for regional cooperative arrangements among medical schools, research institutes, hospitals, and other health institutions to make available to their patients the latest advances and treatment of heart disease, cancer, stroke, and such related diseases as kidney disorders and diabetes. The law also provides for continuing education of physicians in these fields. These steps, momentous as they are, cannot be regarded as solving the problem completely. Further action can certainly be contemplated in these and related fields.

Although the control of chronic diseases still appears difficult, the situation is probably no different from that presented by communicable diseases a half century ago. That problem has been largely conquered. In the light of recent trends we may well look forward to similar results in the field of chronic diseases with the ever increasing knowledge provided by persistent research and the cooperation of the medical, public health, and social professions.

REFERENCES

1. American Public Health Association: Control of chronic diseases in man, New York, 1966, The Association.
2. Mayo, L. W.: Five million people, Public Health Rep. **71**:678, July 1956.
3. Statistical bulletin, Metropolitan Life Insurance Co., **27**:11, Nov. 1946.
4. Bright, M. In Lilienfeld, A. M., and Gifford, A. J., editors: Chronic diseases and public health, Baltimore, 1966, The Johns Hopkins Press.
5. Widmer, C.: Die Neunzigjaehrigen, München, Med. Wschr. **76**:840, 1929.
6. Piersol, G. M.: Medical considerations of some geriatric problems, Arch. Ophthal. (Chicago) **29**:27, Jan. 1943.
7. Planning for the chronically ill. Joint statement of recommendations by the American Hospital Association, American Medical Association, American Public Health Association, and American Public Welfare Association, Amer. J. Public Health **37**:1256, Oct. 1947.
8. Stieglitz, E. J.: The social urgency of research in aging. In Cowdry, E. V., editor: Problems of aging, Baltimore, 1942, The Williams & Wilkins Co.
9. James, G.: Poverty as an obstacle to health progress in our cities, Amer. J. Public Health **55**:1757, Nov. 1965.
10. Prevention of chronic illness, Report of the Commission on Chronic Illness, Boston, 1957, Harvard University Press.
11. Breslow, L.: Prevention of chronic illness, Amer. J. Public Health **46**:1540, Dec. 1956.
12. Davis, N. S.: Factors which may influence senescence, Ann. Intern. Med. **18**:81, Jan. 1943.
13. Ames, W. R., and Longood, R. J.: Home care of the sick—Monroe County acts, New York Health News, p. 4, Mar. 1962.
14. Distribution of health services in the structure of the state government, Washington, 1953, Public Health Service Pub. No. 184.
15. Muller, J. N.: Chronic disease services in local health departments—report of a survey, Amer. J. Public Health **47**:352, Mar. 1957.
16. Knott, L. W.: Components of a chronic disease program, Amer. J. Public Health **52**:2080, Dec. 1962.
17. Development of community programs for the chronically ill, Washington, 1967, Public Health Service.
18. Dunn, J. E.: Public health research in chronic disease, Public Health Rep. **71**:67, Jan. 1956.
19. Getting, V. A.: Multiple screening: organizing a program in chronic disease control, Continued Education Series No. 88, Ann Arbor, 1960, University of Michigan Press.
20. Sargent, E. G.: Detroit VNA's home aid service, Nurs. Outlook **10**:318, May 1962.
21. Pennell, M. Y., and Smith, L. M.: Characteristics of families served by homemakers, Amer. J. Public Health **49**:1467, Nov. 1959.
22. Drenckhahn, V. V.: Educational role of the nurse in chronic disease control, Public Health Rep. **80**:1103, Dec. 1965.
23. Dublin, L. I.: Problems of an aging population, setting the stage, Amer. J. Public Health **37**:155, Feb. 1947.
24. National health forum on chronic disease, Public Health Rep. **71**:675, July 1956.
25. Commission on Chronic Illness: I. Chronic illness in the United States; II. Care of the long-term patient; III. Chronic illness in a rural area; IV. Chronic illness in a large city, Cambridge, 1957, Harvard University Press.
26. Report of the President's Commission on Heart Disease, Cancer, and Stroke: A National program to conquer heart disease, cancer, and stroke, Washington, 1964, U. S. Government Printing Office.

Chapter 21

Public health dentistry*

MAGNITUDE OF THE PROBLEM

Studies of incidence and prevalence of dental ailments carried on during the past two decades have placed problems of dental health clearly in a position of major importance with regard to national health needs. Fortunately the same interval has seen the dramatic development of the field of preventive dentistry and of public health dentistry, something which at the beginning of that period could not have been forecast. As recently as 1938 two of the major contributors[1] to the progress that has since been made stated: "Inasmuch as the etiology of dental caries is unknown, prevention of the disease causing these defects is still in the experimental stage. It is generally acknowledged, however, that the treatment of early carious lesions by the proper placement of chemically and physically stable filling materials will largely prevent carious teeth from terminating in tooth loss, or tooth mortality. A primary purpose of dental health programs becomes, therefore, the promulgation of procedures whereby the early detection and treatment of carious teeth is accomplished, and tooth mortality thereby prevented." Two years later Klein[2] frankly stated, "On the basis of the considerations here discussed, preventive dentistry represents at the present time perhaps more an objective than an accomplished fact." Up to that time the public was certainly aware of their teeth and the ailments to which they were subject. The impression is, however, that the gen-eral attitude was one of fatalism and complacent acceptance of the fact that teeth were a necessary evil and that one necessarily had to expect increasing difficulties with them as one became older. Fortunately, however, and despite obvious difficulties of prime magnitude, that situation did not continue to hold true so that it was possible for Knutson[3] to state before the American Public Health Association in 1953, "I look back over the past ten years and conclude that more has been accomplished during the decade than during the previous fifty years."

Three factors in particular contributed to the tremendous change in outlook which occurred during this period. First was the generally progressive attitude of the dental profession in the United States. This was exemplified by its many inquiries into ways of preventing dental ailments and methods of providing dental care of good quality to large numbers of the people. Second was the tremendous impact which resulted from the military drafting of a fourth of our dentists and particularly the shocking results of the physical examinations of inductees. One of the most startling findings was that, of the first 2 million men examined for service in the armed forces, more were rejected because of dental defects than for any other physical reason. In fact, about 1 out of every 12 men examined was rejected on this basis.[4] The third contributing factor in the progress of recent years is to be found in the brilliant researches and studies that have been made by various investigators and particularly by a small group of dental officers of the Public Health Service. These inquiries into the incidence

---

*For an excellent bibliographic guide, see *A Bookshelf on Dental Public Health,* Amer. J. Public Health **56**:567, Apr. 1966.

and prevalence, dental physiology and pathology, the relationship of various dietary factors and particularly sugars, and the studies of the relationship of fluorides to mottled enamel and the prevention of caries are already considered epidemiologic classics.[5]

In order to appreciate the magnitude of the problem that confronts the dental profession and especially those in public health dentistry one must consider the incidence and prevalence and the backlog and maintenance needs for many types of dental services, including diagnosis, prophylaxis, fillings, extractions, treatment of soft tissue diseases, prosthetics, orthodontics, and special services such as oral surgery, correction of congenital oral deformities, and radiation therapy. Overlying all of these, of course, is the constant need for dental health education.

Many studies have demonstrated that practically everyone in the nation has some type of dental health problem. In 1960, Americans had an estimated total of 700 million unfilled caries. Ten percent of children under 5 years had eight or more cavities. Similarly 10% of children 15 to 19 years had ten or more cavities. Today about 22 million people have lost all their permanent teeth. This is true of 1% of those 15 to 24 years, 25% of those 45 to 54 years, and 60% of those 65 to 74 years of age.[6,7] A study of children 5 to 6 years of age in one state has shown that 87% have dental caries and over 60% have signs of at least mild gingivitis.[8] Twenty percent of school-age children have need of orthodontic treatment, whereas one child in 800 is born with a cleft lip or palate.[9] By middle age about 50% of the population is estimated to have or to have had periodontal disease. This is true of almost all persons who reach the age of 65 years.[6,7]

It leads obviously to a consideration of the size and distribution of the personnel available to serve the dental needs of the nation. In mid-1965 there were about 109,-300 dentists in the United States, which represents a decline from 50 per 100,000 population in 1950 to 45 per 100,000 population in 1965, despite the fact that graduates increased by 20% during the period. Eight new dental schools were established since 1950, making a total of 49 for the nation.[10]

An additional factor to consider in relation to the adequacy of dental resources is that due to improved average economic status and more extensive health educational activities on the part of dentists and health agencies, a much larger proportion of the population now seeks care. Thus 30 years ago about 20 to 25% of the population visited a dentist during the year, whereas at the present time about 36% does so.[11] It is notable, however, that more than 30 million Americans have never visited a dentist. As might be expected, urban dwellers obtain dental care more frequently and readily than do rural dwellers.[12] The ratio of male to female dental visits is almost 1 to 1.3.[13]

Also unfortunate is the fact that dentists are not distributed evenly in relation to population and need. Low ratios of dentists to population are found particularly in the South, in rural counties, and in low-income areas. In 1960 there were 222 counties in the United States that lacked dentists. One state had almost five times as many persons per dentist as the state that was at the other extreme.[14]

Trained dental hygienists and dental assistants have more than proved their worth in recent years. Studies made by Klein[15] brought out that many service hours can be gained and many more patients served through the expansion of operating equipment and the use of dental assistants. He found that the added availability of a dental hygienist or a dental assistant increased the patient load capacity per dentist 33%. If a second chair were added in addition to the assistant, the patient load capacity increased 62%. More recent studies by Knutson[3] and other investigators have substantiated this, especially in relation to the care of children:

An extra dividend of this study was data and experience on the effective utilization of dental assistants. It was found that a dentist can double his out-put with the help of one fulltime and one halftime assistant. In addition, the dentist who uses assistants effectively can give better service at less cost and with less fatigue. The study showed too that once the children are on a maintenance level, one dentist with the help of trained chairside assistants can render service to approximately 1,300 children annually.

Despite the proved value of dental hygienists and dental assistants, we are confronted again by grossly inadequate numbers available, plus very few centers that provide for their training. The American Dental Hygienists' Association reports that in 1965 there were 15,100 registered dental hygienists active in the United States. The average length of the dental hygienist's career is estimated to be about seven years following graduation. About one fifth return after an interval as a homemaker. The number of schools of dental hygiene has increased rapidly in recent years from 37 in 1960 to 56 in 1965. As a result students have increased by 50%. About 1,500 were graduated in 1965. All states now have laws for licensing dental hygienists. With its value proved so conclusively, it would seem reasonable to anticipate much greater expansion of the field of dental hygiene. In addition to increasing numbers of dental hygienists there has developed a large number, now estimated at 91,000, of dental assistants with varying amounts of short-term training usually superimposed upon a high school education. Properly qualified individuals are certified by the American Dental Assistants Association.

A quarter century ago McCall[16] visualized the dentist of the future as a highly trained expert director of a cooperative team that would include a dental hygienist who would place amalgam and other plastic fillings for children, a dental technician who would take impressions or insert and adjust dentures, and a dental assistant. The dentist himself would be free to devote himself to diagnosis, prescriptions for preventive dentistry, operative periodontic and orthodontic treatment, crown and bridge work, and direction of auxiliary personnel. Actually this has come about in the more advanced dental clinics and private practices.

A few words should be said about cost. Despite the inadequacies of dental facilities and personnel, the American public spends about one tenth of its health dollar or almost $2 billion per year for this purpose. In addition, the Veterans Administration pays about $70 million per year more to private dentists for veterans' service-connected dental benefits as well as providing dental care at veterans' hospitals and clinics. If nothing were possible to decrease the incidence of dental disease, it could be estimated that from $5 billion to $10 billion a year would be necessary to serve the dental needs of the American population adequately. One other facet of the cost picture should be mentioned. "Insurance statistics show," as Aston[17] says, "that employees with poor mouth conditions have a greater incidence of illness resulting in absence from work than those with good mouth conditions. Current surveys corroborate this statement, revealing an average of four and one-half days per employee per year lost from work because of toothache or some dental ailment. An industrial manager should have to consider only such figures to see that a dental care program can save the plant money by reducing absentees."

FACTORS INVOLVED IN CARIES

Before considering some of the remarkable developments of the recent past which have led to the possibility of practical and fruitful public health dental programs it may be of value to explore briefly some of the many factors which have been considered to have a relationship to the development of dental caries. Dental caries and the consequences thereof constitute by far the major proportion of the total dental problem. At a workshop at the University of Michigan in 1947 a group of 114 scientists related to the field defined dental caries as follows[18]:

Dental caries is a disease of the calcified tissues of the teeth. It is caused by acids resulting from the action of microorganisms on carbohydrates, is characterized by a decalcification of the inorganic portion, and is accompanied or followed by a disintegration of the organic substance of the tooth.

Innumerable factors have been related at one time or another to the development or lack of development of dental caries. Some of those particularly considered have been pregnancy, chronic debilitating diseases (e.g., diabetes and tuberculosis) endocrinopathies, radiation, psychic trauma, nutritional deficiencies, inadequate dental exercise, inadequate dental cleansing, enzymes, bacteria of various species, and inherited or acquired immunity or susceptibility.

One of the commonest ideas is that the general state of health and nutrition has a close relationship with the presence or absence of dental caries. It is now known that once the teeth have erupted their enamel is thenceforth unaffected by increased intake of calcium, phosphorus, or any of the vitamins. Similarly it has been shown that except in the most extreme instances calcium is not withdrawn from the formed teeth. This disproves one of the oldest and still very common folk ideas of a tooth loss for every baby. As far as can be determined the state of health and nutrition of a mother during pregnancy and lactation have little or no relationship to the subsequent possible development of dental caries in her child. As Florio[19] has stated: "Any woman should have regular dental supervision. It is highly questionable whether there is any particular virtue in having a dental examination and corrections made during pregnancy, unless it is simply easier to impress the mother at such times." He continues, "There are excellent reasons for vitamin and mineral supplement for the mother, but the soundness of the baby's teeth is not one of them."

The group that participated in the Michigan workshop,[18] on reviewing the literature and their own experience, concluded that not only does general health and nutritional status have no significant bearing on the amount of caries but there is also some evidence that malnourished people tend to have a decreased incidence of dental caries apparently as a result of the change in composition, quantity, viscosity, and bacterial or antibacterial nature of the saliva.

Disturbances of various endocrine glands from time to time have been claimed to have an effect on the development of dental caries. The reasoning has been based upon the role which some endocrine substances play in determining the structure and configuration of the dental arch, in their effect on the composition of the saliva, and possibly in relation to the development of resistance or susceptibility to caries. There has been no acceptable substantiation of such claims, and it is generally considered that no relationship exists between endocrine disturbances and the amount of caries. Much attention has been given to the possibility of inherited susceptibility or immunity to dental caries. Hunt and his co-workers[20] were able to breed selectively a strain of rats that were immune to dental caries and another strain which on the same diet were highly susceptible. Many investigators, including Klein, Jay, and Bunting, have reported the existence of families that appear to experience few or no caries. Bacterial and serologic analyses in some of these instances have shown that the lactobacillus was absent from the mouths and digestive tracts of such individuals and that the blood agglutination titer to lactobacilli was high. Despite these various studies, the general feeling is that inherited or acquired susceptibility or immunity to dental caries, if a reality, plays a minor role in the total caries picture and that further investigation is indicated. Marked racial differences, however, appear to exist. Klein and Palmer[21] found the average numbers of decayed, missing, or filled teeth per person of both sexes at 15 years of age to be 6.6 for Hagerstown whites, 6.5 for San Francisco whites, 4.1 for Hagerstown Negroes, 3.1 for Indian children of all tribes studied, and only 1.1 for Navajo Indian children. In other words, at age 15 white children were found to have about 1.5 times more decayed, missing, and filled permanent teeth than Negro children and more than twice the number discovered in Indian children. With regard to the latter, however, it should be noted that the rate for Indian children of the Northwest was higher than for the white children studied, and that the Navajo children lived in a high fluoride area.

Perhaps as a result of highly successful commercial salesmanship, it is widely accepted that various oral hygienic practices will reduce the probability of development of dental caries. Included in this category is the use of the toothbrush, dentifrices, miscellaneous mouthwashes, lozenges, medicated chewing gum, and professional dental prophylaxis. The conclusion of the Michigan Conference on Dental Caries was that, while these agents and procedures are worth while from the standpoint of general oral hygiene, cosmetic effect, and the stimulation of healthier gingival tissues, no evidence exists to indicate that their use bears a relationship to the suppression of caries. Of particular interest was the conclusion that professional dental prophylaxis could not remove all bacterial plaques from the surfaces of the teeth, especially in the pits, fissures, and contact points, and that even where they were removed they tended to reform in a matter of days. Accordingly the conference group stated, "There is no statistical evidence that prophylaxis three or even more times a year will reduce the dental caries attack rate."[18]

Considerable research has been carried on in an attempt to determine a relationship between various microorganisms and the development of dental caries. Most attention has been given to the streptococci, proteolytic bacteria, and acidogenic bacteria. These researches, especially those relating to the lactobacilli, have brough us much closer to the goal of understanding the mechanism of dental caries development and of devising practical preventive measures. By now, it may be considered to have been conclusively demonstrated that there exists a relationship between the formation of dental caries and the number of lactobacilli in the mouth. The careful studies of Jay, Bunting, and their associates, in particular, appear to have settled this question as well as the question of the correlative part which is played by a high intake of carbohydrates, especially free sugars.[22-25]

Because of the long-standing unsolved nature of the problem, it would now appear that much more is known of the nature and cause of caries than is realized by the public in general. Before proceeding to a consideration of some of the other developments of recent decades that have brought us to

the point where a practical preventive dental program is possible, it is worth summarizing, in the words of Easlick,[26] what is now known about the etiology of dental caries:

Somewhat over-simplified perhaps, but nevertheless quite readily understandable, the factors may be outlined which are essential for dental caries. In the first place, the patient must be susceptible to dental caries; very few people are immune. In the second place, the patient must have teeth and the hard tissues of his teeth must be soluble in weak organic acids. In the third place, acidogenic (acid-forming) bacteria, certainly, and apparently aciduric (acid-tolerating) organisms must be present and active in large numbers in the patient's mouth. In the fourth place, the food, the substrate on which aciduric bacteria live, must be made available frequently in the patient's mouth; in other words, the host must ingest fermentable carbohydrate and usually in the form of sugar. In the fifth place, certain specialized "promoters" of chemical activity, the necessary enzymes, must be present in the patient's mouth or must not be inhibited when manufactured by resident bacteria, because at least 13 chemical reactions are required to degrade a fermentable sugar to lactic acid. Finally, in the sixth place, the organic acids, once produced, must be protected from the neutralizing effect of the patient's saliva in order that they may react with the mineral surface of a tooth. A tough, adherent film, the bacterial plaque, therefore, appears essential to the caries process.

These six essential factors, (1) susceptible patient, (2) acid-soluble tooth structure, (3) aciduric organisms, (4) carbohydrate substrate, (5) bacterial enzyme system, and (6) bacterial plaque, deserve careful consideration. They serve as research guideposts since interference with any of these factors, or any combination of them, presents possibilities for prevention or for the reduction of the patient's dental caries.

RECENT DEVELOPMENTS

At the annual meeting of the American Public Health Association in 1953, Knutson,[3] reviewed the events of the preceding decade which presaged a new era in dental health:

At the beginning of the decade we did not have a single practical method for preventing dental caries on a public health basis. To be sure, we had an abundance of evidence of high correlation between the consumption of refined sugars and the prevalence of dental caries. However, the practicability of a preventive program based on reduced sugar consumption had not been demonstrated. Our dental programs were confined largely to the early detection of new carious lesions and the prompt filling of carious teeth.

Detailed knowledge of the characteristics of the disease suggested programs designed to care for the dental needs of children on an incremental basis rather than those which were attempting to deal with the consequences of postponed care. Such dental care programs would minimize needs arising from neglect and would avoid the totally unmanageable problem posed by the accumulation of dental defects over many years. This practical approach to the dental care problem is as sound today as it was then. However, the need for emphasizing care rather than prevention made those early years in dental public health trying, indeed. Because they provided direct dental care, it was difficult to win acceptance of those programs. Public health administrators and dentists were overwhelmed by the size of the problem and the projected costs of a program designed to meet it.

No wonder those of us who lived through the days of the early, limited substance programs appreciate present caries preventive measures which can be applied so effectively and economically on a public health basis.

Of the many advances made in the field of public health dentistry during recent decades, four merit specific mention: (1) the development of a practical method of assessing and stating the dental health status or problem of an individual group, (2) the application of fluorides directly to the teeth or indirectly through public water supplies, (3) the development of public health dentistry as a specialty, and (4) the beginning of an attack upon the economic deterrents to good general dental health.

MEASUREMENT OF DENTAL NEEDS

One of the most important developments of recent decades was the devisement of a practical definitive means of evaluation of dental needs and problems. In order to study the prevalence of caries in the children of various Indian tribes, Klein and Palmer were faced with the necessity of finding some means of defining the overall condition of the teeth of an individual and of large groups. Collins,[27] in compiling data to depict the physical state of school children in 1931, presented the condition of their teeth in terms of the numbers per child that were carious, extracted, and filled. Several years later Messner and associates[28] presented similar data on dental needs and treatment but in terms of the amounts in each category per 100 children specific for age groupings. Klein and Palmer[29] then combined these ideas and developed the D.M.F. (decayed or missing or

filled) concept by means of which they were able to define and statistically handle the prevalence of caries, defining prevalence rate as the number of children per 100 children examined who have one or more teeth decayed or missing or filled. They explained: "The term 'decayed or missing or filled,' which is abbreviated throughout this report as D.M.F., means, with respect to a child, that the mouth contains one or more actively decayed, one or more filled, or one or more missing permanent teeth. It follows that a child having one or more teeth affected in any or all these classes has a D.M.F. or carious mouth. It follows also, that a count of the number of teeth decayed, plus the number filled, plus the number missing, gives a count of the total number of teeth affected by caries which in this report is synonymous with the D.M.F. count." Simple as this concept may appear to us now, its development was a necessity to the advancement of the epidemiology of dental disease. Subsequently Klein, Palmer, and others devised variations in the method of use of the D.M.F. count. Thus the percentage of people with one or more D.M.F. represents the prevalence of caries experience in a group. The number of D.M.F. teeth per person represents the caries tendency of a group of people. The number of D.M.F. tooth surfaces per person represents the total caries tendency. The differences in the numbers of D.M.F. teeth between one point in time and another represents the incidence of caries. By means of these factors it has been possible to depict by use of graphs not only incidence and prevalence, but also expectancy curves.[21]

FLUORIDATION

By far the most dramatic and significant development in dental health has been the discovery of the relationship of fluorides to dental caries. Teeth blackened by minerals or, more correctly, hypoplastic teeth, which in areas of higher fluoride concentration develop posteruptively a characteristic brown stain, were first described two thirds of a century ago by Eager,[30] who studied the condition in a localized area of Italy. Not long afterward, in 1916, Black and Mc-

Kay[31] presented the first of an outstanding series of reports on what was called "mottled enamel" in children in certain areas of Colorado. Repeated searches for the cause of mottled enamel culminated in the report by Smith, Lantz, and Smith[32] in 1931, which definitely implicated a relatively high amount of fluorides in the soil and water. Up to this time and for a number of years thereafter mottled enamel was looked upon exclusively as a pathologic condition and fluorine as its undesirable causative agent.

During the 1930's, however, some investigators not only in the United States but also in Argentina, China, Japan, and South Africa began to notice and question a possible relationship between high fluorine content of soil and water and mottled enamel on the one hand and apparent resistance to caries on the other. Fosdick and Hansen,[33] in their 1936 report on dental changes in Pueblo Indian children, commented, "It is interesting to speculate on the possible relationship of fluorides in fermentation and the reduced susceptibility of mottled enamel to decay." In early 1937 Arnim, Aberle, and Pitney[34] reported on unusual complete freedom from caries in 1,605 permanent incisors of 204 Indian children examined in New Mexico and Arizona. The water used by the tribes contained more than 1 part per million of fluoride. Meanwhile, Armstrong and Brekhus[35] reported a fluorine content of 0.0111% in the enamel of noncarious teeth of individuals from high fluoride areas compared with 0.0069% in carious enamel.

In connection with their 1937 report on dental caries in American Indian children, Klein and Palmer[29] raised the question of the possible beneficial effect of a certain amount of fluoride in the drinking water. They noticed that children of certain tribes in the southwestern part of the United States had much lower caries attack rates than those living elsewhere. They noted that the section involved had been found to be an endemic fluorosis area. They suggested, "This fact may have important implications, and would seem to justify some discussion. Fluorides are well known as

enzyme inhibitors, and it may be suggested that perhaps a measure of the responsibility for low caries attack rates in the southwestern area may be the result of the drinking of fluoride water. Such water may provide an enzyme inhibitor which will operate to limit the chemical degradation of tooth-impacted carbohydrates to organic acids, so reducing the production of local acidity about the teeth, and so limiting an important vector in caries initiation." There followed a large series of investigations by many scientists who compared the fluoride content of the enamel of teeth from different areas and of carious as against noncarious teeth, animal feeding experiments, and many comparative community studies. All substantiated the thesis that while an excessive amount of fluoride in water would produce mottled enamel a certain amount, as low as 1 part per million of fluoride in water consumed during the period of tooth calcification, resulted in a significantly lower incidence of dental caries.

Of significance, especially in view of some antifluoridation arguments, is the recent discovery that rather than harming the skeletal structure and general physiology sodium fluoride does just the opposite. Thus only 3% of females aged 55 to 64 years in high fluoride towns had signs of osteoporosis as compared with almost 21% in low fluoride areas. The study also showed less evidence of hardening of the arteries.[36]

Because of the lack of knowledge at the time with regard to toxicity and costs, the first step to be taken for the practical application of the new knowledge was to apply fluorides directly to the teeth. This procedure was reported independently in 1942 by Bibby[37] and Cheyne.[38] Bibby painted the permanent teeth of children every 4 months with a solution containing 1,000 parts per million sodium fluoride. Cheyne used a solution half that strength of potassium fluoride but at 3-month intervals. Both reported a 50% reduction in caries as compared with the respective control groups. The success of these studies, which were widely publicized, led to a $1 million nationwide demonstration program sponsored by the Public Health Service for the purpose of bringing about widespread knowledge and use of the technique.[39] Another event of this period to which attention should be called was the establishment of the National Institute of Dental Research in 1948 by the Public Health Service. The establishment of this Institute in itself may be considered one of the outstanding developments of recent years. Not only did it represent formal recognition by the Congress of the importance of dental health problems, but it provided funds and facilities for research, research grants, and fellowship programs.

Meanwhile studies underway demonstrated that fluorides in the concentrations being considered were nontoxic.[40-44] The Kettering Laboratory and the Institute of Industrial Health listed over 8,500 carefully analyzed and accepted scientific reports on the subject. The result was summarized by the director of the Institute, Dr. Robert A. Kehoe: "The question of public safety of fluoridation is nonexistent from the standpoint of medical science."[45] At the same time sanitary engineers and waterworks chemists and operators developed policies, procedures, and mechanisms for maintaining within very narrow limits the fluoride levels in water.[46-48] With public sanction a number of carefully controlled community studies were initiated in which fluorides were added to the public water supplies. The results of these studies indicated conclusively that the addition of fluorides up to a concentration of about 1 part per million to the drinking water supply resulted in up to two-thirds reduction in the incidence of dental caries in children who consumed it from birth.[49] If they began to drink it when they were 5 or 6 years of age, the reduction was still 22%.[50] Even those who at 16 years of age had received fluorides for only 6½ years experienced a reduction in expected caries of 18.1%.[51]

The acceptance of the fluoridation of public water supplies as an exceptionally safe, effective, and inexpensive procedure has been disappointingly slow. By the beginning of 1967 only about 63 million people in 3,140 communities in the United States were benefiting from the procedure.

Among the large cities, New York, Chicago, Philadelphia, Detroit, Baltimore, Cleveland, Washington, Minneapolis-St. Paul, St. Louis, Milwaukee, and San Francisco are now included.[52] Four states, Connecticut, Illinois, Kentucky, and Minnesota, as well as Puerto Rico have made mandatory the fluoridation of all public water supplies. Ireland, after much study and debate, now requires by its Health Act of 1960 the fluoridation of all public water supplies. Many other nations have enacted permissive legislation, and no government has prohibited the procedure. Every reputable professional, civic, and governmental organization or agency endorses it.

Despite this, as stated, progress has been much slower than would have been expected. This has been due essentially to the highly successful tactics of a relatively small group of obstructionists—the antifluoridationists. The characteristics, motivations, and methods of these people have interest and meaning for public health workers far beyond the subject of fluoridation. They are the same type and often the same individuals who tend to oppose many progressive and liberal advances be they immunization procedures, pasteurization of milk, civil rights, or international technical assistance. Their personal motivations vary from sincere convictions based upon misunderstanding, religious tenets, or deep-seated cultural factors to what can only be described as fanaticism. Some find the role of professional "anti" economically rewarding. Vice President Hubert Humphrey mentions this in his book, *Cause is Mankind*.[53] He describes the extreme right wing of American politics as composed of a small minority of fanatics who are "against civil rights, against the United Nations, against Social Security, against fluoridation of water, against disarmament" and basically "against people." They have been well analyzed by Hoffer[54] as including certain of the socioeconomically underprivileged, the misfits, the lonely, the innately self-centered and selfish, the bored, the self-accused sinners, and various other groups. He also describes their techniques and unifying forces as including hatred, demagoguery, persuasion and coercion, suspicion, quoting out of context, and guilt by association.* As Paul[56] has pointed out, the arguments of antifluoridationists fall basically into three categories: its benefits are uncertain, it may be injurious, and it violates individual rights. In addition, some object on the basis of added public cost.†

The first two of these have already been commented upon. With reference to economics a simple calculation to compare the per capita, per family or community cost of fluoridation with the tremendous expenditures required to repair carious teeth makes the argument absurd. Perhaps more serious is the charge that fluoridation constitutes enforced medication, thereby violates individual rights, and is illegal.[58-60] Fortunately this charge no longer is valid. The right of communities to adjust the amount of fluoride in their public water supplies as a dental disease preventative has been upheld by courts all the way up to the United States Supreme Court, which has refused review of a number of appeals on the basis that no federal constitutional question was involved. It is of further significance that in 1966 the Michigan branch of the American Civil Liberties Union considered the issue and concluded that there was no basis upon which to consider a violation of personal or civil liberties. One of the problems that have confronted many communities and their health agencies is that antifluoridationists increasingly succeed in placing the issue on the ballot. It has long since been demonstrated that one can obtain sufficient signatures to get practically any referendum before the people and by adroit choice of words so confuse the voters that either they do not vote or vote contrary to their wishes. The question naturally arises whether this type of issue which is in the interests of the general public health should ever be the subject of legislative decision. As stated by Rhyne[61] at the 1966 National Dental Health Assembly, "I think that on the local level the pro-

ponents of fluoridation too frequently go through a referendum without raising the question of whether or not this is a proper issue for submission to the people. . . . I recommend that you think more in terms of presenting this issue to the courts. I think you will find that the courts will hold there is no right to a referendum on a health issue such as this."

PUBLIC HEALTH DENTISTRY
A SPECIALTY

Another significant development during the past 25 years should be mentioned. Because of the growing public and professional awareness of the importance of the problems of dental health and because of the remarkable strides that had been taken in rapid succession and that provided a number of practical measures which could be taken for the solution of those problems, the specialty of public health dentistry was firmly established. Early in the period a Dental Health Section of the American Public Health Association was established, which by 1945 had defined the field of public health dentistry and had established educational qualifications of public health dentists.[62] About the same time the American Association of Public Health Dentists came into being along with a Dental Health Section of the American Dental Association. Annual professional and official conferences of those most directly concerned with programs of dental health were instituted with the establishment of the Conference of State Dental Directors with the Surgeon General of the Public Health Service and the Chief of the Children's Bureau, on the one hand, and the Council on Dental Health of the American Dental Association, on the other. The specialty was formally recognized in 1952 through the establishment of the American Board of Dental Public Health, which is sponsored jointly by the American Dental Association and the American Public Health Association.

PREPAID DENTAL CARE

To plan and provide for adequate dental care of adults is more costly and com-

---

*See also *Comments on the Opponents of Fluoridation*, J. Amer. Dent. Ass.[55]
†For more detailed analysis, see *Fluoridation Facts— Answers to Criticisms of Fluoridation*.[57]

plex than to do so for children. The oral ills of adults are more varied and often require more meticulous and time-consuming work than do those of children. Gruebbel[63] has outlined modern standards of dental care for adults to involve the prevention and treatment of (1) diseases of the teeth, (2) periodontoclasia, (3) anomalies, (4) cysts, (5) malignant and precancerous lesions, (6) oral manifestations of systemic disturbances, and (7) traumatic injuries and the preservation or restoration of mouth function. It is impossible to conceive of any of these being handled on other than a strictly individualized basis. Furthermore, the constantly increasing proportion of older people and the increasing hazards of facial injuries due to automobile and other accidents mitigate against an early lessening of the group needs for some of these services. Even with a marked decrease in the total amount of dental caries, making available a larger proportion of dentists' time for the care of these adult ailments, their very nature makes the cost of remedying them a highly important factor.

The ultimate reasonable solution of adult dental care will depend upon the development of practical, acceptable, and widely available prepayment dental care programs. The first such plan in the United States began in 1867, and by 1900 four others had been established.[64] Since then, development has been slow. Since 1950, some notable developments have occurred.[65] Group practice clinics which employ their own dental staffs began and have been multiplying. Dental service corporations have been formed by a number of local and state dental societies or by groups of dentists by means of which contracting groups receive treatment in the private offices of participating dentists.[66] Some private insurance companies have extended medical prepayment plans to include accidental injury to teeth and major dental surgery. However, it is doubtful that private insurance will ever play a significant role.[67] In addition, several labor unions have sponsored prepaid dental plans with some success. Since 1945 the St. Louis Labor Health Institute has

provided dental services, with the exception of orthodontics, to members on a prepayment basis.[68] A more recent plan is that of the International Longshoremen's and Warehousemen's Union.[69]

Since 1942, the American Dental Association has sponsored numerous studies of prepayment mechanisms. Its original plan[70] proposed to provide family dental service to low-income groups and involved the payment by the subscriber of $1 each month for himself plus an additional $1 monthly for his first dependent and 50 cents per month more for additional dependents. Thus the total fee for a subscriber with two or more dependents amounted to $2.50 per month. Certain services, such as orthodontics and the construction of crowns, bridges, and dentures, were not included. It must be realized that the suggested fees applied to the year 1944.

In 1953 the House of Delegates of the American Dental Association[71] adopted the following set of principles:

1. The plan should be developed, maintained, and promoted to the public with the advice of authorized representatives of the local or state dental society.
2. The plan should foster and encourage the provision of a high quality of dental treatment.
3. The dentist who serves the patient must have complete freedom and responsibility in recommending treatment as his own professional judgment dictates.
4. The patient must have freedom to choose the dentist to whom he may wish to apply for treatment. Similarly the dentist must have the right to accept patients who apply for treatment.
5. The plan should make provision for direct payment to the dentist.
6. All rules and policies that are related to the dental aspects of the plan, including examination, diagnosis, treatment, prevention, and professional education, should be determined by officially designated representatives of the dental profession.
7. Fees for dental services paid to dentists under the plan should be determined by authorized representatives of the dentists who will render the dental services. In all cases payments should be consistent with the provision of high-grade dental service.
8. The plan should designate explicitly both the type and amount of service and the conditions under which it will be provided so that both the patient and the dentist will know

exactly the extent of their participation in the program.

9. Sound and efficient business practices should be used in the management of the plan in order to assure low administrative cost.

One very comprehensive prepaid dental care plan is that of the California Dental Service, a nonprofit corporation that is sponsored by both the California Dental Association and the Southern California State Dental Association. Ninety percent of the dentists in active practice in California are members, and the plan covers more than 1 million persons out of a population of about 20 million. Increasingly, school districts are adopting the plan as a benefit to supplement teachers' salaries.

Despite all these developments, by 1963 in the United States, when prepayment coverage was 145 million people for hospital expenses, 135 million for surgical expenses, and 102 million for regular medical expenses, fewer than 1.2 million people were covered by any type of prepaid dental care program.[72] In other words prepayment for dental services is now at about the same point that medical and hospital prepayment was in the mid-1940's. The extent and rate at which it will develop further will depend upon many factors, not the least of which is much better public understanding of the problem and a wish and willingness to solve it. Germane to the latter is the enormous backlog of existing dental defects which would have to be corrected at great cost in order to achieve a position where continuity of maintenance services would become possible. Add to this the very real shortage of dentists and dental auxiliaries, and the prospect does not appear soluble in the foreseeable future.

PUBLIC HEALTH DENTAL PROGRAMS

In summing up the situation as it existed in 1954, Knutson[3] has stated as follows:

The nature of accomplishments during the past 10 years made this a decade of beginning in the field of dental public health. Water fluoridation, topical fluorides, oral cancer detection and control programs, the team approach to the diagnosis and treatment of cleft lip and cleft palate cases, orthodontic care programs, utilization of chairside assistants, the National Institute of Dental Research, approaches to the epidemiology of dento-facial deformities and periodontal diseases, and principles of prepayment for dental care services—all these are no better than well begun and several are in the budding stage. The objectives of all and the merits of most of them have been firmly established . . .

In view of this it can readily be understood that present-day public health agencies and the relatively few but well-qualified public health dentists on their staffs are in a quite different situation from that which existed but a few years ago, when all they could do was try to devise ways and means of reducing by dental therapy the discouraging flood of accumulating dental needs. By now a practical approach has been unfolded, with some clearly defined and proved preventive measures that, if properly applied, hold promise of reducing the needs for caries correction to a point at which they may be handled reasonably adequately along with the prosthetic, orthodontic, and dental surgical needs of the community.

Easlick[26] has listed the contributions which modern present-day dentistry can make to a child's health. While recognizing that most preventive and promotive dental health activities must be aimed at the child population, his itemization may be generalized and adapted to apply to the total population as follows: Using all modern knowledge available, dentistry and society could prevent and control most dental caries; prevent or control soft tissue inflammation and disease of the supporting tissues of the teeth; with specialist cooperation, correct maloccluding teeth and prevent a relatively small number of the gross tooth irregularities that may interfere with mastication, with the health of the supporting tissues, and with the emotional stability of the individual; with specialist cooperation, can treat the problems arising from anomalies of the oral cavity, e.g., the cleft palate, congenitally missing teeth, supernumerary teeth, hypoplastic teeth, and other developmental dental abnormalities; can treat and restore teeth involved in accidents; can detect oral cancer in the early stages; can prevent and eliminate oral infection which may contribute to body disease.

In reflecting upon how society's existing considerable knowledge may be applied to the successful accomplishment of these goals, the following seven areas of activity would seem to be logically indicated: (1) planning and evaluation, (2) prevention of dental caries, (3) remedial treatment of caries, (4) remedial treatment of other dental and oral defects, (5) public dental health education, and (6) professional development, and (7) development of public and private methods to overcome economic deterrents to obtaining dental health services.

As will be brought out subsequently, the state health departments are the chief governmental agencies which provide dental health services. They operate principally, however, through local health departments which work in cooperation with the dental profession, the schools, and other local organizations. While the state and local health agencies and their public health dentists are often in the position of having to spearhead community activities in this field, the establishment of policies and the development of programs should always be carried out in conjunction with members of the dental societies and for certain components of the program with school health committees, departments of education, and other key groups. A close relationship with the dental profession and schools is particularly important, since their understanding, cooperation, and support are fundamental to a successful dental program.

On the basis of experience acquired in the successful development of a dental health program in Oak Ridge, Tenn., Stroud and Brumback[73] have set down certain guideposts to planning which because of their practicality and good sense are repeated here in part:

1. The first step should be a survey of local needs in order to determine the nature and extent of the problem.
2. A list of resources already available to aid in meeting the needs should be prepared. This should include practicing dentists, official and nonofficial agencies, civic organizations, parent-teacher associations, etc.
3. Resources outside the community should be called upon early in planning. The state public health department can help in many ways. The U. S. Public Health Service has many aids available for use. (To these may be added the state dental society and the American Dental Association.)
4. Local practicing dentists should be active members of the planning group from the start. A committee of dentists should advise the group throughout the inauguration and operation of the program. No action should be taken without approval of the dentists.
5. In planning, representatives of all local organizations having an interest in health should be invited. Their advice can help to avoid many pitfalls and their active interest is essential to a really successful program.
6. If the program operates under the auspices of a lay group as in Oak Ridge, the active administration and supervision should be provided by the local public health department. If funds are to be administered by the lay governing council, this council should be incorporated. Officers responsible for such funds should be bonded and the budget should include an amount to pay for a periodic audit of accounts.
7. Before a program begins operation, policies and procedures should be agreed upon. Personnel policies should be established before employing anyone.
8. In program planning, every opportunity for education should be considered. As many community residents as possible should be encouraged to participate in the organization and operation. In Oak Ridge, several hundred people have taken part in the planning or operation up to the present time. They are members of various community official agencies, private practitioners of dentistry and medicine, housewives, members of clubs and voluntary organizations, scientific workers, teachers, students, businessmen, and private citizens not falling into any of the above categories. Each has made a valuable contribution to the program and all have learned something about dental health.

It is advisable to include in the planning stages of a program provision of a means of its evaluation. Since caries constitutes the bulk of the dental problem and since the chief goal to be attained is a reduction in the amount of dental caries, the prevalence of that condition in the population to be served should be determined. Since the D.M.F. count of adults is closely correlated with that of children, an initial survey of a sample of the child population alone may serve the purpose. Based on the observation that a functional relationship exists between the proportion of children having at least one D.M.F. permanent tooth and the average number of D.M.F. permanent teeth per child, Knutson[74] has developed a simplified method which may be used to determine the initial base line and subsequent evaluation.

Since it has been clearly shown that proper fluoridation of water supplies will decrease dental caries prevalence up to 65%, it is obvious that the primary goal of a public health dental program should be the acceptance and development of this procedure. In order to accomplish this a number of steps should be suggested. Probably the first thing which should be done is to obtain a positive statement of policy on fluoridation by the state dental society and the state health agency. Following this, it will probably be advisable to promote the establishment of a state fluoridation committee to work with the state public health dentists and the state dental society. Such a group may be of considerable value in providing information and data on fluoridation to the general public and the press, to local dental societies, and to state and local nonprofessional organizations and officials. It may also assist by drawing up a sample fluoridation ordinance in conformance with state legislation and by collecting information on costs. On the local level the local dental society might preferably provide the leadership in organizing a local committee and should play an active role in the planning and establishment of the local program.

Despite its greater cost and more difficult method of use, topical application of fluoride to the teeth of children has a place in many if not all public health dental programs. This is especially true in rural areas or where there is shortsighted but effective opposition to fluoridation of public water supplies. Thus, as has been pointed out previously, opposition, procrastination, and scattered populations account for the fact that by 1967 only 63 million people in 3,140 communities had the benefit of fluoridated water. Incidentally it should be noted that now more

than two thirds of the population of the United States lives under urban circumstances.

Another reason for retaining the topical fluoride procedure is that since water fluoridation is most effective during the years of enamel calcification it is advisable that children, whose teeth were already calcified when fluoridation is begun, have topical fluoride applications. Subsequently, as the benefits of fluoridated water become effective, topical fluoride applications may be discontinued gradually beginning with the younger age groups. The extent to which the topical procedure is carried out in the offices of private practicing dentists on the one hand, or through public facilitis on the other, will depend entirely on the local situation. Wertheimer[75] has described some of the difficulties encountered by the program in Michigan, which was one of the first to be established. Of particular interest was the partial solution of the difficult personnel problem by means of summer employment of junior dental students. With proper preparation and demonstration as well as discussions on the place of dentistry in public health, public relations, the group method approach, and the care of equipment, students were found to do a creditable job. Incidentally this approach has reduced the cost of topical fluoride application per child by about 50%. Wertheimer also points out that this approach gives the following additional benefits to the dental students: (1) experience in group method of topical fluoride application, (2) development of skill in handling children, (3) learning about dental conditions of children in communities in contrast to select groups usually seen in dental schools, (4) orientation in public health and the concept that dental disease is a public health problem, and (5) opportunity to observe community action as an approach to the solution of the problems.

It must be recognized that fluoridation of water and topical application of fluorides do not bring about complete caries control and do not eliminate the need for other dental health measures. A certain amount of caries will always develop; hence there probably always will be a need for some remedial treatment of caries. For this and other reasons an essential part of the public health dental program should be the promotion of regular dental supervision as an essential part of individual hygienic living. With a major proportion of caries subject to prevention, it may be possible to repair the backlog of caries on an incremental basis. Even in the face of vast accumulated dental needs, it has been found practical and fruitful in a number of places to restrict caries corrective programs to children in a restricted age span. For example, some programs that began by caring for children from 5 to 10 years of age have found it possible during the second year of the program to add the new crop of 5-year-old children and, in addition, to continue with the 11-year-old children who were in the original group the year before. As each year goes by, new 5-year-olds have been added, and all children previously cared for were continued.

The part of a community dental health program that relates to the remedial treatment of dental and other oral defects, including orthodontics, prosthetics, and dental surgery for congenital defects, would seem to rest largely in the hands of private practicing dentists aided to whatever degree may be possible by the services, facilities, and contributions of public clinics for indigent or low-income groups, philanthropic agencies, and prepayment dental care plans. The scant attention sometimes given to these conditions is in no way indicative of their relative importance. Indeed, as Gruebbel[63] visualizes, "Orthodontic services . . . may some day prove to be high on the list of essential services. The health professions are finding increasing evidence of the value of orthodontic care to the physical and mental well-being and social adjustment of children and youth. It has been estimated that there are approximately 40 million children under the age of 16 years in the United States, of whom 7 to 8 million need major orthodontic care, and of whom less than 4 out of every 100 who need it are actually receiving treatment."

At the present time increasing numbers of underprivileged children with such oral and dental defects that would ordinarily be uncorrected are being cared for by the health components of some of the Economic Opportunity (so-called "Poverty") Programs or by the Comprehensive Health Care section of Title V of the 1965 Amendments to the Social Security Law (P.L. 89-97).

Underlying all the other activities should be a carefully planned dental health education program so varied as to reach all segments of the public, with particular emphasis on "sensitive" groups. For many years those who attend prenatal, well-baby, and other public health clinics have been exposed to dental health educational procedures. It is puzzling, however, to understand why so few hospital waiting rooms and private physicians' offices do anything to encourage their clients to seek dental supervision. In consideration of the numbers of persons involved and the receptive circumstances in which they find themselves this is suggested as a channel of public education worthy of much more intensive exploration and use.

A very important area for dental health education is in relation to the school health program. Those responsible for the community dental health program should work particularly closely with the board of education, classroom teachers, and physical education personnel, assisting them in the preparation of sound and practical information in the field, screening of classroom teaching aids, and obtaining material for them from the various dental and public health associations.[76]

On the state level public health dentists should work closely and in a similar manner with state departments of education, dental schools, and teachers' colleges. Another area worthy of particular attention is that concerned with the school lunch program. The public health dental personnel in collaboration with teachers of nutrition and home economics and with the school lunchroom managers should attempt to bring about a change in lunch and snack habits, particularly with regard to the intake of carbohydrates. With this in mind a great many school systems have discouraged the use and even availability of candy and soft drinks in their lunchrooms and elsewhere on school premises. While it is fully recognized that school children may obtain these products elsewhere, it is at least a partial step in the right direction to bring about a change in the habit pattern at mealtime.

A final and basic part of the community dental health program should be concerned with the improvement of professional standards and practices. This is particularly appropriate at this time, when one considers the many recent developments that have come about since the graduation of many of those now practicing dentistry. Still another reason is the increasing awareness of the relationship of various fields in medicine, economics, and sociology, to the modern practice of dentistry. A number of states have found it very worth while to sponsor postgraduate seminars on subjects related to modern dental practice. Such activities go far in strengthening the local dental society, raising the standards of local practice, and assuring the cooperation and active participation of the dentists of the community. In connection with seminars and postgraduate training it is suggested that the subject matter not be restricted to dentistry or even public health dentistry but include also appropriate aspects of mental hygiene, economics, newer techniques for the diagnosis and treatment of cancer, and other similar subjects.

A previous section of this chapter dealt briefly with the need for and usefulness of dental hygienists and dental assistants. It was pointed out at that time that only a minor percent of practicing dentists are making use of this valuable potential source of assistance. The promotion of the use of dental hygienists and dental assistants is certainly a worth while and legitimate aspect of the community dental health program since its success would be a greater total amount of dentists' time available to the community.

An easily overlooked area of action in a program such as that under considera-tion is related to the solution of the ever present problem of personnel shortages. Those responsible for the program should consider activities in the nature of career guidance to high school and college students as an important responsibility.

REFERENCES

1. Knutson, J., and Klein, H.: Tooth mortality in elementary school children, Public Health Rep. **53:**1021, June 1938.
2. Klein, H., and Palmer, C.: Therapeutic odontotomy and preventive dentistry, J. Amer. Dent. Ass. **27:**1055, July 1940.
3. Knutson, J.: Dental public health accomplishments and predictions, Amer. J. Public Health **44:**331, Mar. 1954.
4. Causes of rejection and incidence of defects, Med. Stat. Bull. **2:**1, Aug. 1943.
5. The epidemiology of dental disease. Collection of papers of Henry Klein and others, 1937-47, Washington, 1948, Federal Security Agency, Public Health Service.
6. Commission on the Survey of Dentistry in the United States, American Council on Education, Washington, 1961, The Council.
7. Health statistics, Series B-22, National Health Survey, Public Health Service, Sept. 1960.
8. Miller, S. L., and Palsgrove, J. E.: Dental disease in preschool children, J. Med. Ass. Alabama **30:**337, Dec. 1960.
9. Grace, L.: Study on incidence of cleft palate, J. Dent. Res. **22:**495, Dec. 1943.
10. Health resources statistics, Washington, 1965, Public Health Service Pub. No. 1509.
11. Preliminary report on volume of dental care, Health statistics from the U. S. National Health Survey, Washington, Mar. 1958, Department of Health, Education, and Welfare.
12. Health statistics, Series B-14, National Health Survey, Public Health Service, Mar. 1960.
13. Bureau of Economic Research and Statistics, J. Amer. Dent. Ass. **62:**627, May 1961.
14. Distribution of dentists in the United States by state, region, district and county, Bureau of Economic Research and Statistics, American Dental Association, 1961.
15. Klein, H.: Civilian dentistry in wartime, J. Amer. Dent. Ass. **31:**648, May 1944.
16. McCall, J. O.: Dental practice and dental education in the future, J. Amer. Dent. Ass. **31:**16, Jan. 1944.
17. Aston, E. R.: Responsibility of the American Association of Industrial Dentists, Public Health Rep. **67:**694, July 1952.
18. Easlick, K. A.: Dental caries, mechanism and present control techniques, St. Louis, 1948, The C. V. Mosby Co.
19. Florio, L. In Leavell, H. R., et al.: Textbook of preventive medicine, New York, 1953, McGraw-Hill Book Co.
20. Hunt, H. R., Hoppert, C., and Erwin, W.: In-

heritance of susceptibility to caries in albino rats, J. Dent. Res. **23**:385, Oct. 1944.

21. Klein, H., and Palmer, C.: On the epidemiology of dental caries, University of Pennsylvania Bicentennial Conference, Philadelphia, 1941, University of Pennsylvania Press.

22. Jay, P.: *Bacillus acidophilus* and dental caries, J. Amer. Dent. Ass. **16**:230, Feb. 1929.

23. Jay, P.: The problem of dental caries with relation to bacteria and diet, J. Pediat. **8**:725, 1936.

24. Bunting, R. W., and Palmerlee, F.: The role of *Bacillus acidophilus* in dental caries, J. Amer. Dent. Ass. **12**:381, Apr. 1925.

25. Jay, P.: The role of sugar in the etiology of caries, J. Amer. Dent. Ass. **27**:393, Mar. 1940.

26. Easlick, K. A.: The caries problem of the school child, Amer. J. Public Health **39**:984, Aug. 1949.

27. Collins, S.: The health of the school child, a study of sickness, physical defects and mortality, Washington, Aug. 1931, Public Health Service Bull. No. 200.

28. Messner, C. T., Gafafer, W. M., Cady, F. C., and Dean, H. T.: Dental survey of school children, ages 6-14 years, made in 1933-34 in 26 states, Washington, May 1936, Public Health Service Bull. No. 226.

29. Klein, H., and Palmer, C.: Dental caries in American Indian children, Washington, Dec. 1937, Public Health Service Bull. No. 239.

30. Eager, J.: Chiaie teeth, Public Health Rep. **16**:2576, 1901.

31. Black, G. V., and McKay, F. S.: Mottled teeth: an endemic developmental imperfection of the enamel of the teeth heretofore unknown in the literature of dentistry, Dent. Cosmos **58**:129, 1916.

32. Smith, M. C., Lantz, E., and Smith, H. B.: The cause of mottled enamel, Science **74**:244, 1931.

33. Fosdick, L., and Hansen, H.: Theoretical considerations of carbohydrate degradation in relation to dental caries, J. Amer. Dent. Ass. **23**:406, Mar. 1936.

34. Arnim, S., Aberle, S., and Pitney, E.: A study of dental changes in a group of Pueblo Indian children, J. Amer. Dent. Ass. **24**:478, Mar. 1937.

35. Armstrong, W., and Brekhus, P.: Chemical constitution of enamel and dentin, J. Biol. Chem. **120**:677, Sept. 1937.

36. Bernstein, D. S., et al.: The prevalence of osteoporosis in high and low fluoride areas in North Dakota, J.A.M.A. **198**:499, Oct. 1966.

37. Bibby, B. G.: Preliminary report on the use of sodium fluoride applications in caries prophylaxis, J. Dent. Res. **21**:314, 1942.

38. Cheyne, V. D.: Human dental caries and topically applied fluorine: a preliminary report, J. Amer. Dent. Ass. **29**:804, 1942.

39. Knutson, J. W.: The nationwide topical fluoride demonstration program, J. Amer. Dent. Ass. **39**:438, 1949.

40. Cox, G. J., and Hodge, H. C.: The toxicity of fluorides in relation to their use in dentistry, J. Amer. Dent. Ass. **40**:440, Apr. 1950.

41. Heyroth, F.: Toxicological evidence for the safety of the fluoridation of public water supplies, Amer. J. Public Health **42**:1568, Dec. 1952.

42. Hagan, T. L., Pasternack, M., and Scholz, G. C.: Waterborne fluorides and mortality, Public Health Rep. **69**:450, May 1954.

43. Geever, E. F., Leone, N. C., Geiser, P., and Lieberman, J. E.: Pathological studies in man after prolonged ingestion of fluoride in drinking water, Public Health Rep. **73**:721, Aug. 1958.

44. Hodge, H. C.: Safety factors in water fluoridation based on the toxicology of fluorides, Proc. Nutr. Soc. **22**:111, 1963.

45. Campbell, I. R., editor: The role of fluoride in public health, a selected bibliography, Cincinnati, 1963, Kettering Laboratory, University of Cincinnati.

46. Tentative standard specifications for sodium fluoride, J. Amer. Waterworks Ass. **42**:899, Sept. 1950.

47. Bull, F. A., Hardgrove, T. A., and Frisch, J. G.: Methods and costs of water fluoridation, J. Amer. Dent. Ass. **42**:29, Jan. 1951.

48. Maier, F. J.: Engineering problems in water fluoridation, Amer. J. Public Health **42**:249, Mar. 1952.

49. Ast, D. B.: Effectiveness of water fluoridation, J. Amer. Dent. Ass. **65**:581, Nov. 1962.

50. Horowitz, H. S., Law, F. E., and Pritzker, T.: Effect of school water fluoridation on dental caries, Public Health Rep. **80**:381, May 1965.

51. Hutton, W. L., Linscott, B. W., and Williams, D. B.: The Brantford fluorine experiment, Canad. J. Public Health **42**:81, Jan. 1951.

52. Dunning, J. M.: Current status of fluoridation, New Eng. J. Med. **272**:30, Jan. 1965.

53. Humphrey, H. H.: Cause is mankind, New York, 1964, Fredricka Praeger, Inc.

54. Hoffer, E.: The true believer, New York, 1958, Mentor Press.

55. Comments on the opponents of fluoridation, J. Amer. Dent. Ass. **71**:1156, Nov. 1965.

56. Paul, B. D.: Fluoridation and the social scientist, J. Soc. Issues, **17**:4, 1, Oct. 1961.

57. Fluoridation facts—answers to criticisms of fluoridation, Chicago, American Dental Society Pub. G 21.

58. Roemer, R.: Water fluoridation: public health responsibility and the democratic process, Amer. J. Public Health **55**:1337, Sept. 1965.

59. Legal note—dental health and fluoridation, Public Health Rep. **77**:639, July 1962.

60. Tobey, J. A.: Water fluoridation and civil rights, Public Health News, New Jersey Department of Health, **43**:121, Apr. 1962.

61. Rhyne, C. S.: Fluoridation and the law, Washington, 1966, Public Health Service Pub. No. 1552.

62. Educational qualifications of public health dentists (revised), Amer. J. Public Health **42**:188, Feb. 1952.

63. Gruebbel, A. O.: Standards of dental care for the different age groups, Amer. J. Public Health **39:**981, Aug. 1949.
64. Penchansky, R., and Safford, B. M.: Prepayment for dental care: need and effect, Public Health Rep. **81:**541, June 1966.
65. Editorial: Current trends in prepaid dental care, Amer. J. Public Health **48:**777, June 1958.
66. The dental service corporation—organization and development, Washington, 1965, Public Health Service Pub. No. 1274.
67. Follmann, J. F.: The role of private insurance. In A symposium on the group purchase of dental care, Amer. J. Public Health **50:**28, Jan. 1960.
68. McNeel, J. O.: Dental program of the St. Louis Labor Health Institute, Amer. J. Public Health **44:**878, July 1954.
69. Report on the dental program of the ILWU-PMA, Washington, 1962, Public Health Service Pub. No. 894.
70. Proposed plan for prepayment of dental insurance, Chicago, 1944, American Dental Association.
71. Transactions of the American Dental Association, 1953.
72. Digest of prepaid dental care plans, 1963, Washington, 1964, Public Health Service Pub. No. 585.
73. Stroud, H., and Brumback, C.: A dental health program for your community, Amer. J. Public Health **40:**1426, Nov. 1950.
74. Knutson, J.: Simplified appraisal of dental health programs, Public Health Rep. **62:**413, Mar. 1947.
75. Wertheimer, F.: Michigan summer topical fluoride program, Amer. J. Public Health **44:**484, Apr. 1954.
76. A dental program for schools, Chicago, 1963, American Dental Association.

Chapter 22

Mental health*

INTRODUCTION

The field of mental and emotional health and illness forms one of the newer frontiers of public health, which has been the subject of considerable exploration and activity during recent years. As a result of increasing attention in both the public and the professional press there has developed an acute awareness of the relationship between mental illnesses of various types and degrees of severity, on the one hand, and crime, juvenile delinquency, prostitution, alcoholism, addictions, accidents, suicides, crimes of violence, marital failures, work inadequacies, and a host of other undesirable social and physical phenomena, on the other. Similarly the public as well as the medical and health professions have become conscious of the increasing mental stresses of urban and especially of industrialized life.[2] Further, the large number of individuals in need of institutional care and the great cost of providing it have become matters of common knowledge and concern.

As with many other problems, preliminary social study and experimentation in this field came about largely out of the interest of a few individuals and private or voluntary groups or agencies. Until relatively recently, mentally ill persons were incarcerated without treatment in filthy goals and other institutions, often in company with criminals and diseased persons; they were exhibited as curiosities or sources of amusement; and they were restrained for long periods of time in chains and straight

jackets, beaten unmercifully, and rendered stuporous by drugs. Some were even burned at the stake on the premise that they were witches or possessed by evil spirits. Their greatest and most courageous champion was Philippe Pinel, who in the 1790's agitated for reforms for their more humane treatment in France. His efforts to remove their chains, to have them considered as victims of illness, and to transfer them from prisons to hospitals were pursued in the face of strenuous opposition and ridicule not only from the public but also from his fellow physicians. About 50 years later a similar movement got under way in the United States due largely to Dorothea Dix. During the late nineteenth century the foundations of the related fields of psychology and psychiatry were laid. These led gradually to consideration of possible preventive and promotive approaches to the problem that eventually crystalized in the form of the mental hygiene movement.

The mental hygiene movement as such may be said to have begun in 1908 with the publication of Clifford W. Beers' book *A Mind That Found Itself*.[3] It presented in dramatic and effective manner the author's experiences as a patient in a number of institutions for the mentally ill. The narrative ended with a plea for drastic reform and public education in mental health. Prompt encouragement and support enabled Beers to establish the first organization of its type, the Connecticut Society for Mental Hygiene. Its purpose was to combat the widespread ignorance about mental illnesses and their causes. One year later, in 1909, the National Committee for Mental Hygiene was organized. Rapid

---

*For a more extensive exploration, see Sanders: Amer. J. Public Health.[1]

growth occurred during the ensuing two decades as evidenced by the organization of 19 state mental hygiene societies as well as societies in 16 different nations. In 1922 the International Congress for Mental Hygiene came into being, and in 1930 it called the first International Mental Hygiene Congress in Washington.

Meanwhile a few local and state governmental units such as health departments began introducing activities in the field of mental health. Usually they were frankly exploratory and experimental and often were integrated with some other activities of the agency rather than identified separately. A great stimulus came in 1946, when the National Mental Health Act (P.L. 487) was passed by Congress. It authorized $7.5 million for the construction and equipment of hospital and research facilities by the Public Health Service as a center for research and training in mental health. Ten million dollars was provided for grants to states to expand their facilities, and an additional $1 million for demonstrations and the employment of personnel. In 1949 these responsibilities were reorganized to form the National Institute of Mental Health. Through this means the Act has made possible much of the expansion of thought and action which since has occurred at all levels of government in the United States and to which subsequent reference will be made.[4]

EXTENT OF PROBLEM

In terms both of incidence and prevalence, on the one hand, and of social and economic implications, on the other, mental illness is one of the most compelling public health problems. So widely do problems of this nature pervade all aspects of community health that Jensen,[5] a sociologist, has claimed: "If it isn't mental health, it isn't public health." Mental illness, like cancer, is not an entity. Rather it is a mixture of a variety of conditions which hamper or destroy the individual's effectiveness. By now about one half of mental disease has been clarified and classified on an organic basis. Much of what remains, including the large area of schizo-

phrenia, is still obscure. Accelerated research, however, is shedding more light on these dark areas. Evidence accumulating indicates increasingly that somatic and psychic functions are so closely related that they operate in health and illness as parts of an entity.[6] As a result the integration of psychiatry with general medicine is considered to be the most significant trend in modern psychiatry. This is evidenced by psychiatrists' increasingly moving out of their hospitals, clinics, and consulting rooms into close relationships with other physicians and groups in the community. Similarly more work is being done on the basis of family and group dynamics.

Each year in the United States over 1 million persons, including 4,000 children and youths, are treated in mental hospitals. While only about 2% of all hospital admissions are for psychiatric disorders, about one half of the hospital beds in the nation are occupied by mentally ill patients. In addition, 1.5 million adults and children visit outpatient clinics and private physicians for psychiatric diagnosis and treatment each year. It has been estimated that about one half of all children and adults who consult private physicians for any reason have some kind of emotional disorder. Similarly it is estimated that of the 20 million patients who go to general hospitals for physical ailments each year about 6 million have illnesses caused by emotional disturbances. There is evidence that at any given time about 1 out of every 10 persons in the country has some form of mental or emotional disorder that needs treatment. Among the many factors contributing to the increase in mental patients are increased stresses of urbanization and industrialization, greater longevity, increased population, improved and more acceptable diagnosis, and increased facilities for diagnosis and care.

Among patients hospitalized for mental illnesses schizophrenia is the most common condition, accounting for 45.6% of the total. The frequency of other important conditions is: mental diseases of the senium, 12.2%; manic depression, 7.6%; syphilitic psychosis, 6.7%; and psychosis with men-

Table 22-1. Hospitalization for mental illness by age, sex, and chance of recovery

Condition	Usual age at first admission	First admissions (%)			Hospitalized mental patients (%)	Chances of recovery
		Men	Women	Both		
Schizophrenia	16 to 35 years	18.6	26.8	22.6	45.6	Poor after age 50; long hospitalization
Manic-depressive psychosis	35 to 50 years	3.1	5.3	4.2	7.6	Poor; long hospitalization
Psychosis with mental deficiency	15 to 44 years	2.7	1.8	2.3	6.0	Poor; long hospitalization
Alcoholic psychosis	25 to 54 years	21.8	5.2	13.7	3.0	Fair; short hospitalization
Involutional psychosis	48 to 58 years	3.0	8.3	5.6	3.0	Poor; die soon; short hospitalization
Senile psychosis	60 years and over	21.1	20.5	20.8	12.2	Poor; die soon; short hospitalization
Personality disorders (nonalcoholic)	15 to 34 years	7.2	3.9	5.6	4.0	Fair; short hospitalization
Psychoneurotic reactions	25 to 44 years	6.3	12.4	9.3	6.0	Fair; short hospitalization
Other disorders, each of low incidence	All ages	16.2	15.8	15.9	12.6	Generally poor; long hospitalization

tal deficiency, 6.0%. Alcoholic and involutional psychoses each account for about 3.0% of those hospitalized.[7]

The incidence of mental illness depends upon many factors. Type of condition in relation to age is especially important. Most mental illnesses have their origins in early childhood but do not become manifest until the developmental or productive years of life. Despite this, schizophrenia is being diagnosed in children with increasing frequency. In general, however, as measured in terms of age at first hospitalization for mental illness, about one half are between 35 and 64 years, about one quarter are between 15 and 34 years, and about one quarter are over 65 years of age, whereas only a little more than 1% are under 15 years of age.

As to type of illness, mental deficiency, epilepsy, personality disorders, and schizophrenia usually appear early in life; alcoholic and manic-depressive psychoses are centered in the middle productive years of life; while involutional and senile psychoses occur during the later years. Mental illness seems to be more frequent among women than among men. About 50% more women than men enter hospitals for schizophrenia and manic-depression than do men. The incidence of psychoneuroses appears to be about twice as common in women as in men, whereas involutional psychoses are three times as high. On the other hand, personality disorders are twice as frequent, and alcoholic psychoses are about four or five times as frequent in males as in females. There is no significant difference between the sexes in the incidence of mental deficiency or of senile psychoses.

These differences by type and age, especially in relation to the chances for recovery, play a determining role in the enormous hospital bed requirements and treatment costs for mental illness. This is indicated in Table 22-1, which presents various mental conditions in the order of their general ultimate importance, considering numbers of persons affected, duration of the illness, length of hospitalization necessary, and chances of recovery.*

Some interesting socioeconomic variations may be noted in the incidence of mental illness. Thus neuroses are twice as common as the more severe psychoses among the wealthy, professional, and top managerial groups. The opposite is true among semi-

*For a more detailed analysis, see Kramer: Amer. J. Public Health.[8]

skilled and unskilled laborers. Another way of looking at this is that neuroses are twice as common in the higher than in the lower socioeconomic groups, whereas severe psychoses occur about twice as frequently in the lower than in the higher socioeconomic groups of the population. Part of these discrepancies may be due to greater awareness of and tendency to seek medical attention for neuroses especially on the part of the economically more privileged. Similarly many in the lower socioeconomic group may not consider neurosis as an illness in relation to the pressures from many other problems.[9,10] On the other hand, some of the causes of the more severe psychoses are more prevalent in the environments and family milieus of the socioeconomically deprived.

At present the most dramatic and effective role is being played by pharmacologic research.[11,12] Indications are that this research will continue to increase. The discovery of the ataraxics or tranquilizers has revolutionized both in- and outpatient care. Many who previously would have been institutionalized now are not because the length of institutional stay has been shortened significantly. Indeed the very atmosphere of mental institutions has changed dramatically. The year 1955 was the turning point. In that year the number of patients discharged from institutions increased sharply and the number of persons institutionalized declined. Further evidence of the effect is that in 1964, while there were 300,000 admissions to state and county mental hospitals, the largest number in history, the number of resident patients on any one day dropped below 500,000 for the first time in 15 years.

The limitations of data restricted to hospitalization are obvious. Many individuals receive some psychiatric guidance through public and private medical facilities other than hospitals, but the amount is unknown. Many more are in need of varying degrees of assistance for relatively minor personality adjustment and psychiatric problems but never receive it. In many ways the latter represents perhaps the greatest social and economic aspect of the total problem.

It has been estimated that the overall annual cost of mental illness in the United States is about $1,200 per patient, or over $4 billion.[13]

The question naturally arises as to the possibility of insuring against the costs of mental illness. Although a number of health insurance organizations and plans that operate their own facilities have psychiatrists on their staffs and some provide mental health clinics, only rarely do they include the costs of psychiatric treatment among their benefits. The few who have attempted to do so have encountered substantial difficulties. Among these, Reed[14] has listed high costs in a setting where all types of health insurance plans are finding their costs expanding; the indeterminateness of these costs, particularly when care over a long period in a hospital or physician's office is required; the question of how mental hospitals in this country should be financed and of demarcation of the respective roles of patient, private insurance, and government in financing mental hospital care; and a rather complete lack of information as to what the utilization of psychiatric services would be if they were available on an insured basis. Meanwhile, following a contract negotiated in 1964 between the United Auto Workers and the automobile and agricultural implement industries under which about 2.5 million workers and their families will receive coverage for psychiatric care, plans have been made for a study of the effect upon the provision and ability of community mental health services.[15]

DEFINITION AND GOAL OF MENTAL HEALTH

Mental health represents a broad field and one that is difficult to define. Potentially there are probably very few areas of public health activity to which it cannot make a real contribution. The increased provision of facilities and the improvement of techniques of treatment of the mentally ill for their own sake are not of course the fundamental interests or ultimate goals of the field of mental health. Rather, its primary concerns may be said to be improved and increased detection of psychiatric and prepsychiatric conditions that may result in personal and social handicaps, the study of their causes, and the initiation of efforts to eliminate as far as possible the factors that bring them about. Thus the goal may be said to be a more satisfying and effective life, free of adverse mental deterrents for more people or, to state it even more simply, the development of emotionally mature people.

Some of the subgoals involved have been presented by Bullis[16] in his description of the program sponsored by the Delaware State Society for Mental Hygiene in which classes on human relations are taught in the public schools. This program, he says, represents "a sincere attempt to help our boys and girls now in school progress toward emotional maturity by developing their ability to make decisions; to accept responsibilities; to learn from their own emotional mistakes; to make and keep friends; to bring their fears out into the open; to carry on to the best of their ability when emotionally disturbed; to accept themselves and depend less on artificial entertainment; to face the past or future without fear; to face up to unpleasant, fearful, or distasteful events of the present; to look at unknown future changes as interesting adventures to be faced."

Nevertheless, as indicated by Lemkau[17] in his excellent definition of the field, the goals, hence the desirable program content, in mental health are two-dimensional. He points out that the vertical or categorical dimension, consisting of early diagnosis and treatment of existing mental ills, as in the case of tuberculosis control, meets several needs: (1) the prevention of the development of more serious and handicapping illness, (2) the removal of sources of stress from family and social environments, and (3) the making available of the services of specialist personnel to the broader horizontal aims of the mental health program. The horizontal goals of mental health he visualizes in terms of the work of every member of the public health department being influenced by mental hygiene principles. The brief consideration of a few of the ways in

which the latter may be attempted is appropriate.

MENTAL HEALTH PROGRAMS

Because of the relative newness of the field and amount of exploration occurring, it is not possible to state clearly what a mental health program should include. However, a consideration of some of the activities that already have been attempted is of some interest. At the present time mental health services of some kind are being carried on by all states. In three fifths of the states the department of health is the responsible agency. In the remainder the program is the responsibility of a department of mental health, a department of welfare, a department of institutions, a special board or commission, or an independent state hospital or laboratory.[18] In these latter instances and even in the cases of a number of the state health department programs the activities are largely limited to diagnosis and psychiatric treatment with little or no effort toward prevention.

The National Mental Health Act passed in 1946 provided for federal grants-in-aid to states for research, training, and assistance in the establishment and development of community mental health programs, particularly for the prevention and early treatment of mental and emotional disorders. A particularly noteworthy result of the act was the establishment several years later of The National Institute of Mental Health at Bethesda, Md. This institute has provided national leadership of high quality. Already significant progress may be noted in having made state public health personnel aware of mental health and in integrating it into various parts of their programs and activities. Within 4 years after the passage of the act, specifically identified bureaus, divisions, or sections for mental health were founded in 28 state public health agencies, and in several others a consultant in mental hygiene served on the staff, usually of the bureau or division of preventive medical services. At the present time the functions of these mental health units variously include the maintenance of lists or rosters of mental health facilities; the gathering of reports or data on mental health needs and problems; the development of and assistance to state and local, lay and professional educational programs; the direct operation of mental health clinics, inpatient facilities, and day-care centers; the promulgation of rules and regulations relating to mental health and the administration of certain aspects of some of them; financial assistance to local agencies; promotional, supervisory, and consultative services to local official and voluntary agencies; and special surveys and research. Mid-1963 saw another milestone in the fight against mental illness in the United States. It took the form of the passage of P.L. 88-164, the Mental Retardation Facilities and Community Mental Health Centers Construction Act. Its purpose was to assist all levels of government to deal more vigorously with the problems of mental illness and mental retardation. In addition to providing more funds for research, it also authorized grants to states for the construction of additional community mental health centers, the extension of community mental health preventive and promotive programs, and the initial staffing of these facilities and programs.[19] The purpose of the act was extended and strengthened in 1965 by an amendment (P.L. 89-105) providing additional support for community-based programs for the care of the mentally ill and encouraging general hospitals to become major community psychiatric resources.

These events on the national level have provided many states with the stimulus to enact legislation for the establishment of Community Mental Health Services Boards, and the provision to them of state matching funds for the extension and coordination of mental health activities on the community or local level.

As in the case of the states, mental health activities on the part of local public health agencies have been somewhat slow to start. Until quite recently few of the official city or county health agencies have endeavored to initiate and to carry on such programs. Part of the reason has been the complexity of the problem, hence the complexity of the

approach to its solution. As a corollary, it has been realized that the solution cannot and must not rest in the hands of one group. This has been pointed out by Felix and Kramer[20]: "Because of the complexity of the problem, effective research on the community aspects of mental illness must be interdisciplinary, combining the skills and knowledge of the psychiatrist, psychologist, social scientist, public health physician and nurse, psychiatric social worker, epidemiologist, and statistician." This was also clearly indicated in the report of the National Health Assembly[21] which stated: "Clergymen, teachers, lawyers, social workers, nurses, recreation and group workers, law enforcement officers, public health personnel, representatives of management and labor, and many others, are constantly presented with opportunities for recognizing emotional problems." A most important omission by each of these listings, and perhaps the key group toward which the efforts of all of the others should be primarily aimed, are parents—both actual and prospective. These important concepts have been clearly illustrated by Blain and Robinson,[22] as shown in Fig. 22-1.

In 1962 more than 1,500 psychiatric outpatient clinics were reported to be in operation in the United States. This is in contrast with fewer than 500 in 1947. To be considered adequate for reporting purposes, it was necessary that a center be staffed at least by a psychiatrist, a clinical psychologist, and a psychiatric social worker. The clinics were located in all states and territories, with the exception of Nevada. However, more than half of the clinics were in the Northeastern states, which have one quarter of the total population. There were more than 200 in the New York City area alone. State governments operated 41% of the clinics, and another 23% received some state aid; 5% were operated by the Veterans Administration.

The relationship between the staff of the mental health center or program and the personnel of the official public health agency sometimes presents an administrative problem. It involves especially the relationship between the psychiatric social

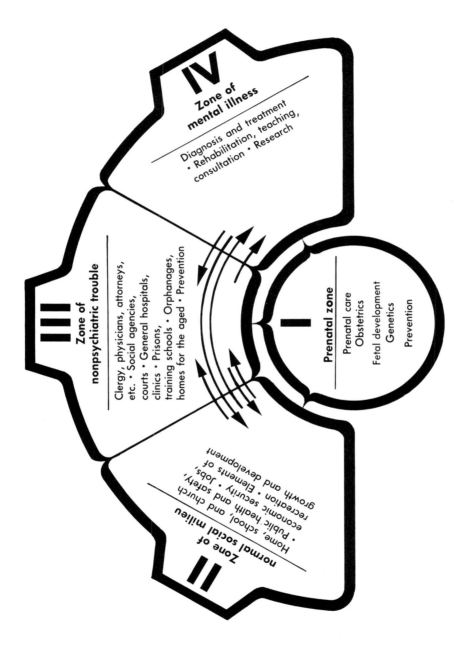

Fig. 22-1. Population and service zones in relation to mental health and illness. (Adapted from Blain, D., and Robinson, R. L.: Personnel shortages in psychiatric services, New York J. Med., Jan. 15, 1957.)

workers and the public health nursing staff. The obvious goal is for the public health nurses and the psychiatric social worker to look upon each other as sources of referral and as a resource for consultation, advice, and in-service education. This can best be accomplished through joint planning, joint conferences, and joint in-service training. Perhaps the key consideration to be kept in mind by the nursing staff is that psychiatric social work is a specialized field in itself. In turn the very limited numbers of psychiatric social workers must recognize that they are physically incapable of making all of the contacts and of meeting all the needs and that public health nurses have wide and well-established contacts and entrée throughout the community. Beyond this, all concerned, including the health officer and the director of the mental health center, should bear in mind that the promotion and maintenance of smooth and fruitful interpersonnel relationships is one manifestation of sound mental health and in turn is a prerequisite to the planning, development, and implementation of an effective community mental health program.[23]

THE ROLE OF THE HEALTH DEPARTMENT

At an Institute on Mental Health in Public Health held in the University of California at Berkeley in 1948[24] it was agreed that one of the most important problems for health departments at that time was to clarify their responsibilities in their communities with respect to mental health in order that citizens and other agencies might know what to expect. It was felt that unless effective organization took place among the various agencies concerned with the problem and unless each understood its specific role and the roles of the others confusion would result. Unhappily a large proportion of health departments have yet to clarify their positions and roles, and confusion still exists. This has also been indicated in the report of the Joint Commission on Mental Illness and Health[25] not only with reference to public health but also in relation to most other types of agencies.

Aronson[26] proposes that the health of-ficer, in attempting to face the challenge of the mental health problem, should turn to well-established patterns used so successfully in the control of communicable disease. First, he looks for broad, well-documented epidemiologic patterns. Then, he searches for elements in existing programs that most nearly meet the needs of those patterns. Finally, he explores ways to use existing personnel in the new areas of activity. He emphasizes the opportunity for the health officer "to act as a catalyst—to be the voice of the community, in calling for the coordination of the variety of services and efforts being made by a number of agencies, in pointing out imbalance and gaps in available services, and in securing the widest community support for a broad spectrum of mental health services consistent with recognized scientific evidence and readily available to all who need them."

Others[27,28] have suggested health department activities to orient and train its own staff and personnel of other community agencies in mental health and illness, to provide diagnostic and referral services, as well as community follow-up after discharge of patients from psychiatric hospitals, to operate community mental health clinics and day-care centers for mentally retarded children, to cooperate with industrial mental health programs, and to educate the public in mental health. In addition, attention is directed to the important psychologic and psychiatric implications of children institutionalized for any reason: geriatric problems, alcoholism, suicide, marital and other family discord, crime and delinquency, and accident proneness. Some of these are discussed elsewhere in this book. For an overview of these and other potential roles for the public health agency in mental health, the reader is referred to a useful handbook developed by the American Public Health Association.[29]

THE FUTURE OF COMMUNITY MENTAL HEALTH

With the ever increasing complexity of our society, the accelerating pace of living and the concentrations of people, it would appear that mental and emotional problems would tend to increase in the years ahead. Offsetting this to a significant extent is the increase in understanding of human behavior and the continuing advances in psychopharmacology. For the immediate future certainly more community based facilities are needed. Felix[30] envisions them as multiservice centers designed to provide preventive services, early diagnosis, and treatment of mental illness on both an inpatient and outpatient basis, and to serve as a locus for the aftercare of discharged hospital patients. He itemizes the spectrum of services to include:

A general diagnostic and evaluation service (precare)
An acute inpatient service and an outpatient service
A day-care service and a night-care service
An emergency service available around the clock
Rehabilitation services
Consultation services
Public information and education services
Supervision of foster homes
Research and training

By means of these, true continuity of mental and emotional care would become possible to the enormous advantage of the patient and of the community of which he is a member.

REFERENCES

1. Sanders, D. S.: A bookshelf on mental health, Amer. J. Public Health 55:502, Apr. 1965.
2. Porterfield, J. D.: Mental health in the environment of the metropolitan area of the future, Amer. J. Public Health 48:489, Apr. 1958.
3. Beers, C. W.: A mind that found itself, New York, 1948, Doubleday & Co., Inc.
4. The national mental health program and the states, Washington, 1959, Public Health Service Pub. No. 629.
5. Jensen, H. E.: Mental health: a local public health responsibility, Ment. Hyg. 37:530, Oct. 1953.
6. Lapouse, R.: Problems in studying the prevalence of psychiatric disorder, Amer. J. Public Health 57:947, June 1967.
7. St. J. Perrott, G., et al.: Care of the long term patient, Washington, 1954, Public Health Service Pub. No. 344.
8. Kramer, M.: A discussion of the concepts of incidence and prevalence as related to epidemiological studies of mental disorders, Amer. J. Public Health 47:826, July 1957.
9. Halpert, H. P.: Surveys of public opinions and attitudes about mental illness, Public Health Rep. 80:589, July 1965.
10. King, S. H.: Perceptions of illness and medical practice, New York, 1962, Russell Sage Foundation.
11. Drugs for the troubled mind, Med. World News Mar. 13, 1964.
12. Kline, N. S., Kris, E. B., Ayd, F. J., and Cameron, W. R.: Symposium on psychopharmacology and community mental health services, Amer. J. Public Health 52: (supp.), Sept. 1962.
13. National Committee Against Mental Illness: What are the facts about mental illness in the United States? Washington, 1957.
14. Reed, L. S.: Health insurance coverage for mental illness, Public Health Rep. 73:185, Feb. 1958.
15. Editorial: Insurance coverage for psychiatric care, Public Health Rep. 80:1118, Dec. 1965.
16. Bullis, H. E.: A positive mental health program, Amer. J. Public Health 40:1113, Sept. 1950.
17. Lemkau, P. V.: Public health administration in mental hygiene, Amer. J. Public Health 41:1382, Nov. 1951.
18. Mountin, J. W. and Flook, E.: Guide to health organization in the United States, Washington, 1953, Public Health Service Pub. No. 196.
19. Felix, R. H.: The national mental health program, Amer. J. Public Health 54:1804, Nov. 1964.
20. Felix, R. H. and Kramer, M.: Research in epidemiology of mental illness, Public Health Rep. 67:160, Feb. 1952.
21. America's health—a report to the nation by the National Health Assembly, New York, 1948, Harper and Bros.
22. Blain, D. and Robinson, R. L.: Personnel shortages in psychiatric services, a shift of emphasis, New York J. Med. 57:257, Jan. 15, 1957.
23. Coleman, J.: Relations between mental health and public health, Amer. J. Public Health 46:805, July 1956.
24. Ginsberg, E. L.: Public health is people, New York, 1950, Commonwealth Fund.
25. Action for mental health, Report of Joint Committee on Mental Illness and Health, New York, 1961, Basic Books, Inc.
26. Aronson, J. B.: Mental health and the local health department, Amer. J. Public Health 51:89, Jan. 1961.
27. Norton, J. W. R., Applewhite, C. C., and Howell, R. W.: Efforts to define and help the health officer to fulfill his role in mental health programs, Amer. J. Public Health 47:812, July 1957.
28. Sparer, P. J.: Mental hygiene in a modern health department program, Amer. J. Public Health 51:892, June 1961.
29. American Public Health Association: Mental disorders: a guide to control methods, New York, 1962, The Association.
30. Felix, R. H.: A model for comprehensive mental health centers, Amer. J. Public Health 54:1964, Dec. 1964.

Chapter 23

Suicide

INTRODUCTION

One of the best-known statements in English literature is the famous soliloquy of Hamlet, in which he muses:

> To be, or not to be,—that is the question:—
> Whether 'tis nobler in the mind to suffer
> The slings and arrows of outrageous fortune,
> Or to take arms against a sea of troubles,
> And by opposing end them?

This is a question that a surprising number of people ask themselves at one time or another, and a distressingly large number act upon it in the form of self-destruction. Regretfully suicide is one of the concealed, untalked about, major causes of disability and death. According to an official report, about 22,000 people die each year in the United States by their own hands.[1] This is greater than the combined annual loss of life from tuberculosis, syphilis, meningitis, poliomyelitis, influenza, and bronchitis. It is almost three times as great as the loss from homicide and half as many as deaths from traffic accidents. However, great as this may seem, suicidal deaths are considered to be grossly underreported; the actual incidence is probably two or three times that which appears in official reports. Beyond this it is estimated that for every successful suicidal attempt, there are probably about 10 unsuccessful attempts. Reconsidering the official report, suicide is currently the tenth leading cause of death in the United States, and in several states its rank is as high as sixth. With respect to age, suicide mortality per 100,000 persons climbs consistently from 0.3 among those 5 to 14 years of age up to more than 24 per 100,000 persons over 75 years of age. Most tragically it is the third leading cause

of death among the young,[2] among college students,[3] and among members of the peacetime armed forces. But Shneidman[4] emphatically states, "Suicide is the *first* leading cause of *unnecessary* and *stigmatizing* deaths."

EPIDEMIOLOGY OF SUICIDE

Much is known about the epidemiology of suicide. It occurs three times as frequently among males as among females, but more women appear to attempt suicide than do men. It is four times as common among members of the white race as among Negroes, although more Negroes appear to attempt suicide than do white persons. It should be noted, however, that suicide rates among Negroes have begun to move upward in recent years. It is much more common among the wealthy and educated than among the poor and uneducated. With reference to occupation, laborers, miners, teachers, and clergymen have low rates, whereas mortality from suicide is high among entertainers, artists, businessmen, and especially professional persons. Among the professions, those in the field of medicine, particularly psychiatrists and psychoanalysts, have the highest rate. Indeed, the annual suicide rate among physicians in America is at least 33 per 100,000, three times that of the population as a whole, whereas for psychiatrists and psychoanalysts the rate is an astounding 70 per 100,000 per year. Great variations may be observed with reference to marital status. Thus between the ages of 35 and 44 years married men have a suicide rate of 16.7, single men 29.8, widowers 81.7, and divorced men 112.6.[5] As might be expected, the tendency to destroy oneself is more common during periods of economic depression. It is interesting, however, that rates drop sharply when a nation is confronted with a military emergency. Many aspects of the environment appear to influence suicidal tendencies. Beginning with geography, the further west one goes in the United States, the higher become the rates. Contrary to what many would expect, the phenomenon is more common in the United States during the months of May and June and on clear sunny days. A similar contradiction is its more frequent occurrence early in the week, on a Monday or Tuesday morning soon after arising, rather than at the end of a possibly long and arduous week. Suicide rates are higher in central cities than in suburbs, which in turn are more threatened than rural areas or small towns, where it is less difficult to be unknown. It is more common among immigrants than among the native born. Religion plays an important role; rates are highest among those who follow Oriental religions, next highest among Protestants and Reformed Jews, low among Roman Catholics, and very low among Orthodox Jews.

INCIDENCE

Among the nations, the United States, with a current rate of 11.1, is by no means the worst. Hungary ranks first with a rate of 26.8. Austria's suicide rate is 22; Germany, 20; Denmark, 19; Sweden, 18.5; Japan, 16; and Great Britain, 12. Ireland, Norway, Spain, Canada, Italy, Holland, and the Latin American countries enjoy consistently low suicide rates.[6] A common error is to relate the welfare systems of the Scandinavian countries with high suicide rates. This is contradicted by the very low rate of 7.9 in Norway, which has the same social welfare program as its Scandinavian neighbors.

METHODS

A wide variety of methods are used by individuals intent upon terminating their existence. An analysis[7] of the methods used by over 20,000 Americans who committed suicide in 1964 is as follows:

Firearms and explosives	47.2%
Hanging and strangulation	14.7%
Analgesics and soporifics	12.4%
Gases	11.5%
Other solid and liquid substances	3.6%
Jumping from high places	3.6%
Submersion (drowning)	2.6%
Piercing instruments	1.8%
Other and unspecified means	2.6%
Total	100.0%

It is interesting that women tend to use nonviolent methods, apparently maintaining some concern about their appearance even unto death.

REPORTING OF SUICIDES

There has been much conjecture as to the reasons for underreporting of suicides and for the general neglect of the subject by scientists and health workers. Without question, many suicides are undetected because the mode of death is not clear from a diagnostic standpoint; thus, was a poison taken by accident or by intent, or was it administered by a second party with homicidal tendencies? By like token a certain number of so-called automobile accidents are actually conscious or subconscious suicides, and some are undoubtedly homicides. Physicians and officials in charge of vital records are understandably hesitant in many instances to call a death a suicide. Furthermore, if they know the patient and his family, they are even more apt to be conservative in their final judgment. This relates in turn to the social stigma placed upon the suicide victim and the members of his family. In this regard, it is interesting that Plutarch wrote of an epidemic of suicides among women in Milesia, who for certain reasons preferred death to matrimony. The epidemic was brought to a stop by a decree that the bodies of those who committed suicide would be displayed naked in the public marketplace. Similarly, in the last century, when there was a rise in suicide in Southern Europe, the rate was cut in half within 1 year by a decree of the Catholic Church that denied the burial of suicides in consecrated ground. Felix[7] places importance upon our Judeo-Christian traditions which teach that life is sacred and can be taken only by a power greater than man himself. According to this viewpoint, since man did not will his beginning, he cannot will his end. Another problem is that in a great many cases the determination of the circumstances of death depends upon careful questioning of friends and relatives of the victim who are usually subject to considerable grief. This often causes the physician or research scientist to avoid inquiries. The fact that some life insurance policies refuse payment in the case of suicide certainly must cause many persons intent upon that act to plan a method difficult of detection; this is also another reason for relatives or friendly physicians to mask the diagnosis.

SUICIDE AND THE PRIVATE PHYSICIAN

Despite the foregoing, there has been a marked tendency even among members of the medical and health professions to regard suicide fatalistically, either as if it was none of their concern or as if nothing could be done about it. By now the relatively few efforts that have been made to attack the problem provide sufficient evidence that much of the suicide problem can be prevented. A number of facts are now known to justify some measure of optimism. Among them are the following: potential suicides do not act impulsively; the majority of them talk about it or give other clues to their thoughts or intentions frequently for a long period of time.[8] Thus in a very detailed study of a significant number of successful suicides Robins and co-workers[9] observe, "One of the most striking findings of this study was the high frequency with which these persons communicated their suicidal ideas, by specific statements of intent to commit suicide, by statements concerning their preoccupation with death and the desire to die, and by making unsuccessful suicide attempts. The statements were made to family, friends, job associates, and many others." In a similar vein Kobler and Stotland[10] view ". . . verbal and other communications of suicidal attempts, as efforts, however misdirected, to solve problems of living, as frantic pleas for help and hope from other people; help in solving the problem and hope that they

can be solved. Whether the individual then actually commits suicide seems to depend to a large part on the nature of the responses by other people to his pleas." Havens[11] also considers suicidal efforts to spring from despair and helplessness. Illustrations of the extent to which these cries for help offer a challenge to the medical profession are frequent.[12] In one study in New Hampshire nearly 50% of individuals who committed suicide consulted a physician a short while before for a wide range of illnesses considered as masks for underlying depressions or anxieties. In a San Francisco study one out of every six suicide victims was known to have seen a physician during the preceding week, and more than two out of five within the preceding 6 months. Shneidman and Dizmang[13] of the Center For Studies of Suicide Prevention of the National Institute of Mental Health insist, "A well-trained and skillful physician should be as able to identify a potentially suicidal patient on a routine examination as he can detect an early heart murmur or slightly enlarged spleen." Similarly they indicate that a past suicidal attempt or history of suicide in a family "must be looked at just as carefully as a history of familial diabetes or previous history of glucose in the urine." In other words, failure by physicians to prevent suicide is due not so much to ignorance of the causes as to failure to recognize the signs and symptoms of impending suicide among those in their practices.

CAUSES OF SUICIDE

What then are the causes of suicide? The actual phenomenon appears to result from the interplay between (1) factors inherent in the patient and (2) factors in the environment. Of the two, the first is without question the most critical. Careful studies have shown that the most significant characteristic of those who attempt suicide is that they are in a state of frank psychosis. For example, Robins and co-workers[9] observe that 98% of the suicides they studied had been clinically ill and 94% of them psychiatrically ill. Of the group, 68% had been suffering from one of two diseases:

manic-depressive depression or chronic alcoholism. None of the individuals in the study had an uncomplicated neurosis (anxiety reaction, conversion reaction, or obsessive compulsive reaction). It is of interest that 73% of the manic-depressives and 40% of the alcoholics had been under medical or psychiatric care for illnesses associated with their suicide during the year preceding their death. Approaching this question from a different direction, as evidence of the significance of mental aberration among would-be suicides are the following observations: Suicide is the most common cause of death among those known to be mentally ill. The method chosen for the actual suicide is very often irrational; individuals have been observed to hang themselves out of a high window instead of jumping. Related to this is the tendency to irrational response. Thus, although the suicidal person cannot be handled adequately by reasoning or logic, he may be influenced often by suggestion: "Come in from that window ledge or I'll close the window!" or "Come aboard this boat or you'll catch a cold!" Another significant observation is that rarely is insufferable pain a factor in suicides. Much more often it is an obsessive hypochondriac concentration on a trivial ailment that of course is not the fundamental cause of the problem. Not infrequently the depression that precedes an actual suicide is out of proportion to the cause of the depression.

DIAGNOSIS OF IMPENDING SUICIDE

In most instances the presuicidal state is temporary. If the condition is recognized and the patient is protected from himself through this critical period, he stands a good chance of being saved. This also provides time for appropriate treatment.

How may the potential suicide be diagnosed? Shneidman[14] states that the suicide syndrome is a constellation of symptoms and lists these under the headings of depressed, disoriented, defiant, and dependent-dissatisfied. The preceding discussion gives some indication of the types of signs and symptoms that should be watched for. As for the type of person to watch, the potentiality of suicide should be kept in mind with reference to (1) all depressed persons, (2) all manic-depressive patients (3) especially all those who have previously attempted suicide—no matter how long ago, (4) those who often speak of suicide with apparent seriousness, and (5) those who have suddenly lost interest in previously important and valued things and events.

A question commonly asked is, "What about those who *think* of suicide?" This in itself would not appear to be dangerous. A number of studies indicate that suicide is considered by the majority of individuals at one time or another. Fortunately, however, only a minor proportion of them act upon the idea and, as indicated previously, because of deep inherent psychologic problems. A number of warning signals are worthy of attention. Among these are evidence of depression, especially with manifestations of guilt, tension, or agitation; insomnia, especially if great concern is expressed about it; severe hypochondriasis; expressions of fear of losing self-control; frequent discussion about and apparent preoccupation with the idea of suicide or death; and, of course, previous attempts. The depths of depression may be judged by an otherwise inexplicable loss of weight, appetite, and sexual desire; a slowing and blurring of speech and action; an unusual hesitancy or unwillingness to meet people; an attitude of hopelessness, often indicated by a drawn and wrinkled facial expression and dullness of the eyes; chronic low back pain that does not respond to appropriate medical treatment; chronic recurring headaches with elusive etiology; vague and frequent gastrointestinal complaints; and interestingly, as Ross[15] has observed, not only peculiar vague sensations and a bad taste in the mouth but actual dental pain and discomfort. Ross gives a good general word picture of such people: "One's first observation may be of a pale faced sallow person sitting huddled in a waiting room chair evidencing little or no spontaneous activity. Further inspection may reveal evidence of weight and sleep loss, perhaps accentuated facial wrinkles and eyelid folds, and lacklustre hair. There may be careless or unkempt grooming." He also calls attention to the manner in which such individuals present complaints to physicians or others. For example, the highly anxious patient may tell his story rapidly and without interruption or be preoccupied with minutiae. "Immobility of facial expression and body," he says, "can communicate underlined discouragement," and notes that "it is remarkable how often the patient presents the notion that things are different for him: his world, his life, his bodily function, his outlook and his habits."

HANDLING OF THE IMPENDING SUICIDE

The question arises, how best to deal with the individual with apparent or frank suicidal intent? First of all, he should be encouraged by "gatekeepers" (spouse, friends, neighbors, clergyman, policeman, bartenders, employer, etc.) to be examined by a physician. The physician in turn should give the patient an opportunity to talk out his troubles and problems, big or small, real or imagined, in his own way. A complete medical examination should, of course, be done since it has been found that a large number of would-be suicides have physical as well as mental complaints and that these are not infrequently interrelated. This also provides the patient and the physician with a specific physical focus of attention and goal. Those who are mildly troubled should be given helpful suggestions. Single and lonely persons should be encouraged to participate in group and religious activities. On the other hand, agitated and depressed patients and those who have previously attempted suicide should be referred promptly to a psychiatrist rather than rely, as so often is the case, on the police or prison or on the county or municipal general hospitals.[16] To the contrary, it is the consensus that such individuals should be immediately referred by physicians for hospitalization in a closed psychiatric ward.[9] This provides the best opportunity for further clinical and psychiatric study, psychotherapy, and whatever drugs or shock therapy might be indicated. After the acute episode is past and the patient is considered eligible for discharge from the psychiatric institution, careful provision should be made for follow-up back into the community. Unfortunately this is the weakest link in the chain and points to the great need for more, competently staffed community mental health facilities.[17]

SUICIDE PREVENTION PROGRAMS

A cursory review of the literature during recent years indicates a growing interest in the subject of suicide and its prevention. This bears out the point by Dublin[18] that while we by no means have all of the necessary answers, the possibility of developing effective programs has been well demonstrated in many countries already and that suicide as a problem lends itself to intelligent public health control efforts. Outstanding in the United States are the experiences of the Suicide Prevention Center in Los Angeles, of Rescue Inc. in Boston, and of the Friends in Miami. Dr. Dublin points also to the work of the Samaritans in England and similarly successful activities in Vienna, Berlin, and Milan. In an address to state and territorial mental health authorities at the end of 1966 Shneidman[19] predicted, "Now at the end of 1966, we stand on the threshold of an efflorescence and burgeoning of suicide prevention activities." He illustrated this by the fact that, whereas in 1958 only two states had programs, by the time of his address 15 states were included. Within the half year following his statement 4 more states were added, but, as he indicated, the total number should be 50. Similar growth has been occurring on the local level, and by now there are approximately 40 suicide prevention centers in cities throughout the nation. Obviously several hundreds are needed.[20] These centers are conducted by a variety of agencies, including hospitals and medical centers, mental health facilities, various official and voluntary social service agencies and religious organizations, as well as some health departments. There are many sources of input for a suicide prevention program. Earlier the term "gatekeeper" was used to describe the wide variety of types of individuals who are in a position to observe and to be alert to the potential suicide and who might refer him to adequate sources of assistance. In addition, there might be listed the major roles possible by private physicians, outpatient clinics and hospitals, mental health programs, poison control centers, accident prevention programs, agencies which deal with juvenile delinquency, alcoholism and narcotic addiction programs, and many other agencies and groups in the community. Generally speaking, on the basis of preventive philosophy, if suicide is essentially a psychiatric problem, it necessarily follows that the earlier the age at which emotional or mental problems might be identified the closer one comes to the inception of the motivating factors for suicide. Because of this, particular emphasis should be placed upon the young person.

On the basis of their various studies of suicide, and in line with what has been presented here, Tuckman and co-workers[21,22] suggest the following as the basis for a community suicide prevention program:

1. Evaluation and referral services for persons showing suicidal thinking and behavior
2. Consultation services for physicians, social agencies, and the community at large with respect to potential suicides
3. Community education, including the preparation of suitable educational materials with emphasis on diagnosis, prevention, and treatment, and the introduction of material on suicide in the medical school curriculum
4. Development of follow-up procedures for attempted suicides with special emphasis on children and young adults
5. Casefinding to obtain a more accurate estimate of suicidal behavior in the community as well as to gather systematically life experience, personality structure, and environmental stresses

To these should be added the need for a type of 24-hour service to which the individual under stress could resort. This is perhaps best illustrated by the Nightwatch part of the Los Angeles program. Callers receive immediate sympathetic consideration with evaluation of the emergency, appropriate counseling, and referral. If indicated, appropriate individuals and teams may be sent to the caller on an emergency

basis. Response to this service has been great, and its success and usefulness have been obvious.[23]

The national center for studies of suicide prevention

An event of great significance in the movement to understand and do more about the problem of suicide was the establishment in 1966 of the Center for Studies of Suicide Prevention in the National Institute of Mental Health. Shneidman,[4] who organized it, considers it to have five basic functions:

1. To serve as the focal point within the Institute to coordinate and direct activities throughout the nation in support of research, pilot studies, training, information, and consultation aimed at furthering basic knowledge about suicide, and improving techniques for helping the suicidal individual
2. To compile and disseminate information and training material designed to assist mental health personnel, clergy, police, educators, and others in obtaining a better understanding of suicidal actions and learning to utilize research findings
3. To assist in developing and experimenting with the variety of regional and local programs and organizational models to coordinate emergency services and techniques of prevention, case finding, treatment, training and research
4. To maintain liaison with studies and programs on suicide prevention undertaken by other agencies, both national and international
5. To promote and maintain the application of research findings by state and local mental health agencies

More specifically, Shneidman lists 10 aspects of a comprehensive national suicide-prevention program to include the following:

1. A program of support of suicide-prevention activities in many communities throughout the nation
2. A special program for the "gatekeepers" of suicide prevention
3. A carefully prepared program in massive public education
4. A special program for followup of suicide attempts
5. An active NIMH program of research and training grants
6. A redefinition and refinement of statistics on suicide
7. The development of a cadre of trained, dedicated professionals

8. Governmentwide liaison and national use of a broad spectrum of professional personnel
9. A special followup program for the survivor-victims of individuals who have committed suicide
10. A rigorous program for the evaluation of the effectiveness of suicide-prevention activities

This 10-point program for suicide prevention is indicated as a mutual enterprise that to be successful will require the active interest, support, and activities of many groups, individuals, and professions in communities throughout the country. Particularly important to this is the development of a group of individuals whom Shneidman has labeled as "suicidologists," who will focus upon the problem as their chief interest. In this regard it is significant that in 1967 the first students of this new profession began a year's fellowship study at the Henry Phipps Psychiatric Clinic of Johns Hopkins University under a grant from the National Institute of Mental Health. Fellowships are offered to qualified members of a variety of disciplines including psychiatry, psychology, social work, anthropology, sociology, public health education and psychiatric nursing. Also in mid-1967 the Center for Studies of Suicide Prevention inaugurated its *Bulletin of Suicidology,* to which reference has previously been made.

In view of the accelerating interest in the subject of suicide and the recent actions that have been taken there is now good reason to anticipate that at last a forthright and intelligent attack will be launched against this major cause of disability and death.

REFERENCES

1. Monthly vital statistics report, April 14, 1967, National Center for Vital Statistics, U. S. Public Health Service.
2. Faigel, H. C.: Suicide among young persons, Clin. Pediat. 5:187, Jan. 1966.
3. Parrish, H. M.: Causes of death among college students, Public Health Rep. 71:1081, Nov. 1956.
4. Shneidman, E. S.: The N.I.M.H. Center for studies of suicide prevention, Bull. Suicidol., Public Health Service 1:2, July 1967.
5. Paffenbarger, R. S., and Asnes, D. P.: Precursors of suicide in early and middle life, Amer. J. Public Health 56:1026, July 1966.
6. International rise in suicide, Stat. Bull., Metro. Life Ins. Co. 48:4, Mar. 1967.
7. Felix, R. H.: Suicide: A neglected problem, Amer. J. Public Health 55:16, Jan. 1965.
8. Bell, J. N.: Lifeline for would-be suicides, Today's Health 45:31, June 1967.
9. Robins, E., Murphy, G. E., Wilkinson, R. H., Gassner, S., and Kayes, J.: Some clinical considerations in the prevention of suicide based on a study of 134 successful suicides, Amer. J. Public Health 49:888, July 1959.
10. Kobler, A. L., and Stotland, E.: The end of hope: A social-clinical study of suicide, Glencoe, Ill., 1964, The Free Press.
11. Havens, L. L.: Recognition of suicidal risks through the psychologic examination, New Eng. J. Med. 276(4):210, Jan. 26, 1967.
12. M.D.s held able to prevent suicides, Medical News, Jan. 2, 1967, p. 19.
13. Discussion on suicide, MD, 11:93, Sept. 1967.
14. Shneidman, E. S.: Preventing suicide, Amer. J. Nurs. 65:111, May 1965.
15. Ross, M.: Talk presented at meeting of Southern Medical Association, 1966.
16. Crocetti, G. M.: Suicide and public health—an attempt to reconceptualization, Amer. J. Public Health 49:881, 1959.
17. Oliven, J. F.: Suicide prevention as a public health problem, Amer. J. Public Health 44:1419, Nov. 1954.
18. Dublin, L. I.: Suicide: A public health problem, Amer. J. Public Health 55:12, Jan. 1965.
19. Shneidman, E. S.: State programs in suicide prevention. Address presented to the Surgeon General's Conference with State and Territorial Mental Health Authorities, Washington, Dec. 6, 1966.
20. Shneidman, E. S., and Farberow, N. L.: The Los Angeles Suicide Prevention Center: A demonstration of public health feasibilities, Amer. J. Public Health 55:21, Jan. 1965.
21. Tuckman, J., Youngman, W. F., and Bleiberg, B. M.: Attempted suicide by adults, Public Health Rep. 77:605, July 1962.
22. Tuckman, J., and Connon, H. E.: Attempted suicide in adolescents, Amer. J. Psychiat. 119:228, Sept. 1962.
23. Litman, R. E., Farberow, N. L., Shneidman, E. S., Heilig, S. M., and Kramer, J. A.: Suicide prevention telephone service, J.A.M.A. 192:107, Apr. 5, 1965.

Chapter 24

Addictive diseases

INTRODUCTION

In addition to the more evident communicable and organic disorders to which man is subject and which in many instances he may share with other creatures, there exists another group of conditions that are peculiarly his own invention. These are behavioral disorders that involve the unreasoned, compulsive consumption of certain chemical substances, some natural and some man-made, to his ultimate physical, psychic, and social detriment. It is interesting that all of these substances have numerous beneficial uses and effects when used properly and judiciously and usually adversely affect only a minor proportion of those who are exposed to their use. Most prominent among these agents is alcohol, a substance of ancient development and widespread consumption. Next in prominence and historic discovery are the narcotizing alkaloids. More recently have been added certain substances, which have been developed synthetically, usually for therapeutic purposes, such as the barbiturates and related drugs, amphetamine, and, to some extent, certain of the so-called tranquilizers, euphoriants, and ataraxics.[1] To these may also be added the psychedelic or psychotomimetic drugs, natural and synthesized, of which mescaline, psilocybin, and lysergic acid diethylamide (LSD-25) are the best known.

Alcohol and narcotics have played a fascinating role in the history of mankind. The production of alcoholic beverages appears to have been one of man's earliest discoveries. The use of alkaloid-bearing plants probably began soon afterward. Because of the physiologic effects they produced, they soon became important adjuncts to social intercourse, religion, and politics and have played an important part in the literature of all cultures. Through the ages there has been much speculation, especially about certain of the psychic effects they produce. They seemed to release the usually pent-up spirit from the tangible body and allow it to wander freely. Sometimes they seemed to bring about the phenomenon of second sight. Such mystical results, coupled with the unusual appearance and behavior of the person affected, inevitably lead to great wonder and awe, especially on the part of primitive peoples. From the beginning, therefore, although these substances appeared to be similar to other materials ingested as food and drink, they were nevertheless considered different and special. Indeed, in many instances they were treated as sacred, to be prepared only by certain persons and to be used only at certain times such as at festivities, religious events, or in instances of individual or group catastrophe.

Undoubtedly early in their use it was recognized that among those who used them were some who developed an uncontrollable necessity for continued use, regardless of the consequences. Thus the drunkard is mentioned in the Old Testament, and hashish was used in India and the Middle East to develop and control groups of assassins. Through time, society typically frowned upon these undesirable results of the abuse of these substances but was at a loss to understand them. Usually they were attributed to innate depravity, some hereditary weakness, or the loss of the soul. Such attitudes have continued down to the present time. Only recently have more enlightened attitudes developed, based upon clearer understanding of the function of the mind, its relationship to the body, and the effects of pressures of society.

ALCOHOLISM*

Alcohol is used in many different situations, i.e., in religious ceremonies, as a food, as a relaxant, as a customary base for many social affairs; by many different kinds of people, i.e., men and women, young and old, well-adjusted and emotionally disturbed; with many different results, i.e., an improved appetite, a warm glow of well-being and conviviality, a blackout, or personality deterioration. More often than not its use and its affects are regarded in terms of a gradient with all persons being distributed along a scale of consumption with a concurrent scale of response. Thus, ordinarily, the less the intake the less the response; the more the intake the greater the response, its consequences, and the probability of becoming an alcoholic. Unfortunately the situation is not as simple as this. There are some individuals who may actually consume, even on a relatively consistent basis, a considerable amount of alcohol yet never become alcoholics. Conversely, there are those whose intake may be significantly less or occasional, yet they may be obvious problem drinkers. The reason for drinking and for continuing to drink has much to do with the making of an alcoholic. Similarly the attitude toward other aspects of life and the world has much to do with deciding whether or not a person is an alcoholic. Still another deciding factor is the relative ease or difficulty of reduction or elimination of the consumption of alcohol.

Definition

The foregoing points up the factors that make alcoholism difficult to define. Nevertheless, the more the problem is studied, the more apparent it becomes that certain types of persons, especially under certain

*For an extensive review of the problem, see the *Annals of the American Academy of Political and Social Science,* vol. 315, Jan. 1958. The entire issue is devoted to the topic "Alcoholism in the United States."

circumstances, do tend to become alcoholics, whereas others do not. The alcoholic has been defined by some as an individual under emotional pressure who drinks to get away from the way he feels but eventually is drinking because of his drinking. This is a practical definition in that it stresses the initial psychosocial trigger followed by the eventual psychophysiologic entanglement.

From an epidemiologic viewpoint, alcoholism may be defined as an acquired chronic progressive disease of adult life involving the compulsive intake of excessive amounts of alcohol and leading in its more advanced stages to certain psychologic, social, and physical deteriorating sequelae. It affects predominantly males to the ratio of about 6 to 1, i.e., adults between 35 and 55 years of age in the most productive period of life to an extent of 85% of cases. This problem is particularly common in certain occupations, such as those involving non-routine, pressure, decision-making, and transiency, is significantly greater in urban areas, and is more frequently found in certain nationalities, especially Scandinavian, Nordic, Celtic, and Polish, in contrast to its infrequency among Italians, Greeks, and Jews.

Extent of problem

The determination of the true magnitude of the problem is also difficult because so many cases never come to definitive social or medical attention and because of the number of individuals at any time who are on the borderline between problem drinking and chronic alcoholism. The Yale Committee on the Study of Alcoholism[2] on the basis of surveys has estimated that there are about 70 million drinkers of alcoholic beverages in the United States. Of these, only an estimated 4.5 million are considered to be problem drinkers, 1 million of them chronic alcoholics. This is a prevalence, however, of 2.4% of the total population or almost 7% of those who drink. Furthermore, since 6 out of 7 are adult males, this means an estimated prevalence of problem drinking in the male population 20 years and over of about 7.5%! To complicate the picture further, this is not a disease primarily of the ignorant or of unskilled labor.

To the contrary, about 80% are regularly employed up to the point of disability and three quarters of them belong to the executive class in large and small businesses, professional men, salesmen, and skilled laborers.[3] The implications of this with regard to social, economic, and professional productivity and morale are obvious. The reality of the problem becomes evident from a number of industrial surveys, notably that of the Western Electric Corporation,[4] that have indicated that the average company can expect about 3% of all its employees to be alcoholics in need of special attention. Little wonder that alcoholism is now included among the seven categories of diseases that cause outstanding numbers of deaths and disabilities and that represent major unsolved public health problems. The others are cardiovascular disease, mental illness, crippling and handicapping conditions, cancer, dental disease, and diabetes. It should be noted incidentally that all of these, including alcoholism, are conditions about which something is known and about which something can be done.

Cost of alcoholism

In view of the foregoing, it is obvious that the cost of alcoholism to society must be very considerable. Many different factors contribute to the cost which is estimated to total about $1.5 billion per year in the United States alone. Absenteeism, high spoilage rates, decreased productivity while on the job due to lowered ability and apparently to avoidance of work situations involving hazard or that are apt to indicate the worker's condition, personnel turnover, and lowered morale of the alcoholic and those working with him account for some of these costs. Added to them is the expense to society of many facilities for grappling with various aspects of the problem, e.g., police, courts, jails, religious organizations, hospitals and medical care, various social and charitable agencies, departments of welfare, domestic relations organizations, visiting nurse agencies, and industrial personnel guidance offices. Less tangible is the ultimate cost of the frequently disastrous effects on other members of the family and circle of friends, e.g., on children at school and

on other adults at work in the home or at the alcoholic's place of employment. Still another social loss due to alcoholism is the amount of crime and prostitution which is related to it as either or both cause and effect. The amount is indeterminate but on the basis of observations by many would appear to be significant.

The relationship of accidents to alcoholism is interesting. Surveys carried out by the Yale University School of Alcohol Studies in 1943 indicated that the estimated 1,370,000 alcoholics employed in industry accounted for 1,500 fatal accidents at work and 2,850 fatal accidents at home, in public places, and in traffic, or a total of 4,350 fatalities.[6] Dr. E. M. Jellinek, the director of the school at that time, pointed out that this was a fatal accident rate of 321 per 100,000 men or more than twice that of nonalcoholic workers in the same occupations. Trice,[7] however, has warned against the common misinterpretation of this data as representing that alcoholics have twice as many work accidents than do others. In fact, he points to studies of his own which indicate surprisingly that as far as work-related accidents are concerned the reverse is true. On the basis of answers given by the subjects he hypothesized that the alcoholic while actually on the job tends to be overcautious, concentrates more upon what he is doing in a deliberate attempt to avoid accidents, is subject to fewer of other types of distractions, develops a well-planned work routine, is sometimes "covered up" by his fellow workers, and, if actually in an alcoholic or hangover state, tends to be absent rather than to risk discovery or a work accident. The only work relationships in which Trice found alcoholics to indulge their addiction and to have work-related accidents were (1) as participants in fellow-worker drinking groups after working hours and (2) on jobs that require geographic mobility, hence separation from protecting or inhibiting influences coupled with greater accessibility to alcohol.

Alcohol-related accidents away from work present a different picture from what happens in the nonmobile work situation. This is best illustrated by the relationship between automobile accidents and alcohol consumption, which has been the subject of many studies. Thus in a review of some such studies it was found that as little as 0.03% of alcohol in the blood reduced driving skill[8] and that the probability of accidents increased consistently with an increase of alcohol in the blood. The risk at 0.10% blood alcohol has been found to be twice that at 0.05%, whereas an increase of the blood level to 0.15% multiplied the risk tenfold.[9] With this in mind, the percentage of automotive accident fatalities with significant blood alcohol levels is illuminating. For instance, in Nassau County, New York, a series of 269 autopsies of driver fatalities showed 52% with blood alcohol levels over 0.10%. Similar recent studies in many places have shown that about 50% of automobile-related fatalities involved significant blood alcohol levels in either or both drivers and pedestrians, if the latter were involved.

It is somewhat more difficult to relate alcohol with home accident fatalities. However, recalling Jellinek's findings that the total fatal accident rate in alcoholic workers was twice that of nondrinkers, coupled with Trice's findings that this was not caused by on-the-job accidents, and recognizing further that in the United States home accidents are about twice as frequent as work accidents and at least four times as frequent as vehicular accidents,[10] it would seem reasonably certain that a close relationship exists between drinking and the probability of home accidents. To paraphrase the slogan "If you drink, don't drive," one might say, "If you drink, don't climb a ladder."

Effects of alcohol

The Alcoholism Subcommittee of the Expert Committee on Mental Health of the World Health Organization has concluded that, although alcohol must be regarded as a drug, it can be classified neither as an addiction-producing drug nor as a habit-forming drug, but that it must be placed in a category of its own, intermediate between these two groups.[11] After ingestion, alcohol is rapidly absorbed directly from the stomach and upper intestine into the blood stream. It is detectable in the blood within five minutes after ingestion and by this medium is distributed throughout the body. The average adult body can oxidize about 10 ml. of alcohol per hour, releasing energy and carbon dioxide and water. Any that is not oxidized is excreted in the urine and through the lungs. Thus, ingestion of excessive amounts gives rise to a build-up in the blood stream and in the tissues, awaiting either oxidation or excretion. Blood concentrations of 0.2% usually result in mild to moderate intoxication, whereas more than 0.3% causes marked effects. Blood concentrations between 0.5% and 0.8% result in death. Repeated and extensive use of alcohol tends to result in increased tolerance.

Alcohol affects all parts of the body, especially the central nervous tissue. Contrary to common belief, it acts not as a stimulant but as a depressant. In so doing it inhibits the controls of behavior in the cerebral cortex. The pulse increases and vasodilation occurs, especially in the skin, and results in decreased body temperature due to heat loss. Because of this, again contrary to common thought, the use of alcohol to warm the body is not physiologically sound. Vision and sense of balance are impaired relatively early. In more advanced states of intoxication the centers in the brain that regulate breathing, cardiac function, and body heat are depressed. As with so many things, the moderate consumption of alcohol actually appears to have little or no effect on longevity. There is good evidence, however, that heavy drinking does shorten life in various ways.

Much of the ill effect of excessive consumption of alcohol is due to malnutrition. The alcoholic typically eats inadequately because of the dulling of the appetite, general disinterest in food, and because calories for energy are obtained from alcohol. Since the latter are so readily available, what food is eaten often is stored unused in the body. Hence many alcoholics, especially in the earlier stages, may become overweight. Most important among the nutritional deficiencies that occur are those involving vitamin B complex. This may result in polyneuritis, so-called beer heart, with cardiac weakening and enlargement with attending edema, pellagra, and the typical skin and ocular manifestations of riboflavin deficiency. Fatty degeneration of the liver may result, probably from a combination of vitamin B deficiency and direct toxic effects of alcohol upon the liver cells. Because of lowered mineral intake, anemia is frequent. Among the more dramatic effects are those relating to the psyche such as delirium tremens, Korsakoff's psychosis, and personality changes due to alcoholic degeneration of cortical tissue. In connection with the latter the advanced alcoholic tends to become socially unstable, careless about his appearance or actions, suspicious, irritable, belligerent and quick to take offense, crafty, over-emotional, and frequently brutal and callous toward those around him, especially those he may love. Much of the latter, of course, is attributable to the very marked guilt complex which is typically developed.

Types of alcoholics

It is important to consider first of all how alcoholics differ from the much larger number of persons who drink but are not alcoholics. As Bacon[12] has indicated, there are many reasons for drinking, such as to fulfill a religious ritual, to be polite, to have a good time, to make friends, to experiment, to show off, to get warm or cool, to quench thirst, to go on a spree, or to flavor food. He states, however:

> None of these is the purpose of the alcoholic, although he might claim any or all to satisfy some questioner. The alcoholic drinks because he has to if he is to go on living. He drinks compulsively; that is, a power greater than rational planning brings him to drinking and to excessive drinking. . . . Most alcoholics hate liquor, hate drinking, hate the taste, hate the results, hate themselves for succumbing, but they can't stop. Their drinking is as compulsive as the stealing by a kleptomaniac or the continued hand washing of a person with a neurosis about cleanliness. . . . It is useful to think of their drinking behavior as a symptom of some inner maladjustment which they do not understand and cannot control. The drinking may be the outward, obvious accompaniment of this more basic hidden factor.

As many psychiatrists have pointed out, if the alcoholic did not drink, unadjusted he would consciously or subconsciously seek some other outlet for his unresolved conflicts and tensions. In addition, there is some evidence that certain physical causes for alcoholism exist. Some feel that the problem drinker may have some abnormal psychologic and physiologic reaction to alcohol that others do not have.[13]

The frank alcoholic is intensely introspective and is disinterested in anything except himself and his problem. He has few if any diversional interests, such as hobbies, entertainment, or social activities. A very large proportion are socially unattached to family or social group. This introspection and social isolation presents a particular difficulty to persons, programs, or agencies that may try to relate meaningfully to them in order to assist them. Sometimes part of the difficulty derives from the sense of failure and guilt which the alcoholic commonly feels and which may even result in a willful rejection of attempts to help. Alcoholics may reject help on the basis that they deserve to be miserable because of their real or imagined failings and because of the compulsive drinking pattern itself, which they developed in relation to their conflicts and failings.

Generally speaking, there are two main types of problem drinkers: The first or primary type is the individual who was maladjusted to begin with, that is, before he embarked upon compulsive drinking. He was what is commonly referred to as neurotic, that is, subject to a sense of constitutional psychoneurotic inferiority. Usually his personality was developed improperly from early childhood with gradual realization of vague and constant feelings of anxiety, apprehension, inadequacy, or inferiority. Often he feels he is defeated before he begins and that he will be unsuccessful in school, in courtship, in work, and in society. He fears such situations and, if at all possible, wants to avoid them. Occasionally such a person finds that indulgence in alcohol brings a sense of release and gives some degree of confidence and apparent success. Perhaps more than anything it makes it possible to forget temporarily his own feeling of inadequacy and dissatisfaction with himself. What is more logical than to repeat the experience? The problem is compounded, however, when the effects of alcohol wear off. There are unpleasant memories or, worse, uncertainties about behavior while under the influence of alcohol, providing additional feelings of anxiety and guilt. This leads to the additional use of alcohol, often the morning after, to overcome the postalcoholic sense of guilt, and a vicious circle is established.

The second type of compulsive drinker begins as an apparently well-adjusted person. He is not neurotic; his personality has not been improperly developed; and in fact he appears to get along well in his family, in his work, and with the group. If anything, he may tend to be an extrovert. He becomes involved in situations and with groups, in connection with either or both his social or his work life, which lead to considerable drinking. He participates with enthusiasm, but is not yet an alcoholic. He is in fact indulging himself without any particular feeling of compulsion. However, the continued use of more alcohol gradually lowers his senses of discrimination and responsibility. He becomes less efficient, careless, and begins to put things off or to let things slide in order to meet the preferred social demands. Almost imperceptibly at first his relationships and behavior at home, on the job, and in society begin to deteriorate. This becomes noticeable to those around him, he becomes aware of it and because of fear or worry drinks more. Meanwhile, his family, friends, and employer, usually indulgent or tolerant at first, become impatient. There occurs a mutual loss of regard and blunt words are exchanged. Because of arguments at home or perhaps a demotion or loss of a job, he begins to feel that everyone is down on him, and with increasing self-pity blames it all on the misunderstanding and intolerance of others or on just plain bad luck. The only thing that provides escape or supports the ego is the very thing which began the process—alcohol. Hence again a vicious circle is begun. As time goes by and the situation becomes worse, he appears on the surface more and more like the primary type of alcoholic. However,

because his alcoholism is not superimposed upon a basic inferiority, his chances of recovery and rehabilitation are decidedly better. Fortunately from society's viewpoint the larger proportion of alcoholics appear to fall into this category.

What can be done

Until recently and even now in far too many places the approach to the alcoholic was to tolerate him if possible; "dry him out" periodically either in jail, a public hospital, or a private sanatorium; or, if he were beyond recovery, to provide him with some type of refuge in skid row or elsewhere in which he could subsist on handouts from friends, strangers, missions, or other charitable organizations during the intervals between employment at usually undesirable types of work. With the relatively recent acceptance of the condition as a disease and on the basis of an increasing amount of social, medical, and psychiatric study and research, a growing number of programs are being established with increasingly fruitful results. Much is still on the basis of trial and demonstration.

It is interesting that the real impetus arose from within the group affected. This took the form of the organization in 1935 of Alcoholics Anonymous. It considers itself "a fellowship of men and women who share their experience, strength, and hope with each other that they may solve their common problem and help others to recover from alcoholism." It states, "The only requirement for membership is an honest desire to stop drinking"; that it is "not allied with any sect, denomination, politics, organization, or institution; does not wish to engage in any controversy, neither endorses nor opposes any causes." The primary purpose of its members "is to stay sober and to help other alcoholics to achieve sobriety."* Since its foundation, A.A. has helped more than 350,000 men and women in the United States, Canada, and many other countries. These people constitute the core of the membership and

---

*For various publications, contact Alcoholics Anonymous, P. O. Box 459, Grand Central Annex, New York, N. Y. 10017.

the nucleus to which others in need of help may relate. There are now about 12,500 groups throughout the world: 7,821 in the U. S., 1,241 in Canada, 2,136 outside of Canada and the U. S., 569 in hospitals, and 677 in prisons.[14] The organization operates on a few simple but sound and effective premises. Participation must be voluntary —there can be no checking up or compulsion. An alcoholic can never indulge in controlled drinking; either his drinking will become progressively worse or he must abstain completely from alcohol and develop a new pattern of constructive living. Belief and faith in God is a fundamental source of strength in the attempt toward recovery. A recovered alcoholic can best understand the problems and motivations of the alcoholic and is therefore in the best position to be of assistance. Group meetings for group therapy and open discussion of problems are valuable in obtaining an understanding of the underlying causes of one's alcoholism. Individual anonymous assistance in the form of moral support is instantly available by visit or phone at all times. The process of trying to help other alcoholics in itself is an important aid to staying sober oneself. Members do not swear off alcohol for life or for any other period in the future, they merely concentrate on the 24 hours of today. Contributions toward recovery and rehabilitation by other groups, such as the medical profession and social agencies, are recognized, and members are referred freely as indicated.

Meanwhile over a number of years an ever increasing amount of knowledge about the psychologic and physiologic causes and effects of alcoholism has been accumulated. One result is the development in effect of three schools of thought with regard to explaining and handling the problem; the social, the psychiatric, and the medical or physiologic. More and more it is recognized that the three are not conflicting but, to the contrary, they are complementary— each approach contributes to the overall solution of the problem. It was not until very recently that attempts were made to apply knowledge as it became available.

In 1944 the Laboratory of Applied Physiology at Yale University established two public clinics in Connecticut, one at New Haven, the other at Hartford, to attract and guide alcoholics and to bring to bear the various resources and approaches to their treatment. Shortly afterward the Yale Summer School of Alcohol Studies for training workers in the field was begun. Subsequently a similar school was begun at Rutgers University. A journal, *The Quarterly Journal of Studies on Alcohol,* devoted exclusively to the subject, appeared.[15] The success of the Yale clinics led to the establishment in 1949 of a pilot program by the Western Electric Corporation, which now estimates that about 70% of their recognized alcoholics are rehabilitated.[4] Since 1949 the number of companies with planned programs for the recognition and treatment of alcoholics is rapidly increasing. For companies without programs, assistance in the form of consultation and information is available through the numerous local committees of the National Council on Alcoholism.

Until 1945 no state had a program for alcoholism. In that year, largely as a result of the success of the Yale clinics, Connecticut began the first state program under an independent commission.[15] Since then a majority of states have established programs. There is no consistency with reference to their organizational location; 11 are in independent commissions, 15 are units of state health departments, 1 is related to a welfare department, 12 are in state mental health agencies, and 3 are in departments of institutions.[16] The programs carried on are various combinations of educational, research, and treatment activities. Until recently, federal interest in alcoholism has been minimal. In 1966, however, President Lyndon Johnson dealt with alcoholism explicitly for the first time in United States history in his health message to the Congress. New legislation has been passed, a National Advisory Committee on Alcoholism has been appointed, and a National Center for the Prevention and Control of Alcoholism has been established within the National Institute of

Mental Health which provides consultation and grants for research and demonstrations to states and through them to localities.

On the local level numerous communities have begun programs. Often these programs consist essentially of treatment clinics. There is a trend, however, toward broadening the base of the approach by utilizing more effectively and extensively the resources and contributions of all fields.[17-19] Considering the magnitude of the problem, none of the existing programs is adequately financed. It is often proposed that a surtax be levied on alcoholic beverages, the revenue from which could be devoted entirely to programs to combat alcoholism. Similarly it has been suggested that the alcoholic beverage industry support the program. It is significant in this light that the industry has already established a foundation for research into the causes and treatment of alcoholism.

Content of programs

Quantitatively the problem is so vast and so complex, with multiple causes, different types of cases, and numerous agencies of potential value, that no standard program is possible or even desirable at this time.[20,21] Certainly, as Vogel[22] has stated:

Treatment of the alcoholic is not the sole province of the psychiatrist, internist, sociologist, minister, or any scientific or lay discipline. Recognition of this is fundamental. . . . A total push is necessary and mobilization of all methods and facilities is necessary to improve results and make help available to more alcoholics. The nonspecificity of present-day treatment should not result in therapeutic nihilism, which is often used by physicians and others as rationalization to avoid this important problem. There are definitely ways to treat the alcoholic.

Basically there is no reason why the approach to the problem of alcoholism should not follow the well-established principles of epidemiology and program planning which have been so successful in many other areas. This should include the gathering of data by survey, reporting, or other means to determine the extent of the problem. The data should be analyzed in order to pinpoint problem areas and problem groups, existing or incipient, and to determine places and circumstances in which alcoholism is or tends to become a problem. Early case finding should be carried out by enlisting the participation of public health and visiting nurses, police, clergy, institutional staff, and many others. Since about one half of the problem drinkers are in the pre-addict stage, special effort should be made to reach them as early as possible for attempts at prevention of progression. Another 30% of problem drinkers are in the early acute addict stage. This group probably represents the combination of the most accessible and potentially most susceptible to rehabilitation. Treatment centers, providing a spectrum of therapies utilizing the services of Alcoholics Anonymous, internists, psychiatrists, sociologists, and others, should be available especially for those in the early acute addict stage. Provision should be made for individual counseling, group therapy, medical treatment as required, and hospital referral if indicated. Increasing use has been made of the drug Antabuse (tetraethylthiuram disulfide) which taken orally produces no effect unless alcohol is subsequently used. In such an event acetaldehyde is formed and causes severe nausea, vomiting, increased pulse rate, and decreased blood pressure. This should always be prescribed and used under medical attention and, if at all possible, should be combined with psychotherapy. Concurrent with the treatment, steps should be initiated for the other aspects of rehabilitation, i.e., social, familial, religious, economic, and the like. In the process the patient's family, especially the spouse, should not be overlooked. The occasional importance of this has been emphasized by Lewis,[23] formerly consultant for the National Institute of Mental Health, in the following terms:

When the wife of an alcoholic remarries, she very often remarries an alcoholic. We often see reciprocal relationships between the alcoholic and his spouse, and as an alcoholic improves the adjustment of the spouse deteriorates. Strange as it may seem, the spouse is often ambivalent about her alcoholic husband's recovery; she frequently derives neurotic satisfaction, which may be unconscious, from his alcoholic binges. The inadequacy of her husband makes her feel needed and more adequate. . . . Wives often resent their alcoholic husband's therapists whom they see as threatening their control of their husbands. A part of this psychological mechanism between husband and wife is the nagging and the pressure which the wife puts on her alcoholic husband, making him feel more inadequate and thus less likely to stop drinking.

Suggestions for meeting this situation are to align oneself with the spouse's positive motivations, to urge her to join Alanon, a group of spouses of A.A. members, or if possible to get her to accept some psychiatric consultation in order that she might better understand her husband's problem and her relationship to it.

Prevention

The development of most cases of alcoholism is so insidious and the causative factors so complex and often buried in the past that prevention is difficult. Experience has shown that prohibition of alcoholic beverages by law is impractical. Even if it could be achieved, the maladjustments and inferiorities which give rise to alcoholism, in the presence of alcohol, would still be there. In a utopian world the elimination of these underlying factors might be anticipated, but under existing conditions this is too much to hope for. Nevertheless, increasing attention to mental health, the greater equalization of social and economic opportunity, and more understanding parents may make some inroads. In the practical sense, however, it would appear that the best chance for prevention still lies along the path of education. This should have as its goal a willingness on the part of all to regard, discuss, study, and deal with alcoholism and its precursors frankly, dispassionately, and intelligently toward the end of combatting the development of the precursors and of seeking in the face of their existence patterns of behavior other than hiding behind the screen of an alcoholic haze. Education in the school can be important, but as Bacon[24] has stressed, "only if (a) the lesson to be taught is realistic, understandable, meaningful to the student, (b) the community is largely in agreement with what is taught and (c) the teachers themselves are taught and properly equipped." It is utterly pointless and farci-

cal for an uninformed teacher to utter prohibitory preachments to students about drinking, when they know that he as well as their own families and friends as well as society in general partake of alcoholic beverages to some extent. Far better for an informed teacher to present the realities of living and upon that basis to discuss its risks and why and how they may be avoided.

Earlier it was stated that one of the most important needs is to recognize alcoholism for what it really is—a disease. Paradoxically, this is still lacking to a considerable degree in the medical profession. Surprisingly few schools of medicine teach to any consequential extent about alcoholism. The average physician and, indeed, the average public health worker still regards the alcoholic as a socially undesirable misfit who refuses to pull himself together. If physicians and public health workers cannot face the problem honestly and properly, how can anyone else? A few recent events serve to emphasize the point. Only within the past few years have some hospitals begun to take alcoholics on their general wards. Only within the past few years have hospitalization insurance organizations begun to pay for hospitalization due to alcoholism. Even yet only about one half of such organizations do so and benefits vary widely. Indeed, it was only in the early part of 1958 that the House of Delegates of the American Medical Association unanimously passed a resolution stating that alcoholism is a disease and that it should be treated by a physician in a hospital setting when necessary. To its credit the Association is now prepared to move rapidly. Its Committee on Alcoholism has prepared a manual on alcoholism[25] distributed to all physicians, is urging the development of uniform legislation dealing with alcoholism based upon scientific fact, is urging hospitalization insurance organizations to allow hospital benefits for alcoholism and most important of all, with its Committee on Professional Education is working toward the much needed improvement in the teaching of alcoholism as a disease in the nation's medical schools. It is to be hoped and expected that schools of nursing and schools of public health will follow suit with regard to improved instruction on the subject.

DRUG ADDICTION

Here again, as in the case of chronic alcoholism, we are dealing with a condition and a situation that appears on the surface to be something quite different from what it really is. Whereas the typical attitude toward the alcoholic is that he is a weakling, lacking in self-control and self-respect, the narcotic addict is usually regarded as an essentially depraved person and a criminal. One might construct an equation to illustrate the typical social and unfortunately all too common medical attitudes that would state something like this: alcoholism is to tuberculosis as narcotic addiction is to leprosy!

Definition

Drug addiction lends itself somewhat more easily to definition than does alcoholism because fewer people regularly use these drugs and because ordinarily they are obtained and used clandestinely. Furthermore, the addiction that results from their use is more clear cut and appears within a relatively short time. The World Health Organization's Expert Committee on addiction-Producing Drugs[26] believes that it is important to distinguish clearly between drug habituation and drug addiction. It defines *drug habituation* (habit) as "a condition resulting from the repeated consumption of a drug," and lists its characteristics as (1) a desire (but not a compulsion) to continue taking the drug for the sense of improved well-being it engenders, (2) little or no tendency to increase the doses, (3) some degree of psychic dependence on the effect of the drug but absence of physical dependence and hence of an abstinence syndrome, and (4) detrimental effects, if any, primarily on the individual. The majority of affinities to synthetic drugs fall in this category.

On the other hand, the Committee defines *drug addiction* as "a state of periodic or chronic intoxication produced by the repeated consumption of a drug (natural or synthetic)," and lists its characteristics

as (1) an overpowering desire or need (compulsion) to continue taking the drug and to obtain it by any means, (2) a tendency to increase the dose, (3) a psychic (psychologic) and generally a physical dependence on the effects of the drug, and (4) detrimental effect upon the individual and a society. The continued compulsive use of the narcotizing alkaloids and of certain synthetic drugs are included herein. For purposes of orientation it should be pointed out that the World Health Organization considers alcohol as intermediate between the addiction-producing and the habit-forming drugs. It points out that alcoholism and drug addiction have certain similarities but also certain important differences. Thus, the severe symptoms which occur on withdrawal of alcohol can be more dangerous to the individual than those which occur when morphine, for example, is withheld. On the other hand, it takes much longer to develop dependence upon alcohol than to develop dependence on narcotics. Also, up to the present time, treatment of alcoholism is much more possible and successful than is treatment of narcotic addiction.[27]

Extent and cost of the problem

There are known to be about 35,000 persons addicted to narcotics in the United States. However, an additional 25,000 are estimated to exist, making a total of about 60,000. This figure has been broken down to 50,000 opiate addicts, 5,000 marijuana users, and 5,000 addicted to opiate-like synthetics.[28] The overall prevalence of narcotic addiction is currently estimated to be about 3.3 per 10,000 of the population. This is a considerable decrease over previous estimates: 25 per 10,000 in 1909, 18 per 10,000 in 1914, and 10 per 10,000 in 1920. This estimate is in line with both production and seizure figures. The World Health Organization notes that worldwide licit production of heroin has dropped from 839 kilograms in 1948 to 132 kilograms in 1954. On the other hand, an estimated 1,500 kilograms of heroin enters the United States illegally each year. This represents less than one half of 1% of the opium produced in the world. Another indication of the magnitude of the problem is that in a recent typical year, United States agents working abroad seized 888 kilograms of raw opium, 128 kilograms of morphine base, and 84 kilograms of heroin destined for the United States.[29]

It is impossible to make even a crude guess as to what drug addiction costs society. Included should be the loss or decrease of production by those afflicted, the costs of hospitals, enforcement agencies, and prisons, losses due to crime stimulated by the search for money with which to purchase drugs, the costs of accidents and illnesses connected with their use, and the cost of the drugs themselves. With regard to the latter it has been estimated that it costs a narcotic addict a minimum of from $10 to $20 per day to maintain his habit. The illegal sale of narcotics is well known to be highly lucrative, hence its attraction to the criminal classes of society. A single kilogram (2.2 pounds) of heroin now costs about $1,000 in Turkey, but by the time it passes through various dealers and peddlers who dilute it, package it, and sell to individual addicts, it may easily bring a total of $1 million. This of course is why illicit dealers so frequently encourage free trials in order to get additional sure customers "on the hook."

Effects of narcotics

Each narcotic produces certain characteristic effects. Generally speaking, they all cause general stimulation, euphoria, and contentment, with release from pain or concerns that arise from worries, neuroses, and conflicts. Various sensory manifestations occur, such as a tingling of the skin, hallucinations, and feelings of ecstasy. All these pleasures, of course, are of temporary and short duration for which the addict pays a high price in continued and progressive misery. Contrary to popular opinion, while these substances act generally as stimulants, they depress certain functions, notably the sexual drive. Continued use produces a marked loss of appetite, resulting in weight loss and nutritional disorders; the typical addict is thin, wan, and undernourished. Severe constipation is common, as is marked itching. The addict suffers

from nervousness, insomnia, and depression, and suicidal attempts are not uncommon, especially during the typical postjag depression. Because of the anxiousness of the addict to experience the drug and because dilution by those who sell it is so common, the addict frequently does not know how much he is actually taking. As a result serious toxic reactions and even death may occur from an overdosage. Another serious aspect of addiction is in relation to infections and other illnesses. Because of lowered resistance, the addict is much more susceptible than the average person to many infectious and organic diseases. Furthermore, one effect of the drug is to dull awareness to pain, fever, and other symptoms. Infections are not infrequently circulated among drug addicts as a result of the use of common materials, especially unsterilized hypodermic needles. Prominent among these are syphilis, malaria, infectious jaundice, and blood poisoning. All told, life expectancy is markedly shortened.

The most unfortunate effect of narcotics is what they do to the morale, morals, and social behavior of those so unfortunate as to become addicted to them. The typical narcotic addict lives only for the next time he can experience the drug; nothing else really matters. As a result, in order to obtain the drug, he will forfeit anything—job, social position, family, self-respect. He will beg, borrow, or steal in order to satisfy his craving and, considering the combination of lowered ability to earn and the high daily cost of the required drugs, much petty crime results. Male addicts commonly turn to picking pockets, shoplifting, burglary, dishonest gambling, and pandering. Women and girls frequently become prostitutes. Very frequently the addict becomes a willing "pusher" of the drug, the riskiest link in the delivery chain, in order to assure his own supply. In effect, the unfortunate addict literally does not own his soul.

Causes of drug addiction

The causes of drug addiction are essentially the same as in the case of alcohol. In fact, not infrequently individuals are found who have passed from alcoholism to drug addiction because they felt that alcohol no longer provided the sought for "lift." Yost[30] has classified drug addicts into the following three groups, to which a fourth may be added:

1. Emotionally well-adjusted individuals who take addicting drugs on medical advice for treatment of pain, sleeplessness, and the like

    (After protracted use they find they cannot get along without them. This type constitutes only 5 in 1,000 of those hospitalized at the Public Health Service Hospitals at Lexington, Ky., and Fort Worth, Tex.)

2. Neurotics who turn to drugs because drugs make them forget their feelings of inadequacy, fear, and the like, making them feel better and more normal, either physically or mentally or both

    (These addicts constitute the largest group.)

3. Psychopaths who take drugs in a deliberate search for thrills and "kicks"

    (These addicts are probably the smallest group numerically.)

4. Otherwise relatively normal individuals, usually adolescents, who try narcotics in order to maintain face with the group

    (This would appear to be a variable group, its numbers depending considerably upon variations and fluctuations in group behavior and fads and upon the extent of law enforcement and availability of supplies.)

Yost applies the apt phrases of "addiction prone" to the second and third categories (neurotics and psychopaths) and of "accidental addicts" to the first group. As might be expected and in line with the experience with alcohol, the first and fourth categories of addicts present the least important and least difficult part of the problem and are much more susceptible to rehabilitation because undesirable underlying personality problems are generally absent. The second and third categories, neurotics and psychopaths, present the core of the problem of addiction in terms of numbers and presence of personality insufficiencies, hence difficulty of cure.

With regard to the type of person who is apt to become an addict a study in 1951 of 260 boys and girls admitted to Bellevue Hospital in New York City is illuminating. It was concluded that there was a striking uniformity in personalities and backgrounds of the boys. The subjects were all nonaggressive and used passive techniques that gave a superficial appearance of ease and poise. Their interpersonal relationships were very weak and superficial, with the notable exception of their relationships with their mothers. They had many acquaintances but few friends, but their relationships with their mothers were extremely close. Often they were their mother's favorite. Many had chosen definitely domestic types of occupations such as cooking or tailoring.

Epidemiology

As with alcoholism, the problem of drug addiction may be approached from the epidemiologic point of view. This has been well illustrated by Jacobziner[31] in connection with the program in the New York City School Health Program.

An epidemic of narcotic addiction must be studied in the same manner as any other outbreak of a communicable disease. The agent, host, and environment and their impact and interrelationship must be studied and investigated. In an epidemic of narcotic addiction the *agent* is perhaps of far lesser significance than the *host* and *environment*. It should be emphasized that drug addiction is not a primary disease entity, but merely symptomatic of an underlying deep-seated disturbance: narcotic addiction being only one of many forms of social maladjustment. Narcotic users are not definitely psychopathic, but in the main, products of an unhealthy and an unhappy environment. Therefore, the underlying causes and motivations must be investigated, discovered, and understood. It is not the *process of addiction* which is important to know, but what causes an adolescent to use a drug or to become socially maladjusted. . . . Two factors are needed for the production of addiction: There must be a vulnerable soil—the individual or host must suffer from a psychological or emotional disturbance—and the drug or agent must be capable of resolving the conflicts, tensions, and anxieties of the maladjusted individual.

From the standpoint of epidemiologic analysis it is interesting to note a predilection for earlier ages than with alcoholism. The most susceptible age group is from 15 to 25 years of age,[32] and about 30% of addicts become addicted before their twentieth year. Although the number of males addicted to drugs exceeds the number of females, they do not nearly predominate to the extent observed with alcoholism. Again most cases are found in the upper and lower socioeconomic thirds of society, tending to spare the middle class somewhat; and again, as would be expected, concentration in urban centers is observed. A major proportion of the problem in the United States is concentrated in the New York City, Chicago, and Los Angeles areas.

Approach to the problem

Any program designed to attack the problem of drug addiction must be multi-pronged and must involve the understanding and cooperation of many disciplines, i.e., medicine, psychiatry, social work, nursing, religion, law and law enforcement, and teaching, to mention only the most obvious. The most logical first step is case finding. Police and other law-enforcement personnel are the primary sources of case finding; physicians are the secondary source. In addition to these, public health and visiting nurses and social workers occasionally learn of addicts from patients and clients. Regardless of the circumstances, on discovery the addict should be regarded primarily as an ill person and not as a criminal. Instead of being dealt with in a punitive fashion, he should be admitted promptly to a hospital or other suitable institution for evaluation and treatment. It is not possible to treat a confirmed narcotic addict as an outpatient. If local facilities are not available or suitable, arrangements can be made for prompt admission to one of the two Public Health Service hospitals specially equipped to handle this type of case; one is located in Lexington, Ky., the other in Fort Worth, Tex.

As to chances of cure, studies of patients after discharge from the Lexington, Ky., hospital revealed that 7% had died, 13% were cured, 40% were using drugs again, and the true status of the remaining 40% was unknown. Usual experience is that three out of every four addicts relapse at some time. Frequently the road to ultimate cure involves a number of relapses.

Thus at Lexington in 1955 there were 3,724 admissions, of which about two thirds were readmissions. There were some who returned as many as six times. However, Kolb,[33] who has been associated with that hospital, feels certain that the majority of addicts want to be helped and would endure almost anything if they thought cure was possible. However, as the Expert Committee of the World Health Organization points out, this does not mean that the average addict will commit himself willingly to an institution for the relatively long period of months necessary. The Committee[34] feels that some legal provisions are necessary because "most addicts require some degree of coercion—preferably civil commitment for medical treatment—to involve them to desist from what is to them often a pleasurable experience."

The high relapse rate points to the most difficult part of the problem, i.e., rehabilitation and follow-up. An important part of the treatment is to make the addict aware of the underlying reasons for his addiction and to help him rehabilitate himself psychologically and socially. Jacobziner[31] stresses the importance of qualified field personnel, public health nurses or social workers, who may obtain pertinent background information about the patient, his family, and his environment. He suggests the importance of repeated visits to the home and environment by such personnel not only before and after the discharge of the patient, but also prior to the patient's admission for treatment. In addition to the patient the family and the community need to be reeducated and prepared for the return of the patient. With special reference to the adolescent, Jacobziner emphasizes, "The importance of good parent-child relationship must be stressed and parents must be made to understand that a poor quality of parent-child relationship is responsible for many forms of social maladjustment." Those close to the patient should be forewarned of the possibility of a relapse and warned not to castigate the patient if this should occur but to contact the appropriate persons or institutions as soon as possible. Attention should be called to the formation in 1949 of an organization known as Narcotics Anonymous, patterned after Alcoholics Anonymous. This is developing into a valuable adjunct in the rehabilitation of narcotic addicts. It has branches in a number of cities and is gaining experience in providing effective resources for addicts. Since a sense of inadequacy and failure often plays an important role, efforts should be made to assist the discharged patient in obtaining employment so that he may develop a feeling of fulfillment and confidence. Much remains to be done toward development of a willingness on the part of most potential employers to give the ex-patient an opportunity and to provide encouragement wherever possible.

A point of considerable controversy at the present time is the advisability and value of the so-called British system, wherein drug addiction is handled primarily by the medical profession with controlled legal distribution of drugs to those who use them. The premise is that by removing the profit motive there is no temptation to resort to crime in order to obtain the drug and there is no incentive to create new addicts. Kolb[33] advocates strenuous attempts to cure the addict during periods of hospitalization but feels that when after several such attempts the patient is apparently not amenable to cure but will get along well with a minimum amount of narcotic (except marijuana or cocaine), he should be given this for the rest of his life under medical supervision. He feels, on the basis of his experience, that the majority of such addicts "would work, support themselves, and create no public problem." This approach is followed in a number of European countries as well, and is advocated on a selective and demonstrative basis by the New York Academy of Medicine.[35] Many object to this procedure on the basis that it removes the incentive for real cure. The Study Group on Treatment and Care of Drug Addicts,[34] called by the World Health Organization in November 1956, discouraged this approach, "While complete withdrawal of the drug of addiction might be deferred in certain circumstances,

the maintenance of drug addiction is not treatment."

Experience in England indicates a recent and significant rise in the prevalence of narcotic addiction. Whether this may correctly be attributed to the system or to more complex sociologic changes is not clear. It has resulted, however, in placing the system in disfavor. As Hess[36] disclaims, "Reference is made to 'the successful British system'. But how can a program be called successful when the addicted population has doubled in the past 10 years? In addition, it has been shown that 35% of a study group in England became involved in crime within a year." Furthermore, as Larimore and Brill[37] point out, not only is the number of known narcotic addicts in England small (about 700), but about one sixth of them were physicians to begin with. They conclude that these factors plus a lower cultural susceptibility to drug addiction on the part of the British account for any difference between the United States and England rather than between the American and British method of handling addicts.

Toward the goal of prevention a number of things should be considered. First, certain legislation is needed (1) to control strictly the importation, production, distribution, and sale of all drugs which potentially may cause addiction, (2) to provide adequate organization and financing for carrying out the foregoing and other activities, (3) to provide for severe punishment of those found guilty of the illicit importation, handling, and sale of narcotics, and (4) to allow for addicts who are apprehended to be turned over to suitable institutions for mandatory treatment without court action. More adequate educational activities are indicated in order to bring about better understanding and cooperation on the part of all those in society who may play a role in attacking this problem. This applies to physicians, nurses, public health workers, teachers, clergy, police, welfare workers, and many others. Most authorities, however, believe strongly that direct propaganda to young people on the subject of narcotics is not only of no value but is actually dangerous. Thus Dr. H. J. Anslinger,* former United States Commissioner of Narcotics, believes that it may only serve to awaken the interest or stimulate the curiosity of potential adolescent addicts. Similarly R. N. Artis, supervisor of the Chicago office of the United States Bureau of Narcotics, has stated:

> We do not recommend or promote direct education on narcotic drugs. In this conclusion, we agree with the conclusions of the 68 nations of the United Nations who passed a resolution on this subject. Narcotic education is open to controversy and great objections. We prefer to educate at the parent-teacher level.

Beyond the activities of adequate legislation and education it is to be anticipated that, as in the case of alcoholism, increased and improved methods in mental health and their wider availability and acceptability will play a significant part in the prevention as well as in the amelioration of the narcotic problem. Added to this are the benefits which are sure to result from constantly improving and equalizing social conditions and opportunities. These in the long run may remove many of the underlying factors which lead some to escape unpleasant realities through the insidious medium of narcotics.

It is regrettable that as yet few official agencies have addressed themselves to the problem of narcotic addiction. A study in 1962 by the American Social Hygiene Association showed that only 28 states had programs.[39] Eight were in state health departments, and most of the remaining programs were in state departments of mental health. In cities with a population of over 100,000 only four local health departments reported programs, whereas another 11 local official agencies other than the health department reported activities. Obviously this is still pioneering territory for public health.

Nonnarcotic drugs

As indicated earlier, there is a variety of substances, both natural and synthetic, which while not addictive are included here for convenience. Among other reasons is the fact that they share certain character-

---

*In *The Bane of Drug Addiction* by Yost.[30]

istics with narcotics: They produce some unusual psychic effects; their use is not ordinarily socially acceptable in most cultures; commerce in them is ordinarily illegal and tends to attract certain socially undesirable types of individuals; and the majority of them have certain undesirable physical or mental consequences. Included are certain drugs with very important legitimate medical uses. Generally speaking, the substances fall into four categories: depressants, stimulants, ataraxics, and hallucinogens.[39]

Depressants include sedatives and hypnotics. Predominant in this group are the barbiturates, the most widely abused of the depressants. These substances are commonly used in medicine for their sedative or calming effect, especially in anxiety states, hyperthyroidism, and high blood pressure, as well as to allay pain and to control convulsions such as occur with epilepsy. When chronically misused, these substances may in some ways become more dangerous than narcotics. Physical dependence upon them may develop, and tolerance is never complete. One habituated to them shows evidence of slurred speech, staggering and even falling from lack of balance, quick temper, and quarrelsome disposition. Overdose produces coma, and pneumonia is not an uncommon complication. When these drugs are withheld from a habitué, the withdrawal symptoms may be as serious and dangerous as those of narcotic withdrawal. Central nervous system symptoms develop, leading possibly to epileptiform convulsions with subsequent delirium and hallucinations similar to delirium tremens. Among persons who use these substances illicitly there is a variety of colorful names, such as goof balls, peanuts, red devils, rainbows, and blue heavens, to mention but a few. In 1963 drugstores in the United States filled 478 million prescriptions for barbiturates. However, a former commissioner of the Food and Drug Administration has testified that enough raw material was produced in 1962 to make over 9 billion doses of barbiturates and amphetamines combined. He estimated that at least half ended up in the illicit market.

The second group of substances to be included here are stimulants. This category includes drugs which directly stimulate the central nervous system, producing alertness, wakefulness, excitation, and sometimes a rise in blood pressure and respiration. The most common substances in this category are the amphetamines, which have been used for the past quarter century in the treatment of a variety of mental diseases and as adjuncts in the correction of excessive weight. They appear to have a specific effect on the appetite center in the brain. They are also valuable in the treatment of narcolepsy and Parkinson's disease. Because of their unusual stimulant action, amphetamines and related compounds tend to be abused by individuals whose occupations require long periods of wakefulness or vivaciousness and by many individuals who attempt to "burn the candle at both ends." A relatively high degree of tolerance can be developed with these substances without necessarily causing physical or psychic damage if dosage is gradually increased. In some instances, however, a true drug psychosis resembling schizophrenia may develop with delusions and hallucinations. Under ordinary misuse, however, the individual appears to be unusually excitable, talkative, restless, with a tremor of the hands and an enlargement of the pupils, sleeplessness, and perspiration. Under certain circumstances a psychic or emotional dependence upon these chemicals may develop. As in the case of the depressants, these materials enjoy many colloquial names including bennies, co-pilots, peaches, cartwheels, hearts, and dexies. The economics of the illicit drug market are well illustrated by amphetamines, which can be purchased wholesale for $1 per 1,000, sold in the illegal market for $30 to $50 per 1,000 and retailed to the individual for as much as 10 to 25 cents per tablet.

The third category of nonnarcotic drugs that tend to be abused are the ataraxics or tranquilizers. These materials introduced during the 1950's are in one sense a type of nervous system depressant. They have revolutionized the treatment of many psychiatric disorders and as such represent a major advance in pharmacology and therapy. Their use under medical direction or otherwise has become extremely commonplace and would appear to be generally lacking in toxic side effects and much less likely to produce habituation among those who use them. More than 1 million pounds are produced and over 60 million prescriptions written for them each year in the United States. The economic value of the tranquilizer market is now measured in the hundreds of millions of dollars annually.

The fourth type of problem, of a nonnarcotic nature, one that appears to be increasing, relates to the use of the hallucinogens. Pharmacologically these are spoken of as psychedelics or psychotomimetics.[40,41] These chemicals exist widely in nature, and a number of them have been synthesized. Most common among them are mescaline, psilocybin, and lysergic acid diethylamide (LSD-25). The latter is an extremely powerful drug, 100 times more potent than psilocybin and 7,000 times more potent than mescaline. Recently an even more powerful hallucinogen has been discovered. The illicit use of these substances, especially by certain psychosocial cults, groups such as beatniks or hippies who attempt to withdraw from society, or mere thrill-seekers on certain college campuses, has been attributed to their mind-expansion effects. It is quite true that many individuals may use these substances with impunity and in the process experience a wide variety of hallucinations that may be greatly stimulating and colorful. On the other hand, ample evidence exists of individuals who under their influence experience overwhelming fears, paranoid delusions about other people, distressing and disturbing distortions with reference to time and place, and intense self-loathing. These and other manifestations have lead to successful as well as unsuccessful attempts at suicide, murder, and other acts of violence. Further evidence of their danger is the fact that in 1966 more than 100 persons were admitted to Bellevue Hospital in New York City suffering from severe LSD-induced psychosis. This is also occurring in numerous other hospitals elsewhere in the country. Specific mention should be made of a much milder but much more widely used hallucinogen, marijuana. The use of this substance has become the subject of much controversy; many claim it is completely harmless and that its use should be legalized. An indication of the growth of its use is evidenced by seizures of the material which have increased from 1,871 kilograms in 1960 to 5,641 kilograms in 1965. Marijuana appears to be used particularly by the juvenile, teen-age, or adolescent drug abuser in an attempt to obtain a quick thrill, to solve life's problems, or to escape briefly from the pressures of the adult world. In this sense, quite aside from any toxic or psychiatric complications that might occur, there is a significant interference with normal development and living and the young user may very easily become psychologically dependent upon the substance.

This leads to at least a brief mention of the use of a number of other substances by children and teen-agers, airplane glue, lighter fluid, gasoline, nutmeg, and ether.[42] Smelling or inhaling these substances tends to provide a momentary sense of exhilaration, euphoria, and intoxication, but all of them have very serious toxic side effects. An important aspect of these materials by adolescents is the fact that very often their use is by a group. Part of the reason is apparently a shared boredom, a lack of definite goals, a revolting against adult rules, and as a manifestation of wanting to belong to a group. Not uncommonly their use begins in a gang or party setting with one of the group introducing the material or practice and the rest responding for fear of appearing to be "chicken" or cowardly. While some of these practices may on the surface appear innocuous, they may lead to criminal acts. For example, while there is no dependable data concerning the number of those who use these materials in the young population, there is mounting police and court evidence of violations of the law by juveniles after having engaged in the practice. These violations extend from breaking and entering and stealing of automobiles to more serious actions. In a recent instance

near our residence the murder and rape of two small twin sisters was committed by a 15-year-old boy who had spent the afternoon sniffing glue. As is often the case, the boy afterwards remembered none of the circumstances.

The solution to these problems is not easy, and, as in the case of alcoholism or narcotic addiction, it requires the interest and joint action of a number of concerned groups. Public education, particularly in the schools, is important. In certain circumstances legal restrictions with reference to the sale of certain materials may have some effect. Development by industry of substitutes for dangerous chemicals that are nonetheless necessary for legitimate purposes may offer some hope. In addition to this is the need for persistent and consistent surveillance of the problem by public health officials, law enforcement officials, and other groups; and the apprehension and prosecution of any who are involved in the sale, dissemination, and use of these dangerous materials for improper purposes is also a critical need.

Fraudulent means of obtaining drugs

It would appear appropriate to include a few words concerning the methods of obtaining dangerous drugs and particularly those that require prescriptions. Certain of the narcotics are smuggled through customs check points into the United States by various devious means. In addition, however, a large amount of potentially dangerous materials legally produced within the country manages to slip into illegal channels of distribution. Normally, drugs move from manufacturer to wholesaler to pharmacist. At each step and point some pilferage or illegal sale may occur. The record of professionals involved in the normal channels of sale and use is excellent. Each year very few arrests are made for illegal sales by pharmacists or physicians. Thus in 1963, despite a total of 300,000 physicians and pharmacists in the country, the Food and Drug Administration recorded only 74 abuses. The three great problem areas are large-scale theft, clandestine drug manufacturers, and individuals who are adept at fraudulently obtaining drugs from physicians and pharmacists. Some concept of the magnitude of theft in transit was indicated by the previously mentioned discrepancies between the amount of barbiturates produced, for example, and the amount legitimately sold. The ability to synthesize certain drugs has lead to large-scale clandestine manufacture of certain of these materials. Usually the counterfeit products appear as exact duplicates of the legitimate drugs, although the product may vary significantly in potency and may be contaminated due to inadequate quality control. In the same category with the clandestine manufacturer is the repackager and the bulk peddler.

A worrisome problem to the ethical physician and pharmacist is the individual user who has become adept at fraudulently obtaining needed supplies through normal channels. A favorite method is the forging of prescription orders. This is done in a variety of ways—by altering legitimate prescriptions, by stealing prescription blanks or having prescription blanks printed illegally, by impersonating a physician either in person or by telephone, and by shopping around from one physician to another. Not infrequently such individuals watch carefully for new young physicians opening practice in the community and take advantage of a combination of the lack of experience and a desire to build up a practice. Such pseudopatients often become proficient in quoting medical journals and relating lengthy medical histories that require stimulants, barbiturates, or narcotics.

Recent legislation

Because of the increase in the problem and growing national concern, Congress passed the Drug Abuse Control Act of 1965 to prevent the misuse and illicit traffic of potentially dangerous drugs (P.L. 89-74). A new Bureau of Drug Abuse Control has been established in the Food and Drug Administration to carry out the intent of the law.

REFERENCES

1. Addiction-producing drugs, Chronicle of the World Health Organization 11:81, Mar. 1957.
2. Jellinek, E. M., and Keller, M.: Rates of alcoholism in the United States of America, Quart. J. Stud. Alcohol 13:49, 1952.
3. Clark, G. A.: The doctor and the alcohol problem, Penn. Med. J. 58:790, Aug. 1955.
4. Moore, P. A.: Western Electric's program on alcoholism, Chicago, Western Electric Co., Industrial Relations Department.
5. Report of the American Public Health Association Task Force, Arden House Conference, Oct. 12-15, 1956, Amer. J. Public Health 47:218, Feb. 1957.
6. Jellinek, E. M.: Phases in the drinking history of alcoholics, Quart. J. Stud. Alcohol 7:1, 1946.
7. Trice, H. M.: Work accidents and the problem drinker, I.L.R. Research, New York State School of Industrial and Labor Relations, Cornell University, 3:2, Mar. 1957.
8. Loomis, T. A., and West, T. C.: The influence of alcohol on automobile driving ability, Quart. J. Stud. Alcohol 19:30, 1958.
9. McFarland, R. A.: The role of preventive medicine in highway accidents, Amer. J. Public Health 47:288, Mar. 1957.
10. United States injury estimates, July-Dec. 1957, Amer. J. Public Health 48:581, July 1958.
11. Alcohol as a drug, Chronicle of the World Health Organization 8:144, Apr. 1954.
12. Bacon, S. D.: Alcoholism, nature of the problem, Federal Probation, Vol. 11, No. 1, 1947.
13. Hirsh, J.: The problem drinker, New York, 1949, Duell, Sloan & Pearce, Inc.
14. World directory of Alcoholics Anonymous, New York, 1966, The organization.
15. McCarthy, R. G.: Public health approach to the control of alcoholism, Amer. J. Public Health 40:1412, Nov. 1950.
16. Membership list, North American Association of Alcoholism Programs, Washington, 1967 (mimeographed).
17. Johnston, M.: Adult guidance center, San Francisco, Public Health Rep. 68:590, June 1953.
18. Zappala, A., and Ketcham, F. S.: Toward sensible rehabilitation of the alcoholic, Public Health Rep. 69:1187, Dec. 1954.
19. Prothro, W. B.: Alcoholics can be rehabilitated, Amer. J. Public Health 51:450, Mar. 1961.
20. Myerson, D. J.: The study and treatment of alcoholism, New Eng. J. Med. 257(17):820, Oct. 24, 1957.
21. Brightman, I. J.: The future of alcoholism programs, Public Health Rep. 75:775, Sept. 1960.
22. Vogel, S.: Psychiatric treatment of alcoholism, Ann. Amer. Acad. Pol. Soc. Sci. 315:99, Jan. 1958.
23. Lewis, J. A.: Alcoholism, Amer. J. Nurs. 56:433, Apr. 1956.
24. Bacon, S. D.: Alcoholism, its extent, therapy and prevention, Federal Probation, Vol. 11, No. 2, 1947.
25. Committee on Alcoholism of Council on Mental Health: Manual on alcoholism, Chicago, 1958, American Medical Association.
26. Drug addiction and drug habituation, Chronicle of the World Health Organization 11:165, May 1957.

27. Alcohol and alcoholism, Chronicle of the World Health Organization **9**:177, June 1955.

28. Winick, C.: The narcotic addiction problem, New York, 1964, American Social Hygiene Association.

29. The challenge of crime in a free society. A report by the President's Commission on Law Enforcement and Administration of Justice, Washington, 1967, U. S. Government Printing Office.

30. Yost, O. R.: The bane of drug addiction, New York, 1954, The Macmillan Co.

31. Jacobziner, H.: Investigating narcotic addiction in shool children, Amer. J. Public Health **43**: 1138, Sept. 1953.

32. Grigg, W. K.: Prevention and control of addiction to narcotics, Amer. J. Public Health **42**:1295, Oct. 1952.

33. Kolb, L.: Narcotic addiction—an interview, Spectrum **5**:136, Mar. 1957.

34. Treatment and care of drug addicts, Chronicle of the World Health Organization **11**:323, Oct. 1957.

35. Drug addiction—III. A Statement by the New York Academy of Medicine, Bull. N. Y. Acad. Med. **41**:825, July 1965.

36. Hess, C. B.: New trends in narcotic addiction control.

37. Larimore, G. W., and Brill, H.: Epidemiologic factors in drug addiction in England and the United States, Public Health Rep. **77**:555, July 1962.

38. Facilities for the treatment and rehabilitation of narcotic addicts, New York, 1962, Amer. Soc. Hyg. Ass. (mimeographed).

39. Fraser, H. P., et al.: Problems resulting from the use of habituating drugs in industry, Amer. J. Public Health **48**:561, May 1958.

40. Cole, J. O., and Katz, M. M.: The psychotomimetic drugs—an overview, J.A.M.A. **187(10)**: 182, Mar. 7, 1964.

41. For detailed reference purposes, see Hallucinogens—a select bibliography, Washington, May 1967, Food and Drug Administration.

42. Mullings, E. B.: Airplane glue, Michigan's Health, Sept.-Oct. 1966.

Chapter 25

Medical and
hospital care

Medical and hospital care has been controversial up to the present and will undoubtedly continue to be so for some time to come. It is not considered within the province of this book to discuss the details of the many legislative bills and proposals of the past and present. Events have been moving so rapidly that any such discussion probably would be out of date at the moment it was written. The intention, therefore, is to present the general problem and the development of attempts at its solution in as unbiased a manner as possible, with emphasis upon the rather dramatic forward movement of recent years.

RELATIONSHIP BETWEEN PUBLIC HEALTH AND PRIVATE MEDICINE

Public health activities cut across a great many other phases of community life and involve contact with the members of most businesses and professions. Among these relationships, one of the most intimate is with the members of the medical profession. There are many reasons for this. In the first place most of those engaged in public health work are themselves either members of the medical profession or of some other profession closely related to it such as nursing. Public health workers and medical practitioners are concerned with the same ultimate goal, health. Furthermore, many of the programs sponsored by health agencies require the active cooperation and participation of private physicians. In fact, one often hears the opinion that every private physician should be in effect a deputy health officer and that his

office should represent, for the families he serves, a branch of the health department. The wish that some day most preventive and promotive as well as therapeutic medicine would be obtained from family or personal physicians seldom meets with argument. Finally, private medical practice and public health activities have a considerable effect, one upon the other. Modern public health programs depend greatly upon coincident effective private practice. Every health officer realizes that the scientific practice of medicine is the foundation of public health. In turn, many public health activities such as laboratories and health education operate to the assistance of private practitioners.

In order to understand adequately the significance of this relationship, which in the light of recent trends is certain to become even more intimate, it is well to review briefly and jointly the development of these two fields, especially as related to and affected by the development of our modern industrial economy and social organization.

EVOLUTION OF MODERN MEDICINE AND SOCIETY

Generally speaking, it is advantageous to consider these developments in three time periods: the period preceding the so-called Industrial Revolution, the period from about 1750 to 1850 during which the Industrial Revolution took place, and the time that has elapsed since. Before the Industrial Revolution, which is usually considered to have begun about 1750, the social

459

and economic structure of the Western world was relatively simple. Few large cities existed, and the economy was essentially agrarian. Economic and social life was limited to the small local community or neighborhood, and while these aspects of life were quite stable, they were on a rather low scale in comparison with the present and involved relatively little personal freedom. Social classes were rigidly stratified and adhered to by custom from one generation to the next. Only with great difficulty could a son pursue a way of life different from that of his father. Industry in the present sense of the word simply did not exist. The family was the unit of production, usually making for itself whatever goods it needed. Manufacturing, to the extent that it did exist, was carried on either through guilds, which provided for the continuous training of a limited number of apprentices by skilled craftsmen, or by means of the "putting-out system." This latter consisted of putting raw materials into the hands of individuals, who, with all of the members of their families, worked on them on a piece basis. Thus the individual craftsman was responsible for the entire process of manufacture and usually was personally acquainted with the source of his materials and the ultimate consumer of the product of his labors.

During this era the practice of medicine was at one of its lowest ebbs. The scientific viewpoint was generally underdeveloped. Medical procedures were based largely upon speculation and superstition, and but little experimentation or planned observation was engaged in. There were no standards of medical education or practice, and healers and physicians were often self-designated. Many of them were charlatans, often unworthy of trust not only with regard to competent medical care but also in terms of private possessions. Since surgeons worked with their hands and often performed surgery as an adjunct to barbering, they were held in particularly low esteem. Treatment consisted chiefly of the use of purgatives and leeches, and considerable attention was given to various aspects of cosmetology. The relatively few

hospitals were essentially pesthouses, consignment to which usually signified impending death. At any rate, the average member of society had little if any contact with physicians since the latter, if not vagrant itinerants, were usually attached to the households of the noble and wealthy classes. They seldom received fixed payments for their services, usually depending on gratuities.

The provision of medical service in a public sense was in its most embryonic form. Social controls and requirements relating to the practice of medicine were either elementary or nonexistent. It is true that during the late Middle Ages the professional behavior and avarice of physicians in some urban centers occasionally led to the legal fixing of fees and to requirements that some arrangements be made for the care of the sick poor. At best, however, these requirements were rare and sporadic and of a very unsatisfactory nature. As early as the thirteenth century, a few European towns employed town surgeons. Town physicians, on the other hand, are not encountered historically until the sixteenth century. From the fourteenth century on, it became not uncommon to require surgeons and later physicians to submit public reports of all injuries they treated as well as cases of certain diseases, notably leprosy, plague, and syphilis. Very gradually physicians became concerned with sanitation and other aspects of public health.

Whatever care, medical or otherwise, provided for the sick, poor, aged, and homeless, the Church was its source. Charity by this time had become a dominant manifestation of acceptable Christian behavior, and medical, nursing, and hospital care became a major interest and activity of many monastic orders. Later, during the sixteenth, seventeenth, and eighteenth centuries these responsibilities gradually began to shift from the Church to the state. As pointed out by Shryock,[1] however: "This humanitarianism, like the clerical form of earlier centuries, largely expressed the benevolence of the upper classes rather than any demand for reform from below."

The Industrial Revolution brought with it tremendous changes not only in methods of manufacturing but also in the modes of transportation and facilities for the communication of ideas and information. Manufacturing was fractionated into component processes, and the laboring class became concentrated in industrial centers of population and organized to work in large factories for the greater profit of management. A new economic and political power came about in the form of the industrialist and economic royalist. To such a height did the desire for high profits soar that all consideration for human welfare and decency was forgotten. No longer were goods made by skilled guild members or craftsmen with pride in their workmanship. No longer was the consumer personally acquainted with the producer. The personal face-to-face relationship between employer and employee disappeared as well. Articles were now produced through the combined efforts of a great many individuals. As might have been expected, the social and economic center of gravity shifted from the agrarian to the urban scene. Rural areas themselves were directly affected. The populations of industrial cities were not self-maintaining because of their appalling death rates. They therefore required continuous replenishment from the rural population.

Interestingly enough it was during this period of cruel industrialization and economic interdependence that the search for scientific knowledge received a much needed impetus. Although it is true that the primary incentive was the development of new techniques for greater economic gains, the results were ultimately beneficial to society. The character of the practice of medicine began to undergo some improvement. A trend toward logical experimentation and observation developed. A system of medical training by apprenticeship came into vogue, and the physician changed his locale from the highway and the manor to take his place as a private entrepreneur in competition with other physicians. For a while this competition resulted in many abuses which led eventually to the necessity

for the reestablishment of a long-dormant code of professional ethics.

With some exceptions diseases were not considered as distinct entities but were classified in terms of their manifestations, such as swellings, fevers, and inflammations. The equipment of the physician was still simple, and his only adjunct was the pharmacy, which in most instances he operated himself. Hospitals more than ever were pesthouses because of the tremendously increased incidence of communicable diseases for which the filthy centers of population served as breeding grounds.

During the nineteenth century the idea of corporate structures developed and resulted in the monopolistic control of each industry and not infrequently of several industries together. The intent, of course, was to achieve still greater industrial efficiency and, not incidentally, the ultimate in profits from the smallest possible cost or investment. Entire geographic regions as well as the workers themselves became specialized in function, and the social distance between producer and consumer was widened even more. Abuse of the laboring class became so flagrant that by 1850 a social reaction began to set in and slowly to swing the pendulum in the opposite direction. Notable in this respect were a number of prominent persons imbued, for that or for any period, with an unusual spirit of humanitarianism. A few among those who might be named were Edwin Chadwick, Robert Owen, Southwood Smith, John Stuart Mill, and Lord Ashley. These and others like them did their utmost to bring into the public consciousness an appreciation of the conditions under which the laboring classes were forced to live and work.

Gradually many social reforms got underway; these reforms dealt with working conditions, poor welfare, housing of the working classes, the care of orphans and the insane, education, and sanitary conditions. Scientific and technologic investigations which had formerly been conducted largely from the point of view of industrial development now began to be pursued for their own sake and for the benefit of humanity as a whole. Despite these trends, economic welfare was still insecure. More than ever, workers earned a living instead of making one. By this time the greatest handicap to industrial expansion was the fact that techniques of distribution of goods lagged far behind techniques of production. The subsequent solution of this was dependent upon the invention of the steam locomotive, the internal combustion engine, and the construction of paved, all-weather roads.

During this period of social revolution tremendous gains were made in the field of medicine, particularly in relation to scientific research and educational standards. There came about a great eagerness for new medical knowledge which eventually led, among other things, to the conclusive proof of the bacteriologic causation of many diseases. Spectacular discoveries followed one another at a breathtaking pace. One result of this was the foundation of preventive medicine and sanitary science. Medical education became formalized with the establishment of schools with increasingly higher standards. Although the general practitioner was still the prototype, many medical specialties began to appear. The construction and use of hospitals was expanded, and they gradually came to be looked upon as places for the restoration of health rather than houses of death. Furthermore, they began to take their place as centers for teaching and research. Professionally trained nurses and scientific laboratories entered the ranks of auxiliary facilities upon which both the public and the medical profession gradually became more and more dependent.

On the economic side of the practice of medicine some interesting changes were coming about. The itinerant physician became a thing of the past. Groups of physicians began to band together to form group practices or private clinics. Medical care was now offered to all components of the population on a competitive fee-for-service basis with a sliding scale as a means of adjustment for varying abilities to pay. A growth of free medical service in hospital wards appeared as one manifestation of the medical profession's acceptance of responsibility for the public welfare. In this manner medicine finally came to be regarded as a social science. Thus in 1847, Dr. Solomon Neumann of Berlin published his book *Public Health and Property* in which he stated that medicine is fundamentally a social science and that as long as it does not correspond to this reality, we cannot taste its fruits and must content ourselves with the rind. A year later Rudolph Virchow declared that physicians were the counselors of the poor and that to a great extent medicine was the key to the social question.[2] Perhaps the most outstanding evidences of the influence of the changing social and economic structure on the form of medical practice were the widening of the breach between the discovery of medical knowledge and its application and the ever rising cost of medical care resulting from the increased investment required for medical education and the rendering of modern medical services by skilled physicians and their auxiliary assistants.

It is interesting that, despite the remarkable medical discoveries of the late nineteenth century such as improved diagnostic and therapeutic techniques, the development of anesthesia, antisepsis and asepsis, and the study of cellular physiology and pathology, to mention but a few, medicine as practiced by average physicians was still scientifically backward. Until the close of the century it was still common to consider illness as fevers, dropsy, inflammations, and the like, and treatment still consisted for the most part of blood letting and the evacuation of "ill humours" by physicking, sweating, diuretics, vomiting, and the formation of blisters. Calomel, the leech, and the lancet were still the important contents of the physician's bag. In fact, leeches were uses literally by the hundreds of thousands each year.

Characteristic of the American physician of this period was Dr. Hiram Buhrman, who practiced in small towns in Maryland and Pennsylvania in the 1870's. His regulation fee was 25 cents for an office call. This included medicines unless expensive drugs were necessary. A house visit within the township was 50 cents without medicine,

75 cents with medicine. The doctor compounded his own prescriptions. In case of death there was a $3 fee, for which he did most of the work of the present-day mortician. All obstetrical cases, regardless of the length of labor, were $5, as were abortions, whereas miscarriages were billed at $1.50. A search through his account books showed that in all but two instances he made only one house visit after delivery, and this on the following day. The fee for setting and caring for a fractured clavicle, including all material used in the dressing, was $5, whereas a fractured thigh cost $10. Lancing an abscess or a felon was 50 cents. Dr. Buhrman also functioned as a dentist. A tooth extraction cost 25 cents, except when several in a row were removed at the same time in which case the fee per tooth was reduced. When chloroform was used for extractions, the total charge was $2. These were the charges, but they were not always collected. When money was needed, the doctor set out in person as a collector of outstanding accounts.

As did other doctors of his day, to visit his patients he traveled on horseback with saddlebags or in a gig or buggy and carried a limited supply of fever medicine, sulfur and molasses, obstetric forceps, and a bag of instruments for emergencies. His major expenses, other than those of his home, involved the stabling and feeding of the horses and the purchase of saddles, horse collars, fly nets, and halters. In this unspecialized small town practice, conducted with few instruments and drugs, on a limited number of diseases, the hospital did not enter into the picture at all.[3]

As a matter of fact, as late as the 1890's much of the most advanced practice was usually carried on in an office which had as its equipment a medicine cabinet, a sofa or an examining table, and a table which could be used as a laboratory. The technical equipment consisted of a thermometer, a stethoscope, a prescription pad, and a sufficient amount of chemicals to determine the presence of albumin and sugar in the urine. A few particularly advanced practitioners had microscopes, and still fewer were able to examine a specimen of blood to determine the leukocyte count and the presence or absence of malarial parasites.

With the beginning of the twentieth century, the practice of medicine began to mature as a science and as a result became much more effective. The speculative theories and traditional practices of the physician of the nineteenth century had failed to win the confidence of the public, and as a consequence many medical cults flourished. With the acceptance and application of the newer scientific knowledge by the orthodox physician in practice and as a result of more widespread public education and understanding, the medical profession has since risen high in the public esteem.

Unfortunately, this has not occurred without accompanying complications. Improvements in diagnosis and treatment have required at the same time the development of highly trained specialists and costly diagnostic and therapeutic tools with a corresponding increase in the cost of medical care. Robinson[4] has emphasized this by comparing two patients admitted to the same hospital with the same heart condition, one in 1913, the other 25 years later in 1938. The first patient was cared for by a visiting physician, an intern, and one specialist, the pathologist-bacteriologist. The completed record covered two and one half pages. The second patient was observed and described by 3 visiting physicians, 2 residents, 3 interns, 10 specialists, and 14 technicians, a total of 32 individuals, and although the record of the case was still incomplete, it already covered 29 pages. He concluded that the more recent case, in its sharp contrast with medicine of the past, presents one of the major social problems facing contemporary medical practice.

ECONOMIC FACTORS INFLUENCING THE NEED FOR MEDICAL CARE

Pertinent to the ability to obtain medical care are a number of related economic factors concerned with the distribution of wealth and its effect on the need for medical care and the distribution of medical facilities. It is obvious that the economic level of a community plays a significant role in determining the degree of its health and illness and in the extensiveness of its facilities to care for them. Since wealth is nowhere distributed equitably, it naturally follows that the state of health of a community or of a nation cannot be uniform. In a very literal sense health and the treatment of illness are purchasable, but the ability to purchase them is not always present. The use of average figures to depict the purchasing power of a community of people tends to be greatly misleading.

Thus, while the median family income in the United States is high, about $6,900 in 1965, there is considerable variation by region, degree of urbanization, and other factors. For example, the mean family income for urban and rural nonfarm families is approximately twice that of the rural farm families. Table 25-1 presents the distribution of families by total money income, before taxes, in 1965 in the United States. It indicates, for example, a variation of from 3% of families with annual incomes less than $1,000 to almost 25% of families with annual incomes between $7,000 and $10,000.[5]

Table 25-1. Distribution of families and unrelated individuals by total money income, United States, 1965*

Total money income	Thousands of families	Percentage
Under $1,000	1,459	3.0
$1,000 to $1,999	2,956	6.1
$2,000 to $2,999	3,583	7.4
$3,000 to $3,999	3,806	7.8
$4,000 to $4,999	3,883	8.0
$5,000 to $5,999	4,502	9.3
$6,000 to $6,999	4,477	9.2
$7,000 to $9,999	11,635	24.4
$10,000 to $14,999	8,342	17.3
$15,000 and over	3,636	7.5
Total	48,279	100.0

*Adapted from Current population reports, Series P-60, No. 51, Jan. 1967, Consumer Income, Bureau of the Census, U. S. Department of Commerce.

The inequity of the distribution of purchasing power is magnified still further when the nation is considered in terms of its constituent parts. It is well known, for example, that physicians tend to cluster in and around cities, especially the large metropolitan centers of population. They do this for many reasons—a better opportunity to develop large active practices; the availability of hospitals, laboratories, ancillary personnel, and other professional aid; opportunities for postgraduate education as well as for teaching; cultural attrac-

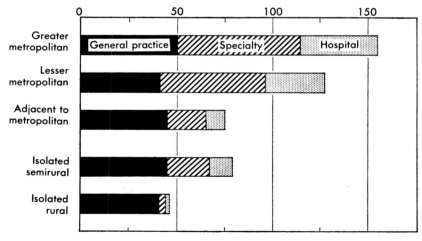

Fig. 25-1. Urban-rural differences in physician supply (active nonfederal physicians per 100,000 population, 1959). (From Indicators, Department of Health, Education, and Welfare, Jan. 1963.)

tions; living comfort; good schools, stores, and other essentials. The result is shown in Fig. 25-1. From it one can note not only the concentration of physicians but especially of specialists in the urban centers of the nation.

This factor combined with another, regional wealth, brings about a geographic variation of considerable dimension. This may be observed in Fig. 25-2, which presents for each of the states the physician-population ratios by specialty and hospital affiliation. It is obvious that the more affluent states have the lion's share not only of physicians but also of specialists. Beyond

this the average age of physicians is significantly higher in the economically less privileged states and areas.[6]

The relative economic standing of the various geographic regions of the nation varies from the well-known disadvantageous position occupied by the Southeastern states to the economically affluent New England and Pacific states. These economic inequities have a marked effect on the distribution of personnel and facilities for the treatment of illness. A direct relationship is readily seen to exist between them and the purchasing powers of the respective regions. Thus the New England states, with an av-

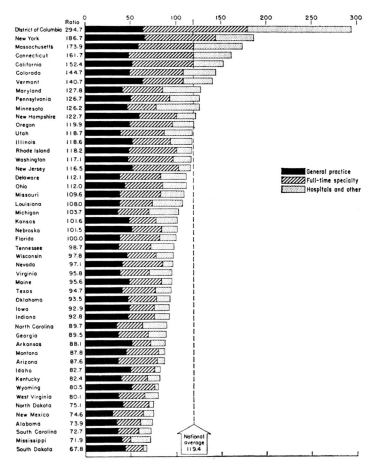

Fig. 25-2. Physician-population ratio in each state and type of practice of physicians (active non-federal physicians per 100,000 civilian population, 1959). (From Indicators, Department of Health, Education, and Welfare, Jan. 1963.)

erage per capita buying income in 1965 of about $3,000, have 1 physician for every 679 inhabitants, in contrast with the Southeastern states whose average per capita buying income of only a little more than $2,000 attracts and supports only 1 physician for every 1,066 inhabitants. If the ages and qualifications of the physicians were considered, these discrepancies would become even more marked. Similarly the more affluent New England states have about twice the number of dentists in relation to population as do the states of the Southeastern region. With regard to the number of acceptable general hospital beds available the same general picture holds true. However, a significant equalization

has been occurring in this regard as a result of the National Hospital Survey and Construction Act (Hill-Burton Act) of 1946.

Another factor which accentuates both the need for medical and hospital care and the disparities which exist among regional resources is the proportion of older persons in the population. Persons 65 years of age and over require more medical attention and hospitalization than any other age component of society. For example, this age group uses about seven days of hospital care per capita per year as compared with less than three days per capita for all other age groups. Furthermore, this is a period of decreased or absent earning power, hence

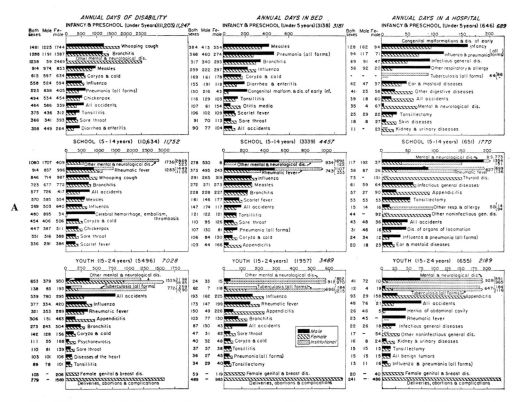

Fig. 25-3, A and **B.** Twelve diagnoses with the highest annual rates per 1,000 population in each of six age groups for days of disability, days confined to bed, and days of hospital care—three household surveys with visits at intervals of 1 to 3 months, covering a total of 37,988 full-time person-years of observation for white persons. (From Collins, S. D., Lehmann, J. L., and Trantham, K. S.: Major causes of illness of various severities and major causes of death in six age periods of life, Washington, 1955, Public Health Service Pub. No. 440.)

much less ability to afford the needed care. Regionally this works especially to the disadvantage of the New England and the Central and Northwestern states.

The unequal distribution of medical personnel and facilities would not be of such serious consequence if the socioeconomic factors causing it did not also have an adverse influence upon the need for them. Numerous studies have shown that the total illness experience of a population follows a more or less definite pattern. Although the average American suffers an injury or an illness about two and one half times a year, there obviously are some who go through the year unscathed while others far exceed the average expectation. Accordingly, in any average current year, out of each million American people

470,000 will suffer no serious illness, 320,-000 will have one illness during the year, 140,000 will have two illnesses, 50,000 will have three illnesses, and 20,000 will have four or more illnesses.

For the general population it is possible to know in advance not only the total amount of illness but also the type. Numerous studies have been carried out for this purpose during recent years. Among them, those of Collins and co-workers[7,8] are particularly instructive. Some of the results of their analyses of five illness and household surveys in the United States are presented in Figs. 25-3 and 25-4. The charts in Fig. 25-3 show annual days of disability, days in bed, and days in a hospital by age and sex for the 12 predominant diagnoses. The charts in Fig. 25-4 show the incidence

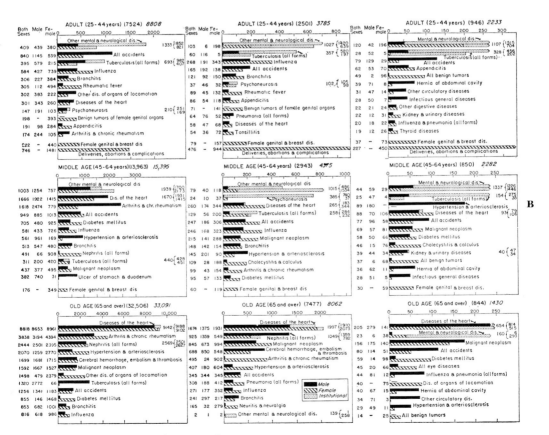

Fig. 25-3, cont'd. For legend see opposite page.

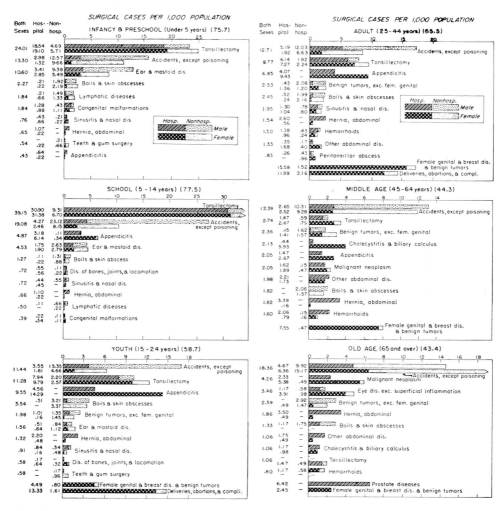

Fig. 25-4. Ten most frequent causes of surgery per 1,000 males and females of five broad age groups, and ten diagnoses with the highest percentage of cases in the same age groups that were treated surgically—white families canvassed periodically in five illness surveys covering 80,768 person-years of observation. (From Collins, S. D., Lehmann, J. L., and Trantham, K. S.: Surgical experience in selected areas of United States, Washington, 1956, Public Health Service Pub. No. 473.)

by age and sex of the most frequent causes of surgery.

The overall pattern of illness in the general population is predictable, whereas the forthcoming experience of the individual cannot be foretold. However, it is known that the lower the individual is on the economic scale, the more apt he is to experience one or more serious illnesses during any year. This is not surprising since pur-

chasing power determines the amount and quality of food consumed, the degree of exposure to or protection from the elements of nature, and the ability to obtain many medical as well as other types of services.

EXPENDITURES FOR MEDICAL CARE

The combined effect of the unpredictability of illness in the individual and the influence of economic factors on the probability of illness and the distribution of medical facilities, therefore, causes a relatively small proportion of a population to bear the major share of the economic burden due to illness at any given time. Furthermore, it is found that this unfortunate fraction of the population includes an unduly disproportionate number of those who are least able, because of their limited incomes, to meet the costs of adequate care.

When the factors of low income and increased tendency to become ill are considered together, it is found that the lower income groups not only have more frequent medical bills, but they also must spend proportionately more of their income for this purpose than the higher income groups; this is true despite their greater tendency toward self-treatment or even their frequent failure to obtain care.

Considering the total picture, attention may be called to the fact that the nation suffers a loss of many billions of dollars each year because of illness. This is made up of expenditures for avoidable medical care, the value of the average 7 working days per year lost by the average wage earner due to illness, and the capital value of the lives that are lost due to causes which in the light of present medical science may be considered preventable (see Chapter 7). These seem like large sums, especially when the relatively small amount of money that would be required to avoid or at least reduce them is considered.

The amount necessary for adequate preventive care and the early diagnosis and treatment of disease becomes almost insignificant when compared with the sums expended by the nation for other purposes. The nation finds it possible to spend enormous amounts in time of war for the destruction of life. World War II necessitated an average daily expenditure by America of $150 million; the total bill for the conduct of the war was slightly less than $300 billion. It is a commentary on our civilization that such expenditures are so willingly made at the same time that appropriations to provide inexpensive immunizations of children or examinations for cancer or heart disease are so often resisted.

Beyond the costs of waging war, expendi-

tures for more routine needs and activities offer an interesting contrast to the amount expended for medical purposes. Table 25-2 presents a breakdown of personal expenditures of the American public during a recent year. It will be observed that the amount spent for recreation is almost as much as the amount devoted to all aspects of medical care. Regretfully, the latter sum is only twice the amount spent for tobacco.

It should be noted that the relative expenditure for medical care has been rising. Thus, in terms of the percent of gross national product, it has increased from 3.7% in 1929 to 6.5% in 1965. However, as will be seen, most of this increase can be accounted for by the rising costs of hospitalization.

How is the medical dollar spent? Table 25-3 presents the proportionate breakdown of medically related expenditures for the period between 1929 and 1965. While in absolute terms, the amount of money spent for all of the items has increased, very significant shifts have occurred among them in relation to each other. By far the most striking change has been in connection with the cost of hospitalization. While the proportion of the medical dollar devoted to payment of physicians and dentists has decreased almost 40% during the past three decades, the proportionate amount expended for hospitalization has doubled. This is especially evident if the proportions for insurance, much of which represent hospitalization insurance, are added to the amounts designated for hospitals. In fact, when this is done the proportionate expenditures for hospitals and insurance combined show an increase from about one sixth of the total medical dollar in 1929 to about one third of the total medical dollar in 1965. Also of interest is the fact that while a large number of complex and valuable new drugs and medicines have been developed and put to use during this period the proportionate expenditure for them has remained about the same. In fact, in relation to percentage of disposable personal income, expenditures for medical drugs and appliances are now about one half of what they were in 1939. The changes that have occurred in expenditures for the

Table 25-2. Personal consumption expenditures, United States, 1965* (in millions of dollars)

Item	Amount	%
Food, tobacco, and beverages (including alcoholic beverages)	106,791	24.8
Housing	63,157	14.7
Household operation	61,877	14.3
Transportation	57,825	13.5
Clothing, accessories, and jewelry	43,427	10.0
Medical, dental, and hospital care	28,120	6.5
Recreation	26,304	6.1
Personal business	22,055	5.1
Personal care (nonmedical)	7,509	1.7
Religious and welfare activities	5,609	1.3
Private education and research	5,585	1.3
Foreign travel and other	3,206	0.7

*Adapted from Statistical abstract of the United States, Washington, 1966, Bureau of the Census, U. S. Department of Commerce.

Table 25-3. Changes in the percentage distribution of medical costs, United States, 1929-1965*

Type of expenditure	1929	1940	1950	1960	1965
Physicians	33	30	28	25	27
Dentists	16	14	11	10	9
Hospitals	14	18	23	26	30
Drugs and appliances	25	27	26	26	22
All other	12	11	12	13	12
Total	100	100	100	100	100

*Statistical abstract of the United States, Washington, 1966, Bureau of the Census, U. S. Department of Commerce.

Table 25-4. Consumer price indexes, all items and components of medical care, United States, 1935-1965* (1957-1959 = 100)

Year	Consumer price index, all items	All medical care	Physicians' fees	Dentists' fees	Prescriptions and drugs	Hospital rates
1935	47.8	49.4	53.9	52.0	69.2	23.8
1945	62.7	57.5	63.3	63.3	73.2	32.5
1955	93.3	88.6	90.0	93.1	92.7	83.0
1965	109.9	122.3	121.5	117.6	98.1	153.3
Ratio, 1965 to 1935	2.28	2.95	2.25	2.26	1.42	6.44

*Medical care financing and utilization, Health Economic Series 1-A, Public Health Service Pub. No. 947-1A, 1967.

various components of medical care, however, are most dramatically indicated by a comparison of them with consumer price indexes. This is presented in Table 25-4, which shows that, while between 1935 and 1965 physicians' and dentists' fees increased at a rate parallel to the general consumer price index and drug price increases actually lagged, hospital rates increased three times as fast. Several other points are of interest in relation to certain items not included in the figures. Expenditures for nursing are about one fifth of the amount paid to private physicians. Also the estimated amount paid to cultists is about equal to the per capita sum expended for public health work.

ATTEMPTS TO SOLVE THE PROBLEM

By the end of the eighteenth century, if indeed not sooner, problems of health and disease were recognized as subjects of social and political concern. In fact by that time it was beginning to be realized that these problems were associated with and part of a social problem of much greater magnitude, i.e., the emerging struggle for the expression of the rights of the common man. This struggle was destined to become a main theme of political appeal, and the health of the masses, particularly of the working classes, became one of the major talking points not only of such humanitarians as Chadwick, Southwood Smith, Shattuck, and others like them but also of the spokesmen for the new political ideologies exemplified by Engels and Marx. Thus the stage of recognition and orientation of the problem was reached. What to do about it, how to solve it, was yet another problem, the solution of which was not to be forthcoming for at least another century and a half.

In order to consider the preliminary attempts to find an answer it is necessary to retrace our steps to some extent. It has been seen that the eighteenth and nineteenth centuries were characterized by a shift from a rural agrarian society to an urban industrialized society, a growing insecurity of personal income, a great increase in the low-income population, a considerably increased risk of sickness due to the social and economic changes, and constantly rising costs of medical care. Rosen[9,10] in his brief but concise discussion of the early attempts to solve the problem, rightly highlights the propositions of three outstanding social thinkers of the times: Defoe and Bellers in England and de Chamousset in France. With the development of statistical methodology and the increasing accumulation and analysis of vital data it became possible, at least in a crude way, to calculate certain types of risks. Marine and fire insurance

were fairly well established and used. Life insurance companies were in the process of acceptance. It is not too surprising, therefore, that even at a relatively early date some thought was given to the possibility of applying this valuable social technique to the risks of illness. Daniel Defoe was apparently the first to make the suggestion, in 1697. In an essay he proposed that the insurance principle be applied to the social problems of the poor, including medical and institutional care and disability pensions. Shortly afterward, in 1714, John Bellers suggested a rather detailed plan for a national health service in England. He believed that the program should be sponsored by government since "it is too great a burden to be left upon the shoulders, or to the care of the physicians alone, no private purse being able to bear the needful charges of it. Especially considering the necessity of many and the indifferency of others of that faculty, further than to procure a plentiful substance for themselves: And how much it concerns every other person, there is more reason to expect, the State should bear a good part of the expense of it."* He therefore proposed the establishment of governmental hospitals for teaching and research, a national health institute, and a plan to provide medical care to the sick poor. Going even further in his social thinking, de Chamousset in 1754 proposed a plan of hospital insurance with a broader population base. Here for perhaps the first time is encountered a concern for others than the traditionally dependent poor, i.e., a concern for the bulk of the population comprising the so-called self-respecting middle class. He argued as follows:

There are asylums available to the destitute, and that is a resource useful to those to whom it is not humiliating to accept the free assistance which charity offers. (But there is) the class of the greatest number of citizens, who not being rich enough to provide sufficient aid at home or poor enough to be taken to an almshouse, languish and often perish miserably, victims of the propriety to which they are subjected by their class of society. Such are the industrious artisans, merchants whose trade is limited, and in general all those valuable men who

*Quoted by Rosen, G. In Galdston, I., editor: Social medicine, New York, 1949, Commonwealth Fund, p. 17.

live daily by the fruits of their labor, and who often for that reason have no recourse to treatment when a disease becomes incurable. The start of a disease exhausts all their resources; the more they deserve help, the less can they bring themselves to profit by the only resources that remain to them, and to find themselves in public asylums.*

Unfortunately little came of these suggestions. Eventually, with no action forthcoming from other directions, workers themselves in some parts of England and a few other countries began to inaugurate schemes at their own expense for protecting themselves against the risks of illness and injury. Trade benefit associations and societies were formed to contract with physicians and surgeons for the care of the members of the group, and each worker was assessed a fixed sum for annual dues or fees. How similar this is to recent events in this country. By the beginning of the nineteenth century there had been formed in England nearly 10,000 societies of this type with a total membership of close to a million workers. So common, in fact, had these plans become, that in 1773 and later in 1789 bills were introduced in Parliament to provide sickness and old-age benefits for the laboring poor. In both instances the bills were approved by the Commons but rejected by the House of Lords. During the same period, there was much discussion in England concerning the possibilty of requiring by law that all workers join privately operated benefit societies, and suggestions were even made that the government should bear part of the cost. Interestingly, such ideas and proposals were vigorously opposed with many arguments similar to those heard much more recently. Note the similarity between this idea and the third of the 12 points of the program suggested by the American Medical Association in early 1949.[11] It proposed that there be "further development and wider coverage by voluntary hospital and medical care plans to meet the costs of illness, with extension as rapidly as possible into rural areas. Aid through the states to the indigent

and medically indigent by the utilization of voluntary hospital and medical care plans with local administration and local determination of needs."

Meanwhile the medical profession was not entirely inactive. Many steps were being taken to clean house by the development of standards, professional licensure, and the improvement of medical education. Public health measures, in the then ordinary but now narrow sense of state administration, of quarantine and public sanitation were generally supported by the medical profession. Opposition to public provisions for vaccination, however, was not unknown. Support was given to the extension of charity relief and medical care to the indigent. Beyond this, except for rare instances, little was attempted by the medical profession to solve the broader aspects of the medical care problem. Occasional private physicians engaged in a certain amount of contract practice whereby for a fixed prepaid sum they provided care to an individual or a family for a year or some other agreed-upon period of time. Even this practice, however, was officially frowned upon, as it still was in the United States only two decades ago.

The most significant attempt to solve the problem of providing adequate medical care for a large population was made in Germany during the second half of the nineteenth century. It took the form of a nationally sponsored and administered plan for compulsory, comprehensive social insurance. Although since frequently pointed to as an autocratic scheme to control the lives and behavior of a people and of the medical profession, it is interesting that the plan was not instituted and enforced merely by Bismarck's will. In all, the plan was the subject of 9 years of argument, debate, and struggle in the Reichstag and when finally adopted represented a considerable compromise. It is also not without interest that it met with relatively little opposition from German practitioners of medicine. The plan provided for sickness, accident, and old-age benefits, supported by contributions from employees, employers, and the state. Despite its past and present critics, so satisfactory was it to those

*de Chamousset, quoted by Rosen, G. In Gladston, I., editor: Social medicine, New York, 1949, Commonwealth Fund, p. 18.

involved that it was retained long after the downfall of the Bismarckian regime. In fact, when Germany was defeated in 1918 and Alsace-Lorraine was returned to France, its population insisted that the German social insurance system be continued for them. Eventually in 1928 a similar nationwide plan was instituted for the rest of the French Republic.

Meanwhile recognition of the problem and attempts to solve it spread not merely throughout the European continent but beyond to many other parts of the world. One nation after another adopted some form of compulsory health insurance, and at the present time practically every major nation has some plan in operation. No two plans are identical, every major aspect of them showing some variation, whether in comprehensiveness of service, population

Table 25-5. Dates of enactment of compulsory health insurance

1883	Germany
1888	Austria
1891	Hungary
1901	Luxemburg
1909	Norway
1911	Great Britain
1911	Eire
1911	Switzerland
1912	Rumania
1917	Estonia
1918	Bulgaria
1919	Czechoslovakia
1919	Portugal
1920	Poland
1922	U.S.S.R.
1922	Yugoslavia
1922	Latvia
1922	Japan
1922	Greece
1924	Chile
1925	Netherlands
1925	Italy
1925	Lithuania
1928	France
1933	Denmark
1936	Peru
1938	New Zealand
1940	Holland
1941	Costa Rica
1943	Mexico
1945	Brazil
1948	England

served, type of administration and payment, or source of funds. Table 25-5 presents a listing of the years in which major compulsory health insurance plans were enacted. At present more than 60 nations have such plans.

The National Health Service, which was initiated in England in 1948, attracted much worldwide attention. This plan, adopted by the government over the strong opposition of the medical profession, now claims 97% enrollment. From its inception it has been very comprehensive in its benefits and services. This resulted in considerable difficulty in its early years because of the public rush to remedy vast backlogs of dental and visual defects. Although it is still criticized on various counts by many outside as well as within the medical profession, there is quite general agreement that it has resulted in more widespread and generally better medical and related services for more people. It is interesting to note, however, that during the first decade of its existence membership in voluntary health insurance plans increased tenfold, from 84,000 in 1948 to 834,000 in 1958.

One basis of difference and disagreement among the prepaid medical care systems which have developed in various countries is the method of payment of physicians. As indicated by Evang,[12] no generally accepted system can be found in Europe at the present time, the following being currently in existence:

1. Payment on a capitation basis (panel system) as in England
2. Payment on a cash basis, as in Germany
3. Fee for service, as in Norway
4. Fixed salaries, as in the U.S.S.R.
5. Basic salary combined with one of the types listed above

DEVELOPMENTS IN THE UNITED STATES

The Western Hemisphere, perhaps because of the tardiness of its discovery and development and because of the usually very localized type of society and government during its early history, was slow to produce any specific thought or action with regard to the problem of the adequate provision of medical care. Provisions for free medical services were scanty and simple and restricted to the very poor. The pattern that was followed varied from one town to another. In some instances a private physician would be engaged, perhaps because of a low bid, at a fixed stipend to provide care to the sick poor. In others stated fees were paid by the town treasurer when bills submitted by a physician were authorized. Not infrequently the fee for each particular case required a special vote. All of these three procedures are still resorted to in certain communities in the United States.

From this beginning there developed the provisions that have been followed for public medical care in the United States. These provisions are still essentially those of charity care of the sick poor, interrelated with and often administered in conjunction with other social welfare benefits such as subsidies for fuel, food, and housing. In most instances, the application of a means test is required. This not too stimulating experience, in addition to being demeaning to the patient, necessarily adds considerably to the cost of administration. In contrast with this is the rather spectacular development of public health measures in the United States. Of most pertinent interest is the extent to which public health programs in this country have repeatedly found themselves in the position of having to assume responsibility for activities that ordinarily might be considered part of the private practice of medicine.

Over the years there has been demonstrated an unfortunate lack of interest on the part of many physicians to render certain types of services. As Davis[13] has stated, tax-supported medical care of the types referred to, for the nonindigent,

. . . has been furnished for a variety of reasons, of which the following have been most evident: (1) because, as in mental disease, only public funds can make the provision necessary for the large number of persons involved*; (2) because certain diseases, as tuberculosis, hookworm, and trachoma, frequently involve, or lead to, incapacity for self-support; (3) because only a public authority can pro-

vide care in a manner which will protect the rest of the community, as in the case of acute communicable disease; (4) because, as in poliomyelitis and some orthopedic conditions among children and in early tuberculosis among young adults, the diseases if untreated, are likely to make permanent dependents of those who, with proper care, could be self-supporting; (5) because, as in eye, ear, throat, and dental defects among children, the education and the usefulness of future citizens are threatened unless these conditions are corrected; (6) because, as with the diseases of babies and of the puerperal state, the widespread public interest in maternity and infancy devolves some responsibility for them upon a public agency; and (7) because, as in the case of syphilis or cancer, the relative costliness of diagnosis or treatment renders many self-supporting persons unable to meet the expense.

The public pressures upon public health agencies to take the leadership for more complete protection and promotion of the health of all of the people have resulted in greatly expanded and more personalized programs. The evolution of this process has been described in a statement of the Joint Committee on Medical Care of the American Public Health Association and the American Public Welfare Association[14]:

Public Health has its historical roots in the long recognized necessity of invoking governmental authority to protect the community against the spread of communicable disease. From these limited beginnings, the increasing interdependence of individuals living in a highly industrialized and urbanized society has brought major advances in both areas of governmental responsibility for individual well-being. . . . Public health has also been undergoing a definite evolutionary trend toward a broadened concept of governmental responsibility. Whereas its earlier functions were primarily concerned with measures related to community sanitation and regulatory control of infectious diseases, public health activities have increasingly entered the area of services directly concerned with the personal health of individuals. With advances in medical science, the arbitrary line between prevention and treatment has narrowed and the distinction between community and individual health has become less sharply defined. Society has increasingly placed on public health an obligation to assure the availability of essential health services. This trend has been translated into broadened programs of prevention, diagnosis, and treatment for the principal communicable diseases; programs for the protection of the health of mothers and infants; school health programs; health education; and programs for the prevention, detection, and correction of dental, visual, hearing, and other defects.

Health Departments also provide an increasing

---

*Note that only 2% of patients hospitalized for mental illness in the United States are in private hospitals.

range of services designed to help control such chronic diseases as cancer, heart disease, diabetes, arthritis and rheumatism, and to rehabilitate children crippled by orthopedic, cardiac, orthodontic, and other conditions. Programs have been developed in the fields of mental hygiene; hospital planning, construction and licensure; hygiene of the aging; as well as, in some states, general medical care for needy individuals.

In a brief but excellent review Anderson[15] has traced the development of interest in and agitation for medical care insurance in the United States. He divides it into three broad periods. The first, from 1910 to 1920, was notable for the activities of the American Association for Labor Legislation which were instrumental in bringing about the widespread enactment of workmen's compensation laws. On achieving this success the Association selected medical care insurance as its next cause. It established a Committee on Social Legislation, which at first was supported by and participated in by the American Medical Association. Eventually, when a number of bills were introduced into state legislatures, many of the previously interested and cooperative groups including medical societies and pharmaceutical companies, as well as insurance companies and cultists turned against it. In 1920 the House of Delegates of the American Medical Association enunciated a basic policy of unequivocal opposition to any type of compulsory contributory insurance against illness.

The second period, from 1921 to 1933, is described by Anderson as "a quiet one devoted to the study of basic facts and problems only superficially comprehended in the first period." It saw the establishment of the Committee on the Costs of Medical Care, financed by six foundations and consisting of 42 persons representing medicine, public health, institutions, economists, and the general public. Its many studies and reports between 1928 and 1932 resulted in a final report, the conclusion of which has been summarized by Falk[16] in the form of five basic recommendations:

1. Comprehensive medical service should be provided largely by organized groups of practitioners, organized preferably around hospitals, encouraging high standards, and preserving personal relations.

2. All basic public health services should be extended to the entire population, requiring increased financial support, full-time trained health officers and staffs, with security of tenure.
3. Medical costs should be placed on a group payment basis through insurance, taxation, or both; individual fee-for-service should be available for those who prefer it; and cash benefits for wage loss should be kept separate.
4. State and local agencies should be formed to study, evaluate, and coordinate services, with special attention to urban-rural coordination.
5. Professional education should be improved for physicians, health officers, dentists, pharmacists, registered nurses, nursing aids, midwives, and hospital and clinic administrators.

A minority report was submitted. It agreed with recommendations 2, 4, and 5 above, but took strong exception to recommendation 1 on the organization of medical services and to recommendation 3 on group payment for medical service. The degree of concern of some of the opposition is illustrated by the tone of the editorial comment of the American Medical Association at the time.[17]

The alinement [sic] is clear—on the one side the forces representing the great foundations, public health officialdom, social theory—even socialism and communism—inciting to revolution; on the other side, the organized medical profession of this country urging an orderly evolution guided by controlled experimentation which will observe the principles that have been found through the centuries to be necessary to the sound practice of medicine.

The third period, beginning in 1933 and continuing into the present, represents again an action period similar to the first. Replacing the initiative of an unofficial labor legislation association, however, has been action by the federal government, strongly supported by well-developed and organized labor groups. Progress was served initially by the exigencies of the economic depression. The necessity to provide medical care as well as the other basic needs of food, clothing and shelter to the many individuals who were on unemployment relief was recognized and accepted by the American Medical Association as well as by other groups. However, this did not lead to inclusion of medical care insurance in the subsequent Social Security Act. The A.M.A. fought and defeated this but, as

Falk[16] points out, "at the price of insuring the enactment in 1935 of Title VI of the Social Security Act which inaugurated federal grants to states for public health services and the federal funds for a research program out of which the National Institutes of Health have burgeoned."

The passage of the Social Security Act was followed promptly by the 1935-1936 National Health Surveys of illness and underlying social and economic factors, and by the Presidential appointment of the Interdepartmental Committee to Coordinate Health and Welfare Activities. Its Technical Committee on Medical Care recognized the need for a general program of medical care and insurance against loss of wages due to sickness. A National Health Conference was called in July 1938 to consider the Technical Committee's findings and recommendations, with wide representation and discussion by all possibly interested parties. Legislation for a national health program was introduced the following year by Senator Robert Wagner, and extensive hearings were held. In addition to federal grants to match state expenditures for public health the bill proposed to offer "services and supplies necessary for the prevention, diagnosis and treatment of illness and disability." This prompted the A.M.A. to call an "emergency" meeting in St. Louis, as a result of which there was formed the National Physicians' Committee for the Extension of Medical Services. The subsequent history of action by this committee belied its name; whether because of great pressure from the National Physicians' Committee or for reasons of political expediency, President Roosevelt late in 1939 withdrew his support of the bill, and it died in Congress. Then the nation entered World War II. The large number of young men who were found unfit for military service because of physical defects obviously contradicted the claim that the American people were receiving adequate medical care. Furthermore, millions of young men and women who served in the Armed Forces were exposed to a system of medical care operated by the government that served their needs promptly and effec-

tively. Beyond this, while the war was in progress, a public opinion poll by *Fortune* magazine in 1942 indicated that three quarters of the people of the nation were in favor of national health insurance. Because of these and other factors, Senator Wagner in company with Senator James Murray and Representative John Dingell, Sr., in mid-1943 sponsored another bill more far reaching than his earlier bill. It proposed comprehensive medical, hospital, dental, and nursing home care for practically the entire population to be paid for out of a special fund based on equal contributions from employers and empolyees. The A.M.A. called it "the most virulent scheme ever to be conjured out of the mind of man," and again was successful in causing the bill to die in committee. As the war approached an end, President Truman asked that a new health insurance bill be prepared with careful consideration given to the rights of the public and the medical profession. As a result a new Wagner-Murray-Dingell Bill was filed which according to the A.M.A. would "mean the end of freedom for all classes of Americans." This bill, like its predecessors, was also killed.

In 1949, Governor Earl Warren of California unexpectedly sent to his state legislature a compulsory health insurance bill which was almost identical to one that had been proposed by the California Medical Association a decade earlier. Now, however, the latter organization took a completely opposite stand and employed a public relations firm to carry the attack. Ironically the attack took the form of encouraging, as a substitute, membership in Blue Cross, Blue Shield, and commercial health insurance plans, programs that up to this time the A.M.A. had also been attacking as "socialized medicine." The idea in back of this tactic was to prevent compulsory governmentally sponsored health insurance by offering voluntary insurance. An intensive propaganda campaign was conducted at a cost to the California Medical Association of a quarter of a million dollars, as a result of which the California bill was defeated. In 1946, with the war at an end, Senator Robert A. Taft, widely known as a conservative, decided to solve the problem by means of a bill that provided matching grants to states for medical care for those who on the basis of a means test could be proved to be indigent. The bill appealed to no one and it is interesting that the A.M.A. called even this "socialized medicine." A year later another Wagner-Murray-Dingell Bill was introduced. No one expected it to get any further than its predecessors. However, apparently on the basis of President Truman's reelection, the A.M.A. called it a crisis and assessed every member $25 to establish a $3.5 million "war chest" and to finance the largest lobby in American history. The assessment received wide publicity and was the subject of great criticism. More or less typical was the statement by Bishop G. Bromley Oxnam, "The assessment put upon every American doctor to raise a propaganda fund that today is being used to misinform a nation is a national disgrace." The A.M.A. engaged the same public relations firm that had been successful in California and the same approach was decided upon, voluntary health insurance instead of governmental compulsory health insurance. On deciding to do this it is interesting that the A.M.A., despite its earlier opposition, now claimed that it had been one of the first originators and supporters of the voluntary health insurance idea. Again the bill in Congress was defeated.

In 1948 another National Health Assembly was held, out of which came a statement of the principle that contributory insurance should be the basic method of financing medical care for most of the American public. Agreement was not reached however as to implementation. This was followed by a decade or more marked by (1) the continuation of the introduction of various types of medical insurance bills, (2) the acceptance and implementation of all of the recommendations of the Technical Committee on Medical Care of the President's Interdepartmental Committee with the exception of the general medical proposal, (3) a growing and marked concern and awareness by the general public regarding problems of medical care, its distribution, and costs, (4) a considerable extension of group medical practice, (5) a significant development of labor and union medical care programs, and (6) a remarkable growth of voluntary medical and hospital insurance. With respect to the latter, by 1965 an estimated 150 million people in the United States or 78% of the civilian population were covered by voluntary hospitalization insurance. Of these, an estimated 139 million also had surgical expense insurance, and 105 million had regular medical coverage. During 1964 an estimated $8.6 million were paid by more than 1,800 separate organizations, 903 commercial insurance companies, 77 Blue Cross plans, 72 Blue Shield plans, and nearly 800 independent health care organizations.[18] Unquestionably the interest and activity of government in the problems of medical care since the 1930's served as a major stimulus to the development and extension of voluntary prepaid medical care insurance plans and their acceptance and endorsement by organized medicine. However the growth of these plans was also undoubtedly indicative of a need and desire for action on the part of the public. Meanwhile the American Dental Association forthrightly addressed itself to the difficult problem of dental insurance. By 1964 about 1.3 million persons were covered by dental care insurance and the A.D.A. estimates that this will increase to 15 million by 1970.

Experience has indicated that voluntary plans are not without their problems. Furthermore, they have a number of significant limitations. They are rarely comprehensive, being limited essentially to hospitalization and medical services while in the hospital. Only a few provide preventive and diagnostic services, and certain illnesses such as tuberculosis and mental disease are generally excluded from coverage. Frequently hospitalization for long-term catastrophic illness is not adequately provided. Much of the population, including a large part of the low-income group and the aged, those with the greatest need, are not covered. As time went on, particular concern developed with reference to the older component of the population. It was increasing in numbers and percent. Because of their greater longevity, a disproportionate number of the aged were women; women seek medical and hospital care more than do men. Increasingly, older persons were forced to retire whether they wished to or not, thereby limiting their incomes severely. Not infrequently the combination of limited financial resources, increased medical needs, and aloneness have brought about the development of a vicious cycle wherein the older person delays obtaining necessary medical care, economizes on food, which in turn results in malnutrition, and thus has more medical problems, which require eventually more money.[19] From an actuarial viewpoint very few voluntary insurance companies or plans have shown interest in trying to solve the problems of the aged, and from an individual viewpoint only an exceedingly small proportion of the elderly can afford effective voluntary medical insurance. The situation was unequivocally expressed by Dr. Basil MacLean[20] as recently as 1960, when he retired as President of the Blue Cross Association, which had attempted to find some solution to the medical insurance needs of the aged. He stated the following:

A lifetime's experience has lead me at last to conclude that the cost of care of the aged cannot be met, unaided, by the mechanisms of insurance or prepayment as they exist today. The aged simply cannot afford to buy from any of these the scope of care that is required, nor do the stern competitive realities permit any carrier, whether non-profit or commercial, to provide benefits which are adequate at a price which is feasible for any but a small proportion of the aged.

It is interesting that, although 78% of the population is now covered by some form of medical and hospital insurance, only about 25% of the total expenditures for medical care is in the form of insurance payments. Furthermore, as Reed[21] has pointed out, a significant amount of health insurance is written by companies on an individual basis, a form of insurance that results in about one half of the premiums going to selling costs and overhead rather than to medical service. Similarly coverage by voluntary insurance has done nothing to prevent occasional excessively high medical fees or to effect economical hospital practice or to encourage sound hospital fiscal procedures.

The critical situation the nation was getting itself into was pointed out by Somers and Somers[22] in 1962, indicating the inability of insurance companies and private payment plans to provide in any adequate sense for the aged or other poor-risk groups. Presaging the events of the following few years, they observed that the atmosphere had become one of impending impasse and indecision—a clear reversal of the optimism and dynamism that had characterized private health insurance for several decades. They noted that this had led to various forms of public intervention already but that even here the problem had been found to be beyond the abilities of local and state governments alone to solve to any degree of satisfaction. Increasingly they noted that the public and local governments had been forced to look to the federal government for a solution.

Meanwhile, because of the lack of progress on the Wagner-Murray-Dingell Bill and the growing concern over the problems of the aged, Wilbur Cohen and I. S. Falk, who had drafted the preceding bills, decided on a more limited approach: a medical care plan for the aged that might possibly be acceptable. It took the form of a bill which was introduced in April 1952 by Senator Murray and Congressman Dingell to provide 60 days of hospital care each year as needed for all those on Social Security pensions. The number estimated to be eligible at that time was 7 million of the approximate 13 million people over 65 years of age. The financing would be by means of a slight increase in the Social Security assessments. Modest though it was, the bill was defeated, as it was again in 1953 and still later in 1955. The latter year, however, witnesses the merger of the American Federation of Labor and the Congress of Industrial Organization. This resulted in a single union with more than 16 million workers, the vast majority of whom not only had family members who voted but also who tended to be liberal. Promptly the AFL-CIO adopted health insurance for the elderly as a major concern. One of the union's key officials, in company with a representative of the Social Security Administration and Cohen and Falk, cooperated in the preparation of a new and much broader bill to provide medical care for Social Security beneficiaries. Not only did it cover hospitalization costs, but it also included costs of surgery and nursing home care. As had been true with all previous and subsequent bills, it was careful to allow for freedom of choice by both physician and patient. Again it was proposed that costs be financed by means of increasing the Social Security payments by employers and employees. Congressman Aimé Forand agreed to sponsor the bill and introduced it on August 27, 1957. Despite attempts to the contrary by the A.M.A., both the American Nurses' Association and the American Hospital Association endorsed the principle on which the bill was based. Hearings on the bill were held both in 1958 and 1959, but no legislation was forthcoming.

Growing concern, however, about the problems of chronic and degenerative diseases, especially among the older members of the population, caused the Senate Committee on Labor and Public Welfare to establish a Subcommittee on the Problems of the Aged and Aging. Senator McNamara was made chairman, and he proceeded to conduct public hearings in a number of cities throughout the nation. The attendance was considerable, and Senator McNamara followed a practice of first listening to experts and then making the microphone available to anyone in the audience. Large numbers of older citizens responded and told in dramatic form of their problems. It became quite apparent to the nation through these firsthand statements that, contrary to the avowals of the A.M.A., their needs were not being met. When the Subcommittee submitted its report to the Senate in February 1960, its first recommendation was that the Social Security program be expanded to include health service benefits for all persons eligible under the program. Congress now began to be deluged by letters concerning the Forand Bill, 2 to 1 in favor

of it. This forced the Ways and Means Committee of the House to vote on it, but it was defeated. By now various political writers referred to medical insurance for the elderly as the most critical political issue in the nation. Mail now overflowed the post offices of the House and Senate, 30 to 1 in favor of the Forand Bill. This forced its reconsideration. It also resulted in the Eisenhower Administration's finally presenting a bill of its own called the Medicare Program for the Aged. The name was borrowed from a previous measure that provided free medical care for dependents of servicemen. If viewed superficially, the administration bill seemed to go even further than the Forand Bill. However, when the various deductibles and exceptions were considered, very few elderly people could benefit much. As a result it received little support from any quarter. Nevertheless, it had a significance: It indicated that by this time both political parties manifested an obligation on the part of the federal government to somehow provide medical care for the indigent and elderly. Meanwhile the Forand Bill was again defeated in Committee.

Soon afterward the House passed a bill which had been introduced by Congressman Mills and provided for the federal government to make grants to states to provide medical care for the elderly poor. It was not, however, to be financed through the Social Security system. This was quickly followed by a bill in the Senate under the sponsorship of Senator Kerr, the intention of which was to assist the aged who were neither poor enough to be on welfare nor wealthy enough to pay their own medical expenses. Again financing would be by federal grants matching state expenditures. Wilbur Cohen, who drafted the bill for Kerr, adroitly included in it much of the intent of Congressman Mills' bill. It passed both houses with little opposition, and in mid-September 1960 the President signed what became known as the Kerr-Mills Act. It lacked many things. It was estimated that actually only about 2 million people would be assisted by it. Interestingly, while the A.M.A. did not oppose it apparently on the basis of the lesser of two evils, it included many principles to which that organization had been objecting over the years. It consisted of two parts: (1) extension of the Old-Age Assistance Program which had originated with the 1935 Social Security Act; the limit of federal participation was increased from $65 per person per month to $77 and later to $85, and (2) a new section known as the Medical Assistance for the Aged Program; the intent of this was to provide medical expenses for elderly citizens who previously were ineligible for aid, in other words the so-called medically indigent who were over 65 years of age and who, while not on relief, could not meet the cost of medical services. The legislation placed no ceiling on federal support for this part of the act, the federal government paying a flat percentage of total outlays ranging from 50% for high-income states to 80% for poorer states. It was entirely up to the states to determine whether they wished to participate in the program. Furthermore, individual states could set not only their own income limits and deductibles but also all the conditions for the provision of care. The overall result was that many states did not elect to participate in the Kerr-Mills Act and the conditions established by those that did presented all possible variations. While the A.M.A. during the next several years spent large sums of money to try to convince everyone that the Kerr-Mills program was actually meeting the needs, it became apparent very shortly that this was not the case.

When Senator John Kennedy became President-elect, he let it be known that one of the first items on the agenda for his administration would be the enactment of a health insurance bill for the aged. Shortly after he took office, Representative King and Senator Anderson served as co-sponsors of what became known as the Medicare Bill. Its provisions were extensive, and again it was proposed to be financed by an increase in Social Security assessments. It called forth the usual and expected accusations and cries of alarm from the A.M.A., which promptly established the American Medical Political Action Committee in order to raise several million dollars with which to fight it. The bill had a great deal of support however, not only from the public but also from organizations such as the National Council of Churches, the Y.W.C.A., the American Nurses' Association, the American Hospital Association, and the American Public Health Association. In addition, a number of groups of physicians in several places in the nation disassociated themselves from the A.M.A. in order to form endorsing groups. Despite this the bill was defeated in the Senate by a close vote. It was reintroduced in 1963 at President Kennedy's request, but his assassination brought hearings on the matter to a halt. As eventual successor to the Presidency, the then Senator Lyndon Johnson had already made clear his support of the Medicare idea. Hearings on the bill in the Ways and Means Committee of the House were begun again; but progress was very slow. In the Senate the Social Security Act was the subject for amendment, and in the face of many obstacles the Medicare concept was attached to the bill that eventually was passed by the Senate only to be held up in the Conference Committee by the representatives of the House.

After election in his own right, when President Johnson gave his State of the Union address on January 4, 1965, at the opening of the Eighty-ninth Congress, he called for action on a Medicare Bill as the first order of business. Senator Anderson introduced S. 1, and Representative King introduced H.R. 1—identical bills very similar to those they had introduced in the previous Congress. In short order a number of other bills were introduced, among them one by Representative Byrnes which provided for subsidies to pay for private health insurance policies and one to expand and liberalize the Kerr-Mills Act. To the surprise of everyone Representative Mills, as Chairman of the Ways and Means Committee of the House, suddenly resolved the problem by deciding on a meld of the King-Anderson Bills, the bill to expand and liberalize the Kerr-Mills Act, and Representative Byrnes' bill. As

tern, one that first became very clear in Germany. Increased industrialization creates the need, be cause it increases the social insecurity of growing numbers of the population. A second factor is found in the phenomenon that under the pressure of industrialization the working class organized into militant political parties that present a threat to the existing order. This was the case in Germany when the Social Democratic Party was founded in 1869 by Bebel and Liebknecht; in 1875 it absorbed the conservative Lassalle group. The Paris Commune of 1871 created a great scare in all conservative circles of Europe because it showed that socialism was not a parlor philosophy but might well become a tangible reality. A conservative statesman, Bismarck stepped in and with social insurance created a corrective mechanism to the system that he wished to perpetuate.

The very same pattern can be traced in England, the next large country that enacted national social insurance in the beginning of our century. At that time the impact of the second industrial revolution was being felt. The number of wage earners increased as a result of it and so did their insecurity. In 1900 the Independent Labor Party, the Fabian Society, and the Trade Unions joined to organize the Labor Party, which was in no way revolutionary but nevertheless had great potentialities in a highly industrialized country. In the election of 1906 the Labor Party won 29 seats and England changed from a two-party country to a three-party country. The Russian Revolution of 1905 broke down as the Paris Commune had done thirty-five years before, but it again reminded conservative groups that socialism was not dead. Lloyd George and Winston Churchill began to promote social legislation, culminating in the National Insurance Act of 1911, which included sickness and unemployment benefits. Like the German system, it had all the weaknesses of a compromise, was not comprehensive enough, and suffered from a considerable lack of uniformity, as it had to take into account the vested interests of a great number of private benefit societies and insurance companies.

World War I created a new and very strong stimulus to the enactment of social legislation. It was the first war in which the industrial potential of a group of countries proved to be the decisive factor. Industrialization was intensified in every warring country and the Russian Revolution of 1917 created a totally new situation. Not only France, but a number of other countries adopted systems of health insurance, and it was recognized that no nation could enjoy the benefits of industrialization without providing a corrective mechanism for the hardships and insecurity it created. This became particularly apparent during the protracted economic depression that followed the crisis of 1929 when all over the Western world millions of people were unemployed. At that time social insurance bills were introduced increasingly in the American republics. Chile introduced health insurance as early as 1924, and by 1942 nine Central and South American countries had some form of health insurance. In the United States, following the National Health Conference of 1938, various bills were introduced into Congress that had the purpose of completing the social security legislation of the Roosevelt era by developing a national health program that would include health insurance. So far no bill has been passed, but the need remains and some solution will have to be found because the attitude of medicine to society has changed and the view is generally accepted that in a civilized commonwealth the benefits of medical science should be available to all people.

REFERENCES

1. Shryock, R. H. In Galdston, I., editor: Social medicine, New York, 1949, Commonwealth Fund.
2. Sand, R.: Health and human progress, New York, 1936, The Macmillan Co.
3. Buhrman, H. M. F.: Leaves from a doctor's notebook of seventy years ago, Milit. Surgeon **86:**547, June 1940.
4. Robinson, G. C.: The patient as a person, New York, 1939, Commonwealth Fund.
5. Current population reports, Series P-60, No. 51, Jan. 1967, Consumer Income, Bureau of the Census, U. S. Department of Commerce.
6. Physicians for a growing America. Report of Surgeon General's Consultation Group on Medical Education, Washington, 1959, Public Health Service Pub. No. 709.
7. Collins, S. D., Lehmann, J. L., and Trantham, K. S.: Major causes of illness of various severities and major causes of death in six age periods of life, Washington, 1955, Public Health Service Pub. No. 440.
8. Collins, S. D., Lehmann, J. L., and Trantham, K. S.: Surgical experience in selected areas of United States, Washington, 1956, Public Health Service Pub. No. 473.
9. Rosen, G.: Provision of medical care—history, sociology, innovation, Public Health Rep. **74:** 199, Mar. 1959.
10. Rosen, G.: In Galdston, I., editor: Social medicine, New York, 1949, Commonwealth Fund.
11. Editorial: J.A.M.A. **139:**529, 1949.
12. Evang, K.: Medical care in Europe, Amer. J. Public Health **48:**427, Apr. 1958.
13. Davis, M. M.: Public medical services, Chicago, 1937, University of Chicago Press.
14. Editorial: Tax-supported medical care of the needy, Amer. J. Public Health **42:**1314, Oct. 1952.
15. Anderson, O. W.: Compulsory medical care insurance, 1910-1950, Ann. Amer. Acad. Polit. and Social Sci. **273:**106, Jan. 1951; also in Committee on Medical Care Teaching of the Association of Teachers of Preventive Medicine: Readings in medical care, Chapel Hill, 1958, University of North Carolina Press.
16. Falk, I. S.: The committee on the costs of medical care—25 years of progress, Amer. J. Public Health **48:**979, Aug. 1958.
17. Editorial: J.A.M.A. **99:**1952, Dec. 3, 1932.

18. Med. World News, Mar. 26, 1965.
19. The aged and aging in the United States: a national problem. A report of the Subcommittee on the Problems of the Aged and Aging to the Senate Committee on Labor and Public Welfare, Washington, 1960, U. S. Government Printing Office.
20. Somers, H. M., and Somers, A. R.: Doctors, patients, and health insurance, Washington, 1961, The Brookings Institution.
21. Reed, L. S.: Group payment since the Committee on the Costs of Medical Care, Amer. J. Public Health **48**:992, Aug. 1958.
22. Somers, H. M., and Somers, A. R.: The paradox of medical progress, New Eng. J. Med. **226**(24):1253, June 14, 1962.
23. Galdston, I., editor: Social medicine, New York, 1949, Commonwealth Fund.

Chapter 26

Rehabilitation

INTRODUCTION

It is only relatively recently that the concept of community responsibility for the consequences of so-called acts of God, chance, and Mars has become a reality. One has to turn back but few pages in human history to find an attitude of rather complete social irresponsibility even for disabled veterans who were accorded their day of acclaim, followed by a bitter lifetime as dependents or outcasts. Recent years, however, have brought increasing discussion of the problems of the handicapped and what might be done to make their lives personally more satisfying and economically more fruitful. It is only in the past few decades that the disabled began to be considered as fellow human beings, subject as any other to sensitivity, pride, and ambition, and as potential social and economic assets rather than liabilities.

On arriving at this point there developed the problem of the definition of a handicap or a handicapped person. Adequate definition, of course, is fundamental to the determination and conduct of a comprehensive and satisfactory program of rehabilitation. As might be expected, attention and effort were focused first upon the visibly most obvious physical defects, i.e., the traditional lame, halt, and blind. Gradually other physical handicaps began to receive attention in the public consciousness. Tuberculosis was established as an etiologic entity, and its physiopathology became understood. In the absence of other means, intensive rest and supportive care were instituted as a cure. Eventually it became evident that it was difficult to determine where cure ended and rehabilitation began. At

any rate, high relapse rates soon emphasized the importance of rehabilitation, at least in this and a few other diseases. Such circumstances provoked further reconsideration and redefinition. There resulted a realization that there also existed such conditions as mental, emotional, psychologic, or personality crippling which might be just as devastating to the individual and as costly to society as a physical defect. In addition, it has come to be appreciated that mental or psychologic handicaps and physical handicaps are frequently related. As a result the present trend is to look upon rehabilitation in very broad terms, as a need applicable to practically all types of ills and of as much concern to society as to the individual.

SOURCE OF THE PROBLEM

There are many reasons why the field of rehabilitation should command attention at this time. For a long period it was ignored or overlooked because of the magnitude of other problems, many of which have been eliminated or abated, thereby allowing more time and effort for attention to other things. With the development of practical social and medical tools there occurred a movement away from the complacent fatalistic attitude that there were many conditions for which nothing could be done. The results of examinations for eligibility in the armed forces at the beginning of World War II came as a shock to most people and spotlighted the enormous numbers of ills, mostly chronic, among the supposedly most healthy segment of our population. Despite our high standard of living, it was found that 40%

of men called up for possible military service had to be rejected because they could not meet standard requirements. At the same time, because of ensuing manpower shortage it became necessary to draw upon the reservoir of disabled persons who were not eligible for the armed services. This brought out the surprising fact that many of all types of handicapped persons were capable of making very significant social and economic contributions if they were given an opportunity to readjust themselves and their disability to the demands of working and living situations. In other words the rehabilitation needs of the nation and its communities represented a vast but diffuse frontier of preventive, therapeutic, and promotive medicine and community action which was waiting to be discovered.

Beyond this, however, is the fact that the number and proportion of disabled persons have increased considerably in recent years. Our society has become more keyed up, more centralized, more industrialized, more complex, and faster moving, with an accompanying increase in accidents, cardiac and hypertensive disease, and mental illness. Recent wars have involved increasing numbers of people and have been more devastating, directly and indirectly, to the people on both the battle and the home fronts. Crippling diseases such as multiple sclerosis and, until recently, poliomyelitis, have increased. Finally, and despite the foregoing, the average life-span has increased remarkably during the past half-century. As a result our population has been aging, with many more people reaching advanced years with accumulations of handicapping effects of chronic diseases, many of which had their origins in preventable illnesses which occurred earlier in life. While all these events and changes were occurring, certain sociologic and cultural changes were coming about. Especially pertinent was society's gradual assumption of the responsibility for doing something about the needs and problems of the handicapped, which heretofore were considered to be essentially private burdens, responsibilities of the individual and his family. In the presence of such a vast vacuum, assistance to individuals began to be given by the many voluntary and philanthropic agencies which sprang up, often on the basis of very personal motivations. In recent years, however, governmental agencies have gradually entered more and more into the picture.

These various events and revelations necessitated the reexamination of existing concepts of physical fitness, disability, and rehabilitation. It has been realized that the term "physical fitness" must refer not only to the physical ability and endurance of the military man in combat but also to the ability of the worker and the family breadwinner to perform productive and continuous work. It is a term which is key to the correct understanding of the whole problem of the crippled and disabled. False concepts of physical fitness have had an important influence on our social, economic, industrial, and military life. Fitness, disability, and rehabilitation are now recognized to be terms with many political and economic implications. Vague and unsatisfactory standards and definitions have often been created, sometimes by law, which have in effect branded those with physical or psychologic defects as unproductive and socially useless and have committed them to the bleak outlook of permanent dependency.

Numerous attempts have been made to describe and define the field of rehabilitation. Rusk[1] referred to it as the third phase of medicine, saying:

> We now talk about the third phase of medical care, the first being obviously prevention, the second, definitive medicine and surgery, and the third that phase between the bed and the job, what you do after the fever is down and the stitches are out to allow the chronically ill or the physically disabled person to live a self-supporting, self-respecting life with dignity.

Sensenich[2] viewed the field in terms of what should be done:

> The problem of rehabilitation of an individual involves a twofold effort—on the one hand, to lessen and minimize through medical treatment his physical handicap, and on the other, to help the individual develop his strength and his abilities so that he is better equipped to meet and live on comfor

able terms with the physically able of the community.

Another definition, succinct but useful, was developed by a group[3] who studied the field:

Rehabilitation is the process of assisting the individual with a handicap to realize his potentialities and goals, physically, mentally, socially and economically.

MAGNITUDE OF THE PROBLEM

One strange aspect of the problem of the disabled is that the reaction of the public often appears to be that of seeing but not comprehending. This is to say that, while in the majority of instances the disabled are visually very much in evidence, the public tends not to react by grasping the total significance to society of the implications of vast numbers of disabled individuals. Perhaps the reason is that to many the thought of disability is unpleasant, so they thrust it out of their consciousness. Yet even a cursory analysis indicates forcefully the great magnitude of the problem and the enormous economic loss to society which it entails.

In terms of impact upon the public mind probably the most effective picture of national disability resulted from the National Health Survey of 1935-1936.[4] Information was secured on illnesses that were present during the preceding 12 months in a sample of 800,000 families in 83 cities and 23 rural areas of 19 states. From the findings, which had been demonstrated to be reliable, the following national estimates were developed[5]:

1. 4.4% were disabled on the day of the survey visit
2. 1.2% were disabled the entire preceding twelve months
3. 17.7% were reported as having a chronic disease or impairment
4. 1.1% of workers (15 to 64 years of age) were reported to be "unemployable" by reason of disability

Not long afterward the nation became involved in World War II, and large numbers of young men were examined for military service. As previously mentioned, the nation was shocked by the high proportion

with defects and in need of rehabilitation. Since the war ended, other surveys have been conducted, in February 1949 and in September 1950,[6] followed later by the National Health Survey, which began in 1957 and is continuing through the 1960's. These surveys have all reported on the number of persons between 14 and 64 years of age who were unable to carry on their usual activities because of some illness or other medical condition. The figures vary from about 3.6 million to about 5 million. Most of the variation is due to disabilities of short duration, 1 month or less, many of which are probably seasonal. On the other hand, the incidence of disabilities of 3 or more months' duration was generally similar in each of the various surveys.

In 1948, Rusk and Taylor[7] prepared a concise summary of the extent of the problem based upon a review of recent literature. They reported about 2.6 million persons with orthopedic impairments of which 341,000 were incapacitating; approximately 900,000 amputees, almost one half of which were major; almost 400,000 registered crippled children; an estimated 336,000 persons with cerebral palsy; and somewhere between 500,000 and 1.5 million cases of epilepsy. Among additional impairments they called attention to between 9 million and 10 million persons suffering from diseases of the heart and arteries; an estimated 2 million diabetics; approximately 300,000 clinically significant, active cases of tuberculosis plus 150,000 convalescents who would benefit from rehabilitation services; an estimated 2.4 million persons in need of hearing aids, only one third of whom have them; and about 230,000 blind. These figures substantiated the statement that 88% of all disabilities were due to disease, 10% to accidents, and 2% to congenital conditions.[8]

A few years later, with specific reference to children, Lesser and Hunt[9] called attention to 500,000 under 18 years of age who suffered from rheumatic fever or its effects; about 64,000 with cleft palate or cleft lip or both; at least 60,000 with visual handicaps so serious as to need special educational help (with facilities at the time for only 8,000); from one-quarter to one-half million children with serious hearing loss; and about 1.5 million children between 5 and 20 years of age with speech handicaps unrelated to hearing, cerebral palsy, or cleft lip or palate, of which about one half were functionally serious. An analysis[10] of those served by crippled children's programs in 1964 throughout the United States showed 276,297 children with only one condition and 55,274 with multiple conditions in need of rehabilitation. Overall there were 5.9 conditions requiring rehabilitation per 1,000 children under 21 years of age. The conditions for which children received rehabilitation services were as follows:

1. Congenital malformations — 27.3%
2. Diseases of bones and organs of movement, excluding congenital malformations — 18.1%
3. Cerebral palsy — 8.4%
4. Poliomyelitis — 6.8%
5. Diseases of the ears and mastoid processes — 6.1%
6. Diseases and conditions of the eyes — 5.7%
7. Accidents, poisoning, and violence — 4.5%
8. Diseases of nervous system and sense organs (excluding 3, 5, and 6) — 3.3%
9. Rheumatic fever and heart disease — 3.2%
10. Other disorders — 9.8%
11. Provisional or deferred diagnoses — 6.8%

Disability related to military service is dramatic and tends to attract attention more readily than handicaps from other sources. However, it is important to realize that they constitute only a minor proportion of the problem. During World War II there occurred about 17,000 amputations in the United States Army. During the same period there were 120,000 major amputations in the civilian population attributable to disease and accidents. It has been estimated that there are about 2 million civilian men and women of working age in the United States so severely disabled by physical or mental impairments that they cannot support themselves or their families. Furthermore, the total number of disabilities grows at the rate of about 250,000 per year because of accidents, illness, or congenital causes.[11]

Table 26-1. Medical reasons for Selective Service rejection, 1953-1958*

Diagnostic category	Prevalence per 1,000 examinees
Disorders of bones and organs of movement	25.4
Psychiatric disorders	21.1
Diseases of circulatory system	19.1
Eye diseases and defects	18.3
Anthropometric reasons (mostly obesity)	11.5
Diseases and defects of ear and mastoid	10.0
Diseases of digestive system	9.2
Allergic disorders	8.6
Infective and parasitic diseases	7.1
Neurologic diseases	7.1
Congenital defects	6.2
All other reasons	25.1
Total	168.7

*Karpinos, B. D.: Qualification of American youths for military service, Washington, 1962, Medical Statistics Division, Office of the Surgeon General, Department of the Army.

An indication of the prevalence by age of various disabilities is presented in Fig. 26-1, which presents selected data from the current National Health Survey.[12] As still another indication of the need for rehabilitative services are the results of more recent selective service examinations of young men between 1953 and 1958 (Table 26-1). A current summarization[13] is that about 28 million people in the United States have some degree of disability. This represents about 1 in 6 of the population. More than 17 million of them are limited in their activity as workers, students, or housewives by chronic conditions. Almost 5 million are confined to their homes and cannot move about freely or have trouble doing so without assistance. Beyond this it is estimated that more than 2 million need and would profit from vocational rehabilitation services.[14]

ECONOMICS OF THE PROBLEM

Certain general economic aspects of illness and death were discussed in Chapter 25. It may be pertinent to add here some comments on the economic implications of disability and what may be gained by re-

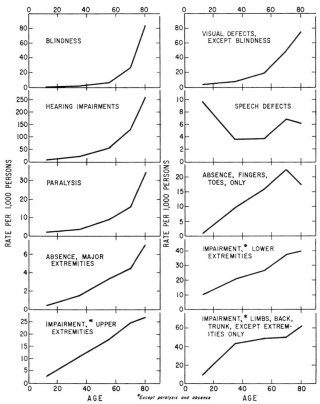

Fig. 26-1. Impairments per 1,000 persons by type and age, United States, 1958. (From Health statistics, Public Health Service Pub. No. 584-B9, Apr. 1959, p. 3.)

habilitation efforts. Society pays in many ways for its failure to prevent and to care for disabilities among its constituents. A few of the more obvious ways are through insurance payments and therefore higher rates, wage losses, production losses, employees' disability compensation, and a significant part of the relief load. Considering the labor force alone, estimated at about 75 million people fully employed, the loss due to compensable disability during 1 year approximates $4.5 billion. Add to this the production loss of about twice the lost wages and the total is a staggering $13.5 billion per year. It must be recognized, of course, that much of this loss is due to temporary, self-eliminating disability and that it is dependent upon fluctuating employment opportunities, strikes,

and similar factors. However, a great deal of it represents, without question, needless and stupid loss.[15] With reference to those between 15 and 54 years who have never worked due to severe chronic physical or mental disabilities, Allan,[14] using 1 million as the lower end of their estimated number, calculated a possible economic contribution. If only one half could be partially rehabilitated to a point where they could earn only $35 per week, they would add over $900 million to the purchasing power of the nation.

To approach the premise from the positive direction, the results of some of the limited efforts at rehabilitation of the handicapped are available. During 1948 successful rehabilitation services were made available under joint federal-state sponsorship to 53,000 persons.[16] Of these, 13% had never been employed, and an additional 74% were not employed when they began rehabilitation; 7.7% had been in or eventually entered professional or semiprofessional work; 37% in managerial, clerical, sales, or service activities; 7.9% in agriculture; 30.9% in skilled or semiskilled work; 9.3% in unskilled work; and 7.2% in family work or housewifery. Many had been on public assistance at a cost of $400 to $700 per year as compared with an average cost for rehabilitation of $460 per case— a single rather than an annually recurring expenditure. Their average annual wage after rehabilitation was $1,623 in contrast with $321 before. This small group of 53,000 persons rehabilitated in 1948 increased the national purchasing power by $69 million and paid over $5 million in federal income taxes in addition to state and local taxes. It has been shown that for every dollar spent by the federal government on rehabilitation, the average rehabilitated person will eventually pay $10 in federal income tax. This is based on the rate of earnings at completion of rehabilitation and on employment for only 85% of the individual's work life expectancy.

An analysis of handicapped people rehabilitated during 1955 showed that they have since increased their earnings from $15 million to $105 million per year and have added more than 100 million man-hours to the nation's productive effort. Almost 20% or about 11,000 of those rehabilitated had been receiving public assistance which amounted to $11 million annually. These rehabilitated persons are now paying about $8.5 million each year in federal taxes. At this rate within 3 years they will have repaid the total investment of $25 million made in them. In terms of their working life expectancy, it may be considered that, on the average, they will pay $10 in federal income taxes for each dollar spent for their rehabilitation.[17] During 1959 state vocational rehabilitation agencies assisted 80,739 persons. Before rehabilitation their median annual wage was a mere $464 or a total of $61.4 million. After rehabilitation their median annual

wage had increased to $2,292 and the total yearly earnings to $157.3 million.[18] It is estimated that within 4 years the cost of their rehabilitation will be repaid in taxes. Beyond this, of course, they and their communities will be spared the cost and the indignity of welfare existence.

Employment of handicapped workers, therefore, is far from a charitable proposition. It has been shown[19] that many of the physically or mentally handicapped are able to perform efficiently about 3,500 different jobs or tasks and in general have better volume of production, higher attendance rates, better safety records, and better stability and dependability than nonhandicapped workers.

PROGRAM NEEDS AND GOALS

Many communities already have many rehabilitation services available for their handicapped citizens. Most of these, however, are scattered throughout many public and private agencies and often are unrelated. They have developed as part of the communitywide social services, beginning usually as isolated entities, e.g., as programs for special handicaps or diseases or as services to particular age groups. As might be expected, more often than not a state of confusion in the field of rehabilitation, with some difficulty and inefficiency and a lack of services for certain types of cases or individuals, has resulted. Thus in one large city where the problem was studied preparatory to efforts toward coordination there were 37 agencies which were significantly active in some phase or other of rehabilitation. This did not include the various businessmen's service clubs or many of the church groups.

Rehabilitation is actually a complex of many component parts of which the physical or medical aspects of the handicap is only one phase. The individual's emotional acceptance or rejection of the handicap must be taken into account and treated, and his home and job environment, his mental attitude, his vocational skills, aptitudes, and training must also be considered. Attention must be given to all of these and other factors on a coordinated interrelated basis with respect to the total individual in order that he might become self-reliant and fill a useful place in society.

This philosophy requires a unified approach if it is to serve adequately the needs of all types of handicapped persons. It is just as important for the restoration of a patient with multiple sclerosis as for a double amputee. It applies equally to the less severely and to the more severely handicapped. It brings all the skills of a number of professions to bear upon a common effort to restore the individual to a position of maximum usefulness and satisfaction in his society. It places each phase of the approach in its proper relationship to every other phase of treatment or education. The development of this philosophy is so recent that not many really adequate centers have yet been established. Some, such as those at the Bellevue Institute of Rehabilitation and Physical Medicine, the Cleveland Rehabilitation Center, the Detroit Rehabilitation Institute, and the District of Columbia Hospital, provide excellent comprehensive rehabilitative care on an in- and outpatient basis. By following this approach of broad training for self-care, these institutions have conclusively demonstrated the achievement of considerable economies in addition to far more successful patient care. Thus during the year prior to the formation of the department of rehabilitation of the District of Columbia Hospital, orthopedic patients spent an average of 55 days in the hospital. After the new program was instituted, the hospital stay of similar patients was reduced to 33 days, a saving of $122,000 for orthopedic patients alone.[20]

The challenge that faces at least the moderate to larger sized communities was indicated by Taylor[21] in a study he carried out in one of the major cities. He concluded as follows:

The greatest need . . . is the development of a single large center with sufficient staff and facilities to furnish rehabilitation services to all persons with physical disabilities regardless of the medical condition which has caused those disabilities.

He suggests that patients be referred to this community rehabilitation center from any physician, whether in private practice, industry, public agency, or elsewhere, and that the primary medical responsibility for the patient should remain with the referring physician. Following evaluation, if the patient is accepted, the medical director of the center could assume the primary responsibility for the prescription and supervision of the physical medicine and rehabilitation services only. Such a procedure is similar to that customarily followed in the referral of patients for specialized care in other areas of medicine. A center of this type should have facilities for inpatients as well as outpatients. In fact, Taylor suggests that eventually a large proportion of the hospital beds in a city might gradually be allocated for convalescents and patients being rehabilitated, up to a level of 1 bed for each 1,000 of the population. This could be accomplished, at least in part, by the decreasing need for beds for communicable diseases and as a result of shortened hospital stays for many conditions.

The community rehabilitation center should operate under the leadership of a physician whose training qualifies him for certification by the American Board of Physical Medicine. The Baruch Committee on Physical Medicine recommends the organization of such a center under two primary divisions, i.e., a medical services division and a vocational services division. The medical services division should include a physical medicine branch with an occupational therapy section, a physical therapy section, and a physical education section; and a psychosocial branch with a clinical psychologic section and a social service section. The second of the primary divisions, that dealing with vocational services, should provide branches for vocational testing and guidance and for special education. In addition, in order to meet the graded needs of various degrees of disability, the vocational services division should conduct a sheltered workshop program, a curative workshop program, and a homebound program.

Sponsorship and support should be looked upon, especially at this stage, as variable. In many communities the reha-bilitation center may undoubtedly begin as a result of the initiative of a forward-looking public health agency in focusing attention on the total problem, drawing together all interested groups and perhaps providing the basic care of the center to which the others may make additions. There are few fields in which it is as easy to contemplate true community-wide inter-est and action involving public agencies, voluntary agencies, industry and labor. It should be realized, however, that there is no single pattern that will be acceptable and successful everywhere. In the absence of a community rehabilitation center a few communities have developed central rehabilitation diagnosis and referral cen-ters. This has usually been done under the sponsorship of health and welfare councils. The purposes are to provide preliminary screening and diagnosis, sometimes elemen-tary therapy, social service, and referral and follow-up. Other aims are to ensure that the patient neither gets lost among the several agencies that may contribute to his rehabilitation nor gets captured by any single one. The best of these agencies have multidisciplinary staffs available for the consideration of the various aspects of the patient's problem.

Commendable rehabilitation centers have been instituted and operated exclu-sively by voluntary agencies, industrial concerns, insurance companies, and labor unions. The goal of course should be a truly cooperative well-integrated and com-prehensive program which serves all com-ponents of the community and for which all parts of the community have a re-sponsibility and concern. It is in this re-gard that the official public health agency can bring into play its important role of catalyst. If many public health workers have not considered it, workers in other fields have. After considering the many community agencies interested in the hand-icapped, the director of a prominent vol-untary agency[22] commented:

Some place major responsibility for leadership in community organization for rehabilitation on the hospital-medical school, others on the Bureau of Vocational Rehabilitation. The Health Department might logically be asked to exhibit leadership· even in an area of health concern where its current ser-vices are minor. A more realistic approach would seem to be one of accepting leadership where one finds it. This jibes with the nature of rehabilitation, a drawn-out process which uses many professional skills as it shifts emphasis from the original medi-cal to the later vocational aspects.

In a somewhat similar vein, Notkin[23] states as follows:

In recent years, vocational rehabilitation and public health groups have been widely expounding both their ideas and the scope of their operations. Although autonomous operation is probably still desirable at this stage of progress, it may be wise to start thinking of vocational rehabilitation as part of the broader concept of public health which is prevalent today.

So it would appear that here is a public service frontier calling for effective coor-dinating leadership which some people outside of the field believe might well be provided by a community's official health agency. Whether this frontier will be de-veloped or lost by default will be interest-ing to watch and will be of intimate con-cern to many thousands of disabled persons who are waiting for an opportunity to live their lives properly.

REHABILITATION PROGRAM CONTENT

For its part the American Public Health Association has expressed concern with the disparity between the high degrees of ex-isting rehabilitative skills and the custo-mary level of their application to those in need of them. It feels that rehabilitation should be everyone's concern, command-ing the concentrated efforts not only of the public health field but all other major professional health and related groups.[24] With this in mind its Program Area Committee on Chronic Disease and Re-habilitation has enunciated the following general principles as a basis for a more effective national rehabilitation philos-ophy[25]:

    I. **Local, regional, state, and national legislation and program planning should embrace all the disabled.**
        Planning should be comprehensive in scope, embracing all categories of disa-bility, all degrees of disability. It is recog-

nized that rehabilitation work may be done by categories, special groups, and by priorities.

The skills, services, and facilities needed for independent living or for decreasing the disability of the chronically ill of all ages are very similar to those needed for rehabilitation of persons with foreseeable vocational goals. These include medical, psychological, and social (including educational and vocational) evaluations and a combined overall evaluation of these reports to determine a suitable goal for each disabled person.

II. Significant data needed for planning.

It is necessary to determine more accurately the nature and extent of disability in the population so that the scope of the problem can be appreciated and the magnitude of the measures needed may be foreseen. Resources for rehabilitation must be evaluated in each community and their actual availability to persons needing them documented.

III. Services must be centered on the individual and his family, and all aspects of a given individual's disabilities and capabilities must be considered.

Failure to look at any one individual's total situation—whether it be the medical, social, psychological, educational, environmental, or vocational facet—may allow an apparently reasonable program to proceed to the point at which all the efforts may have to be abandoned or reconstructed because of failure to reckon with limitations, lack of job opportunity, and so on. Individual-centered services also require the availability of comprehensive services. Particularly in smaller communities it is most unlikely that one disability can be planned for and serviced satisfactorily by itself. Characteristically the chronically ill suffer from multiple disabilities. . . . The categorical appeal for funding and for educational efforts may have to be continued or strengthened, but the categorical approach should not necessarily apply to the rendering of service to individuals.

IV. Services must be provided early in the course, or in anticipation, of disability.

Early provision of services is a self-evident approach to avoidance of disability induced by prolonged bed rest or altered functions. It also serves to minimize psychological, social, and work pattern changes due to unnecessarily prolonged disuse, disability, and displacement. It avoids social and psychological dependency through unnecessary impoverishment of contact and feelings of productivity.

V. Specific services must be under the appropriate responsible skill.

Rehabilitation, involving a continuum and a variety of services and professional skills, requires careful teamwork and careful direction in order to insure the earliest and most effective result. In any phase, the decision as to the most desirable supervision must be based on the professional area of the patient's paramount problem at that time.

VI. Recognition and mutual respect for the contribution of the various disciplines and public and private agencies that participate in this problem are essential.

The three major national groups currently showing concern are health, vocational rehabilitation and social welfare. They have approached the field of rehabilitation from different viewpoints of their disciplines over the years. . . . For any one individual, no matter what his basic disability, both the medical and social-vocational skills are involved and innumerable other skills may be. The provision of rehabilitation services should not be the competitive, but rather the coordinated, use of the various services or skills, depending on the kind of rehabilitation problem involved.

VII. Rehabilitation is such a large field that many agencies must share the responsibilities, for it is unlikely that any one agency can or will be given the authority to encompass all of the activities concerned.

It is unreasonable to expect that all aspects of rehabilitation and all skills involved in the rehabilitation effort can or need be centered in one agency—be it voluntary or official. . . . The job is so huge that many agencies will be concerned, and many have already officially been given responsibility for different segments of the problem. . . . All agencies that have designated responsibility must develop their area of responsibility so their professed deeds are competently performed. When gaps appear at the local level in providing services to the individual, one of these agencies or even a new one may have to be created to fill this gap.

VIII. Location, administration, and responsibility for rehabilitation services.

If services are to be quantitatively and qualitatively adequate, responsibility must be clearly assigned. At least three levels of organizational pattern—national, state, and local—must be considered, whether the responsibility for services is to be governmental, voluntary, or professional. Local communities are where people live, and in so far as possible the community should provide the services required for rehabilitation of their citizens. . . . Some highly specialized or more expensive services may require support or even administration at the regional, state, or national level. . . . State and local organizations should also be responsible for providing consultation to help establish quality standards and to help the evaluation of locally provided services. . . . National responsibilities include appropriate financial support for other levels, recommendations relating to service standards, the provision of nationwide channels of communication and exchange of ideas, and the major burden of research, professional training, and establishment of facilities.

REFERENCES

1. Rusk, H. A.: America's number one medical problem, Proceedings of the Forty-Second Annual Meeting of Life Insurance Association of America, Dec. 9, 1948.
2. Sensenich, H.: Team work in rehabilitation, Amer. J. Public Health 40:969, Aug. 1950.
3. Van Riper, H. E.: Rehabilitation interests of a voluntary agency, Amer. J. Public Health 44:744, June 1954.
4. The National Health Survey, list of publications, Public Health Rep. 57:834, May 29, 1942.
5. Britten, R. H., Collins, S. D., and Fitzgerald, J. S.: The National Health Survey, Some general findings as to diseases, accidents and impairments in urban areas, Public Health Rep. 55:444, Mar. 15, 1940.
6. Woolsey, T. D.: Estimates of disabling illness prevalence in the United States, Washington, 1952, Public Health Service Pub. No. 181.
7. Rusk, H. A., and Taylor, E. J.: Physical disability: A national problem, Amer. J. Public Health 38:1381, Oct. 1948.
8. Hearings before Subcommittee on Health of the Committee on Labor and Public Welfare, U. S. Senate, Eighty-Third Congress, Second Session, on "President's Health Recommendations and Related Measures," Mar. 30, 1954.
9. Lesser, A. J., and Hunt, E. P.: The nation's handicapped children, Amer. J. Public Health 44:166, Feb. 1954.
10. Crippled children's program: Statistical highlights, 1964, Washington, 1966, Children's Bureau.
11. Number of disabled persons in need of vocational rehabilitation, Washington, 1954, Rehabilitation Service Series No. 274, Office of Vocational Rehabilitation.
12. Health statistics, Impairments by type, sex and age, Public Health Service Bull. No. 584-B9, Apr. 1959.
13. National Health Survey, Series B-11, Washington, July 1959, Public Health Service.
14. Allan, W. S.: Rehabilitation, a community challenge, New York, 1958, John Wiley & Sons, Inc.
15. Strow, C. W.: The extent and economic cost of disability, Research Council for Economic Security, Chicago, 1947, Pub. No. 23.
16. Brass tacks, Office of Vocational Rehabilitation, Washington, June 1949.
17. Annual Report—1955, Washington, 1957, U. S. Department of Health, Education, and Welfare.
18. Health, education and welfare trends, Washington, 1961, U. S. Department of Health, Education, and Welfare.
19. Editorial: Public health workers and rehabilitation, Amer. J. Public Health 38:1455, Oct. 1948.
20. Rusk, H. A.: Rehabilitation in the hospital, Public Health Rep. 68:281, Mar. 1953.
21. Taylor, E. J.: Unpublished study, 1950, Health Council of the Council of Social Agencies of Metropolitan Detroit.
22. Wenkert, W.: Community planning for rehabilitation, Amer. J. Public Health 42:782, July 1952.
23. Notkin, H.: Vocational rehabilitation and public health, Amer. J. Public Health 41:1100, Sept. 1951.
24. American Public Health Association: Chronic disease and rehabilitation—a program guide for state and local health agencies, New York, 1960, The Association.
25. Rehabilitation—everyone's concern. Report of Program Area Committee on Chronic Disease and Rehabilitation of the American Public Health Association, Amer. J. Public Health 53:294, Feb. 1963.

Chapter 27

Environmental control*

INTRODUCTION

Activities aimed at the preservation and improvement of the environment will always represent a major part of community health programs. In Chapter 2, which dealt with history, mention was made of the many sanitary installations that remain as evidences of the degree of sanitary consciousness attained by Minoan, Grecian, Roman, and other early civilizations. Similar reference was made to the problems which concerned the early public health organizations of this nation. It will be recalled that most of them related to problems of the physical environment, particularly of the growing urban communities. The essential similarities among the sanitary concerns of ancient civilizations, those of our founding fathers, and those of the present time are striking. This has prompted Hollis[2] to comment as follows:

> The need for a healthful environment is common to all peoples; it cuts across boundaries of occupations, race, class, and politics. If it differs from neighborhood to neighborhood, and from region to region, it differs not in fundamentals but only in complexity.
>
> It is in this setting that we are beginning to perceive the framework of the new concept of environmental health. Its foundation rests on the essentials of existence—man's need for and man's use of air, water, food, and shelter. The protective lining of this foundation is sanitation. . . . Since sanitation is basic to community existence, it is understandable that the pioneers in public health gave primary attention to cleanliness. Water supply, waste disposal, and food and milk received top consideration.

Whatever the reason, activities in environmental health tend to be the most firmly

established, most readily supported, and most vigorously demanded of the many constituent parts of the community health programs. Because of this, newly established local health departments have often begun operation with various phases of a sanitation program before proceeding to some of the other aspects of a well-rounded health program that might be less readily understood, less evident in results, or more controversial.

Many of the public health or epidemiologic accomplishments in the United States and certain other countries can be attributed to the sanitary measures which have been instituted. Included among these have been the spectacular reductions in typhoid fever, cholera, dysenteries, summer diarrheas, the control of many of the milk-borne and food-borne infections, the control of malaria, and the elimination of yellow fever. It was not until the beginning of the present century that the chains of events involved in the transmission and perpetuation of these diseases became unraveled. Prompt steps were taken to break links in these chains. At first, activities in the field of sanitation were concerned primarily with the abatement of noisome nuisances. Gradually the provision and supervision of sanitary water supplies and sewage disposal facilities were added as the first well-defined and scientific measures. Meanwhile the Rockefeller Sanitary Commission, established in 1909 to combat hookworm disease, led to programs by state health departments with emphasis upon the eradication of hookworm and other enteric infections in the rural population. These activities laid the foundation for

---

*For a general bibliographic guide, see Jacobson: Amer. J. Public Health.[1]

the eventual establishment and spread of full-time county health departments in the United States.

In this regard the noteworthy surveys, demonstrations, and epidemiologic investigations of the Public Health Service, particularly those by Lumsden, should not go unmentioned. Throughout this formative era of the modern sanitation and public health program much emphasis was placed upon the construction and use of sanitary privies as a practical means of preventing the spread of enteric disease, and it was one of the chief functions of public health workers of that period to assure the sanitary disposal of human excreta. This has prompted some to indicate the sanitary privy as a primary factor in the development of the tremendously significant public health movement.

CONTENT AND PURPOSE OF ENVIRONMENTAL CONTROL

It is essentially true that the initial phases of sanitation activities centered on keeping human excreta out of the diet. By comparison the field today covers an imposing spectrum of responsibilities and activities, for most of which sound technical and scientific reasons have been demonstrated. This has been emphasized by numerous recent groups particularly notable among which are the Task Force on Environmental Health of the National Commission on Community Health Services[3] and the Program Area Committee on Environmental Health of the American Public Health Association. In discussing the present definition and scope of the field, the latter group has indicated that the administration of today's environmental health programs has become so complex that it must weigh, balance, and take action on situations involving, in varying proportions, air pollution, water pollution, surface-water and ground-water disposal; food protection, occupational health, solid waste collection—its transportation and disposal; housing conservation and rehabilitation; radiation protection, insect and rodent control; institutional sanitation, subdivision control, hospital sanitation, ac-

cident prevention, sanitation and safety supervision of swimming pools; planning and zoning, recreation, flood control, topography, road networks, transportation, traffic, budgeting, tax jurisdictions, and neighboring communities and special districts. It must also place the economic, legal, sociologic, and political factors in their proper perspective in relation to the technical factors.[4]

The trend has been to draw away as much as possible from activities which involve repair, correction and enforcement toward programs of a positive or promotive nature. In other words, until relatively recently, public health activities have been based upon negative concepts, upon definitions of ills, environmental as well as human. This resulted in programs designed to attack things that have gone wrong, i.e., the isolation of an infected person, the filling of a decayed tooth, the purification of polluted water. We have now reached the point in many areas where we can begin to think and act in positive terms. We can begin to base our planning on a definition of good health rather than of illness, on the maintenance of cleanliness and salubrity instead of continually cleaning up an environment allowed to become insanitary. This trend has led to the consideration of man, his environment, and their interrelationships in both a positive and total sense.[5-7] In other words it is a recognition of the fact that man is affected by his environment and his environment can affect him, and that preventive and promotive measures may be applied to all aspects of man's environment as well as to man himself. Thus a recent Task Force[8] established by the Secretary of Health, Education, and Welfare to consider the broad problem recommended that the purpose of environmental control be regarded as the assurance "that every American can thrive in an attractive, comfortable, convenient, and healthy environment by controlling pollution at its source, reducing hazards, converting waste to use, and improving the aesthetic value of man's surroundings."

It is also a recognition of the fact that man, his psyche as well as his physical being, is inseparable from his total environment and that much more emphasis must be placed upon the total ecology of man. For this reason it has been recommended that there be established a Council of Ecological Advisors on the federal level, as a supra-cabinet organism advisory to the President on all problems, proposals, or activities which relate to the complex interrelationship of man and his total environment.

Finally, the trend is a recognition of the synergistic and cumulative effects of a spectrum of environmental hazards. Because of the usually slow development of the consequences of environmental abuse our society has failed to recognize the full impact of environmental hazards on human health and welfare. This has led to sporadic and fragmentary efforts to meet only some of the most flagrant of environmental problems. Thus not only should the rate and direction of environmental pollution be changed, the citizenry also needs protection from a conglomerate total of environmental health threats—not only air and water pollutants, but also combinations of these, plus noise and crowding, safety hazards, and other factors. It must be recognized that an individually acceptable amount of water pollution, added to a tolerable amount of air pollution, added to a bearable amount of noise and congestion can produce a totally unacceptable health environment.

It is entirely possible that the biological effects of these environmental hazards, some of which reach man slowly and silently over decades or generations, will first begin to reveal themselves only after their impact has become irreversible. Because of this, the Task Force on Environmental Health and Related Problems insisted that an effectively coordinated environmental health protection system is necessary. It should be predicated on the basic premise that the environment affects man's mental as well as his physical health and welfare. Any approach toward environmental health protection which is limited to concern for less than the total range of hazards that do or may exist in man's environment must be viewed as inadequate.

The concept of a coordinated, total en-vironmental health protection system has also been presented by Stead[9] in a clear and perceptive manner. In line with the thinking of the APHA Program Area Committee on Environmental Health he subdivides the field into four basic sectors: water sanitation, food sanitation, air sanitation, and shelter sanitation.

Water sanitation includes consideration of the quantity, quality, and safety aspects of water from the stages of planning, development, transportation, storage, treatment, distribution, and use on through the stages of treatment and disposal or conservation, reclamation, and reuse of waste water for sewage. As he indicates, public health concern must go beyond the provision of potable water. It must also extend to the use of water for recreation, irrigation, and food processing as well as the potential for vector breeding.

Food sanitation encompasses the entire chain of events from production of food on land or sea, its processing, distribution, storage, and marketing down to the actual preparation and serving of meals and the disposal of wastes. Stead summarizes this sector with the neat phrase that the food sanitation program must "follow the food" back to its source and forward to its ultimate consumption.

Air sanitation is concerned with the physical, chemical, and biologic quality of air as a natural resource. Problems vary from its transparency to its radioactivity, and programs should be alert to air quality at home, at work, during travel and recreation, and outdoors as well as indoors.

Shelter sanitation is regarded as encompassing not only the field of housing as related to dwelling units, apartments, hotels, public buildings, trailers, and camps but also the general artificial and natural environment for work, play, and general living. It includes the whole field of protection of human beings from rigors of the elements as well as the onslaught of insects, rodents, dust, dirt, odors, noise, radiation, accident hazards, and other detrimental impacts of the environment on man. Stead properly considers that omission of any of the four sectors briefly described results in an unbalanced environmental health program.

The four basic levels of concern with the environment are listed in the order of program preference:

1. Insuring the elements of simple survival
2. Prevention of disease and poisoning
3. Maintaining an environment suited to man's efficient performance
4. Preservation of comfort and the enjoyment of living

As Stead analyzes it, each of the four levels of concern (survival, disease prevention, efficient performance, and enjoyment) necessitates programs in each of the four program sectors (water, food, air, and shelter), which requires four program stages (research, field investigation, analysis and planning, and the action program).

To assist in the planning of broadly comprehensive environmental health programs, the Public Health Service has developed an excellent Environmental Health Planning Guide[10] which, if used as extensively as is merited, is certain to contribute to the improved development, performance, and evaluation of programs in this field.

REGIONAL DIFFERENCES

Although the basic objectives are universal, the details of the environmental health program have not developed uniformly throughout the communities and states of the nation. Furthermore, as will be discussed later, all activities in this field have not necessarily been centered in health departments. The more rural agricultural South and Midwest are faced with rather different problems than the urban industrialized Northeast, the fringe of the lower Great Lakes, or the West Coast. As a result certain activities are stressed more in one area than in the other, and dependence is placed upon somewhat different categories of personnel. The congregation of large numbers of people in the many cities of the northeastern, western coastal, and Great Lakes states necessarily has led to their emphasis on the construction and operation of sanitary engineering facilities and to the employment of many sanitary and public health engineers.

In other more rural parts of the country, particularly in the southern states, the opportunity for centralized sanitary control has been limited essentially to a few moderate sized towns and a handful of larger cities. Chief emphasis in this area, therefore, is placed upon a somewhat simpler and more individualized approach. Here much more patient and persistent attention had to be given to such matters as privy and well location and construction, dairy barn sanitation, screening, and the like. To many, these may appear prosaic, elementary, and nontechnical. However, a background of technical knowledge of no small degree is necessary for the solution of such environmental problems. Furthermore, they provide a measure of community health protection quite comparable to that resulting from the more complex and sophisticated structures of municipal sanitary engineering. For example, during the period from December 1933 to July 1942 a total of about 3 million sanitary privies were constructed in 38 states and in Puerto Rico through the cooperative efforts of the federal work-projects agencies, the state health departments, and the Public Health Service. This figure does not include the many others constructed privately or under the sponsorship of the agricultural and farm agencies.

A further point to be remembered here is that while the turning of a valve in a water treatment plant or the flushing of a toilet in the urban or surburban areas involves no particular educational impact for the individual citizen, this is not true on the rural scene. This was dramatically emphasized by Mustard in a poignant statement that it is fortunate that sanitary safety is more easily attained in warm, comfortable indoor bathrooms than in drafty, outdoor privies. The observation has been made in connection with the Federal Community Sanitation Program that in view of the many persons employed in "selling" 3 million privies it was necessary to explain to at least 15 million persons the reasons for sanitary disposal of excreta. It cannot be doubted that this program during the 1930's contributed significantly to the public understanding of this and, in fact, of a number of other important phases of environmental sanitation and public health.

One of the great difficulties of course is found in the differences in means, abilities, and willingness to finance sanitary improvements. Thus, as Hollis[11] points out:

Government is ordinarily held responsible for financing public health services in the city. This is not so in the country. Sanitation of food and premises is clearly a public problem in the village and other rural centers such as the school, church, and grange or community hall. But in most rural areas in the United States, sanitation is ordinarily regarded as an individual or private concern, even though many individual rural families cannot finance sanitation by themselves. If there is the will to bring rural demands for environmental improvement into balance with the demand for cars and electricity, however, the economic devices that provide cars, telephones, and power are capable of financing pipes and drains as well.

In the city, the danger of contagion has created awareness of community responsibility. In rural areas, the danger of contagion is less apparent. It is recognized mainly in the enforcement of sanitation on dairy farms, in the effort to protect the safety of fluid milk produced for the urban market. Hygienic milk production is probably the heaviest single contribution of its kind to rural environmental health in the United States.

He concludes therefore:

Three major factors in the lag in rural sanitation are the relatively high cost of water and sewage systems for isolated structures, the usual necessity to finance each installation individually at relatively high rates, and the absence in many rural areas of a strong public health authority. These factors have less force in the village than on the farm.

An important variation with regard to the foregoing is found in the relationship between the environmental health problems and programs of decentralized suburban and urban fringe areas as against core cities. Indeed, it is perhaps here that a solution may be found to some of the differences which exist between rural and urban opportunities for environmental health. Board and Dunsmore[12] have carried out a particularly interesting analysis of this increasingly frequent type of situation in which they have indicated many of the similarities and differences among urban, suburban, transitional, and rural problems, as well as the many agencies which may contribute to their adequate solution.

An administrative benefit for which the rural sanitation program may be given credit has been the development of a spirit of cooperation between the officials of the health agencies on the various levels of government. Thus it may be said with little exaggeration that it was in this field that the state health departments and the Public Health Service first learned to work together as did, to a considerable degree, the state and local health organizations. Furthermore, the successful pursuance of the program necessitated the integration of activities and therefore cooperation between public health departments and other agencies on the same governmental level such as the agricultural and farm organizations.

SANITATION NEEDS

Although the United States is already the most sanitized nation in the world, much unfinished business remains. In a review of the past and an examination of the present, in order to enunciate aims and objectives for the future, Hollis[13] reached the following conclusion:

As we look back on environmental health over the past fifty years, we see that despite our great achievement there lies before us a whole continent of unfinished business. To our credit, we have shown some intelligence about clearing a few health barriers ahead of orderly national growth. This was true to a great degree of municipal water supply and liquid waste collection. It is true also of certain aggressive actions in the past ten years against insect-borne diseases.

However, he continues:

We cannot be smug or comfortable about the history of milk sanitation, shellfish sanitation, and sanitation of bathing waters. There are no grounds for congratulations on the national record on controlling water pollution, on school and institutional sanitation, and unsolved questions of food sanitation. What, one may ask, is the national health plan on air pollution including control of irritating pollens, the hygiene of housing, and home accident prevention? What do we know about unhealthful aspects of faulty community planning, substandard recreational facilities, and abnormal noise? Most certainly we cannot view with pride our progress in rural sanitation—more than 25 million of our rural population who have been able to obtain electric power are still without running water and water-carried waste systems. These are but examples.

Numerous surveys and evaluations of environmental health needs have been made by various organizations and agencies. They have resulted in a number of useful reports that have influenced to varying degrees public opinion, legislation, programming, and organization in the field.[3,8,14-21] In 1947 the Public Health Service conducted a detailed inventory[22] which illustrated the extensive sanitation needs at that time. It pointed out the following significant accomplishments:

1. More than 14,000 systems provide water to about 85 million people, and the quality of the water furnished is generally excellent.
2. More than 70 million people are served by sewerage systems, and more than 5,500 treatment plants have been installed, which serve about 42 million people.
3. More than 70 per cent of our market-milk supply is pasteurized.
4. Practically all of our larger cities, and a constantly increasing number of the smaller ones, provide regular collection service of garbage and refuse, and disposal methods have been improved.

On the other side of the ledger, many unmet needs of great proportions were found to exist. They were summarized as follows:

1. Approximately 2,360,000 people in 5,710 communities with no public waterworks systems need such facilities. Almost 15,000 communities with over 79 million people have waterworks which need improvements or extensions. In rural areas where community systems are impracticable, 27 million people need either new or improved water supplies.
2. More than 9,100 towns with 6,360,000 people need complete sewerage systems. Some 9,900 additional communities with almost 80 million people have systems which need improvements. In rural areas, more than 33 million people lack satisfactory sewage or excreta disposal facilities of even the simplest type.
3. In 8,300 communities with 70 million people, there are needs for better facilities for collecting and disposing of garbage and other municipal refuse.
4. More than 36 per cent of the community needs are either ready for construction or in the planning stage. Two-thirds of the work which is ready for construction, and more than half which is being definitely planned, is in cities of 100,000 or more. In cities of over 5,000 population almost half of the needed work is at least at the planning stage. In the smaller towns much less advance planning has been done.
5. Much of this needed construction is a backlog of work which developed during and after the war. Materials shortages, rapidly rising construction costs, and an unwillingness of local governments to enter into competition for materials and labor necessary to meet the acute housing shortage, have made most communities continue to defer all except emergency work. As conditions in the construction industry return to more nearly normal, this backlog of needed work should proceed at an increasingly rapid rate.
6. The cost of needed water supply and waste disposal facilities for the United States is estimated at $7,834,581,000.
7. The per capita cost of needs varies from $23 in Rhode Island to $107 in New York State and averages about $60 for the nation as a whole.
8. The per capita cost of needs is greatest in the smallest communities and in the largest ones. In towns of less than 1,000 population, needs exceed $100 per capita, while in cities of over 1,000,000 they approach $120 per capita. However, a much larger proportion of income will be required in the smaller towns than in the wealthier big cities.
9. In the fringes of most of our metropolitan areas, houses with inadequate sanitary facilities are being built which promise to become the slums of tomorrow. State legislation to enable counties to adopt and enforce suitable zoning laws are badly needed, as well as additional personnel in the local and State health departments who can deal with the sanitation problems of these rapidly growing areas.
10. Educational work and technical advice are needed to assist the small communities in obtaining the water and sewerage facilities they should have. This will require additional personnel in the State health departments. In some States improved laws are necessary to facilitate the formation of sanitary districts. In other States the laws providing for revenue financing of sanitation facilities need revision to make them more usable. Financial assistance in the form of low-interest loans would give impetus to the installation of needed community facilities. These small towns and the rural areas deserve special attention since it is in them that the incidence of the filth-borne diseases is highest and serves as focal points of infection from which these diseases can spread.
11. It is in the rural areas beyond the reach of any practicable community facilities that the greatest shortage of sanitation facilities exists. Although this is due to some extent to a lack of money, it is also due to a lack of realization of the dangers involved. Local health departments are lacking in many of these areas and are understaffed in most of them. Extension of adequate local health services to these areas is a prime necessity.

While it is true that significant strides have been taken since this study was made in 1947, the combination of population growth, continued urbanization and suburbanization, and industrial expansion has easily offset any additions and improvements in sanitary facilities. As merely one example, there are still about 5,500 communities with inadequate or no sewage treatment facilities and the cost of remedying just this problem is estimated at more than $2 billion. Similarly it is questionable if the air and water pollution problems and the housing problem have improved significantly if any since the survey was made.

In the light of recent developments in public health dentistry there should also be added to the foregoing the fluoridation needs of the nation. There are about 17,000 public water supplies in the United States, of which about 15,000 contain no natural fluorides. By 1966 only about 60 million people in 2,848 communities in the nation were benefiting from this valuable procedure. As Knutson[23] once said, "At the present rate of progress in the fluoridation of public drinking water supplies it will take 150 years to complete the task ahead." However, with the pattern of implementing chlorination of water as a guide, fluoridation of water may proceed more rapidly.

With this general background and the statement of sanitation needs a consideration of the most important present concerns in environmental health is indicated.

WATER SUPPLIES

Water is one of the prime necessities of human existence, so much so that, given dire enough circumstances, even the most educated individual will resort to the consumption of water from grossly polluted or dangerous sources. Beyond its importance for human consumption, water serves many purposes: as a source of fluid for animals; as a medium of transportation; as an agent for cleansing and cooling the body, objects, or the environment; as a means of recreation for swimming, boating, and fishing; as an agricultural irrigant; as an adjunct to innumerable industrial processes; as a conveyor for the disposal of human and industrial wastes; as a means of air conditioning; as a fire extinguisher. The per capita domestic use of water from public supplies has grown from about 90 gallons per day in 1890 to approximately 175 gallons per day at the present time. With regard to total use it is estimated that munici-

pal water consumers use about 20 billion gallons of water each day, rural consumers about 5 billion gallons, private industry about 130 billion gallons, and about 160 billion gallons are used for irrigation.

Our chief concern here is with the consumption of water by humans for domestic purposes. At the moment most of the other uses of water are of interest to us insofar as they affect the salubrity of the water that humans drink. Water supply systems may be classified as public and private. About two thirds of the population are served by public water systems. However, about 10% of the families living in about 7 million homes in communities so served do not have water outlets readily available. In addition, there are still 2.5 million people living in 5,700 communities of 200 to 500 population without a public water system. In rural areas about 27 million people need improved pure water facilities.

Public water supplies are derived from various sources, i.e., streams, lakes, cisterns, deep wells, and springs, and their nature differs according to their source. Atmospheric waters which are caught in cisterns are by far the most pure, both bacteriologically and chemically. However, they constitute only a very minor proportion of all public water supplies and only in very small communities. Surface waters such as streams and lakes which depend for replenishment upon repeated run-offs under most circumstances do not have as high a chemical content as do ground waters from deep wells and springs. However, while the latter tend to be more pure bacteriologically, surface waters, because of their more extensive exposure, are more apt to become bacteriologically polluted. Similarly, underground waters in general are clear, while surface waters ordinarily contain considerable amounts of suspended matter which must be removed before they can be considered suitable for human consumption. These differences in source, hence composition, necessarily give rise to differences in approach to administrative control. Streams and lakes in general do not lend themselves to adequate control of the watershed. On the other hand, some impounding reservoirs are subject to control from the standpoint of prevention of further pollution of the water. Increasing public pressure for recreational facilities is resulting in more liberal access to both the reservoir and the surrounding watershed. In any case, in view of the high factor of safety in relation to cost, surface waters should probably always be subjected to filtration, chlorination, and fluoridation. Rapid sand filtration is the usual method of choice. Recent improvements in sanitary engineering have resulted in filters with rates up to four gallons per square foot per minute, about double the previous usual rate, without any sacrifice of safety.

The provision of a safe and satisfactory public water supply to a community involves the following procedures:

1. If a surface water, the watershed should be protected and controlled insofar as is practical.
2. The intake should be located properly with regard to all possible sources of contamination and pollution.
3. If necessary and practical, provision should be made for primary sedimentation and purification by means of storage reservoirs and exposure to air and light.
4. Bacteria, algae, and any residual turbidity should be removed by the addition of a coagulant (usually alum) and settling out of the coagulated particles, and then passage through a rapid sand filter.
5. Residual and subsequent bacterial contaminants are combatted by the addition of a disinfectant, usually chlorine, to a concentration of from 0.2 to 0.5 parts per million. This is a most important procedure.
6. A concentration up to from 0.7 to 1.5 parts per million of fluoride should be achieved by the addition of sodium fluoride, sodium silicofluoride, or hydrofluosilicic acid for the prevention of dental caries. The ultimate concentration will depend upon the average water consumption per individual.
7. Use of the water by all the population of the community should be assured by low water rates, adequate distribution systems, and housing requirements.
8. Contamination of the purified water should be prevented by initial disinfection of the distribution system pipes and by prevention of cross-connections and back-siphonage.

In order to achieve these ends the cooperative action of a number of community agencies is necessary. Among these are the health department, the department of public works or the water department, the tax or finance office, possibly the park police, the plumbing department, the housing commission, the dental society, and possibly others.

The assurance of safe water to the rural population poses a completely different set of problems. The sources are usually relatively simple and primitive wells, often shallow and unprotected. Hence they are easily subject to pollution not only from the surface but also through seepage from poorly placed privies, improperly constructed septic tanks, or nearby barnyards. Contamination over greater distances may occur if fissures or other subterranean passages exist in the substrata. Offsetting these hazards is the fact that the use of each small rural water supply is characteristically limited to a very small group of people, often only one family.

The solution of this difficult problem lies essentially in persistent rural health education programs coupled with sanitary consultation from the local health department. The objectives of these efforts should be encouragement of proper locating of wells and excreta disposal facilities, proper construction of wells, and installation of a pump in a tightly sealed, curbed, and drained well top.[24]

STREAM POLLUTION CONTROL

Although pure water for drinking purposes is of paramount public health concern, the many other uses of this precious commodity make it desirable to regard the development, protection, and use of water resources as a unit. By now 75% of our population lives and works in metropolitan centers with resultant concentration of tremendous burdens of human and industrial wastes on the bodies of water to which they are related. The magnitude of this water pollution was brought out by studies covering 226 river basins in the United States, of which 146 are interstate. The summary of these studies[25] indicates that there are more than 22,000 sources of stream pollution in the country, including 11,800 municipal sewer systems and 10,400 industrial waste outlets. Of the latter, one half produce organic wastes which markedly increase the biologic oxygen demand, and others discharge wastes that are toxic or give rise to tastes and odors which detract from the subsequent usefulness of the water by humans. Despite the reduction of pollution by 9,300 treatment plants, 6,700 municipal and 2,600 industrial, the wastes still being discharged into rivers and lakes are equivalent in biologic oxygen demand to those from over 150 million people. It is estimated that to solve this problem adequately, 6,600 more municipal sewage treatment plants or additions to present plants and 3,500 more industrial waste treatment plants or additions will be necessary at a cost of from $9 billion to $12 billion of public and private funds.

Increasing concern with the problem led to the enactment of Water Pollution Control Acts in 1948 and in 1956. Whereas Congress recognized the primary responsibilities of the states in the matter, the Water Pollution Control Acts authorized and directed the Public Health Service to take the initiative in developing or adopting comprehensive programs for the solution of water pollution problems in cooperation with the states, interstate agencies, municipalities, and industries. The Acts stated that comprehensive programs were to be developed for surface and underground waters, giving due consideration to all water uses—public water supply, propagation of fish and aquatic life, recreation, and agricultural, industrial, and other legitimate uses. They provided for federal grants to the states and interstate agencies to help them carry out industrial waste studies, and for loans to municipalities to assist in the

construction of needed abatement work. The Acts further provided for federal research and technical and consultative assistance to state and interstate agencies, municipalities, and industries, and for the encouragement of uniform state laws, interstate compacts, and cooperative state activities in the field of water pollution control. Initial responsibility for enforcement of pollution control measures was left with the states; federal authority was to be exercised only on interstate waters, only after the efforts of the states had been exhausted, and only with the consent of the states.

To carry out its responsibilities, the Public Health Service instituted a water pollution control program with field units in each of the ten large drainage basin areas. Each unit was staffed with engineers and scientists with extensive experience in water pollution control to work closely with officials of the various state governments. The Robert A. Taft Sanitary Engineering Center in Cincinnati served as the research center for the work. In 1962, Congress further supplemented this program by providing for the establishment of a series of water pollution research laboratories throughout the nation. As indication of its growing concern and impatience, Congress subsequently passed the Water Quality Act of 1965, the Water Resources Planning Act of 1965, the Public Works and Economic Development Act of 1965, and the Clean Water Act of 1966. In the process it established a Federal Water Pollution Control Administration in the Department of the Interior and transferred the water pollution control responsibilities of the Public Health Service to it. This new authority is to encourage state action through grants, loans, contracts, advice and consultation, research demonstrations, and training programs.

There are two particularly important conditions for successful control of stream pollution. The first is planning on a regional basis since few situations involve only one state. While it is important that each state develop its own programs based upon its own legislation, it is fundamental, as Klassen[26] has described, to plan and coordinate the various state water pollution control programs and, insofar as it is possible, the laws upon which they are based, in order to bring about a practical program which will serve the needs of the drainage basin in question.

The second condition is a recognition of the fact that while the chemical and physical characteristics of human wastes do not vary significantly, it is rare that industrial wastes, even those from similar enterprises, are the same. Hence each stream pollution problem, especially if it involves industrial wastes, is a case study in itself. Therefore, as Eliassen[27] says, while the sanitary engineer is most adequately fitted in education and experience for water pollution control work, he cannot go it alone. He must have qualified sanitary chemists and sanitary biologists as members of his team. With the right combination of talents in these three major realms of sanitary engineering this team can give distinguished service to industry and government in the abatement of stream pollution by the control and treatment of industrial wastes.

WASTE DISPOSAL

Closely related to the problems of water sanitation and stream sanitation is that of satisfactory waste disposal. The waste materials of present-day households consist of human excreta, garbage, and refuse. In urban areas there is also added an increasing amount of industrial wastes. Until recently each of these was considered to be a somewhat separate problem. In urban communities, however, they have become increasingly interrelated. In some instances, garbage and refuse are collected and disposed of together. Also there is a trend toward the grinding of garbage in the household and disposal along with excreta and other household wastes through the plumbing and sewerage system. Industrial wastes may also be discharged into the sewerage system or directly into bodies of water which also receive raw or treated sewage.

There are various methods of disposal of waste products of human societies. These may be listed as: (1) discharge into bodies of water, with or without treatment, (2) discharge onto the surface of the ground, (3) discharge onto the surface of the ground, (3) discharge onto the surface of the ground, (3)

burial in the ground, and (4) incineration. No one of these offers the perfect solution since each has some disadvantages or hazards and each may be more applicable than the others in specific situations. Ehlers and Steel[28] have listed the following goals or requirements which should be applied to the choice of satisfactory disposal methods:

1. There should be no contamination of ground water that may enter springs or wells.
2. There should be no contamination of surface water.
3. The surface soil should not be contaminated.
4. Excreta should not be accessible to flies or animals.
5. There should be freedom from odors or unsightly conditions.
6. The method used should be simple and inexpensive as to construction and operation; this applies particularly to rural areas where the farmer may construct his own facilities.

It is not within the province of this book to describe and assess the various methods of waste disposal since those details are readily available in a number of excellent books devoted specifically to the field of sanitation and sanitary engineering. An excellent overview of the complexities, needs, and methodologies in this field is available in a recent report by the National Academy of Sciences and the National Research Council.[29] The intent here is merely to present a general background picture of certain factors which must be considered with regard to a public health agency's interest and responsibility in the problem.

Social and environmental circumstances are of particular significance with regard to the disposal of human excreta which is by far the potentially most dangerous type of waste material. The pertinent situations, hence the methods of approach, are three in kind. The simplest situation is that in which no water carriage is possible; this applies particularly to rural areas. Under such circumstances resort may be made to the pit privy, the bored hole latrine, the vault privy, the chemical toilet, the septic privy, or the box and can toilet. A second situation is that found most commonly in suburban areas and some small communities where a supply of running water is available thereby making water carriage of excreta possible, but where no public sewerage system exists. Under such circumstances, individual cesspools or septic tanks are commonly used. Finally, there is the situation where both a public water supply and a public sewerage system make possible not only water carriage but also water disposal of human excreta. Here new problems arise in that there is a concentration of tremendous amounts of human wastes, the complication of plumbing hazards in the form of possible cross-connections and back-siphonage, and the frequent addition of garbage and industrial wastes. Some attempts have been made to dispose of sewage by making use of it for irrigation purposes in so-called sewage farms. The success and practicability of this approach have been very limited in the United States.[30,31]

Generally speaking, therefore, and because of the large amount of water it contains, sewage is usually disposed of in a body of water. This may be done with or without treatment. The dangers of the discharge of raw sewage into streams or lakes are obvious, and increasingly it is becoming important and necessary to treat sewage for the following reasons:

1. Public health reasons—to prevent the pollution of drinking water, fish and mollusks, and bathing places
2. Aesthetic reasons—to prevent the formation of foul odors, and the development of streams and shorelines made unsightly by solid or suspended waste matter
3. Economic reasons—to prevent the killing of commercially valuable fish life, the infection of livestock and other animal life, and the deterioration of land values
4. Salvage reasons—to make possible the recovery of commercially valuable fertilizer, grease, gases, and other products[32]

The objectives of the various methods of sewage treatment have been summarized as follows[33]:

1. To diminish the amount of solid materials discharged into a stream, in order to lessen the demands on its purifying properties, and to prevent the formation of sludge banks and the appearance of objectionable floating materials.
2. To decompose, through the agency of biological methods, the organic matter in sewage, and to transform it into simpler organic compounds, and into gases and liquids. In this way, the burden of the final purification which takes place in a stream will be greatly diminished.
3. To stabilize the organic matter in sewage through the agency of biological methods operating under aerobic conditions, so that the purifying properties of a stream into which the treated sewage is ultimately discharged will be taxed to a minimum.
4. To diminish or destroy the bacteria present in sewage, particularly the pathogenic varieties capable of producing disease.

These objectives are accomplished in different situations by combinations of the following procedures: (1) screening and/or sedimentation, (2) anaerobic digestion of settleable solids in a septic tank, Imhoff tank, or separate sludge digestion tank, (3) oxidation of nonsettleable organic matter by filtration, activated sludge, or irrigation methods, (4) disinfection with chlorine or other disinfectants.

Although the operation of public sewerage as well as water systems is a local responsibility,[34] the overall routine control of these matters is largely a state concern. The state health department is the official agency with major responsibility, but in nearly three fourths of the states the responsibility is shared with other departments or special commissions. Among these are departments of public works, labor, education, and industry; special state sewage, stream pollution or sanitary boards or commissions; state universities and laboratories. Among the functions for which the state commonly has responsibility are the promulgation and enforcement of laws, rules, and regulations; approval of plans and installations; examination and licensure of treatment plant operators; periodic inspection of installations; provision of consultation services to localities; provision of grants-in-aid to local sanitation units; and the promotion of satisfactory local facilities.

Authority for the supervision of semipublic waste disposal systems is more apt to be shared among several agencies than in the case of public supplies. Thus, if the system involves educational institutions, parks, or industries, for example, the departments of education, parks, industry, or labor are almost certain to be involved in practically all instances. This shared responsibility and authority, however, does not alter the fact that the state health department must play the primary regulatory and supervisory role with respect to the sanitary aspects of the situation. Often, of course, these responsibilities are met in collaboration with or through the local public health structure if it is adequately staffed.

The weakest link exists in relation to supervision and control of individual private waste disposal systems in rural areas. Where a local public health department exists, it almost invariably includes some form of activity in the field of human excreta control. The basis of the activity usually consists of a persistent health educational approach on a personal basis augmented by general educational measures, consultation from the state health department, and sometimes actual assistance in the financing and construction of private sanitary privies or septic tank systems.

FOOD AND MILK SANITATION

The majority of the cases of epidemic gastrointestinal infections which occurred up through the first quarter of this century were attributable to impure water. Because of the remarkable strides that have been made since that time in providing safe water to the majority of the people, water no longer plays an outstanding role as a transmitter of disease in the United States. Since 1923 the Public Health Service has compiled and analyzed reports of milk-borne epidemics from data submitted by state health departments. Since 1938 these analyses have also included outbreaks traced to water and to other foods. An analysis of these data (Table 27-1) presents an interesting and significant picture.

As recent as 1938 to 1942, water not only caused many outbreaks but was most important in terms of persons affected. While the average annual number of outbreaks caused by water and milk was roughly the same and in each case only about one fourth of the number caused by other foods, the number of persons affected by water-borne epidemics was about three and one half times the number affected by other foods and about eleven times the number affected by milk and milk products.

However, when the data for the period since 1942 are considered, a marked shift is found to have occurred. Comparing the two periods, it is seen that although the average annual numbers of epidemics attributable to water and to milk and milk products have been cut in half, those due to other foods have doubled in number. Furthermore, while the average annual number of persons affected in the recent years by milk and milk products was one

Table 27-1. Changes in food-borne and water-borne disease outbreaks, United States, 1938-1960*

Time period	Water		Milk and milk products		Other foods	
	Outbreaks	Cases	Outbreaks	Cases	Outbreaks	Cases
1938-1942—Number	247	103,441	208	9,114	902	29,095
Annual average	49	20,688	42	1,823	181	5,819
1943-1951—Number	208	32,342	205	7,259	2,769	101,466
Annual average	23	3,594	23	806	308	11,274
1953-1957—Number	33	3,043	55	1,539	1,081	53,469
Annual average	7	609	11	308	216	10,694
1958-1960—Number	22	2,535	29	538	740	27,954
Annual average	7	845	10	179	247	9,318

*From Dauer, C. C.: 1960 Summary of disease outbreaks and a 10-year résumé, Public Health Rep. **76:**915, Oct. 1961.

half of what it had been and for water only one sixth of what it had been, with regard to outbreaks due to other foods, the number of persons affected doubled. The more recent period, 1953 to 1960, has witnessed a decline in all three types of epidemics. However, the decline is most marked in the instances of water-borne and milk-borne epidemics which declined both in number of epidemics and number of persons affected. Indeed, although the average annual number of epidemics borne by foods was about one third less in the period from 1953 to 1957 than in the period from 1943 to 1951, the number of persons affected remained essentially the same.

These figures illustrate two facts with reguard to the present time: (1) Foods are easily the most important and an increasing cause of gastrointestinal infections in the United States. (2) Although milk and milk products are potentially the most perishable and most dangerous foods and despite their ever increasing use, they now are a relatively unimportant cause of disease when compared with other foods. This is explainable on the basis that their very perishability has focused so much attention upon means of ensuring their safety. In order to promote scientifically sound standards and uniform legislation the Public Health Service in 1924 developed a standard milk ordinance. Since then, there have been nine revised editions of the Milk Ordinance and Code Recommended by the United States Public Health Service. Each one represents the pooled opinions and experience of public health officials, the milk and dairy industry, veterinarians, agriculturists, scientists, consumer representatives, and others. By 1962 it formed the basis for regulation and practice in 37 states and is enforced statewide in 16 states. Adopted by 512 counties and 1,435 municipalities on a voluntary basis, the ordinance and its accompanying code now protect a majority of the urban and much of the nonurban population.[35] It is recognized as the only fluid milk regulation approaching a national standard and has been accepted by many states as the basic regulation for an interstate certification program and an industry-wide

education program. More recently there has been developed a Frozen Desserts Ordinance and Code Recommended by the Public Health Service. Of particular effect on the maintenance of the safety of milk and milk products is the widespread application of the pasteurization process. Pasteurization of all market milk is compulsory in 5 states, 15 counties, and 152 municipalities. In addition, 346 towns and cities require pasteurization of all except certified raw milk. As a result, about 90% of the fluid milk consumed by the urban population in the United States is protected by pasteurization.

Effective supervision and control of the many complex factors involved in the production, processing, and sale of milk and milk products has resulted from cooperative action on the part of public health agencies, departments of agriculture, and the responsible representatives of the milk and dairy industry. The actual control programs are administered by sanitarians and veterinarians on the local level supported by the state departments of health and agriculture and by the industry. On the state level authority may be vested in either the the state health department or the department of agriculture, and sometimes in both.

From the analysis of epidemics presented it is obvious that foods other than milk are a matter of considerable concern to public health agencies as an increasing source of preventable disease. An analysis[36] of the food-borne outbreaks of 1960 gives a more complete picture of the problem. Of the 182 food-borne outbreaks reported, the diseases involved were gastroenteritis, 84; staphylococcal food poisoning, 51; salmonellosis, 16; shigellosis, 5; botulism, 4; noxious plant illness, 4; chemical poisoning, 4; trichinosis, 3; typhoid, 2; streptococcal infection, 1; hepatitis, 1; and others, 4. The types of establishments known to be involved were public restaurants, 46; schools and colleges, 14; hospitals and institutions, 10; labor camps, 3; trains, 2; private homes, 44; private clubs, 8; social gatherings, 30; and picnics, 7. Dauer points out that the last four types of establishments, involved in 89 outbreaks, are of a private character but the remaining 73 (40% of the total) are public or semipublic food places that should be subject to control by health authorities.

The first efforts of the federal government to bring about control and supervision of the quality of foods occurred in 1879, when a bill was introduced in Congress to prohibit the adulteration of articles of food and drink. This and a number of subsequent efforts came to naught, and 27 years passed before June 30, 1906, when Theodore Roosevelt signed a bill that prohibited the manufacture and sale of adulterated and misbranded food. For 20 years it was administered by the Bureau of Chemistry of the Department of Agriculture. During this period several other acts were passed relating to proper weights, packaging, labeling, food purity, meats, and standards for butter. In 1927 the Secretary of Agriculture recommended the establishment of a Food and Drug Administration to administer all of these various acts. Between 1927 and 1933 additional legislation was passed dealing with canned foods and inspection of seafood plants on invitation. Meanwhile attempts were made to revise and bring up to date the original Food and Drug Act of 1906. On June 25, 1938, President Franklin D. Roosevelt signed a bill that established the present Federal Food, Drug, and Cosmetic Act. Two years later the Food and Drug Administration was transferred from the Department of Agriculture to the Federal Security Agency (now the Department of Health, Education, and Welfare), where it is part of the Consumer Protection and Environmental Health Service.

The situation on the federal level is somewhat complicated by the retention of meat inspection responsibilities by the Department of Agriculture, and by the obvious concern of the Public Health Service for all matters dealing with the salubrity of foods. In general, all three federal agencies concerned with different aspects of the food problem work in close collaboration, each fulfilling certain responsibilities. On the state level the situation is even more confused. All but 4 states have some food control agency, but there is no uniformity

among them. The agencies involved are departments of agriculture, 23 states; departments of health, 20 states; food or food and drug commissions, 2 states; state chemist, 1 state; and public service department, 1 state. Since 1939, efforts have been under way to revise state laws to bring them into conformity with the Federal Food, Drug, and Cosmetic Act. This has been more or less accomplished in about one third of the states.

Practically all municipalities and a great many counties carry out some form of food control activities, usually by personnel of the local public health agency. The personnel vary in quality from untrained inspectors to well-qualified sanitarians and veterinarians. In general the activities consist of inspection, rating, and certification of food processing and dispensing establishments, sampling and analysis of foodstuffs, physical examination and training of food-handlers, and local prosecution of infringements of food ordinances and laws. In carrying out these activities, the local personnel work closely with and are supported by personnel of the various interested state and federal agencies.

Particular attention is given by local public health authorities to sanitary conditions in restaurants and taverns and bars. Many different types of inspectional and rating forms have been developed, and many types of action such as certification, licensing, and awards of merit have been used. In order to bring about some reasonable and sound basis for uniform action, the Public Health Service in 1934 began the development of a suggested procedure. After several experimental editions, the Ordinance and Code Regulating Eating and Drinking Establishments Recommended by the Public Health Service was published in 1943. By 1962 it had been adopted by 37 states and more than 1,100 county and municipal jurisdictions. It now protects over 100 million people.[37] Fuchs,[38] who has played a major role in its development and use, explains: "The question of enforcement methods was settled by offering two different forms of the ordinance, one a grading type which permits enforcement by degrading or permit revocation or both, the other a nongrading minimum-requirements type enforceable by permit revocation only. In the grading type the competitive effect of grading on public patronage tends to improve conditions in eating establishments, thereby aiding in enforcement."

In a number of fields public health interests and private enterprise have found themselves in the same arena. In some instances they have unfortunately acted at cross-purposes. Sometimes business and industry have looked upon public health workers as interfering, unrealistic, and restraining and have pointed, with considerable right, to the maze of conflicting requirements, ordinances, codes, and standards with regard to the same article or process in different communities or states. Public health workers on the other hand have sometimes accused private enterprise of being completely mercenary and without social conscience. Fortunately in recent years industry and public health have made a number of sincere attempts to get together in an amiable and intelligent manner to arrive at mutually satisfactory conclusions and recommendations. In the field of environmental health, and especially with regard to food sanitation, this led to the establishment in 1944 of the National Sanitation Foundation. This is an independent, nonprofit corporation financed entirely by business and industry and governed by a board of directors comprised of individuals from private enterprise and public health. Its purposes are (1) to bring together representative industrialists, businessmen, and public health workers to define and outline mutual problems, (2) to finance research in fields of mutual concern and interest, (3) to promote a program of personal and community health to acquaint employees and the general public with the needs for good sanitary practices and community cleanliness, and (4) to provide a testing laboratory, similar to the Fire Underwriters Laboratory, for materials of sanitary and health-promoting value.

The Foundation sponsors Joint Committees on Standards with representatives from interested national professional organizations. "Task committees" set up by industry prepare preliminary standards for consideration with the Joint Committees. After repeated conferences and revisions, if agreement is reached, the standards may be approved by the Joint Committee. After final review and approval by the Foundation's Council of Sanitation Consultants the standards are published. Equipment which meets the standards is then awarded the Foundation's seal of approval. The procedure, although long and complex, assures the careful study and consideration of all aspects of the problem at hand and when completed, concurrence of public health workers, scientists, and industrialists is certain. So far, standards for soda fountain equipment, general food service equipment, dishwashing equipment and numerous other items have been satisfactorily developed and adopted. In addition, the Foundation carries out significant activities in public sanitation education and has conducted a number of worthwhile symposia and in-service training courses for representatives of public health agencies, business and industrial groups, and public officials.

Somewhat similar to these efforts are the increased activities on the part of business and industry toward "self-policing." Among the examples of this are the programs of the National Canners' Association, the Ice Cream Merchandising Institute, the Food Industries Sanitarian Association, and the American Institute of Baking. These are all good signs which point toward a more fruitful and mutually more agreeable method of cooperative action from which the public cannot help benefiting. This is in conformity with one of the recommendations of the National Commission on Community Health Services, which states, "Industry and commerce [should] assume more responsibility for self-policing and control of their products, services, and operations in relation to associated environmental health problems; and health agencies [should] encourage and assist them in so doing."[3]

ATMOSPHERIC POLLUTION

During recent years public and health officials have become increasingly aware of the atmosphere as the important medium in which we live and of the possibility and consequences of overloading it with waste products of human activity. Thus concern has been mounting in relation to air pollution similar to that which exists with reference to stream pollution. Increasingly it is recognized that the layer of air above us is thin, is not limitless, and must stop being used as an aerial sewer. Pound for pound man consumes at least 10 times as much air as water. Although there has been for many years concern over the purity of the water used by human societies, little attention has been given to the quality of the air which constantly is breathed into the lungs and absorbed into the bloodstream. Historical records do exist, however, that indicate at least momentary concern with the problem and even related legislation. As a result of the widespread use of soft sea-coal for fuel in English towns and cities, a smoke abatement law was passed as early as 1273 by Edward I. He banned the use of coal as being prejudicial to the public health. Shortly after, Parliament in 1306 formed a smoke-abatement group whose recommendations resulted in a royal proclamation which prohibited the use of coal in the furnaces of artificers. Record has it that in 1307 one offender was actually executed for violating the regulations.[39] In 1661 a report entitled *Fumifugium* claimed that almost one half the deaths in London were "phthisical and pulmonic distempers" resulting from polluted air.[40]

Even now the most common complaints about air pollution relate to smoke content and odor. A smoky or sooty atmosphere obviously results in dirty clothes and buildings, less sunlight, damaged vegetation, and sometimes impaired breathing. However, there are a number of other reasons for concern, including particulate and gaseous chemicals, dusts, and irritating pollens. Recognition of this has resulted in a change in name and emphasis of many agencies and associations from "smoke abatement" to "atmospheric pollution control."

The atmosphere may be polluted from many sources. Smoke results whenever fuel or other material is incompletely burned, i.e., industrial, commercial, or domestic heating facilities, incinerators, brush fires, dumps, and automobile motors. In urban areas especially, automobile motors are a major generator of toxic gases.[41] In rural and suburban areas irritating pollens and toxic agricultural sprays and dusts are apt to be particularly prevalent. Industrial contaminants represent a particularly complex and important source of atmospheric pollution.

In general, air pollutants fall into two classes: (1) particulate matter or aerosols, and (2) gases and vapors. The most common types of the former are metallic oxides, sulfur trioxide, fumes, mists, fogs, carbon, tar, and fly ash. Sulfur dioxide and carbon monoxide probably are the most common of the gases and vapors. In addition, it has been shown that ozone which may be produced by photochemical reactions can give rise to irritating proportions as well as aid in the development of additional irritants by its oxidizing action on other pollutants. The complexity of industrial, automotive, and other sources that may pollute air is well illustrated by the studies reported by Magill[42] and by Larson[43] of the qualitative constitution of smog in Los Angeles. Analysis of samples of air in that area have indicated the presence of the following contaminants:

Aerosols

Ether-soluble aerosols	Lead
Sulfuric acid mist	Aluminum
Carbon	Calcium
Silicon	Iron

Gases and Vapors

Acetylene	Methyl chloride
Aromatics	Nitric oxide
Benzene	Nitrogen dioxide
Isobutane	Nitrous oxide
n-Butane	n-Pentane
Butenes	Phosgene
Carbon tetrachloride	Propane
Ethane	Propylene
Ethyl benzene and xylene	Sulfur dioxide
Formic acid	Toluene
Methyl cellosolve	Trichlorethylene

Unsaturated hydrocarbons ranging from C_5H_8 to $C_{12}H_{24}$.

Products of oxidation of the above unsaturated hydrocarbons (aldehydes, peroxides, ketones, and organic acids).

It is obvious that in addition to the discharge of contaminants into the atmosphere there are certain fixed or variable meteorologic and topographic factors that may determine whether or not a nuisance will develop, the degree of its concentration or extension, and the acuteness and severity of its result. If a community is situated within a topographic bowl, natural dispersal of atmospheric pollutants will be somewhat limited and there may result a considerable concentration of soot and noxious gases. The role of weather was summarized by the 1951 Technical Conference on Air Pollution[44] as follows: "The average distribution of contaminants in a city is governed by wind, rain, atmospheric stability, and topographic features. The contaminants in their turn influence rainfall and fog occurrence and persistence." Baynton[45] has pointed out that insufficient attention is given to these factors until they combine under special circumstances to cause dramatic disastrous situations such as those at Donora, the Meuse Valley, and elsewhere. He urges that any program relating to atmospheric pollution must take into account a study of winds, atmospheric stability, and precipitation as they are related to seasonal variation, diurnal variation, surface temperatures, and many other meteorologic factors.

Pollution of the atmosphere may result in economic loss to individuals and to the general population in a variety of ways. Losses may take the form of damage to livestock and vegetation, corrosion of metals and structural materials, damage to clothing and other fabrics, damage to the finishes of automobiles and houses, disruption of communications and increased artificial lighting requirements, depreciated real estate values, and last, but by no means least, the acute and chronic harm done to humans. Not including the effect on humans, the national economic loss due to atmospheric pollution has been estimated at from $2 billion to $4 billion or about $10 per capita per year.[46] On the other hand, one can cite many examples of industrial establishments which, by installation of control procedures, have actually netted from modest to substantial profits from the recovered materials. For example, one chemical company in Los Angeles spent $40,000 for equipment to prevent atmospheric contamination. As a result it is now recovering 15 barrels per day of lead oxide worth $90,000 per year. This is not meant to imply, however, that air pollution control precedures necessarily result in profit because that is by no means the case.

For our purposes, of course, it is the effects upon human life that are of greatest interest and importance. The question of the effect of air pollution on the health of the individual or of a community under ordinary circumstances is so insidious that an answer is as yet impossible. Base lines, standards, and methods of measurement necessary to determine adequately the physiologic or histologic effects of substances in the air still leave much to be desired. Even when a relatively severe short-term exposure occurs, such as that at Donora, conclusive answers are usually not obtained because the investigations take place after the fact and not before and during the incident. Nevertheless, much has been learned during recent years as a result of studying "epidemics" of air pollution, continuous smog situations, long-term effects on workers constantly exposed to certain substances, and laboratory experiments.[47]

The "epidemic" situation, of course, is the most dramatic, and a number of facts of value have resulted from their investigation. Four of these occurrences merit special mention. During 1930 the heavily industrialized area in and around Liege in the Meuse Valley of Belgium was subjected to 4 days of continuous fog saturated with industrial smoke and fumes. Many thousands of people became ill, and 63 died. While studies indicated significant amounts of sulfur dioxide, sulfuric acid and other chemicals in the air, no single substance was found in a concentration sufficiently high to have caused the damage by itself.[48]

A similar tragedy occurred in 1948 in Donora, Pa., a small town of about 14,000 inhabitants. Because of its location in a valley and because of its industry, polluted fogs are very common in Donora. Usually the sun and wind dissipate the fog during the early hours of the day. Occasionally, however, it may remain throughout a day. On October 27, 1948, a thick fog settled down in the valley and remained for $4\frac{1}{2}$ days, meanwhile becoming more and more polluted by the smoke, fumes, and gases from the town's industrial plants. During the period, 20 individuals died and about 6,000 others, or 43% of the population, became ill in varying degrees. The episode and the circumstances were studied exhaustively for a year by the Pennsylvania Department of Health assisted by the United States Public Health Service.[49,50]

As in the case of the Liege disaster, although a large number of gases and fumes were identified in the atmosphere, it was concluded that no single contaminant was responsible. In both instances it was felt that a combination of irritating and toxic materials, of which sulfur dioxide undoubtedly was one, acted synergistically to produce the illnesses and deaths. In both instances the deleterious conditions were observed to affect the population selectively. Almost all the victims who were affected fatally and many of those who became ill but did not die suffered from respiratory or cardiac difficulties. The prolonged and intensive pollution of the air harmed the aged, the infirm, and enfeebled infants earlier than it affected the remaining more vigorous fraction of the population. Among other things, this indicates the need for a completely different set of tolerance levels of toxic substances for a community as a whole as against those used heretofore. Most of the latter are based on the tolerance of industrial workers.

A third disaster of this type occurred on November 24, 1950, at Poza Rica, Mexico, where 320 persons were hospitalized, 22 of whom died.[51] This case differed from the Liege and Donora episodes in that it was

possible to point to a single toxic agent. A gasoline refinery at the site discharged a number of aerial contaminants, one of which was hydrogen sulfide. A combination of relatively localized unusual meteorologic phenomena resulted in a very high concentration of hydrogen sulfide gas around the plant.

The city of London, England, has experienced a number of sudden increases in the death rate due to atmospheric pollution. Its situation is somewhat different from the others described in that unlike the others the problem is not primarily related to industrial contaminants. Severe fogs with stasis and lethal concentration of atmospheric pollutants occurred particularly in 1873, 1880, 1892, 1948, 1952, and 1962. In the 1880 incident, the death rate of 896 per million was about 50% above normal expectancy. In fact, it was significantly higher than the rate of 876 recorded for the worst week of the great London cholera epidemic of 1866. Despite this, the events of December 1952 and especially of the 5 days December 5 to 9 were even more spectacular. It has been shown conclusively that during the total period of the first 3 weeks of December about 4,000 deaths were caused by the polluted fog. Although the very young, the aged, and the infirm were affected most, it is interesting that all age groups contributed to the increased mortality. The mortality of infants doubled, deaths of children 10 to 13 years of age increased by a third, and deaths of young adults increased almost two thirds. Deaths from bronchitis which were eight times normal and deaths from pneumonia which were three times normal accounted for about one half of the total increase in mortality. Other causes of death for which marked increases were observed were pulmonary tuberculosis and cancer, coronary disease, and myocardial degeneration.

The cause of the phenomenon was a prolonged absence of wind and a low temperature which produced a low altitude inversion whereby the normal upward air currents came to a stop. As a result the usual air contaminants of the area accumulated to unprecedented concentrations. For example, the summer daily average concentration of smoke is about 0.12 mg. per cubic meter of air and of sulfur dioxide about 0.07 parts per million. On December 8, 1952, these figures rose to 4.46 mg. per cubic meter and 1.339 parts per million, respectively.[52,53] In December 1962 during 4 days, 1,000 persons were hospitalized and about 100 died from the effects of a similar, but shorter, episode.

More difficult than "epidemic" situations is the problem of determining the chronic effects of atmospheric contaminants. Attempts have been made to study this problem, but inherent difficulties have made them incomplete and inconclusive. The best work has been in relation to the chronic smog problem of Los Angeles.[54,55] There, the outstanding effect has been eye irritation. At first, sulfur dioxide, an outstanding air contaminant, was assumed to be the cause. This was because of its known irritating effect, and perhaps because of the ease of identifying it. However, control procedures which significantly reduced the amount of SO_2 in the area did not result in appreciable relief. This led to a discovery that certain hydrocarbons, including gasoline vapors, could be oxidized in air and light to form ozone and other compounds which cause all of the observed deleterious effects, including eye irritation.

By its very nature, atmospheric pollution is difficult to control. Its causes are many and complex, really adequate standards and means of measurement are still in the process of development, and an extensive number of public and private agencies, businesses, and industries have important interests in anything that is done. The atmosphere surrounding a present-day community is bound to be contaminated. Obviously a completely pure atmosphere is unattainable. Numerous compromises must be made. Not the least of the problems facing those interested is where to draw the line. It would seem that control must depend upon legislation, public as well as industrial education, the further development of standards and measurement techniques, the further development and application of practical mechanical devices for controlling the aerial waste products of industry, and the development and application of new sources of heat and power. Recognition of air pollution as a health and social problem has resulted in the enactment of legislation at all levels of government. Enabling legislation to permit local jurisdictions to act against specific problems was passed in California in 1947. This was followed in 1955 by legislation which permitted regional control programs. In addition to establishing a control authority and providing for continuous study and research, it placed a limit on the dusts, fumes, and sulfur which may be discharged by industry and requires approval of plans for any installation that might add to the pollution of the atmosphere. An increasing number of cities have enacted ordinances dealing with various phases of air pollution. Since the mid-1940's, Pittsburgh and St. Louis particularly have brought about spectacular improvements. In St. Louis, for example, the sulfur dioxide concentration in the air in 1950 had been reduced 83% below the level of the winter of 1936-1937, and the downtown concentration was no higher in 1950 than it had been 20 miles out of the city 15 years before. In Pittsburgh, between 1945 and 1948, the average number of hours per month of heavy smoke during the heating season decreased more than 50%, from 158 to 77. During the same period visibility at the airport improved 75%.[47] These improvements were due essentially to the enforcement, coupled with community education, of an ordinance which declared the production or emission of dense smoke a nuisance to be summarily abated; made it unlawful to import, sell, or use any solid fuel for hand-firing or surface-burning types of equipment which did not meet the standards of a smokeless fuel; and specifically included control of smoke from locomotives.

Federal legislation in 1955 authorized and supported research and technical assistance on the federal and state level. In 1959 the California legislature required the promulgation of ambient air quality standards and emission standards for motor vehicles. This led to the California Motor Vehicle Pollution Control Act of 1960, which required the installation on motor vehicles of devices to reduce emissions. This affected the entire automobile industry, and exhaust control devices became applicable on all new cars in the United States in September 1967.

The 1955 federal air pollution control legislation was strengthened by the passage of the Clean Air Acts of 1963, 1965, 1966, and 1967. These are administered by the National Air Pollution Control Administration, which is part of the Consumer Protection and Environmental Health Service, Department of Health, Education, and Welfare. The goal of the Clean Air Acts as described by MacKenzie[56] is the creation of an expanded national program based upon strong and capable state and local efforts and aided by a federal program empowered to provide assistance through broadened technical, financial, and legal authorities. The acts emphasize the primary responsibility of state and local governments. In addition to increased research and training the acts provide substantial financial support on a matching basis for the creation or improvement of state and local air pollution control programs.

With reference to the legislative aspects of the air pollution problem Dyktor[57] warns against the tendency to go to extremes and by means of legislation to "throw the whole book" at both industry and all fuel users. He advises the following:

> Legislation must be of the 'performance' type without specifying the means of attainment of the 'performance.' In other words, one should be concerned principally with the discharge from the stack and the potential violator should be given a free choice of means to avoid an actual violation.

He concludes with particularly sound advice well worth repetition here:

> Human experience teaches that a policy of adjustment and flexibility is the best policy in the long run. This applies particularly well in air pollution control. Litigation is to be avoided because the democratic process demands careful preparation of the facts plus considerable time spent in court, and

this energy can be used to better advantage in a cooperative effort which will give more permanent results. Therefore, in practice, the provisions of legislation must be applied with a great deal of judgment, and sight must not be lost of the fact that only a compromise can be arrived at in most instances.

RADIOLOGIC HEALTH

One of the newest and very important aspects of environmental health relates to problems arising from the use of fissionable materials.[58] Increasing amounts of radioactive isotopes are being used for medical diagnosis and treatment, for industrial research and materials testing,[59] and for food preservation.[60] Already a number of ships as well as electrical power plants using nuclear energy have been constructed. The potential of fallout from nuclear weapons testing or attack compounds the situation. In several instances accidental spillage of fissionable material has presented health agencies with new challenges.[61]

The chief concern of the public health agency is protection of the community and the nation from damaging radiations, whether due to misuse, accident, improper disposal of fissionable waste materials, weapons testing, or military attack. Understandably the last two possibilities are dominant in the public's mind largely due to extensive discussion in the public information media. It is important to realize, however, that they do not represent the major threats. Bugher[62] emphasized this in the First Annual Bronfman Lecture. He pointed out that studies by the National Academy of Sciences and the National Research Council have shown that fallout from weapons testing in the atmosphere represents only a small fraction of the total radiation exposure of the public in contrast with the large part of the total exposure from the diagnostic and therapeutic uses of X rays. He went on to predict that "With the rapid development of nuclear power and the expanding employment of radioactive materials and nuclear reactions in industry, agriculture, and medicine, we may anticipate that maintaining control over these potential hazards will become more complex rather than less."

Among the radiologic control activities in which various health agencies have become involved are the determination of the amounts and effects of natural or background radiation[63]; the prohibition of shoe-fitting fluoroscopic machines; the testing of x-ray and fluoroscopic equipment in medical and dental offices, hospitals, and clinics[64] as well as in industry[65]; the surveillance of fluctuations in atmospheric radiation; the testing of milk,[66] water,[67] and other substances for levels of radioactive contamination; consultation in the construction of nuclear-powered ships[68] and electric power plants[69]; planning for civilian protection in case of nuclear attack[70]; and the disposal of radioactive wastes.[71] With reference to the latter and in line with Bugher's observations previously quoted it has been indicated that when worldwide nuclear-powered industry becomes fully developed, its accumulated waste products will represent more radiation than would be released in any atomic war.[72]

These new responsibilities have made it necessary for increasing numbers of public health workers to familiarize themselves with totally new areas of knowledge. To facilitate this, the Division of Radiological Health of the Public Health Service, the Atomic Energy Commission, the Department of Defense, and many universities have provided special continued education and in-service training courses and have engaged in the development of various specialized technicians in this field. Of assistance to the general health worker is a recently published handbook by the American Public Health Association.[73] Furthermore, because of the extensive geographic, social, political, as well as biologic ramifications of this field, it has become increasingly necessary for public health workers to involve themselves in interdisciplinary, interorganizational, and intergovernmental relationships quite different from the past.[74,75]

Actually, governmental concern about radiation is not new. Its history in the United States may be considered to have begun with the standardization by the National Bureau of Standards of radium for medical uses in 1913, the concerns in relation to radium poisoning of watch-dial painters as well as radium water tonics and rejuvenators, leading eventually to the formation in the late 1920's of the Advisory Committee on X Ray and Radium Protection, later renamed the National Committee on Radiation Protection. In 1946 the Atomic Energy Act was passed, which provided for the distribution of radioactive isotopes on the basis of strict health and safety standards. In the late 1950's the Public Health Service established a Division of Radiological Health and designated an Advisory Committee on Radiation. It has cooperated with the Atomic Energy Commission, the Food and Drug Administration, the Department of Defense, and various other agencies. In the process it has carried out many studies on the decontamination of radioactively contaminated waters, the treatment and disposal of radioactive wastes, the standards necessary in the industrial and transportation uses of atomic power, and the evaluation of varying degrees of hazards associated with radioactive elements. In 1960 a further step forward was taken by the enactment of P.L. 86-373 which established the Federal Radiation Council. A major purpose has been to examine all scientific evidence, as it develops, regarding the biologic effects of radiation, leading to the development of broad guidelines for national policy.

Accompanying national action and greatly stimulated by it has been the development of programs of varying degrees of extensiveness throughout the states and major cities of the nation.[76,77] In the process of developing and carrying out these programs, one of the most difficult problems which confronts the public health worker is the maintenance of an appropriate balance between the benefits that may result from the use of radioactive materials and equipment and the risks that might possibly be entailed.[78] No one would suggest that the use of X rays be ceased because of some measure of risk. Similarly it would be ill-advised to deprive man and his societies of the tremendous benefits to be reaped from the application of radiation to industry, food preservation, power development and the like. Bugher[62] has put the question well, "Nearly all of us of this scientific generation have been brought up on the concept that all changes produced by ionizing radiation are deleterious in general and that in the genetic sense any biologically beneficial effect is outweighed by the handicaps that are introduced. We find it difficult to conceive that absorption of radiation may not be followed by permanent cell changes. It is possible that we neglect to consider that all life on this earth has come to its present state through continuous contact with a radioactive environment. There has been not a single living cell in all the history of life on this planet that has not been subjected to radiation from both without and within its substance."

The challenge then is for public health workers to deal with problems of radioactivity with a balance of respect and reason based upon sound proven scientific data and not emotion or fear of the unknown. In order to provide a practical measure of protection from unnecessary emissions from x-ray equipment, television sets, and other electronic devices, Congress passed the Radiation Control for Health and Safety Act in October 1968.

HOUSING AND CITY PLANNING

In discussing the need for public health interest in housing Winslow[79] commented as follows:

The filth epidemics of the Nineteenth Century have been conquered in civilized and relatively prosperous lands like ours. We can now think in terms of health rather than in terms of disease; and, from this standpoint, such problems as nutrition and housing come to the forefront. The slum of today is no longer a hot-bed of cholera and typhus fever as it was seventy-five years ago. It remains, however, one of the major obstacles to that physical and emotional and social vigor and efficiency and satisfaction which we conceive as the health objective of the future.

Many attempts have been made to estab-

lish a conclusive relationship between unsatisfactory housing and ill health. Several of these have been referred to earlier in the discussion in Chapter 5 of the sociologic aspects of public health. However, because the dwellers in poor housing are subjected to so many other undesirable factors such as low economic income, malnutrition, limited education, and the like it is impossible to determine with exactness what is cause and what is effect. The difficulty and its proper interpretation has been well summarized by Anderson[80] as follows:

Of the many newer aspects of environmental sanitation, the standards of housing seem to rest on an especially insecure epidemiological foundation. I would not question the potential health significance of housing, and yet epidemiological data on which to base this belief are virtually nonexistent for poor housing cannot be separated from other attributes of poverty.

This inability to secure epidemiological support for housing standards should not discourage us from attempts to improve housing conditions or even to do so by regulation. Almost every community has houses that by no stretch of the imagination can be defended as desirable for human habitation. An appreciable fraction of our population lives under conditions that are undesirable socially, morally, and hygienically. Housing needs no defense nor need await epidemiological support.

The history of the movement to provide decent housing for people has been briefly traced by Catherine Bauer[81] on a basis which should not be disregarded by public health workers. She reminds us that the housing movement may be viewed not only as a significant chapter in scientific and public health history, "but also as a very lively and important chapter in political history." She points out that without exception, "every major step in housing progress in the past century has involved some public action," and suggests that "political philosophy—the motivating forces behind public action and the application of scientific knowledge—is not secondary or incidental, but paramount." Of particular significance to our present consideration, she traces the gradual development of enlightened political philosophy, dating from the English Poor Laws of the early nineteenth century, with its expanding concepts of individual rights—to due process of law, to health, to education—to the more recent concept of the right of individuals to a decent home. She proceeds then to provide us with a sound basis for future thought and action in proposing that henceforth our interest is "not just a question of 'minimum standards,' to allay disease or prevent divorce or save the taxpayers money, or of sporadic housing programs tied to one emergency kite or another, to provide employment or increase the birthrate or improve the physical qualities of soldiers or lessen the danger of revolution, but good housing for all, to be provided by public action where private enterprise could not do the job, on the fundamental democratic principle of equal opportunity."

The production of housing in the United States has depended essentially on the law of supply and demand. The demand, however, has been closely linked to the economic ability of individuals and families to afford the product. Thus, even in the relatively prosperous year 1929, a third of American families had incomes under $1,200 and an additional third had incomes from $1,200 to $2,000 per year. Budget experts believe that a family should not expend more than about one fifth of its income for housing. The inability of a considerable proportion of the population to afford good housing entirely on their own was pointed out to public health workers a number of years ago[82]:

> The slum dweller is the real problem, not the slum. The basic inescapable fact is that a substantial part of our urban population cannot pay for decent housing. In an Atlantic seaboard city like New York, private capital cannot possibly build and maintain decent housing for rent at less than $30 per room per month. No family of a size requiring a three-room apartment can afford to pay such a rent on a family income of less than $5,000 a year. It is true that gouging landlords are, in some instances, obtaining huge incomes from subdivided tenements and cellar dwellings. To expect, however, the private landlord to be able to meet the housing needs of the $2,000-income families with children is a fantastic dream. The submerged one-tenth of the population of New York and of other large cities, who have incomes of $2,000 or less, can pay only $30 per month for the whole dwelling unit.

It was for this very reason that our federally subsidized low-rent housing program was initiated; it can provide a most economical type of basically decent housing and provide it to the needy tenant for a price of $30 per month for an average household. The far more extensive development of this program is an essential precedent to the elimination of the slum dwelling.

An important consideration is that private housing is constructed largely during periods of economic upswing when building costs are also going up. Furthermore, during periods of economic depression, the cost of houses does not go down to the extent that salaries and incomes decline. During the depression years of the 1930's, despite ever growing needs due to population increase and continued movement toward cities, construction of homes lagged considerably. The postdepression spurt was then thrown off balance by the exigencies of the war effort. By the end of World War II, a tremendous backlog of housing needs had developed. Since that time we have observed the greatest building boom in our history. Despite this, about one quarter of the nation's dwellings are still considered to have basic health deficiences. Of over 58 million housing units reported in the 1960 census, more than 8 million were deteriorating, and almost 3 million were dilapidated. Overcrowding and deficient lighting, ventilation, and heating were not included among the criteria.

The components of healthful housing have been studied over a number of years by the Committee on the Hygiene of Housing which was established in 1937 by the American Public Health Association. In the course of its work the Committee has issued a series of important documents[79,83,84] that have filled an important need not only of public health but of other disciplines. It has also produced a Proposed Housing Ordinance which has been widely used as a model. Under four broad headings the Committee has listed the following thirty basic principles which must be considered with regard to healthful housing[83]:

Fundamental physiologic needs
1. Maintenance of a thermal environment which will avoid undue heat loss from the human body

2. Maintenance of a thermal environment which will permit adequate heat loss from the human body
3. Provision of an atmosphere of reasonable chemical purity
4. Provision of adequate daylight illumination and avoidance of undue daylight glare
5. Provision for admission of direct sunlight
6. Provision of adequate artificial illumination and avoidance of glare
7. Protection against excessive noise
8. Provision of adequate space for exercise and for play of children

Fundamental psychologic needs

1. Provision of adequate privacy for the individual
2. Provision of opportunities for normal family life
3. Provision of opportunities for normal community life
4. Provision of facilities which make possible the performance of tasks of the household without undue physical and mental fatigue
5. Provision of facilities for maintenance of cleanliness of the dwelling and of the person
6. Concordance with prevailing social standards of the local community

Protection against contagion

1. Provision of a water supply of safe, sanitary quality, available to the dwelling
2. Protection of the water supply system against pollution within the dwelling
3. Provision of toilet facilities of such a character as to minimize the danger of transmitting disease
4. Protection against sewage contamination of the interior surfaces of the dwelling
5. Avoidance of insanitary conditions in the vicinity of the dwelling
6. Exclusion from the dwelling of vermin which may play a part in the transmission of disease
7. Provision of facilities for keeping milk and food undecomposed
8. Provision of sufficient space in sleeping rooms, to minimize the danger of contact infection

Protection against accidents

1. Erection of the dwelling with such materials and methods of construction as to minimize danger of accidents due to collapse of any part of the structure
2. Control of conditions likely to cause fires or to promote their spread
3. Provision of adequate facilities for escape in case of fire
4. Protection against danger of electrical shocks and burns
5. Protection against falls and other mechanical injuries in the home
6. Protection of the neighborhood against the hazards of automobile traffic

The achievement of these goals involves action on three fronts: first, *prevention* of accelerated rates of deterioration of dwellings and their environment, thereby forestalling the formation of new blighted and slum areas; second, *rehabilitation* of existing substandard housing, if salvage is economically feasible, and its demolition—which is part of rehabilitation in its broader sense—of substandard dwellings that are beyond repair; and third, *production* of enough new housing to provide for population increase, for families now overcrowded, for replacement of demolished and decayed structures, and for the normal vacancy cushion.[85]

As is indicated by several of the preceding criteria, adequate housing is now considered to involve circumstances which extend beyond the physical structure of the dwelling. Many of the objectives are unattainable if the surrounding neighborhood or indeed the entire community is allowed to develop in a completely hit or miss fashion. It is necessary, therefore, to give consideration to the overall living needs of the neighborhood and to the planning of the community as a whole. This involves the development of long-range programs of neighborhood and community improvement, land use and traffic planning, with attention to street and freeway layouts, parks and playgrounds, sites for schools and other public buildings, shopping center, and the location of business and industrial enterprises. A serious mistake would be to consider the dwelling alone without reference to its use, its surroundings, and its community service connections. Thus Molner and Hilbert[86] list the following items as important if an optimum residential environment is to be achieved:

1. Space for light, air, and recreation
2. Adequate water supply
3. Proper sewage and waste disposal facilities
4. Drainage
5. Freedom from accident hazard
6. Clean air
7. Freedom from unnecessary noise and disturbances
8. Insect, rodent and nuisance control
9. Suitable recreational facilities
10. Building codes
11. A land use plan
12. Zoning

Beyond this is the need for increased attention by public health workers and others to fringe areas and suburbs which surround municipalities. Here some of the worst housing problems exist today. O'Harrow[87] points to much of the American population which lives under these circumstances. He points out that, "In 1950, the census counted approximately 20,900,000 people living in this 'no man's land'—more than the combined population of our five largest cities." In 1962 the number was estimated at 30 million persons. While not all, of course, live under substandard conditions, many do. Three reasons are given by O'Harrow for subdivisions going sour and giving rise to difficulties. In the first place they may be premature, with land subdivided before there is a real need. Beyond the economic loss which results from much of the land lying unused the situation invites the development of suburban squatter slums. A second reason for failure is that subdivisions may be poorly designed by promoters butchering the land into inadequate sized lots in an uncompromising gridiron pattern, with no concern for recreation, parking, or other public spaces. Finally, subdivisions and fringe areas are very apt to suffer because of no plans for, much less provision of, water, sanitary or storm sewers, street lights, fire hydrants, or grading and surfacing of streets. Woodbury[88] insists that the dispersal of people and their housing is not basically at fault. To the contrary, he points out that the nineteenth century city, which still determines much of our urban thinking and planning, was a product of a time, culture, and technology quite different from ours. As he says, "Nothing could be more illogical and more disastrous for our increasingly metropolitan civilization than to let the problems of urban sprawl drive us back to a pattern of city building that, on balance, is definitely worse, even if the new version of that pattern would be largely in metal and glass in place of brick, stone, and wood." The problem then is twofold—the inadequacy of our archaic cities and the unplanned manner in which our suburbs are being allowed to develop.

Any reasonably adequate solution of the tremendous and complex problem of housing obviously requires the combined and coordinated efforts of private enterprise, the local, state, and federal governments, and various professional and civic groups. Governmental action on all levels involves participation by many different agencies and departments including those concerned with health, building inspection, plumbing, water, legal counseling, schools, recreation, traffic engineering, fire protection, public works, tax enforcement, public welfare, public housing, and redevelopment. This is not a job to be done by the official health agency alone.

Several administrative approaches have been tried. Traditionally, in this country responsibility for the quality of new housing has been vested in housing officials who have been primarily concerned with protection against fire and structural collapse. Of somewhat secondary interest have been requirements relating to the water supply, plumbing, heating, lighting, and ventilation. Once housing is constructed and occupied, responsibility for the supervision of its quality is usually transferred to the local health department. This is perhaps because the health department is in the best position to use effectively the police power and other legislative measures[89] and because of the multiplicity of interests of public health agencies. Thus many local health departments have long been active in various fields directly related to housing. Among these are the enforcement of requirements with regard to heating, lighting, and ventilation, control of atmospheric pollution, supervision of water supplies, plumbing and sewerage systems, rodent and vermin control, nuisance abatement, accident prevention, and sanitary education.

The contributions of the local health department to the solution of the broad problem of housing may be in several fields which include:

1. Development and promotion of the acceptance of local desirable housing and neighborhood standards
2. Participation in the enactment and

enforcement of proper building codes and housing ordinances

3. Measurement of the quality of existing housing and neighborhoods
4. Participation in the remedying of existing housing deficiencies, through rehabilitation and slum clearance
5. Participation in the proper control and direction of new housing, through zoning, city planning, and the issuance of various permits and licenses
6. Education of the public in the hygiene of housing

Mood[90] cautions however that in assuming a leadership role public health officials should be cognizant of the fact that the involvement of health agencies in housing programs is not revolutionary in nature but rather that it is evolutionary.

The need for concentrating the responsibility for administering laws or regulations relating to housing is emphasized by Johnson[91] who advocates the formation of a Housing Board responsible to the administrative head of the community. He suggests that it consist of the heads of departments directly concerned with the various aspects of the housing regulations, plus one or two others who are vitally concerned: "For example, a typical board might consist of the commissioners of the building, fire, and health departments, along with the executive director of the Housing Agency or the slum clearance and redevelopment agency, and the head of the planning department. In some communities the commissioner of police and the director of welfare may be added to, or substituted for, one of the above representatives."

It must always be remembered, however, that while laws and regulations may provide a basic background and a legal means of requiring conformance to housing standards they have never in themselves provided or maintained a decent dwelling. One of the greatest areas of neglect has been in health education as it relates to housing. If adequately pursued, it would undoubtedly bring about the correction of more housing deficiencies than could ever be accomplished by laws.

Major consideration of necessity has been

given to the situation and possibilities on the local level. A few words should be said about the position of the state and federal governments. They may provide types of assistance and service which individuals, communities, and organizations are unable to provide for themselves. State governments may provide funds and consultation for the planning and construction of public housing, for slum clearance and redevelopment, and for regional planning. In a few instances, statewide housing legislation has been enacted and enforced. The federal government through legislation may assist by the insurance of mortgages and of deposits in home loan banks, by the subsidization of slum clearance, redevelopment and low-rent public housing, by rent controls, grants for farm housing, by research, and by the collection of statistics on housing, labor, and materials.

In 1949 Congress passed the Federal Housing Act. It established a Housing and Home Finance Agency as part of a major national housing instrument, the Federal Housing Administration. The functions of the Agency were gradually expanded by subsequent amendment. The agency establishes standards and requirements which qualify local governments for grants and loans for surveying, planning, and correcting substandard housing and environmental living conditions. To qualify, the local government must submit a plan of action designated as the "workable program." It should give consideration to seven basic elements:

1. Enforcement of sound local housing and building codes; an end to tolerating thousands of illegal, degrading, unhealthy, substandard structures and areas where many people have to live
2. General master plan for the community's development; an end to haphazard, thoughtless planning and growth; a road map for the city's future in a planned framework for the region, metropolitan, or intercity urbanization of which it is a part
3. Basic analysis of neighborhoods and the kind of treatment needed; an inventory of blighted and threatened

areas to form the basis of a plan of treatment to stop blight in its tracks

4. An effective administrative organization to run the program; coordinated activity toward a common purpose by all officers and arms of the local government

5. Financial capacity to carry out the program, using community revenues and resources to build a better city for the future instead of continuing to pay heavily for past mistakes

6. Rehousing of displaced families; expanding the supply of good housing for all income groups, through new construction and rehabilitation so that families paying premium prices for slums can be rehoused

7. Full communitywide participation and support; public demand for a better community, and public backing for the steps needed to get it

In 1965 the functions of the Federal Housing Administration became the nucleus of a new Cabinet entity, the Department of Housing and Urban Development.

VECTOR CONTROL

As pointed out in Chapter 17, which deals with the control of communicable diseases, those pathogenic organisms which involve nonhuman hosts or vectors at any stage of their life cycles offer an additional point of potential control. The number of such diseases is very large and the numbers and types of vectors impressive. Vectors of particular public health concern are rodents and arthropods. Of the former, rats, ground squirrels, and prairie dogs are most important, especially in view of their role in the spread of plague. Among the innumerable arthropods, certain mosquitoes, flies, fleas, roaches, lice, mites, and ticks are of impressive significance. It is all too easily overlooked by residents of the United States that insects exact a far greater toll of health and life than any other thing. Malaria is still the world's leading cause of death, and many other insect-borne diseases are far from rare. Furthermore, considerable numbers of the insect vectors of many of those diseases are present in many parts of the

United States. Accordingly, the control of insect vectors of disease is still and will long continue to be an important phase of environmental health programs in many places.

The possibility of controlling disease-transmitting insects became a reality at about the turn of the century. Life cycles of many organisms and of many vectors became known. Experiments and demonstrations of various methods of control of breeding places and of protection against adult insects were carried out. The use of courageous administrative procedures for the widespread use of these methods established Havana and Panama as famous landmarks in public health history. Destruction of mosquito breeding places was accomplished by drainage and fillings; larvae were killed by fish and by the spreading of oils; adult insects were destroyed or repelled by fumigants and smudges and were excluded from living and sleeping quarters by screening and bed nets. Subsequent decades brought cheaper and easier larviciding with Paris green, and pyrethrum became widely used as an insect adulticide. It was not, however, until World War II presented the terrible risk of action in far-flung disease-ridden areas that insect control really came into its own. Some of the older materials like pyrethrum were made more effective by refining their insecticidal principles and applying them with aerosols as the medium. Remarkably efficient new repellents were also developed. It was the development of DDT and other potent insecticides and their widespread use against mosquitoes, lice, and other disease vectors, however, that really opened a new epidemiologic era. The numerous successes of these compounds against the vectors of a large number of diseases in many places represent a real triumph of man over his environment.

The control and destruction of rodents is of importance because of two diseases in particular, i.e., plague and murine typhus. In the United States, plague-infected wild rodents have been spreading eastward from the west coast at a rapid rate, necessitating intensified control procedures in order to prevent epidemics. Murine typhus is endemic in a number of southeastern and some western states. In this instance rats and mice which infest households are the rodents of consequence. Other mammalian hosts of diseases dangerous to man that in certain areas assume importance are wild monkeys and some ruminants (in relation to yellow fever) and dogs, wolves, foxes, and bats (in relation to rabies).

Many urban and rural local health departments, as well as state health departments, have established vector control activities, usually in conjunction with their environmental health programs. Activities that are variously included are educational and promotional activities, vector surveys, research with regard to vectors, materials, and control measures, direct application of insecticides and rodenticides, licensure and supervision of pest eradicators, studies on or supervision of garbage disposal, rat proofing in relation to the housing program, and elimination of mosquito breeding by spraying, drainage, filling, or variation of impounded water levels. To perform these various functions adequately, a variety of types of personnel is required, i.e., sanitary engineers, laboratorians, sanitarians, sanitary inspectors, and sometimes biologists, zoologists, and chemists. Of particular importance are entomologists and ecologists, to whose services and abilities increasing attention is being given by public health agencies.

MISCELLANEOUS SANITATION ACTIVITIES

In addition to the areas of environmental health already discussed there is a varied array of miscellaneous activities and programs which may be carried out by health agencies. No more than passing mention will be made of them here since most of them are of specialized and restricted importance, interest, and responsibility.

Of specific federal concern is the supervision of the salubrity of vehicles of interstate and international traffic, i.e., buses, trains, boats, and airplanes. The Public Health Service, which is responsible for these activities, has developed standards for each.[92-94] The maintenance of a sanitary environment in connection with parks, rec-reation areas, and trailer camps may be a concern of a local, state, or federal health agency depending upon the particular situation. Usually the responsibility is shared with another branch of government, such as those concerned with highways, recreation, or conservation. Related to these problems but more exclusively the responsibility of the public health agency is the supervision of the quality of swimming pools and bathing places.

PERSONNEL IN ENVIRONMENTAL CONTROL

Because of the regional differences which exist with regard to types of problems, degree of urbanity, and availability of funds, facilities, and trained personnel, a certain amount of difference of opinion has resulted concerning the types of persons needed in order to carry on a satisfactory environmental control program. Generally speaking, the rural areas and small towns have found it necessary to depend upon nonengineering personnel, often with no training except perhaps for a few weeks' indoctrination and orientation provided by the state health departments. In contrast, by virtue of the complexity of their problems, urban centers have characteristically employed persons with professional training in civil or sanitary engineering to provide the leadership for their environmental control programs. These, of course, must be augmented by a cadre of qualified sanitarians. Engineering is concerned essentially with design, construction, and operation. Although benefits of great significance to public health result from sanitary and civil engineering, their practitioners are primarily interested in the design and construction of a waterworks system, a sewage treatment plant, or a garbage incinerator and focus their attention much more upon construction materials, hydraulics, rates of flow, and heat losses rather than upon potential morbidity decreases and other responses of those served.

Sanitary inspection, as has been pointed out, antedated sanitary engineering by a considerable period. Its efforts have been directed toward more local and personal environmental factors that were thought to exert a possible deleterious or unpleasant effect upon living. Much of it was, and still is, based upon supposition rather than scientific knowledge and to a considerable degree it may be regarded as largely concerned with aesthetics. Interestingly enough the swing of the pendulum has resulted in a renewal of interest in the aesthetic aspects of environmental sanitation. The engineer in a public health agency finds his responsibilities more comprehensive than either of the foregoing fields. Actually he is concerned with the public health aspects of both sanitary engineering and sanitary inspection. The prestige and potential of this specialty which is sometimes referred to as public health engineering is based upon the intimate dependence of human beings on their environment and the fact that control and adjustment of the environment in all its aspects involves the application of engineering principles. It has been defined as including the public health aspects of all types of environmental conditions whose control is based upon engineering principles regardless of the magnitude or technical difficulty of the individual problems involved. It may also be considered that environmental sanitation problems, whether small or large, simple or complicated, are fundamentally engineering in character.

The answer to the question regarding the types of personnel that should be employed in environmental control programs would appear to involve the provision, wherever possible, in one way or another, and on all levels, of planning and supervision by professionally trained engineers. On the national and state levels this does not present a problem since the advisory and policy-making functions on those levels imply the employment of engineers. The difficulty arises chiefly on the local level. Even here most municipalities of any significant size now employ engineers who may plan and supervise the total environmental control program including its inspectional phases as well as those of a more complex engineering nature. In rural areas, however, as typified by the usual county health department, the employment of engineering personnel is relatively rare. This is due to a number of factors among which are insufficient funds for adequate salaries and lack of enough job interest to attract and to hold well-qualified engineers in the face of personnel shortages elsewhere. As a result dependence for the sanitation program in rural areas has been placed upon sanitary inspectors or, what is far better, upon sanitarians who have received formal training to qualify them as Registered Sanitarians.

Under either rural or urban circumstances local health departments, functioning on the direct service level, must for reasons of economy and efficiency supplement the services of professionally trained workers by assigning specific functions to auxiliary workers who, through training and experience, have demonstrable ability to perform those functions adequately under supervision. This policy has been found practical and justifiable in other phases of the public health program, as well as in medicine and engineering, and there is ample reason to follow it in the field of environmental control.

Where the needed professional personnel does not exist on the local level, supervision, as well as planning and direction, should be provided by the state health department. Fortunately there is an increasing appreciation by engineers on the staffs of state health departments of their responsibility for the guidance and supervision of the local sanitation program. This makes for a more comprehensive program in the field and enables the local sanitarian to assist with certain difficult and technical activities which formerly were handled exclusively by the state. Among these may be named the supervision of water supplies and sewage disposal systems of towns and small cities, the surveillance of milk sheds, participation in programs of industrial hygiene, and the prevention of stream pollution. When the state health department endeavors to fulfill these functions alone, it is essentially an attempt at remote control. By bringing the local staff into the program the supervision and services are rendered on a day-to-day basis rather than at monthly or yearly intervals. This acknowledgement by the state of the responsibility to provide the local personnel with technical assistance and direction is expanding the usefulness of the local sanitarian considerably and is making it possible for the local health department to provide much more adequate service to the public than would otherwise be possible.

Theoretically some of the need for supervision of the local environmental control personnel should be met by the local health officer who, after all, is ultimately responsible for all phases of the community health program. In some instances, however, this is neither attempted nor possible since all too many local health officers unfortunately appear to lack the inclination, interest, or ability to assist their environmental control staffs with their problems. This provides further evidence of the need for rather extensive postmedical training in public health for physicians who aspire to become directors of public health programs. Recent trends indicate more and more reason for closer association between the health officer and the sanitation staff and for mutual attack upon problems that are really of common concern. Where formerly sanitarians may have restricted their activities to the inspection of wells, privies, and restaurants, they now, in addition, engage in many functions which cut across the direct interests of the medical health officer. Among these are intensive programs of school sanitation and education, typhus fever and malaria control, and the epidemiologic control of food and milk. Attention is called in the chapter on public health nursing to the recent introduction in some schools of public health of courses for medical health officers in the administration and supervision of public health nursing. Under the circumstances the development of similar courses relating to the responsibilities of the health officer in the field of environmental control would also appear to be indicated.

PRESENT ORGANIZATION OF ENVIRONMENTAL CONTROL PROGRAMS

As has been implied by previous comments, responsibilities and functions in environmental control are ordinarily divided among the different levels of government ac-cording to a more or less typical pattern. Generally speaking, the supervision of public water supplies and sewage disposal systems and the prevention of stream pollution are responsibilities of the federal and state governments. The federal concern, through the Public Health Service, is based largely upon responsibility for interstate sanitation and interstate and international public carriers, although in recent years the introduction of federal grants-in-aid to states and localities is a factor of great potential significance. State precedence over local communities in these matters results from legislative direction, the potentiality of intercommunity problems, and the availability of professionally qualified engineers in the average state health department.

In the matters of food and milk control there exists in most instances a division of functions and responsibility between the Food and Drug Administration, the Department of Agriculture, and the departments of health. Federal interests are concerned with research, the development of standards, and the promulgation and enforcement of various laws relating to pure food. The states are concerned with the establishment of state standards, the formulation and enforcement of state policies and regulations, and the promotion and general supervision of local programs. In some instances state agencies engage in the field inspection activities necessary for the implementation of the standards and regulations, but more often this is left to the local health department.

The developmental history of local health units in a state has much to do with the functional relationship which exists between the state and local agencies in matters of environmental control. Those states that were slow to promote the establishment of local health units still tend toward the centralization of sanitation activities in the state health department, even though they may now contain ample city and county health departments.

In contrast with public water and sewerage systems, those private facilities that are designed to serve single or small groups of families are practically always left to the supervision of the local health department. In many instances these small private facilities are inspected only upon request or complaint or when they are related to epidemiologically significant circumstances such as dairies or food processing or handling establishments. Between these two types of facilities, public and private, are some that are termed semipublic. These are found in tourist camps, roadside parks, comfort stations, rural schools, hospitals, and other institutions. Since they serve a number of unrelated persons of diverse origins, they constitute an obvious public health responsibility. In some areas this is met primarily by the state, whereas in other areas the local health departments provide most of the supervision.

Aside from the variations in responsibilities for environmental control that relate to the different levels of government, the organizational and administrative picture is further complicated by the spreading of health functions, and especially environmental control functions, throughout a number of agencies of government on each level. Although true on all levels, it is most evident in the states. Usually the state health department is designated as the regulatory agency responsible for public water and sewerage systems, although in some instances other departments of government, particularly state universities and special sanitary authorities, commissions, or boards, enter into certain phases of the program. This relatively well-defined distribution of authority, however, does not apply to other activities in environmental control. The situation was very well described by Mountin and Flook[95] in the following terms:

The acme of complexity in sanitation activities occurs in that portion of the program which involves food and drug control (including milk and shellfish sanitation) and restaurant supervision. Confusion is due to disagreement regarding what should be covered, who should be responsible and how the desired results should be attained. As a result, the division of authority and variation in procedures are so heterogeneous that they almost defy classification and description in accordance with any pattern that could be devised. Functional overlapping and interweaving apply principally to the health departments and the departments of agriculture. To a lesser degree, they involve many other State agencies among which the dairy and food commissions, hotel and restaurant commissions, livestock sanitary boards, departments of labor, departments of conservation, boards of pharmacy, state universities and colleges, and independent state laboratories are outstanding. Control methods of agencies other than the health department are usually limited to inspections, laboratory analysis of suspected products, and law enforcement.

Similar variation is found in connection with most other sanitary activities including the control of stream pollution, industrial safety and hygiene, insect and pest control, resort sanitation, and many others.

It is hoped that one of the long-term results of the various governmental reorganizations and of the deliberations of the various professional associations concerned with the field will be the ultimate unification of programs and the clear-cut definition of responsibilities. A significant step was taken on the federal level by the establishment in mid-1968 of the Consumer Protection and Environmental Health Service as one of the three components of the reorganized Public Health Service. This new agency brings together in close organizational, planning, and operational relationships the Food and Drug Administration, the National Air Pollution Control Administration, and the Environmental Control Administration. It represents, perhaps for the first time, a federal agency charged with concern for the ecologic interface between the total man and his total environment.

REFERENCES

1. Jacobson, A. R.: A bookshelf on environmental health, Amer. J. Public Health **52:**559, Apr. 1962.
2. Hollis, M.: Environmental health needs in a dynamic society, Public Health Rep. **67:**903, Sept. 1952.
3. Changing environmental hazards, challenges to community health. Report of The Task Force on Environmental Health of The National Commission on Community Health Services, Washington, 1967, U. S. Department of Health, Education, and Welfare.
4. Description of environmental health, Amer. J. Public Health **65:**928, June 1965.
5. Environmental determinants of community well-being, Scientific Publication 123, Washington, 1965, Pan American Health Organization-World Health Organization.
6. Marquis, R. W., editor: Environmental im-

provement, Washington, 1966, Graduate School, U. S. Department of Agriculture.

7. Kates, R. W. and Wohlwill, J. F., editors: Man's response to the physical environment, J. Social Issues, Vol. 22, No. 4, Oct. 1966.
8. A strategy for a livable environment. Report of the Task Force on Environmental Health and Related Problems, Washington, 1967, U. S. Department of Health, Education, and Welfare.
9. Stead, F. M.: Levels in environmental health, Amer. J. Public Health 50:312, Mar. 1960.
10. Environmental health planning guide, Washington, 1967, Public Health Service Pub. No. 823.
11. Hollis, M.: Environmental health in a rural economy, Public Health Rep. 68:1108, Nov. 1953.
12. Board, L., and Dunsmore, H.: Environmental health problems related to urban decentralization, Amer. J. Public Health 38:986, July 1948.
13. Hollis, M.: Aims and objectives in environmental health, Amer. J. Public Health 41:264, Mar. 1951.
14. Man and environment, report of a conference, Public Health Rep. 73:1073, Dec. 1958.
15. Urban sprawl and health. Report of the 1958 National Health Forum, New York 1959, National Health Council.
16. Report of the Committee on Enironmental Health Problems, Washington, 1962, Public Health Service Pub. No. 908.
17. Man—his environment and health. Report of a conference, Amer. J. Public Health 54: (supp.) Jan. 1964.
18. Special report on water supply and pollution control—are we ready for the future?, Water Works and Wastes Eng., Vol. 2, 1965.
19. Environmental pollution, a challenge to science and technology. Report of the Subcommittee on Science, Research and Development, to the Committee on Science and Astronautics, House of Representatives, Eighty-ninth Congress, Second Session, Serial S, Washington, 1966, U. S. Government Printing Office.
20. Restoring the quality of our environment. Report of the Environmental Pollution Panel, President's Science Advisory Committee, Washington, 1966, The White House.
21. Research needs in environmental health, Washington, 1966, National Academy of Science.
22. Nation-wide inventory of sanitation needs, Public Health Rep. (supp. 204), Apr. 1948.
23. Knutson, J. W.: Tasks of state health departments in developing fluoridation, Public Health Rep. 67:180, Feb. 1952.
24. Individual water supply systems, recommendations of the Joint Committee on Rural Sanitation, 1950, Public Health Service, Department of Health, Education, and Welfare.
25. A water policy for the American people, report of the President's Water Resource Policy Commission, Washington, 1950, U. S. Government Printing Office.
26. Klassen, C. W.: Integrating a state water pollu-

tion control program with a regional water resources plan, Amer. J. Public Health 43:438, April 1953.
27. Eliassen, R.: Abatement of stream pollution caused by industrial wastes, Public Health Rep. 68:44, Jan. 1953.
28. Ehlers, V. M., and Steel, E. W.: Municipal and rural sanitation, ed. 4, New York, 1950, McGraw-Hill Book Co.
29. Waste management and control, report to the Federal Council for Science and Technology, Washington, 1966, National Academy of Sciences-National Research Council.
30. Greenberg, A. E., and Gotaas, H. B.: Reclamation of sewage water, Amer. J. Public Health 42:401, Apr. 1952.
31. Rudolfs, W., Falk, L., and Rogotzkie, R.: Contamination of vegetables grown in polluted soil, Sewage and Industrial Wastes, Mar.-Aug. 1951.
32. Rudolfs, W.: Salvage from sewage, Engineering News-Record 119:1055, July-Dec. 1937.
33. Prescott, S. C., and Horwood, M. P.: Sedgwick's principles of sanitary science and public health, New York, 1935, The Macmillan Co.
34. Statistical summary of 1962 inventory of municipal waste facilities in the U. S., Washington, 1964, Public Health Service Pub. No. 1165.
35. The recommended milk ordinance, Public Health Rep. 78:267, Mar. 1963.
36. Dauer, C. C.: 1960 summary of disease outbreaks and a 10-year résumé, Public Health Rep. 76:915, Oct. 1961.
37. Food service sanitation, Washington, 1962, Public Health Service Pub. No. 934.
38. Fuchs, A. W.: Restaurant sanitation program of the United States Public Health Service, Public Health Rep. 62:263, Feb. 21, 1947.
39. Isaac, P. C.: Air pollution and man's health—in Great Britain, Public Health Rep. 68:868, Sept. 1953.
40. Environment and health, Washington, 1951, Public Health Service Pub. No. 84.
41. Prindle, R. A., and Yaffee, C. D.: Motor vehicles, air pollution, and public health, Pub. Health Rep. 77:955, Nov. 1962.
42. Magill, P. L.: Techniques employed in the analysis of Los Angeles smog, Proceedings of the First National Air Pollution Symposium, Stanford Research Institute, 1951.
43. Larson, G. P.: Air pollution and man's health—in Los Angeles, Public Health Rep. 68:873, Sept. 1953.
44. Proceedings of the United States Technical Conference on Air Pollution, New York, 1952, McGraw-Hill Book Co.
45. Baynton, H. W.: Environmental studies—meteorological aspects, Public Health Rep. 67:668, July 1952.
46. National conference on air pollution, Public Health Rep. 78:423, May 1963.
47. Heimann, H.: Status of air pollution health research, 1966, Arch. Environ. Health 14:488, Mar. 1967.
48. Firket, J.: Sur les causes des accidents survenus

dans la vallée de la Meuse, lors des brouillards de décembre 1930, Bull. Acad. Roy. Med. Belg. 11:683, 1931.

49. Townsend, J. G.: Investigation of the smog incident in Donora, Pennsylvania, and vicinity, Amer. J. Public Health 40:183, Feb. 1950.

50. Ciocco, A., and Thompson, D. J.: A follow-up of Donora ten years after, Amer. J. Public Health 51:155, Feb. 1961.

51. McCabe, L., and Clayton, G.: Air pollution by hydrogen sulfide in Poza Rica, Mexico, Arch. Industr. Hyg. Occup. Med. 6:199, Sept. 1952.

52. Logan, W.: Mortality in the London fog incident, 1952, Lancet 7:336, 1953.

53. Scott, J.: Fog and deaths in London, December, 1952, Public Health Rep. 68:474, May 1953.

54. Technical and administrative reports on air pollution control in Los Angeles County, Air Pollution Control District, County of Los Angeles, Calif.

55. Ludwig, J. H., and Steigerwald, B. J.: Research in air pollution: current trends, Amer. J. Public Health 55:1082, July 1965.

56. MacKenzie, V. G.: The Clean Air Act and its implications, Amer. J. Public Health 55:901, June 1965.

57. Dyktor, H. G.: The community problem. In-service Training Course in Air Pollution, Ann Arbor, Feb. 6-8, 1950, University of Michigan School of Public Health.

58. Policy statement on radiological health, Amer. J. Public Health 50:885, June 1960.

59. Eisenbud, M.: Industrial uses of ionizing radiation, Amer. J. Public Health, 55:748, May 1965.

60. Goresline, H. E., and Desrosier, N. W.: Preservation of foods by irradiation, Amer. J. Public Health 49:488, Apr. 1959.

61. Longood, R. J.: Radiation accidents—the public's right to know, Amer. J. Public Health 56:1751, Oct. 1966.

62. Bugher, J. C.: Health perspectives of our radioactive world, Amer. J. Public Health 52:727, May 1962.

63. Gentry, J. T., Parkhurst, E., and Bulin, G. V.: An epidemiological study of congenital malformations in New York State, Amer. J. Public Health 49:497, Apr. 1959.

64. Gerusky, T. M., Lubenau, J. O., Roskopf, R., and Lieban, J.: Survey of radium sources in offices of private physicians, Public Health Rep. 80:75, Jan. 1965.

65. Gorman, A. E.: Environmental safety for industrial uses of radionuclides, Public Health Rep. 72:1107, Dec. 1957.

66. Campbell, J. E.: Radionuclides in milk, J. Agric. and Food Chem. 9:117, Mar.-Apr. 1961.

67. Thomas, H. A.: The public health implications of radioactive fallout in water supplies, Amer. J. Public Health 46:1266, Oct. 1956.

68. Godwin, R. P., Eddy, P. P., and Longaker, R. K.: Safety on the nuclear ship Savannah, Public Health Rep. 74:669, Aug. 1959.

69. Davies, S., and Thompson, M. H.: Protecting the environment around a nuclear power reactor, Amer. J. Public Health 52:1993, Dec. 1962.

70. Kinsman, S.: Radiological defense, Public Health Rep. 71:181, Feb. 1956.

71. Lieberman, J. A.: Engineering aspects of the disposal of radioactive wastes from the peacetime applications of nuclear technology, Amer. J. Public Health 47:345, Mar. 1957.

72. Editorial: Atomic radiations, Amer. J. Public Health 46:1147, Sept. 1956.

73. American Public Health Association: Ionizing radiation, New York, 1966, The Association.

74. Anderson, E. C.: Administrative aspects of nuclear energy, Public Health Rep. 73:811, Sept. 1958.

75. Hutton, G. L.: Public control of radiation emitters, Public Health Rep. 69:1133, Dec. 1954.

76. Blatz, H., and Lynch, D. E.: Radiation control problems faced by a large city, Amer. J. Public Health 53:882, June 1963.

77. Committee on Local Control of Ionizing Radiation of the Conference of Municipal Public Health Engineers: The responsibility of local health agencies in the control of ionizing radiation, Amer. J. Public Health 53:1136, July 1963.

78. Brodsky, A.: Balancing benefit versus risk in the control of consumer items containing radioactive material, Amer. J. Public Health 55:1971, Dec. 1965.

79. American Public Health Association Committee on the Hygiene of Housing, Winslow, C.-E. A., chairman: An appraisal method for measuring the quality of housing: Part I, Nature and uses of the method, 1945, The Association.

80. Anderson, G. W.: The present epidemiological basis of environmental sanitation, Amer. J. Public Health 33:113, Feb. 1943.

81. Bauer, C.: The provision of good housing, Amer. J. Public Health 39:462, Apr. 1949.

82. Editorial: The shame of the slums, Amer. J. Public Health 43:621, May 1953.

83. American Public Health Association: Basic principles of healthful housing, ed. 2, New York, 1950, The Association.

84. American Public Health Association: Guide for health administrators in housing hygiene, New York, 1967, The Association.

85. Johnson, R. J.: Health departments and the housing problem, Amer. J. Public Health 42:1583, Dec. 1952.

86. Molner, J. G., and Hilbert, M. S.: Responsibilities of public health administrations in the field of housing. In Housing programmes: The role of public health agencies, Geneva, 1964, World Health Organization.

87. O'Harrow, D.: Subdivision and fringe area control, Amer. J. Public Health 44:473, Apr. 1954.

88. Woodbury, C.: Impact of the urban sprawl on housing and community development, Amer. J. Public Health 50:357, Mar. 1960.

89. Ascher, C. S.: Regulation of housing: hints for health officers, Amer. J. Public Health 37:507, May 1937.

90. Mood, E. W.: Health and housing programs in large cities, U.S.A., 1965, Amer. J. Public Health **56:**1540, Sept. 1966.

91. Johnson, R. J.: Housing law enforcement, Public Health Rep. **66:**1451, Nov. 1951.

92. Handbook on sanitation of railroad and passenger car construction, Washington, 1951. Public Health Service Pub. No. 95.

93. Handbook on sanitation of vessels in operation, Washington, 1951, Public Health Service Pub. No. 88.

94. Handbook on sanitation of airlines, Washington, 1953, Public Health Service Pub. No. 306.

95. Mountin, J. W., and Flook, E.: Distribution of health services in the structure of state government, Pub Health Rep. **57:**948, June 19, 1942.

Chapter 28

Occupational health*

GENERAL CONSIDERATIONS

The existence of a common ground of concern and responsibility between public health and private enterprise has become increasingly evident in recent years. Public health's concern with private enterprise is based upon a number of factors. A fundamental consideration is that health is everybody's business. Perhaps the most obvious interest of public health agencies in the affairs of private enterprise relates to products manufactured and sold. Certain industrial products have far-reaching potential consequences for the buying public; therefore tax-supported public health agencies bear a responsibility. The production, handling, processing, and circumstances of sale of a large number of food products are well established as big business. The paths of public health workers and private entrepreneurs, therefore, have long since crossed in relation to the supervision of the sanitary aspects of these products. This subject has been considered in Chapter 27.

Another obvious and early reason for public health interest in private enterprise relates to problems brought about by the conditions of work in industry. At times workers have been exposed to grievous physical and chemical risks. There are four types of recourse against undesirable conditions of work: strikes, disability compensation, labor-management arbitration, and cooperative preventive planning and action by public health agencies, labor, and indus-

try. The latter has led to the development and use of safety devices, and provision for the diagnosis, treatment, and prevention of occupational diseases and injuries. It is this phase of the problem which constitutes the chief concern of this chapter.

A further reason why public health agencies should be concerned with conditions of employment is the fact that a large segment of the population spends a significant amount of their time in the work environment. Not only may they be affected by it, but they may also be reached and influenced for public health purposes through their place of employment This circumstance has been used to considerable advantage in preservice and in-service physical examinations, health education and nutrition programs, mass diagnosis, and illness and disability surveys. As one authority[2] has written, "People are employees and employers only part of the day. The remainder of the time they are plain everyday citizens." Their influence on community action is tremendous and worth consideration in planning and providing community services essential to the maintenance of health. Hence in any community planning for health all groups should be represented. Moreover, this planning should be for total community health and not merely for health services in the place of employment. The greatest opportunity for lifesaving, and the prevention of disease and disability lies, at the present time, in the age and social class represented by the wage earner. This is also the point of greatest social and economic productivity and potential. The approach through industry, business, and labor unions to the health

---

*For a series of interesting presentations of various aspects of the subject, see Occupational Health, 1914-1964, Pub. Health Rep.[1]

of the wage earner offers the same administrative advantages inherent in school health programs, i.e., large numbers readily accessible and, from the community standpoint, a group whose health is vitally important and peculiarly at risk.

Finally, if proper relationships are developed, support of the general public health program of no small magnitude and significance may be obtained from those in positions of responsibility and authority in private business and industry, as well as in labor unions. The nature of industrial hygiene activities requires accessible service and a close relationship between the public health administrator and the industrialist. Through an effective and profitable program of industrial hygiene and product sanitation the health officer is in a position to meet and influence the industrialists and businessmen of his community on their own terms with the importance of the total public health program. The health officer should always bear in mind that businessmen and industrialists are citizens too and that business and industrial enterprises produce the economic lifeblood of the modern community.

Programs and activities concerned with the well-being of workers exist under numerous labels in various times and places, i.e., industrial or occupational health, hygiene, safety, engineering, welfare, or medicine. As a result of the gradual coming together and synthesis of the various interests implied by these designations and the ever broadening view of the many factors that are involved in the well-being and efficiency of workers, there has come about a tendency to refer to the entire area of interest as occupational health. In general it appears that the label and definition given to the field has depended essentially upon the profession of primary interest or background of the discussant. In this regard Hussey[3] has very appropriately written the following:

This whole subject of occupational health and medicine is analogous to a three-legged stool, one leg representing medical science, one representing engineering and chemical science, and one representing the social sciences. . . . Up to the present we have been trying to balance ourselves on two legs and in some instances on one leg. It is a very uncomfortable position and one that cannot get us very far and certainly will lead, as it has, to fatigue.

With this in mind the following definition by the Council on Industrial Health of the American Medical Association[4] is presented:

Occupational Medicine deals with the restoration and conservation of health in relation to work, the working environment and maximum efficiency. It involves prevention, recognition, and treatment of occupational disabilities and requires the application of special techniques in the fields of rehabilitation, environmental hygiene, toxicology, sanitation and human relations.

BACKGROUND

Ramazzini is usually considered to be the father of occupational health, based upon the publication in the early eighteenth century of his treatise *Diseases of Tradesmen*. Modern occupational health is an outcome of the industrial revolution in nineteenth century England. As a result of the rapid development of deplorable work conditions, in general, and the exploitation of women and children, in particular, numerous laws were passed for the protection of workers. Following a short lag period, there came about what Legge[5] referred to as the "American Industrial Renaissance." During this period America profited by the events, researches, and measures that had previously occurred in England, even to the extent of adoption by some states of some of the earlier English legislation. In 1908 Congress passed the Federal Employers' Liability Act, which made railroads and other interstate carriers liable for industrial injuries sustained by their employees. At that time the Wainwright Commission in New York showed that only one out of every eight injured men was awarded any compensation and that he actually received only about a third of what was awarded. The other two thirds went for insurance adjusters, legal advice, and commissions. Various states had previously enacted workmen's compensation laws, but these early laws were declared unconstitutional by the courts. The year 1911, however, marked the beginning of the first valid state workmen's compensation laws, and no less than 10 states passed legislation in that year alone. There followed an era of compensation medical service, and employers were made increasingly responsible for the medical and surgical care of workers who became injured or ill at their jobs and for payment of accident and disease compensation.

Meanwhile increasing attention was being given to the identification, definition, and diagnosis of occupational diseases, i.e., silicosis, plumbism, anthrax, benzol and radium poisoning, and many others. There resulted a separate development of occupational disease compensation laws, among the earliest of which were California and Wisconsin (1919), North Dakota (1925), Minnesota and Connecticut (1929). Unfortunately many of these compensation laws were hastily promulgated during a period of considerable public stimulation and concern, with the result that many were extreme, ill advised, and impractical. Under the circumstances extensive subsequent amendment is not surprising. At the present time workmen's compensation laws exist in all 50 states.

As Hatch[6] has indicated, the period 1910 to 1920 witnessed the firm establishment of occupational health as a specialty. The Department of Labor was established as a separate Cabinet entity, the Bureau of Mines of the Department of the Interior and the Office of Industrial Hygiene and Sanitation (later the Division of Occupational Health) of the Public Health Service came into existence, an Industrial Hygiene Section was established in the American Public Health Association, and the National Safety Council was organized. Two of the most significant events were the organization in 1915 of the American Association of Industrial Physicians and Surgeons (now the Industrial Medical Association), and the adoption of minimum standards for medical service in industry by the Committee on Industrial Medicine and Traumatic Surgery of the American College of Surgeons. Some years later, in 1937, the American Medical Association created the Council on Industrial Health to coordinate all medical efforts in the industrial

health field. The Journal of Industrial Hygiene and the first specialized teaching of the subject appeared in schools of public health at about the same time. Whereas all such schools now give courses in the subject, the University of Pittsburgh and the University of Michigan give it particular attention.

Prior to the passage of the federal Social Security Act of 1935, little progress had been made by state health agencies in occupational health. Up to that time only five states engaged in any activities designed for the benefit of industrial workers. The first were instituted in 1913 in New York and Ohio. The Act made funds available for the expansion of state and local programs as well as other forms of activity, with the result that by 1950 all of the states and Alaska, Hawaii, Puerto Rico, and the District of Columbia were engaged in some type of activity for the improvement of health and safety of workers in gainful occupations.[7] These are but a few of the many landmarks in the development of this important field.*

BENEFITS

Serious attention to and support of occupational and public health activities carry with them many benefits to private enterprise. Three of the greatest items of loss to business and industry are labor turnover, absenteeism, and liability compensation for occupational illness and injury.

Among the tangible profits of good community and industrial health programs are remedies against these three sources of loss. A healthy worker is a happier, more dependable worker with high morale and pride in his work. He will tend to remain in his position rather than to roam in search of another.

According to statistics of the National Safety Council[10] for the year 1966, there occurred 2.2 million work-related disabling injuries. Of these, 14,500 resulted in death

*For excellent illustrated outlines of significant events the reader is referred to Man, Medicine and Work, Public Health Service Pub. No. 1044[8] and Fifty Years of Occupational Health, Public Health Service Pub. No. 1171.[9]

and about 90,000 resulted in permanent disability. In addition to the liability compensation involved this constituted a work loss to industrial production and an estimated total economic loss of $6.8 billion. Manufacturing industries have gained the most, with a reduction in their occupational death rate of about 40% during the past 15 years. In fact, it is interesting that the work-related death rate during 1966 for manufacturing occupations was only 10 per 100,000 workers in contrast with 23 per 100,000 workers in nonmanufacturing employment. It is further significant that during 1966 the overall on-the-job death rate was 20 per 100,000 workers in contrast with an off-the-job death rate of 54 per 100,000 workers. The improvements noted have been largely due to the efforts of the National Safety Council, the National Association of Manufacturers, and the Industrial Conference comprised of 160 top safety experts. In return, a reduction in absenteeism of 20% to 30% has been noted.

Several factors are involved in such striking results from occupational health programs:

1. Industrial health personnel has done much to control environmental hazards, thereby providing built-in safety measures which in turn result in a greater sense of security and employment satisfaction in the worker.
2. Industrial health personnel is more apt to make the worker realize that his welfare and employment career are partly dependent upon his own sense of responsibility for maintaining his health, safety, and working ability.
3. A sound occupational health program makes possible a gradual and selective return to work consistent with the degree and speed of recovery.
4. Competent industrial medical and nursing personnel has had a desirable persuasive effect upon patients and their physicians, which often results in the seeking of early preventive and curative private medical care and in a demand for private medical service of high quality.
5. Industrial health personnel has developed effective and appropriate techniques for the detection and handling of occasional malingerers.
6. Occupational health services form a link between the workers' total health problems and the community health and social services.

Other benefits to business and industry are a diminution in employee grievances, improved employee relations and consequently improved public relations, increased worker and community pride in the company and its products, and the enhanced appeal and advertising value of a clean plant, healthy, contented employees, and a sanitary product. Out of 1,625 companies completing questionnaires concerning the value of industrial health programs, only 5 companies failed to report to the National Association of Manufacturers that they considered their health program a paying proposition.

The important point is that health problems and responsibilities are always present in the plant or in the office, whether or not industry and business want to recognize them, and whether or not they wish to do anything about them. If they do accept these responsibilities, they not only perform an important public service but, as already pointed out, may also turn that recognition and action to their own financial advantage. On the other hand, if they refuse to recognize their health problems and responsibilities, it automatically becomes incumbent upon official public health agencies, acting in the public interest, to step in and do something about the situation. However, from the standpoint of official agencies, there is much to be gained by interesting private enterprise in meeting their own problems.

In the past private enterprise, business, and industry traditionally have been looked up to by the public. During recent years the public has also developed an intense interest in matters of personal and community health. This is indicated by the findings of investigators at the University of Minnesota who have studied shifts in social prestige occurring over the past three decades. They report the most notable change to be the replacement of the banker and businessman by the physician as the individual enjoying the highest prestige in America today. Here, therefore, is a situation in which business and industry may work with another high prestige group to mutual advantage, in providing valuable community leadership and achieving even greater public esteem as well as efficiency in the process. Many large companies and industrial concerns have already seen the value of following this line of action and not only are cooperating actively with official public health agencies but, in addition, on their own initiative are engaging in personnel health programs, plant safety, and product sanitation activities of considerable consequence.

In summary, therefore, occupational health programs bring many benefits—to the employee, to the employer, and to the community. For the employee and his dependents it means better personal health and sustained earnings, lower personal medical and hospital expenditures, increased and prolonged productive capacity, and the enjoyment and security that comes with good health and job satisfaction. For the employer it means decreased production costs because of lower labor turnover, less absenteeism, fewer disability payments, lower insurance, and more capable and more alert workers. It also brings higher worker morale and desirable labor-management relations. All of these result in diffused but extensive benefits to the community in increased prosperity, decreased welfare costs, less labor-management strife, and increased pressures for and support of high quality medical, hospital, and public health services.

INDUSTRIAL HEALTH PROGRAMS

It is appropriate to preface a discussion of the objectives and content of industrial health programs by a pertinent comment made by the Director of Industrial Hygiene of one of the world's largest industrial corporations.[11] "Business," he has pointed out, "is conducted on a practical, or profit and loss, basis and when losses equal or exceed profits, you do not stay in business long. Industrial hygiene programs that are not basically sound are not likely to survive the test of time."

A good industrial health program is designed primarily for the benefit and welfare of the workers. Its objectives, as listed by Cameron,[12] are the following:

1. Assessment of a worker's physical and psychological assets, as well as his liabilities, to facilitate proper selection and placement
2. Prevention of occupational and nonoccupational illnesses
3. Provision of treatment, the type and extent of which depends on the policy of the organization
4. Fostering of a personal, physical, mental, and social ability to work and enjoy life beyond the mere absence of disease or infirmity

The inclusion of psychologic, mental, and social factors merits particular note. There are indications that up to 30% of absenteeism is due to emotional disturbances resulting from interpersonal problems in the plant, in the home, and in the community.

Many factors influence the nature and extent of an industrial health program that a business or an industry may find it worthwhile to carry out. Among these are the type of industry or business; the nature of its product and of the ingredients and equipment used in its manufacture; the disposition of the product; the size and location of the establishment; the complex attitudes and relationships among top management, labor unions, the community and and its medical profession, public health agency, and government; and the organizational status of the unit responsible for the activities. For these reasons it is obvious that a detailed standard pattern is impossible. To the contrary, each program must be more or less tailored to fit the needs and circumstances of the particular situation. It is possible, however, to state certain fundamental principles which should apply in general. Thus the Council on Industrial Health of the American Medical Association[13] lists the objectives of an occupational health program to be (1) to protect individuals against health hazards in their work environment, (2) to ensure and facilitate the suitable placement of individuals according to their physical capacities and their emotional makeup in work which they can perform with an acceptable degree of efficiency and without endangering their own health and safety or that of their fellow employees, and (3) to encourage personal health maintenance.

The statement goes on to describe in more detail the scope of services that the Council considers should be provided by the medical department of an industry. They include the following:

1. Regular appraisal of plant sanitation
2. Periodic inspection for occupational disease hazards
3. Adoption and maintenance of adequate control measures
4. Provision of first aid and emergency services
5. Prompt and early treatment for all illnesses resulting from occupational exposure
6. Reference to the family physician of individuals with conditions needing attention, cooperating with the patient and physician in every practical way to remedy the condition
7. Uniform recording of absenteeism due to all types of disability
8. Impartial health appraisals of all workers
9. Provision of rehabilitation services within industry
10. The conduct of a beneficial health education program

Adequately expanded and developed, and adapted to the particular circumstances, these areas of activity would provide a satisfactory occupational health program in most situations.

Recently an entirely new relationship has been introduced in the field of industrial health. During the war years, when wages were more or less frozen as an anti-inflationary measure, organized labor took the opportunity to press for other types of benefits such as group health and sickness insurance. An increasing number of unions have succeeded in having benefits of this nature included in the terms of their agreements with employers. It should be noted, however, that in many instances this represents a substitution of union-administered plans for previously existing employer-administered plans. In fact, a number of concerns have extended their industrial medical services to include general medical care for their employees and in some instances for the families of employees as well.

Because of the large numbers of employees involved, many of the larger business and industrial concerns find it practical to operate most or all of their employee health and safety programs themselves. The great problem arises in connection with small plants and businesses, which are in the majority and which taken together employ the major proportion, 60%, of workers. Individually they are usually too small to afford or justify the employment of even a single full-time nurse, much less a physician. Up to the present day they have been largely left out of the picture except for essentially token services rendered by the industrial hygiene divisions of state and occasionally local health departments. To overcome the problem, there has been a trend toward the joint employment, by groups of small industrial plants, of full-time health personnel who devote the necessary number of hours a week to each plant in the group. This plan has proved of value in a number of locations. For the supervision of the environmental hazards of small plants various types of portable or mobile equipment have also been used to advantage.

THE ROLE OF GOVERNMENT

Since the occupational environment is part of the total community to which the public health agency is responsible, it is to be expected that the latter have appropriate interest in the field. Reference has been made to the relatively slow growth of occupational health programs in governmental agencies, beginning with the initiation of activities in 1913 in New York and Ohio. Activity and interest accelerated with the passage of the Social Security Act in 1935 and again during the period of the Second World War. In 1940 more than a

Chapter 29

Accident prevention

EMERGENCE OF THE PROBLEM

In the discussion of the philosophy and content of public health, its ever broadening vista and the constant extension of its activities were described. It was pointed out that the present-day public health agency must be interested in the well-being of the total individual and the total community life. Accordingly it concerns itself wherever feasible with all factors which may adversely affect any phase of the physical and mental health of the community and its population. As a result we find ourselves involved more and more in what some might consider fringe activities. Actually to consider them as such is erroneous. Merely because certain problems require joint action with other community agencies or groups, they are not necessarily of a fringe or tangential nature. Indeed, it should be realized that joint or community action is the very essence of public health programs. Accident prevention represents a good example.

If there is ever a tendency for people to consider disease or disability fatalistically, it is most apt to be in relation to accidents.[1] In fact, the average person in even the most advanced societies tends to define the word accident as something due to chance, over which the individual has very little, if any, control. This negative attitude explains to a considerable degree why so little concerted attention has been given to the problem until quite recent years. Gradually, however, a number of factors have captured the attention of certain groups in society. Each has attempted, in its own way and for various reasons to explore approaches to solution. Some partial progress has resulted.

The large life insurance companies were perhaps the first to give attention to this problem. With a major portion of the population in the United States now covered by some type of life or disability insurance it has become increasingly important to these companies that everything possible be done to decrease the extent of accidental disability or death. At the same time it is of importance to the policyholder, not only from the standpoint of avoiding suffering or death but also in terms of lowering the costs of policies. As a result some of the best health educational work and promotion of home safety has been conducted by the large insurance companies. For somewhat similar reasons, although companies that ensure against losses due to fire have the reduction of material losses as their primary interest, they nevertheless have also been involved in the prevention of fire injuries and deaths. Industries, particularly the larger industries, have carried out safety programs of considerable magnitude involving the installation of various safety devices and careful worker selection, placement, and education. Increasing costs of tax-supported service for fire prevention, emergency care, and hospitalization have caused public officials to look for means of reducing the extent of accidents from all causes. Finally, as mentioned above, public health workers have become aware of the ever growing threat of accidents to well-being and of the relationships of certain types of accidents to various mental or physiologic factors with which they were already concerned. Gradually, therefore, the fatalistic attitude that accidents are events that just happen has been changing. Increasingly, individuals

537

and agencies have been getting together to see if something positive could be done about the problem.

EXTENT OF THE PROBLEM

Currently about 113,000 people are killed each year by accidents in the United States. This amounts to about 13 deaths each hour. The number of nonfatal accidents is more difficult to determine since many of them never come to official attention. On the basis of reports, insurance claims, and the like the National Safety Council has estimated that there are about 100 injuries for each fatality, or a total of almost 12 million.[2] However, the National Health Survey,[3] through its household interviews, determined a total of 46,919,000 nonfatal injuries of all types and degrees of severity during the year July 1957 to June 1958. (In 1966 almost 51 million injuries were estimated.) Slightly more than half, or 27,614,-000, required restricted activity; 11,246,000 of these required convalescence in bed, 1,-715,000 of which were hospitalized. These accidents resulted in 424.1 million days of restricted activity, including 113.7 million spent in bed at home or in a hospital. Altogether the cost of accidents in terms of lost wages, medical expenses, and other factors has been estimated by the National Safety Council to amount to a staggering total of about $20 billion in 1966. Although three fifths of all the accidents involved males, there is an interesting sex variation by age. Male accidental death rates exceed those in females of all ages except the most advanced. Accidental death rates for males are only slightly in excess of rates for fe-males up to about the fifteenth year of life, after which male accidental death rates increase sharply and remain high from then on. By contrast, accidental death rates for females remain relatively low until about the sixty-fifth year, following which they rise sharply and exceed those in males at age 85 years. An unusual study[4] of 50,000 child-years of accidental injury in which 8,874 children were followed for 16 years showed that the rate for all medically attended nonfatal injuries was 246 per 1,000 children per year. Boys had more injuries than girls at all ages, and their injury rate increased with age, whereas for girls it went down. It was also noted that children with high rates at one age tended to have high rates in subsequent periods of childhood.

The carnage occurs in all parts of our environment—in automobiles, on the streets, in the home, at work, and on the farm as well as in the city. About five eighths of nonfatal accidents are urban, two eighths are rural nonfarm, and one eighth is rural farm. Because of their dramatic nature, accidents involving public or private vehicles tend to monopolize the public attention. These, however, are only a part of a much larger problem. Accidental injuries and deaths by place of occurrence present an interesting picture (Table 29-1). Whereas the home is the most dangerous locale in terms of frequency of accidents, motor vehicles are most dangerous in terms of serious injury or death.

Motor vehicle accidents rose sharply following World War I and have continued high. Annual deaths from this cause were about 12,500 in 1920 but by 1930 had risen

Table 29-1. Annual distribution of accidental injuries and deaths by location

| Location | Injuries | | | Deaths | Deaths per 1,000 injuries |
	Total	Activity restricted	Hospitalized		
Motor vehicle	4,702,000	3,004,000	890,000	40,000	8.5
Home	19,137,000	10,974,000	469,000	27,700	1.4
Work	8,150,000	4,228,000	123,000	11,300	1.4
Other	14,930,000	9,408,000	233,000	16,000	1.1
Total	46,919,000	27,614,000	1,715,000	95,000	2.0

to about 33,000. They have continued to climb more slowly but constantly, except for the tire and gasoline rationing period of World War II. By 1966 motor vehicular deaths reached 53,000. During the period since World War I, however, the death rate from motor vehicle accidents per ten thousand motor vehicles registered has dropped markedly. Thus in 1920 it was about 13.5 deaths per 10,000 cars registered, whereas now it is only about 5.5 deaths per 10,000 cars registered. Similarly in terms of vehicular deaths per 100 million miles traveled, the rate has dropped from about 14.0 in 1925 to 5.7 in 1966. Nevertheless, both in terms of absolute numbers of deaths and deaths per thousand injuries, motor vehicle accidents are by far the most serious part of the problem.

Occupational injuries and deaths have been subjected to a considerable reduction. For example, in terms of injuries per million man-hours, the frequency in 1926 was 32 as against about 7 now. Work-related accidents do not appear to be so severe in terms of fatalities as do motor vehicle accidents, deaths per thousand injuries for the former being about one sixth those of the latter.

Accidents in the home are particularly important because of their frequency which approaches one half of all accidents. However, in terms of severity, as measured by deaths per thousand injuries they are on a par with occupational accidents. In recent years there has been considerable study of home accidents which has brought out numerous facts of interest. Of social significance is the fact that among females the highest home injury rate is in the lowest income group whereas among males it is just the opposite, with the home injury rate in the highest income group being twice the rate among males in the lowest income group. It is interesting that, whereas the kitchen is the locale of the highest percent of all home accidents (26%), the bedroom is the most fatal place, accounting for 40% of all accidental deaths in the home. This is attributable to the many toxic drugs kept there plus the dangerous habit of some to smoke in bed. Other fatal accidents in the home occur in living rooms, 10%; in kitchens, 12%; on stairs, 4%; in dining rooms, 3%; and in bathrooms, 3%. By type of home accident, falls are the most frequent cause of death, accounting for 40% of accidental deaths. Fires account for 23%, suffocation for 8%, and poisoning for 6%.[2]

Accidents should also be considered from the viewpoint of their relative position as a cause of death. Although more than 3,000 infants die accidentally each year, there are numerous other conditions which contribute more to the infant mortality. Once the first birthday is approached and passed, however, the picture changes dramatically. Accidents constitute the leading cause of death in age groups 1 to 4, 5 to 14, 15 to 24, and 25 to 34 years. From 35 to 44 years and from 45 to 54 years accidents are in second place; from 55 to 64 years, fourth place; and beyond age 65, sixth place as a cause of death. Certainly a problem of this magnitude cannot be ignored.

COST OF ACCIDENTAL INJURIES

It is difficult, of course, to determine with accuracy the economic loss due to accidents. The magnitude of estimates depends upon the extent to which accidents and injuries are reported and the items that are included in the calculations. The National Safety Council[2] has carried out perhaps the most accurate analysis which attempts to take into consideration all possible cost factors that might legitimately be involved. The result is summarized as follows:

1. Wages losses due to temporary inability to work, lower wages after returning to work due to permanent impairment, and present value of future earnings lost by those totally incapacitated or killed — $5,900,000,000
2. Medical fees and hospital expenses — $2,000,000,000
3. Insurance administrative and claim settlement costs — $4,300,000,000
4. Property damage in motor vehicle accidents — $3,300,000,000
5. Property destroyed by fire — $1,496,000,000
6. Property destroyed and production lost due to work injury accidents — $3,000,000,000

The total of all these factors comes to about $20 billion per year, which, as has been pointed out, approximates the annual appropriation for conducting the war in Vietnam.[1]

PROGRAMS TO OFFSET THE ACCIDENT TOLL

The Governing Council of the American Public Health Association in 1960 put in the form of a policy statement[5] its growing concern about accidents as a public health problem and challenge equal in scope to the prevention of infectious diseases and the control of chronic diseases. The Council recommended that:

Accident prevention be recognized as a major public health problem and that all component units of the American Public Health Association cooperate to improve accident prevention activities at the local, state and national level;

State and local health departments, the Public Health Service, and the Children's Bureau increase the size and scope of their accident prevention activities to be more commensurate with the magnitude of the problem and with the level of activity that has been or is being achieved in the field of infectious and chronic disease;

All state health departments and large local health departments provide that: Their accident prevention programs be headed by a full-time administrator qualified by training and experience to discharge this responsibility adequately and that a wide range of consultant services be made available to the administrator and

Active educational efforts be designed to dispel ignorance about the basic causes of accidents and the role people play in their causation, devised and carried out in cooperation with other interested agencies and organizations, and

Research efforts be significantly increased in number, scope, and depth and embrace the study and control of all types of accidents regardless of their place of occurrence, and

Greater attention be directed to identifying the human factors involved in accidents, and to developing active methods of coping with them, and that in this concern full consideration be given to the structures, implements, and conditions created by man himself which make accidents more likely to occur, and

Increased efforts be made to enlist the cooperation of physicians and state and local medical societies in accident prevention activities;

Increased cooperation be promoted by official agencies with the National Safety Council and state and local safety councils, which have played so important a role in accident prevention; and

Additional funds be provided for the Public Health Service and the Children's Bureau to encourage and support additional research efforts and to assist state and local health departments in developing more effective accident prevention programs.

There are many reasons why public health agencies and workers should be concerned with the problem of accidents. The absolute and proportional magnitude of the problem which has been described is, of course, one reason for concern, as is also its economic significance. Beyond these, however, there are actually a great many activities of public health agencies which do, or may be made to, impinge upon the problem. Emphasizing this are a number of excellent manuals that have been issued to assist the public health worker in the development of accident control programs.[6,7,8,9] Among the various activities that may make significant contributions are public health statistics,[10,11] health surveys and studies, community health and safety education,[12] child health,[13,14] industrial hygiene, housing, and mental hygiene.[15] The latter is mentioned specifically in view of the growing body of knowledge about accident proneness and the development of techniques for its determination.[16,17,18] Increasingly workers in the fields of public health and preventive medicine have been relating these general activities or methods of approach to accident prevention. In a number of communities accidental injuries as well as deaths are reported to the public health agency for study and analysis to determine improved and more fruitful avenues of attack. In many other communities surveys have been carried out for the same reason. In still others the recording of and educational activities about home accidents have been incorporated as part of the public health nursing function. In the overall sense, some excellent epidemiologic studies have been made of the problem.[19-26]

Of particular interest and value are some studies on program analysis and cost-benefits carried out by the Public Health Service.[27] One of these relates to motor vehicle and passenger injury prevention. The problem was examined exclusively in terms of human factors. Three major factors in the vehicular accident complex—law enforcement, road design, and traffic engineering— were for the most part excluded. Thus the problem was limited to considerations traditionally within the purview of health agencies. Six alternative programs were examined in terms of the program cost per death anticipated to be averted if an effective program were adequately financed and carried out. The results were as follows:

Program	Cost per death averted
1. Seat belt use—to encourage people to use seat belts	$87
2. Restraint devices—to educate people to obtain and use additional safety restraining devices	$103
3. Pedestrian injury—to educate accident prone pedestrians how to cross the street	$666
4. Motorcycle injury—to encourage motorcyclists to use helmets and eye shields	$3,336
5. Reduce driver drinking—to educate people not to drink and drive	$5,824
6. Driver licensing—to establish a medical screening program for licensing and to exclude drivers with certain conditions	$13,801

Through the efforts of workers in the field of environmental health, more and more accident prevention measures are being built into the standards, specifications, and requirements for house and city plans. Such measures coupled with persistent public educational measures form the core of the attack on home accidents.[28,29] Reference has been made to the significant decline in occupational accidents. This has resulted in large part from activities in industrial health and safety programs, involving inspections and surveys, improved plant and machine design, development and use of safety devices, preemployment examinations, and worker education.

Many state health departments engage in some activities relating to accident prevention at the present time. Accident prevention educational activities are carried on by almost all state health departments. In addition, many of them are attempting to stimulate local accident prevention programs. Special conferences, short courses, and workshops are held for local health department personnel and for representatives of other official and nonofficial local agencies. Also various state health departments cooperate with other official state agencies such as those concerned with mines, industry, labor, and traffic safety in carrying out cooperative programs in those areas.

On the federal level increased interest and concern has been manifest by research, education, and encouragement of and grants to state and local health agencies. The Eighty-ninth Congress during 1965 played a most significant role by the passage of three pieces of legislation aimed at three different aspects of the accident problem. The Traffic Safety Act (P.L. 89-542) provides for highway safety, research and development, certain highway safety programs, a national driver register, and a highway accident research and test facility. The Auto Safety Act (P.L. 89-563) provides for a coordinated national safety program and for the establishment of safety standards for motor vehicles in interstate commerce. The Child Protection Act (P.L. 89-756) bans hazardous toys and articles intended for children and other articles too dangerous to be in the household regardless of labeling.

In the final analysis, of course, the prevention of accidents depends upon the individual, and efforts in order to be fruitful must take place especially on the local level. "Public apathy to the mounting toll from accidents must be transformed into an action program under strong leadership. This can be accomplished by the methods employed to bring poliomyelitis and other epidemics under control, and to make frontal attacks to conquer cancer, heart disease and mental disease. . . . Basic to this unified approach is identification of the individual citizen with a means by which he can satisfy the inherent desire to serve his fellow man."[1]

No single satisfactory pattern has yet been devised or adopted. It is certain, however, that there must be involved some of the basic epidemiologic approaches and techniques that have proved to be effective in many diverse fields. Among these are (1) development and improvement of data on the prevalence and incidence of accidents through reporting, surveys, and studies, (2) education of the public through effective pertinent channels, (3) improvement and extension of safety devices in the home, public buildings, industry, vehicles, and farm machinery, (4) inclusion of training in accident prevention in schools of public health, public administration, and architecture, (5) improvement of structural safety through the general inclusion of accident prevention factors in building codes, (6) improvement of city planning, traffic studies, and highway design, (7) improved driver training, education, and supervision with consideration given to physical and mental factors that may indicate accident proneness, and (8) improvement of the functional design of toys, household equipment, and furniture with consideration given to the peculiar needs and behavior habits of the very young and of the handicapped and elderly.

Only through the cooperative efforts of many community agencies, one of which is the health department, in attacking along all of these and many other fronts, will the toll of accidents be lessened eventually. In the process, because of its all-embracing interest in all aspects of safe and healthful living, it is the official public health agency which is best fitted to serve as a catalyst and rallying point.

POISON CONTROL

A special type of accident hazard is presented by the extensive and increasing number of toxic materials to be found in the modern home.[30] In recent years industrial chemists and pharmaceutical research have developed many wonderful products which have contributed greatly to our way of life. Their widespread availability, however, has not been without danger. No longer is it possible to use a "universal antidote." The highly complex nature of many new pharmaceuticals and household products re-

quires a knowledge of their chemical constitution in order that a quick and effective remedy may be used in case of toxic ingestion.

It is estimated that each year about 600,000 individuals in the United States, many of them children, accidentally ingest a wide variety of household aids and about 1,700 die. This is approximately the number of deaths from appendicitis. The nature of the substances ingested is of interest. In a study of accidental poisonings in children under 15 years of age in New York City, Jacobziner[31] found the causes shown in Table 29-2.

Particular attention should be called to poisonings from lead. Most of these occur in young children from low-income families who live in old housing, the interiors of which have been painted with many layers of lead-containing paint. The problem is complicated by the frequent casual attitude of many parents who accept pica as normal behavior in young children and by the frequent absence of supervision of children in such socioeconomic circumstances.[32]

As a result of the growing concern over accidental poisoning an increasing number of communities have been developing poison control centers.[33,34] There are now about 460 centers in all but two states and the District of Columbia. To varying extents they compile and keep up to date a readily usable file on pharmaceutical, house-

Table 29-2. Accidental poisonings of children under 15 years of age, New York City, 1956

Type of poisoning	Percent of total
Aspirin, barbiturates, and other internal medications	26
Bleach, furniture polish, lye, and other household preparations	20
Lead	10
Iodine and other external medications	9
Insecticides	7
Turpentine and other solvents	6
Cosmetics	5
Rodenticides	3
Miscellaneous	15

hold, industrial, and other substances with data about their composition, toxicity, and antidotes; they provide laboratory analytic service and treatment; they answer telephone requests for first aid information and carry out educational activities for the professions and the public. Some provide follow-up by means of public health nurses or other types of investigators or educators.

One interesting question that calls for more study is the relationship of mental health to so-called accidental poisoning. Unquestionably a certain number of such "accidents" actually represent either conscious or subconscious attempts at suicide or homicide. With regard to the latter is the possible factor of withheld or avoided supervision, warning, or prompt treatment by some parents, older children, or spouses.[35]

SHEET PLASTIC

Another special problem has resulted from improvements in the packaging of goods. The development and inexpensive production of polyethylene plastic have prompted its widespread use for packaging many types of foods, household materials, and equipment and for use as a protective covering of clothing. Concurrent with its widespread use has been a rise in the number of young children who have suffocated as a result of having their faces covered by this material. Since the sheet plastic tends to build up a considerable amount of static electricity, it is particularly apt to adhere tightly to the skin. Already a number of states and communities are exploring the possibility of limiting the use of the material. Meanwhile extensive programs are being conducted to educate parents concerning the potential dangers of sheet plastic.

REFERENCES

1. Accidental death and disability, the neglected disease of modern society, Washington, 1967, National Academy of Sciences, National Research Council.
2. Accidents facts, National Safety Council, Chicago, 1967, The Council.
3. Health statistics, persons injured by class of accident, U. S., July 1957-June 1958, Washington, Feb. 1959, Public Health Service Pub. No. 584-B8.
4. Manheimer, D. I., Dewey, J., Mellinger, G. D., and Corsa, L.: Fifty thousand child-years of accidental injuries, Public Health Rep. 81:519, June 1966.
5. Policy statement on accidents—a public health problem, Amer. J. Public Health 51:122, Jan. 1961.
6. Home accident prevention text, for use by local health departments, Washington, 1957, Public Health Service Pub. No. 564.
7. American Public Health Association: Accident prevention, New York, 1961, McGraw-Hill Book Co.
8. A guide to the development of accidental injury control programs in a local health department, Washington, 1965, Public Health Service Pub. No. 1368.
9. Tiboni, E., editor: Development and operation of an accident control program through a local health department, Ann Arbor, 1967, School of Public Health, University of Michigan.
10. Service statistics for home accident prevention programs, Public Health Rep. 72:494, June 1957.
11. Brightman, I. J., et al.: Mortality statistics as a direction finder in home accident prevention, Amer. J. Public Health 42:840, July 1952.
12. Zindwer, R.: An educational project in childhood accident prevention, Amer. J. Public Health 45:438, Apr. 1955.
13. Jacobziner, H.: Home safety and accident prevention in a child health conference, Amer. J. Public Health 44:83, Jan. 1954.
14. Dietrich, H. F.: Clinical application of the theory of accident prevention in childhood, Amer. J. Public Health 42:849, July 1952.
15. Boek, J. K.: Driver behavior and accidents, Amer. J. Public Health 47:546, May 1947.
16. Weinerman, E. R.: Accident-proneness, a critique, Amer. J. Public Health 39:1527, Dec. 1949.
17. Webb, W. B.: The illusive phenomena in accident proneness, Public Health Rep. 70:951, Oct. 1955.
18. McFarland, R. A., and Moore, R. C.: Human factors in highway safety, New Eng. J. Med. 256:792, Apr. 25, 1957; 256:837, May 2, 1957; 256:890, May 9, 1957.
19. Press, E.: Epidemiological approach to accident prevention, Amer. J. Public Health 38:1442, Oct. 1948.
20. Gordon, J. E.: The epidemiology of accidents, Amer. J. Public Health 39:504, April 1949.
21. Roberts, H., Gordon, J. E., and Fiore, A.: Epidemiological techniques in home accident prevention, Public Health Rep. 67:547, June 1952.
22. Chapman, A. L.: Epidemiological approach to traffic safety, Public Health Rep. 69:773, Aug. 1954.
23. Beadenkopf, W. G., et al.: An epidemiological approach to traffic accidents, Public Health Rep. 71:15, Jan. 1956.

24. Braunstein, P. W.: Medical aspects of automotive crash injury research, J.A.M.A. **163**:249, Jan. 26, 1957.
25. McFarland, R. A.: Epidemiological principles applicable to the study and prevention of child accidents, Amer. J. Public Health **45**:1302, Oct. 1955.
26. Iskrant, A. P.: The epidemiological approach to accident causation, Amer. J. Public Health **57**:1708, Oct. 1967.
27. Program analysis, selected disease control programs, Washington, 1966, Office of the Assistant Secretary for Program Coordination, Department of Health, Education, and Welfare.
28. Kent, F. S.: Engineering aspects of home accident prevention, Amer. J. Public Health **39**:1531, Dec. 1949.
29. Kent, F. S., and Pond, M. A.: Public health consideration on housing design and home accident prevention, Public Health Rep. **66**:1461, Nov. 9, 1951.
30. The public health problem of accidental poisoning, a symposium, Amer. J. Public Health **46**:951, Aug. 1956.
31. Jacobziner, H.: Accidental poisoning among children, Amer. J. Dis. Child. **93**:647, June 1957.
32. Bradley, J. E., and Bessman, S. P.: Poverty, pica, and poisoning, Public Health Rep. **73**:467, May 1958.
33. Press, E., and Mellins, R. B.: A poisoning control program, Amer. J. Public Health **44**:1515, Dec. 1954.
34. Cann, H. M.: Control of accidental poisoning—a progress report, J.A.M.A. **168**:717, Oct. 11, 1958.
35. Schulzinger, M. S.: The accident syndrome, Springfield, Ill., 1956, Charles C Thomas, Publisher.

Chapter 30

Vital statistics

INTRODUCTION

Vital statistics, the bookkeeping of public health, is an essential activity of every public health agency on every level of government. Not only is it a legal responsibility of health agencies, but it also provides the foundation upon which all other parts of the public health program are constructed. It is impossible to imagine a sound program of maternal and child health, communicable disease control, environmental health, or even laboratory services in the absence of this invaluable adjunct. Its influence, if properly used, permeates every part of the organization. At one point it determines what visits should be made by staff nurses or sanitarians; at another it assists in deciding matters of policy for the top administrator.[1]

When satisfactorily organized and conducted, the vital statistics office may serve literally as the brain center, continually giving answers to "What is the score?" and "What next?" Its constituent parts taken in toto present the composite life history of a community, state, or nation. It is the storehouse of indispensable information which reflects the strengths and foibles, successes and failures, joys and sorrows of the group. It is the key that opens the door to a competent, sound, and efficient community health administration. The applications of statistics in public health have been summarized to include (1) population estimation and prediction, (2) surveys of population characteristics, health needs, and problems, (3) analysis of health trends, (4) epidemiologic research, (5) treatment and program evaluation, (6) pro-

gram planning, (7) budget preparation and justification, (8) operational and administrative decision making, and (9) health education.[2]

It is difficult, if not impossible, for a public health worker to be either successful or satisfied without an intelligent and sympathetic appreciation of the vital data of the area he serves. Unfortunately too many regard this activity as a chore or necessary evil to be delegated to a few inadequately trained clerks working in an out-of-the-way office. It should be realized that although the real material of statistics may appear to be scraps of paper containing crooked little integers each represents a human interest story which with its fellows leads to a critically important end product—a philosophic plan for the alleviation of human misery and the attainment of health for all.

The compilation of vital statistics is of ancient origin. Enumerations of people were carried out long before the birth of Christ, notably in China, Egypt, Persia, Greece, and Rome, primarily for purposes of taxation and to determine the military manpower. Data relating to births, deaths, and marriages were recorded in elementary form in the old church registers of England. The oldest known copy of these so-called "Bills of Mortality" can be seen in the British Museum and is dated November 1532. These bills were compiled by parish priests and clerks for more than a century before John Graunt in 1662 published his book *Natural and Political Observations Mentioned in a Following Index and Made Upon the Bills of Mortality.*

Vital statistics in the modern sense can be considered to have originated from the publication of this book.

The late eighteenth century saw the beginning of the modern national census. Priority is somewhat open to question. The outstanding claims are Canada, 1666; Sweden, 1749; and England and the United States, 1790. Regardless of the earliest claim it may be stated that the United States Census had a tremendous influence on the spread of the idea throughout the rest of the world. The institution of a national census in America has, with good reason, been called a political accident, since the provision for our decennial enumeration arose from the conflict between the small and large states. The former demanded equal representation in the national legislature, whereas the latter felt that their larger populations justified more power. The compromise solution was to establish a bicameral legislature consisting of the Senate, in which states were equally represented, and the House of Representatives, with representation in proportion to population. This compromise solution made necessary some provision for the periodic inventory of the population. As a result the following was included in the Constitution: "Representatives shall be apportioned among the several States according to their respective numbers, counting the whole number of persons in each State, excluding Indians not taxed. The actual enumeration shall be made within three years after the first meeting of the Congress of the United States, and within every subsequent term of ten years, in such manner as they shall by law direct."* It should be noted that all that was required was a simple count. From this basic purpose and requirement there has developed a national census of great complexity and detail which provides data of great value far beyond what was envisioned by the framers of the Constitution. Similarly the value and use of vital data in general now extends far beyond the original intent and

*Article I, Section 2, Paragraph 3, modified by the Fourteenth Amendment.

purpose. Very few parts of our social, political, economic, and industrial systems could possibly operate without it.[3]

It is significant that the collection and analysis of vital statistics or more specifically public health statistics are considered to be one of the basic functions in public health. With substantial reason it may be stated that all of the other functions depend essentially upon the adequate fulfillment of this primary function for their success. Statistics have come to be regarded as an indispensable administrative tool for the proper planning, performance, and evaluation of any modern business or public program.

SOURCES OF PUBLIC HEALTH STATISTICS

The most fundamental information upon which activities in public health must be predicated is a knowledge of the quantitative and qualitative characteristics of the population to be served. This implies some form of a count or estimate of the people within a jurisdiction. On the surface it would appear that the decennial census, to which reference has been made, would supply whatever data is necessary. This was the case in the more stable or immobile societies which preceded the era of paved highways, rapid transportation, and industrialization. Reasonably adequate intercensal populations could be estimated by means of rather simple arithmetic or geometric projections. The situation has been drastically changed in recent years however, particularly as a result of World War II. In 1940 a very detailed census was carried out. However, within little more than a year the nation became engaged in an international conflict of great magnitude requiring the enlistment and draft of several millions of citizens. In addition, new and old industries underwent spectacular expansion, necessitating the movement of additional millions of persons in order to serve them. Many communities within a short space of time found their populations doubled or trebled, whereas others were noticeably depleted. It soon became evident that neither the 1940 census data, which by this time had been released, nor any estimates based upon them could serve much valuable present purpose. Many attempts were made to find suitable substitutes in the form of school attendance records, work records, or food ration card applications. Of the group, the latter was probably the most useful during the World War II years. Currently, Social Security registration provides an additional measure of the population with the handicaps, however, of not including children and certain groups of the employable and not giving an indication of population movement. It was hoped that the confused situation would be of a temporary nature, but soon statisticians, economists, and public health workers were convinced that our national mode of life had been so deeply affected as to require some new form of population determination and analysis. During the same period of time a new business and social study technique, the sample survey or poll, came upon the scene and began to serve a valuable purpose. The ultimate answer to the population data problem will probably take the form of relatively simple, easily made enumerations, such as those the framers of the Constitution had in mind, augmented by frequent representative sample surveys in order to determine the internal characteristics of the total enumerated population.

Next in importance to the population base are data obtained from administrative registration and reporting procedures. Responsibility for this function in the United States rests with the respective states. The most significant of these activities relate to the vital events of birth, death, and morbidity. Again, in order that these data may be of value in the planning of public health programs, there must be some assurance of their qualitative and quantitative dependability. This need led to the establishment of birth and death registration areas by the Bureau of the Census. The death registration area was organized in 1900 and included the states of Connecticut, Indiana, Maine, Massachusetts, Michigan, New Hampshire, New Jersey, New York, Rhode Island, Vermont, and the District of Columbia. At that time

these areas contained about 40% of the total population of the United States. The birth registration area was established in 1915 and included originally Connecticut, Maine, Massachusetts, Michigan, Minnesota, New Hampshire, New York, Pennsylvania, Rhode Island, Vermont, and the District of Columbia, accounting for 31% of the total population. By 1933 all states had become members of both the birth and the death registration areas. Membership is based upon two criteria: satisfactory state registration laws, and at least 90% completeness in reporting.

Certain limitations are found in relation to the value of birth and death reports. The most obvious is the fact that as yet some of these events may be unrecorded. This has become relatively unimportant in recent years. An analysis in 1950 by the Bureau of the Census indicated that after 35 years of birth registration 97.8% completeness had been achieved, although each year in the United States an estimated 50,000 babies are born who are not registered. Much of this discrepancy, however, is remedied by late registration when individuals enter school, the armed forces, or apply for a Social Security number in the process of employment. Other problems are related to the inadequate reporting of stillbirths and babies born out of wedlock.[4]

Efforts to secure better reporting of both live and stillbirths require constant vigilance on the part of registrars and directors of vital statistical offices. Many different approaches have been used and it would appear that no one alone is satisfactory. Education of the public, of attendants at birth, and of hospitals must be conducted constantly. In addition to this is the use of many types of checks. Hospital records, baptismal records, and, of much less value, newspaper announcements have been recommended for this purpose. Probably the most common and accurate check of completeness of birth reporting is that of deaths of infants under one year of age. When corrected for residence, this group constitutes a more or less representative sample of the infants born in the area. Other groups that have been used are entering school children in states requiring a birth certificate for school attendance, and children attending well-baby or child hygiene clinics. In some states, especially where most births occur in hospitals, an arrangement has been made with many of the hospitals to prepare a birth certificate at the time the prospective mother enters the hospital, complete except for the date of birth, sex, and name of the child, which can be readily filled in after birth at the time the physician signs the certificate. In addition to producing very satisfactory results, this procedure has added value in that the certificates are usually typed and therefore are more legible than they otherwise might be.

The problem of reporting illegitimate births has been approached in three different ways by the various states.[5] The first of these is to make mandatory provision for the attendant at birth to file the birth certificate of an illegitimate child directly with the state office of vital statistics rather than to have it pass through the hands of the local registrar. Some feel that this weakens the local registration system and is therefore undesirable. The second approach, found in many states, is the provision that the certificate of an illegitimate child not differ from that of a legitimate child— once the child in question has been adopted or legitimized. The objection that has been raised against this is the necessity of preparing new certificates. The third and least desirable method is to delete the item of legitimacy entirely. This has been successfully promoted in a few states by welfare agencies and certain other groups. The objection, of course, is that this precludes knowledge concerning the extent of illegitimacy and of the many social and health problems relating to it and may give rise to a number of legal complications.

Two compromises should be mentioned that offer perhaps the best solutions up to the present. Many states have removed the item of legitimacy from the certificate proper and have placed it on a supplementary portion. Perhaps more satisfactory is the policy of a few states of including the item on the certificate but eliminating it

on certified copies of the certificate, usually by the general use of an abbreviated copy of the certificate.

One other phase of birth reporting that causes difficulty is delayed registration of births. This problem came to a head during the first half of the 1940's when a birth certificate, as evidence of citizenship, was required for employment in the large numbers of war industries. As Bailey[5] has put it, "The system has undergone its baptism of fire and, in general, has emerged unscathed." Two outstanding questions have arisen: What evidence should be required to support the application for delayed registration of a birth? Should this evidence be reviewed by the registrar or by the courts? The manual on Uniform Procedures for Delayed Registration prepared jointly by the American Association of Registration Executives and the National Center for Health Statistics seems to provide the answers as to the nature of acceptable evidence. Since routine court evaluation is unwieldly, particularly by virtue of the numbers of applications involved, most states now have the evidence reviewed by the state registrar, with recourse to the courts in case of a rejection. This seems to be a satisfactory and advisable pattern.

Because of burial requirements, deaths are reported to a greater degree of completeness than are births. The value of death certificates is impaired, however, not only by some inadequate reporting but also by the subjective nature of much of the data requested on the form. It is still not rare for the cause of a death to be misstated deliberately in order to circumvent potential social stigma. This occurs not only in relation to suicides and syphilis but also in some degree to tuberculosis, cancer, and some hereditary ailments. Incorrect diagnoses present a constant problem to the vital statistician. Numerous studies have been made regarding the degree of accuracy of the physician's statement of cause of death. The figure varies considerably by time and place. The magnitude of this error is subject to steady reduction by virtue of improved medical education and the development and use of new laboratory and clinical diagnostic techniques. Beyond this, the most that can be hoped for at present is that each jurisdiction for its own purposes attempt some estimate of this source of error by means of checking with autopsy reports and by consultations. Even the most conscientious physician is faced with the difficult problem of deciding the primary cause of death as against contributing causes. This problem has been partially solved by the publication and wide adoption of the World Health Organization's International Classification of Diseases, Injuries, and Causes of Death which presents primary and secondary causal preferences for all possible combinations of diseases.

With but two exceptions, responsibility for the collection and processing of reports of births and deaths is delegated to the state health department, and in the majority of instances the state health officer is designated by law as the state registrar of vital statistics. In Massachusetts the secretary of state and in Alaska the state auditor are the officers responsible. In all the states and territories collection is accomplished through local registrars who receive reports directly from attending physicians, midwives, undertakers, and others. With regard to the definition of local registration areas and the appointment of local registrars, Mountin and Flook[7] in their analysis of state health department organization found the following:

The basis upon which local registration districts are formed and the method by which local registrars are appointed are prescribed by State law. For the most part, political subdivisions of a county constitute the basis for establishing local vital statistics registration districts. Cities, villages, towns, townships, election districts, magisterial districts, or similar minor civil divisions form the local registration areas in 42 States. In the remaining States, geographic rather than political characteristics are the factors which determine the boundaries of local registration districts. Convenience of communication, transportation facilities, and mail service are items usually considered under this plan. There is even greater variation with respect to the method of appointing local registrars. In over two-fifths of the States, either the State board of health, the State health officer, or the director of the bureau of vital statistics makes the appointments; in a dozen more, they are appointed locally by the board of county

commissioners, the local health officer, the board of town trustees, the mayor, or board of aldermen; in 10 States the duties of city or town clerk or of local health officer automatically include the collection of vital statistics; while in the remaining half dozen States, the office is elective—by popular vote of the community.

The routing of reports of births and deaths is subject to much variation. In some states certificates are either filed with the county health officers, who transmit them to the state health departments, or are routed by the local registrars through the county health departments. More commonly, local registrars send the certificates directly to their state health departments. In one state the local registrars also send copies to the county health departments for their use. In about one half of the states the two procedures described above are combined. Certificates are forwarded by local registrars directly to the state health departments, except that in counties or districts with full-time local health departments certificates are sent to them for transmission to the state office.

In all but two states birth and death certificates are forwarded to the state health department once a month. One state receives them but once a year, a practice conducive to error and inadequate use. The other exception requires that certificates be forwarded weekly. Among other values this makes it possible for the public health nursing service of that state health department to establish educational and other contact with families in which there is a new baby, within 1 or 2 weeks of delivery. It would appear desirable that, whatever routing procedure is followed, four basic principles should be adhered to:

1. Certificates should be made promptly by medical or other attendants.
2. There should be a system of routine checking by registrars of all certificates for correctness and completeness.
3. Certificates should be forwarded to the state agency at intervals of not longer than one month.
4. Pertinent data on certificates should be made readily and promptly available to local health departments, preferably by means of their acting as in-

termediaries in the transmission of certificates from local registrars to the state department. If this is not provided for, much of the value of the reporting is lost.

Morbidity reporting presents a very difficult problem. Information relating to the incidence of disease in a community is obviously necessary for a public health program of any logical design. Upon this data depend whatever steps the organization may take in many of its other activities. The incidence of various types of disease points to the extent of hospital, laboratory, and home nursing facilities needed. The prevalence of enteric diseases gives an index of the adequacy of the environmental sanitation and the food and milk control programs. Information concerning disease is one of the most potent items in the armamentarium of the health educator. With increased interest in problems of older citizens, data depicting their illnesses are fundamental to the crystalization of a program for their benefit.

Completeness of morbidity reporting is subject to great variation, depending upon the state laws and local regulations, the presence or absence and adequacy or inadequacy of local health departments, the types and severity of diseases common in the area, the professional and social attitudes of the physicians practicing in the area, and the customs and economy of the people.

There is great variation among the states both in the total number of diseases reportable and in the specific diseases included. The total number varied from 28 in Virginia to 66 in Iowa. Reports of occupational diseases are required in addition in many states. All states require the reporting of conjunctivitis, diphtheria, measles, meningitis, poliomyelitis, scarlet fever, smallpox, syphilis, typhoid fever, tuberculosis, undulant fever, and whooping cough. Similar variation has been noted with respect to morbidity reporting procedures.[8] Only two requirements are uniform in all the states. First, every state requires that cases of notifiable diseases be reported by the attending physician or in the absence of a physician by

householder, head of the family, or person in charge of the patient. Second, the reports are to be made to the local health authority. Of the 50 states, 46 use report cards. Seventeen use the same card for all diseases, 13 have a special card for tuberculosis, and 29 have a special card for cases of venereal diseases. Format varies from no regular form (4 states), to single (27 states) and multiple (9 states) case penalty cards, stamped cards (2 states), cards requiring postage (3 states), and forms other than a postcard (4 states).

The usual practice is to route morbidity reports through the local health department to the state health department. Some states require only that copies of daily, weekly, or monthly summaries be sent to the state health department. A few states follow the unreasonable practice of requiring physicians to send reports both to the local and to the state health departments.

Certain factors must be considered in the use of morbidity data. Fundamental is the need to prepare and educate those in the community from whom reports are expected to be obtained. The most important of these are private physicians, hospitals, and schools. Two other sources worthy of mention are the dental profession and industry. Too often there is an inclination to require reports of too many diseases and in too much detail, whether or not any practical use can be made of the information. Physicians and other reporting agencies soon form a conclusion concerning the practicality of the request and the use made of it. If they decide that the information is merely received and filed away, they soon become careless in their reporting. In all fairness, they can hardly be blamed if no one takes the trouble to explain the purpose of the items requested.

An additional important factor is the amount of work involved in making the report. Busy practitioners are loath to spend much time in writing out details of cases for official agencies. The problem of red tape is very real. The average physician practicing in an American community today finds it necessary to have readily available an increasing number of different official and semiofficial report forms which must be filled out for births, deaths, communicable diseases, premarital examinations, medical care, acts of violence, workmen's compensation, veteran's benefits, and insurance examinations, to mention but a few. The least that can be done is to standardize and simplify some of these forms insofar as possible. In the case of morbidity reporting, requirements and methods should be reduced to the barest essentials. Thus an increasing number of official health agencies accept reports of cases of communicable diseases in the form of telephone calls or preaddressed postcards, requiring only the diagnosis and the name, age, and address of the person affected. It is significant that the patient's name, address, and age and the name of the disease are the only items common to the morbidity report forms of all of the states.[8] From there on it is the responsibility of the public health personnel to obtain what further details appear necessary for the adequate public health management of the case.

West,[9] in an analysis of the completeness of morbidity reporting, found that, whereas physicians were the most important and in some areas almost the only source, in other areas hospitals, schools, visiting nurse associations, industrial plants, health department clinics, staff members, and householders were also valuable reporting sources. Within given areas she found that some diseases, particularly scarlet fever, were reported almost entirely by physicians whereas other sources were more important for certain other diseases, notably tuberculosis. As a result she suggests the use of certain indices for the estimation of the level of reporting of various diseases. In the areas studied it was found that for the childhood diseases—chickenpox, diphtheria, German measles, measles, mumps, scarlet fever, and whooping cough—the level of reporting of cases included in the school records furnishes useful information as to the completeness of reporting.

For meningococcal meningitis, pneumonia, and poliomyelitis the completeness of reporting of cases in general hospitals provides a very useful index. For diseases for which there is available no one source representative of the population at risk, an index representing an upper limit to the completeness of reporting can be obtained by combining the available data in the form:

$$\frac{\text{All reported cases}}{\text{All reported cases} + \text{Unreported cases from all relevant sources}}$$

In the case of rheumatic fever, for instance, no single source was found to be satisfactory. Here an upper limit based on data from hospital, school, and death records provides an index. For tuberculosis an upper limit based on the reporting of cases found in hospital, sanatorium, death certificate, and health department data provides the most useful index.

It is concluded that it is impossible to devise any final or universally applicable index since such shifting factors as the occurrence of an epidemic or a change in the population will temporarily alter the level of reporting of particular diseases. However, West[9] states, "The need of the local health officer is not for refined figures which could be developed from protracted study, but for approximate figures which will assist him in interpreting and evaluating the morbidity program of his own department and in planning the better utilization of reporting sources."

Since 1925 there have been many proposals for the establishment of a morbidity reporting area similar to the birth and death registration areas. As yet no definite steps have been taken. It has been increasingly suggested that public health agencies obtain morbidity data for administrative planning by means of special detailed studies and sample surveys rather than to depend upon routine reports that are subject to so many limitations.[10] This approach to the problem has already been put into effect in a number of instances, notable among which are the Hagerstown studies and more recently the United States National Health Survey.[11] The use that has already been made of the data collected in these two instances has more than justified their cost and points to the need for further application and development of these techniques. Langmuir[12] has stated the following viewpoint:

> The morbidity survey is a particularly useful epidemiological tool in that data on both the sick and the well are obtained concurrently. The problems arising from underreporting of cases, from arbitrary classifications of causes of death, and from unknown shifts of population between census years are largely eliminated. . . . Its unique advantage lies in the detailed information that can be collected about the population. Frequency rates, specific for a wide variety of social and environmental factors, can be determined. Such comparisons are not obtainable by matching routine morbidity reports and death certificates with census figures.

He further points out the interrelationships between the simple survey and the special study:

> The simple morbidity survey has one inherent limitation—only general data can be obtained. The questions asked by the interviewers must be simple and understandable to the informants. Few specific diseases can be adequately counted by this method. Special studies are necessary to collect such definitive epidemiological information.

In order to obtain vital data for the nation as a whole, states routinely transmit the information they obtain to the National Center for Health Statistics in the Public Health Service for collation, analysis, and publication. Numerous useful documents are prepared and made available. Among them are the annual *Vital Statistics of the United States*[13] and the *Morbidity and Mortality Weekly Report,*[14] which present data for the nation as a whole and for each state, including comparisons with the year before and indications of trends. In addition, the weekly report includes descriptions of unusual or particularly important epidemiologic occurrences. The National Center in its turn submits its data and analyses to the World Health Organization for inclusion in the development of the worldwide picture[15,16] and for epidemiologic intelligence purposes.

ADMINISTRATIVE USES OF VITAL STATISTICS

The collection and analysis of public health statistics are at best costly and difficult tasks. The only real justification for performing it is the administrative use to which the resulting information may be put. Reports of vital and of related events, such as the services rendered by the personnel of a health department, constitute important legal records. Their personal value arises in connection with proof of citizenship, the right to attend school, to vote, to marry, to enter the armed services, and to draw benefits of many types. Records of births and deaths are of particular significance in the establishment of inheritance rights and in the prevention of capital crime. Not infrequently health department service records play an important role in litigation relating to property use and condemnation.

Of particular importance are the uses to which statistical data may be put in the administration and management of the public health program. For statistical data to be of real value in the public health program, efforts far beyond the strict legal responsibilities imposed upon public health agencies are required. Too often the minimal acts of registration and reporting have been conducted as the sole activity in this field. Registration may be relegated to an untrained clerk who routinely accepts, transcribes, and files the documents after a most cursory examination. This procedure can make statistics nothing but "dead" in the most literal sense. When, on the other hand, all the statistics available to a health department are correlated, they become of fourfold value in that they make possible (1) the definition of the problem, (2) the development of a logical program for its control, (3) the planning of records and procedures for the administration and analysis of the program as it progresses, and (4) the evaluation of the results of the program.

An example may serve to illustrate these points. The crude number of deaths occurring in a community is of relatively little value. It must be fixed to some standard, the most convenient and useful being a unit of population. This involves an appreciation of the adequacy of reporting and the availability of a dependable population count or estimate. The death rate may then be found to be 9.5 per 1,000 inhabitants. A series of questions now arise: Is this high or low? Comparison must be made with the rates of other communities of a comparable nature or adjusted for the differences. If it is decided that the single figure is relatively low, is that true of all groups in the community? Age is one basis for grouping. Calculation of age-specific death rates may show a much higher than average mortality under the age of one year. Further breakdown may localize the problem in the neonatal period, involving particularly infants born prematurely. What can be done to alleviate the situation? Perhaps an analysis of certain other factors may point the way. Correlation of birth and infant death certificates may point to premature infants born at home or in a particular hospital as accounting for a majority of the deaths. The health department may then strive for the installation of special facilities, incubators, and specially trained nurses in the hos-

pital in question. In order to include those born at home, it is imperative that birth certificates be sent to the local health department within 24 hours after birth, in which case they should be routinely screened for prematures. A somewhat better solution would be the arrangement of a discussion of prematurity with the local medical society and the adoption of a policy of phoning the health department immediately upon delivery of a premature infant in the home. In either of these ways, it becomes possible for the health department to detail a public health nurse to the care of the infant within the first few crucial days of life.

Perhaps analysis of the statistical data relating to births and infants deaths indicated a higher incidence of prematurity and premature death among certain racial or nationality groups. It then becomes the task of the public health staff to study the habits and customs of these groups in an attempt

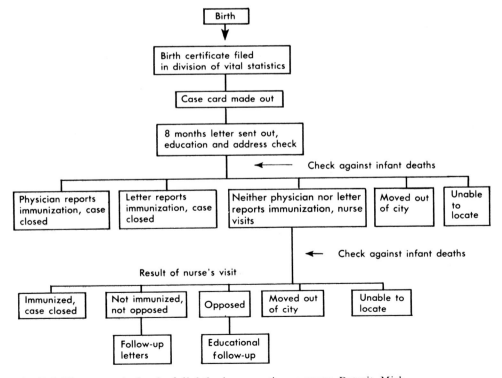

Fig. 30-1. Diagrammatic sketch of diphtheria prevention program, Detroit, Mich.

to discover causal relationships. If such relationships are discovered, a difficult but fascinating task is laid before the health education and public health nursing staffs.

Fig. 30-1 presents another example, this time of the use of the birth certificate in the diphtheria prevention program of one city. It should be noted that the birth certificates represent the key to the approach and also that for public relations reasons a constant running check is made against reports of infant deaths.

PRESENTATION OF VITAL DATA

Of increasing importance in the planning and operation of modern public health programs is the use of fractionated data and of certain graphic devices. There is nothing particularly new or difficult about the breakdown of crude or general data into its component parts. The possible number and types of such breakdowns are practically infinite, and the public health worker must decide which are going to be most useful. With all statistical analyses, much depends upon the form in which the material is arranged for study and presentation. A mass of figures is generally incomprehensible. It is desirable, therefore, to depict the data in some manner which makes it possible to grasp the total picture and all of the details. One of the most common methods is the simple spot or pin map which gives an instant overall answer to the question of where the problem is located. An example is presented in Fig. 30-2, which shows for a large city the residences of persons who died from tuberculosis known to the health department as of a certain date. Since the information is based upon a constantly moving point in time, this should preferably be in the form of a pin map. This would make possible the shifting of pins as cases are added or dropped and would also allow for the use of different-colored pins to indicate the present status of each case as to severity and hospitalization.

By itself a spot map of a disease or other single item is limited in that it does not indicate the extent to which the group is affected. One general approach to this

problem is to distribute the data on the basis of various personal characteristics such as age, race, sex, or economic status. Fig. 30-3 illustrates one method of doing this. The city to which the figure relates has a low tuberculosis death rate. But note how this analysis and presentation point specifically to tuberculosis as an important cause of death in one particular age group. A few of the many other facts it brings to the surface are that cancer and heart disease are important even as early as the young adult years, that the greatest risk of death is during the first year of life particularly because of prematurity, and that accidents are of great significance throughout childhood and young adulthood. Naturally information of this sort will largely determine the nature of the public health program of the area.

An effective and easily comprehended method of relating specific problems to other factors and to the group is by means of transparent overlay maps. This is particularly useful if there is available for use as a base a map such as Fig. 30-4, which shows the distribution of the population of the area. Thus if spot maps such as Fig. 30-2 are of the same size and are made on transparent material such as Pliofilm, they may be successively superimposed on the population map or on each other for visual correlation.

In recent years public health administrators have come to realize that the health programs of large cities are best administered through decentralized neighborhood health centers. These centers are usually decentralized administrative units of the central health department and are often planned to serve populations of about 200,-000. Merely to determine the best locations of the health centers, it is necessary to have detailed information concerning the various subdivisions of the jurisdiction. It is strange that, while data have long been available for small villages and towns, this has not been generally true of the neighborhood units of large cities until the 1940 census. Too often programs have been based upon data limited to the incidence of cases and deaths and have totally ignored the composition of the matrix among whom the cases and deaths were occurring. To be of more than limited use and significance these vital statistics must be related to the places people live, the way they live, the kinds of work they do, and the problems they face. Because of this, the Bureau of the Census during recent years has broken down and made available much of the enormous fund of information it gathers on the basis of census tracts.

A census tract is a small area with defi-

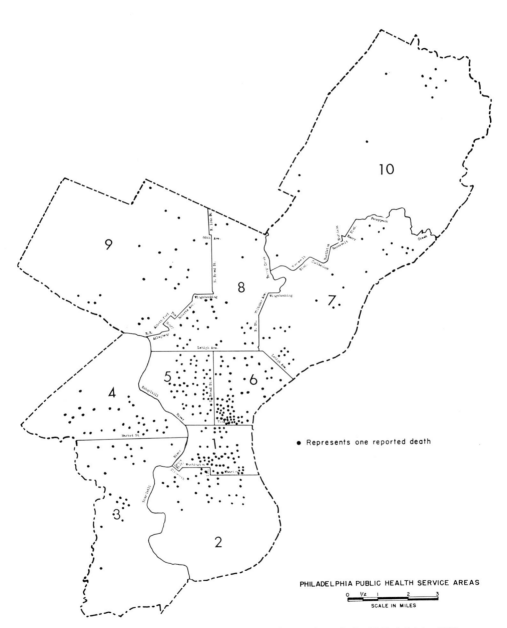

Fig. 30-2. Spot map. Distribution of reported deaths from tuberculosis, Philadelphia, 1957.

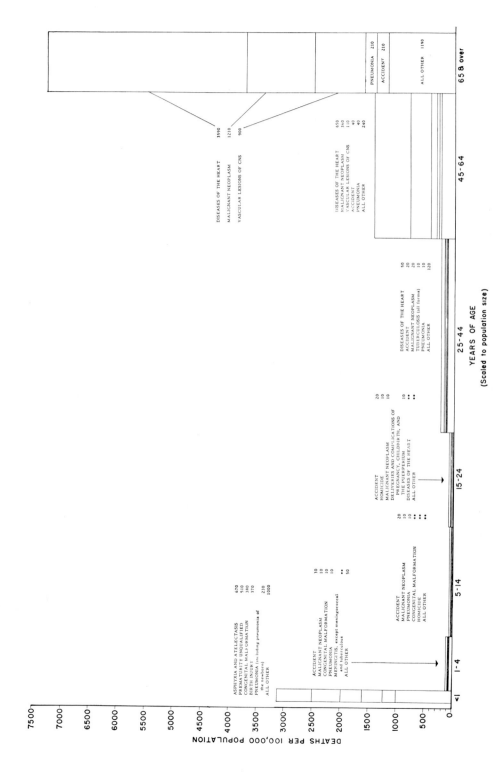

Fig. 30-3. Five principal causes of death by age group per 100,000 estimated population, Philadelphia, 1957.

nite and permanent boundaries, including a population of between 3,000 and 6,000. It is usually fairly homogeneous with respect to race, nativity, economic status, and general living conditions. This has made it worthwhile for public health administrators in turn to tabulate the vital statistical data of their jurisdictions on the basis of smaller administrative areas. The correlation of these two sources of infor-

mation has two great advantages: (1) health statistics compiled on a census tract basis serve to show the geographic distribution of health problems, and (2) health statistics compiled on a census tract basis may be related to other social and economic factors also available by census tracts. As Dunn[17] has well stated, the ability to spot births, deaths, communicable disease cases, nurses' visits, and other perti-

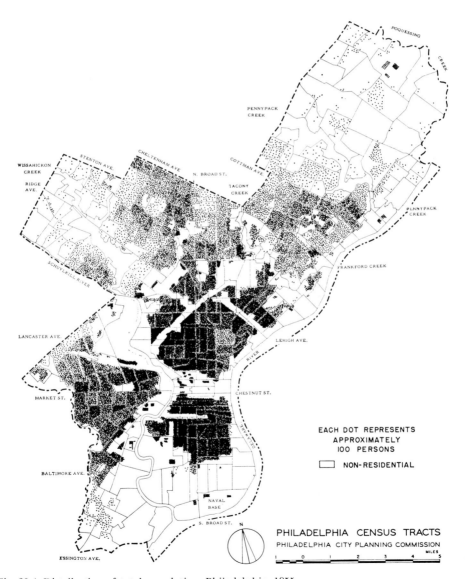

Fig. 30-4. Distribution of total population, Philadelphia, 1955.

nent data on a tract map shows the health administrator where his business is. Classes for mothers should be organized in areas where births are most frequent. There should be special effort and specific preventive measures in areas where stillbirths and infant deaths predominate. Well-baby clinics should be located in the areas where the babies live. Venereal disease and tuberculosis clinics should be located in the areas where venereal disease and tuberculosis cases are concentrated. Similarly public health education programs on venereal disease and tuberculosis should be stressed in these areas. Special preventive measures should be taken in areas where certain other communicable diseases occur. Accident prevention programs should be stressed in areas where most accidents occur and where persons who are involved in accidents reside. Outpatient hospital clinics should be located in areas where the people who use them reside. Nurses' areas should be designed according to the distribution of demand for nurses' services. Housing inspections and inspections of food establishments are presumably made on a citywide basis. It is a good idea to design inspectors' areas by census tracts and to keep inspection records on this basis. Problem areas may be easily spotted and special attention can be given these areas.

It is not practical, of course, to establish a health center or clinic in each census tract. Furthermore, because of the small numbers of births, deaths, and cases of disease occurring in each tract, any rates computed in this relatively small population base are of doubtful significance. In using the information, therefore, the health officer usually finds it desirable to recombine the census tract data in a manner most convenient and best suited to his needs. The usual practice is to form health or sanitary districts, the boundaries of which coincide with those of a number of census tracts. It is then possible to compute statistically significant rates and ratios that may be presented in one or several of a number of ways as has been done in Fig. 30-5.

A particularly valuable and illustrative method of presentation of fractionated data for administrative purposes is in the form of what has been called the epidemiologic master chart. This type of chart makes possible the presentation at one time of the most complex yet comprehensible pictures of the total public health situation. An example is shown in Fig. 30-6, which presents a detailed and interrelated analysis of a great many important factors bearing on the public health program of the city of Philadelphia. It presents vital data in a form which makes it possible to compare the health districts of the city with one another and to gain a composite view of a large number of factors within each district. The total width of the bars represents 100% of the population of Philadelphia. The width of the 10 subdivisions in each bar indicates the percentage of the total population residing in each district. The numerical percentage is indicated for each district, at the top of the first bar. The height of the two bars for race and age groups represents 100% of the population that resides in each district, the subdivisions indicating the percentage of persons in each age and race group. In the remaining bars are shown rates of birth, death, infant deaths, and deaths from important causes, with the scale placed at the left of each bar. On the right, opposite the title of each bar, is noted the rate for the city as a whole, this being shown further by a horizontal line drawn across each bar.

Although it is in no sense the purpose of this chapter to discuss statistical methodology, there are several computations that public health workers have found particularly useful in judging their programs and in gauging their problems. The simplest of these is the crude death rate. This commonly used rate is merely the number of deaths occurring within a certain time period, usually one year, relative to a convenient unit of population, usually 1,000 persons. Thus a community of 23,460 persons which experiences 220 deaths during a year has a crude death rate of $\frac{220 \times 1,000}{23,460} = 9.4$

Text continued on p. 564.

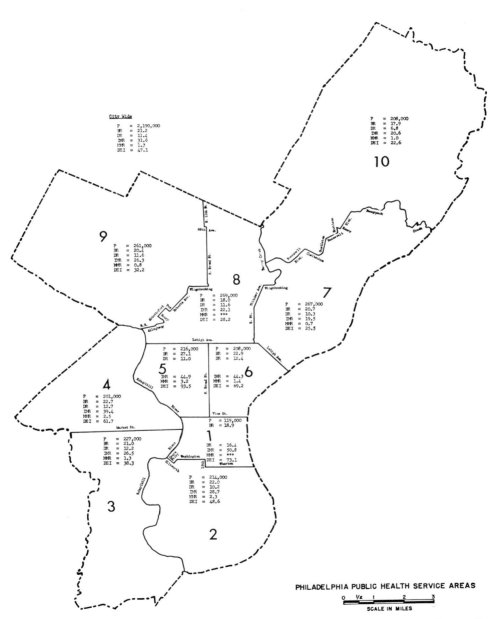

City Wide
```
P   = 2,190,000
BR  =    21.2
DR  =    11.4
IMR =    31.6
MMR =     1.2
DEI =    47.1
```

```
P   = 208,000
BR  =   17.9
DR  =    6.8
IMR =   20.6
MMR =    1.0
DEI =   22.6
```
10

9
```
P   = 261,000
BR  =   20.4
DR  =   11.6
IMR =   26.3
MMR =    0.8
DEI =   32.2
```

8
```
P   = 269,000
BR  =   18.0
DR  =   11.6
IMR =   22.1
MMR =   ***
DEI =   28.2
```

7
```
P   = 267,000
BR  =   20.7
DR  =   10.3
IMR =   19.5
MMR =    0.7
DEI =   25.5
```

5
```
P   = 216,000
BR  =   27.1
DR  =   11.0
IMR =   44.9
MMR =    3.2
DEI =   93.5
```

6
```
P   = 208,000
BR  =   22.9
DR  =   12.4
IMR =   44.3
MMR =    1.4
DEI =   69.2
```

4
```
P   = 201,000
BR  =   22.7
DR  =   12.7
IMR =   39.4
MMR =    2.5
DEI =   61.7
```

```
P   = 227,000
BR  =   21.0
DR  =   12.2
IMR =   26.5
MMR =    1.3
DEI =   38.3
```

1
```
P = 119,000
BR = 18.9
DR  =   16.4
IMR =   50.8
MMR =   ***
DEI =   73.1
```

```
P   = 214,000
BR  =   22.0
DR  =   10.2
IMR =   28.7
MMR =    2.3
DEI =   48.6
```

3

2

PHILADELPHIA PUBLIC HEALTH SERVICE AREAS

0   ½   1   2   3

SCALE IN MILES

Fig. 30-5. Estimated population, birthrate, death rate, infant mortality rate, and maternal mortality rate, and death from diseases of early infancy by health district, Philadelphia, 1957. *P*, Population; *BR*, birthrate; *DR*, death rate; *IMR*, infant mortality rate; *MMR*, maternal mortality rate; *DEI*, diseases of early infancy.

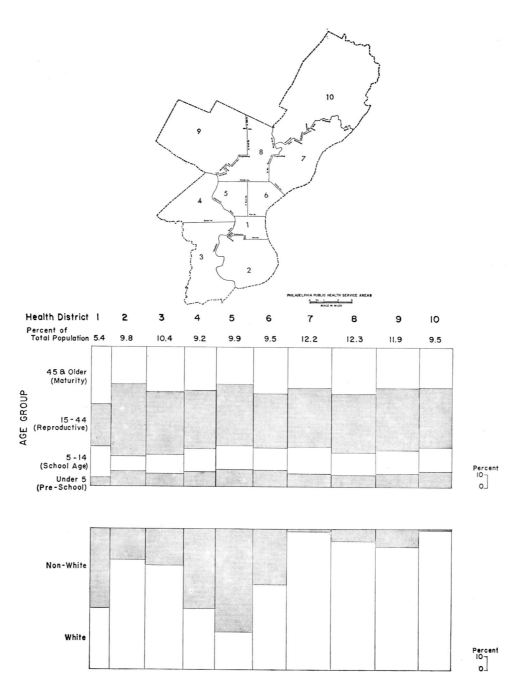

Fig. 30-6. Epidemiologic master chart, Philadelphia, 1957.

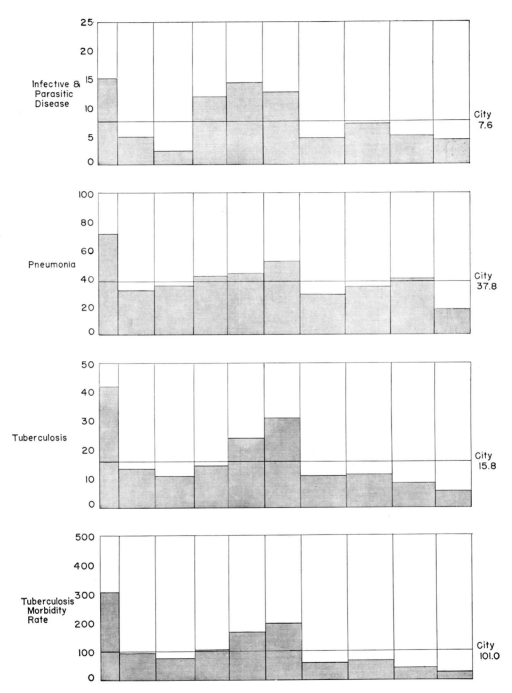

Fig. 30-6, cont'd. For legend see opposite page.

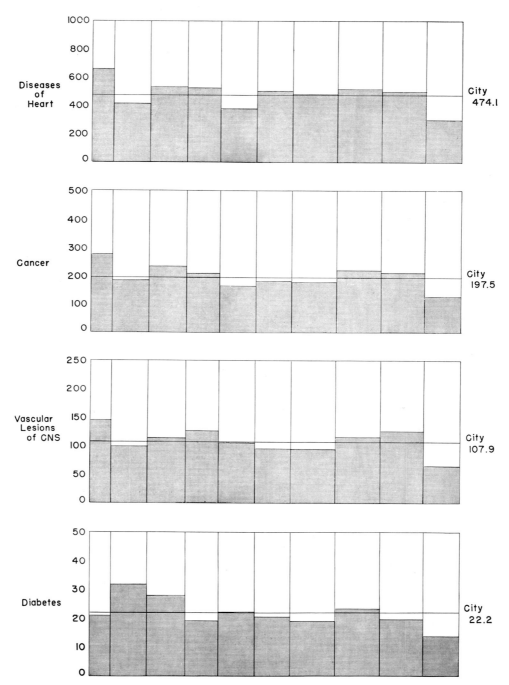

Fig. 30-6, cont'd. For legend see p. 560.

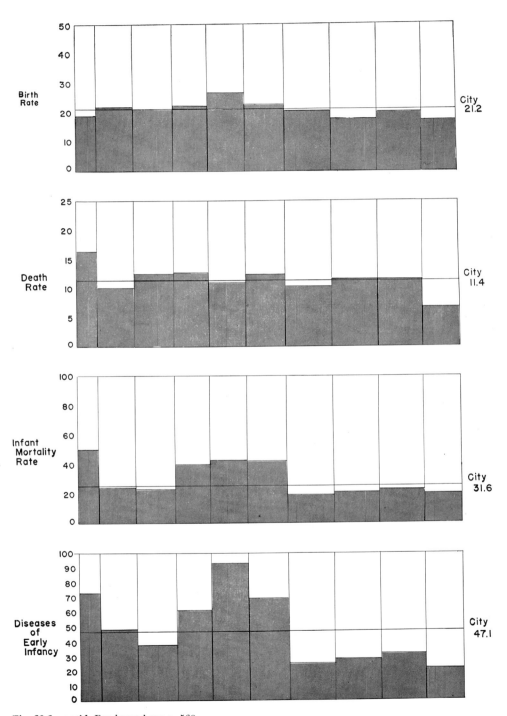

Fig. 30-6, cont'd. For legend see p. 560.

deaths per 1,000 population. This figure has obvious limitations, all of which arise from the many factors its innate crudeness may conceal. It is easily possible, for example, for a community to have a low crude death rate and yet experience serious mortality from certain particular diseases. Similarly one community may have a lower death rate than another, merely by virtue of a greater proportion of young adults in its population. Despite these handicaps, however, the crude death rate is still the single most commonly used basis for comparison by time and place.

Less commonly used is the vital index or birth-death ratio. This is obtained by dividing the number of births by the number of deaths occurring during a year and multiplying by 100 as a base. If this ratio exceeds 100, the population is growing; it it is less than 100, the population is decreasing due to biologic factors alone. One limitation of the figure is that a prolific community may have a vital index of more than 100 in the face of unhealthy conditions and many deaths, while the index of another and perhaps healthier community may be low merely because of small families or an older average age of the population.

An interesting rate not commonly used in most countries is the discratic index. It presents the relationship between the infant mortality rate and the mean age at death. It is considered a good measure of the state of well-being of a community since it takes into consideration both the tendency of death during the sensitive first year of life in relation to the total number born and the average length of life of the total dynamic population, which is necessarily influenced by all sanitary measures and preventable causes of death along each phase of life. The population under one year of age is subject to all of the conditions that tend to raise or lower the infant mortality. If the mean age at death is low, it indicates that diseases are destroying life in the younger age groups of childhood and early adulthood where preventive medicine and public health measures offer the greatest benefits up to the present

time. The discratic index is defined by de Shelley-Hernandez[18] as "the reflection of the sanitary condition of the community as seen through the observed relation between the mean age at death of the inhabitants and the force of infant mortality. It is obtained by dividing for a given year the coefficient in terms of 1,000 live births of the infant deaths, by the mean age at death or average duration of life of the inhabitants of the same community." For the practical application of this interesting and useful index, de Shelley-Hernandez has suggested the following standards:

Discratic index	Sanitary and health conditions
1	Very good
2	Good
3	Almost good
4	Almost bad
5	Bad
6	Very bad

Another type of statistical index of fundamental importance to health officers is the endemic index. This may be developed in several ways. If one wishes to compare the current frequency of a disease with some standard for the community in the recent past, the experience for several years might be averaged to obtain a mean. If for the previous 5 years the experience of each calendar week is averaged, there results a 5-year moving mean. If a disease demonstrates cyclicity, as does measles, an endemic and epidemic moving mean may be calculated and graphed for comparison with the current experience and for estimating to a certain limited degree the probable anticipated incidence. Similarly an endemic median and a 3-, 5-, or 7-year moving median may be obtained. Fig. 17-4 presents several charts of this type.

An increasingly important use of vital statistics is in connection with the allocation of federal funds to state health departments and of state funds to local health departments. Various aspects of this subject have been discussed in Chapter 8. It will suffice here to call attention to the bases upon which such grants-in-aid are made. Just as population serves as the basic factor in the computation of incidence and death rates, population or per capita data form the most significant single factor in the allocation of public health funds. Beyond this, many fiscal formulas include provisions for supplemental grants beyond the per capita grants based upon special problems. The existence of these is determined by morbidity data, prevalence rates, facilities available or needed, mortality, natality, and rate of population increase.

Statistical data are of further administrative importance in the sense that they provide a measure of the degree of compliance of local health departments with established standards and a means for the evaluation and comparison of the programs of health departments.

Elsewhere it has been stated that every progressive health department has a responsibility to accept research as one of its functions. The word research almost automatically makes one think of statistics. They are mutually interdependent. Unfortunately, too few official health departments on either the state or local level engage in special statistical research projects. The potentialities here are very great. To conduct such investigations obviously requires highly trained statistical personnel. When they are available and engaged by the health department, a problem arises as to their relationship with the rest of the personnel of the vital statistics unit. This logically calls attention to the question of the organization of statistical services in public health agencies.

ORGANIZATION OF STATISTICAL ACTIVITIES

In rural counties and small communities the local health officer is usually designated as the registrar of vital statistics. Ordinarily he in turn delegates this responsibility to some member of his office staff who, although seldom specifically trained, in some instances is referred to as a statistical clerk. This person acts as a sort of combination record clerk and clearing house for the reports that come to the health department. Certificates of birth and death are received, checked, transcribed, indexed, and filed. His analytic activities are usually confined to the compilation of simple tabulations for the annual report. He also receives the reports of cases of morbidity which are transmitted to the health officer or whatever person is responsible for their control. In connection with this, he often maintains files and registers of active and closed cases. In most instances he has no responsibility for the service and activity records of the health department personnel who usually take care of their own. Where systems such as the family or household folder are used, however, he is often put in charge. The general picture, therefore, is one of simplicity and almost informality, brought about by the combination of small staff, proximity to problems, and lack of statistically trained personnel and of funds to employ them.

When the public health departments of large cities and states are considered, one would expect to find a more or less uniform plan of statistical organization since the needs and problems are essentially similar in such situations. Interestingly enough this is not the case. From the viewpoint of organizational principles the statistical activities of these larger units are of two types: functional or line (in the sense of the routine collection, preservation, and transcription of vital statistical documents) and staff (in the sense of the activities related to studies, research, consultation, fiscal and program control). Herein lies the origin of most of the organizational problems and variations.

The patterns found on the state level may be used for purposes of illustration since data concerning them are conveniently available and since the state is ultimately responsible. An analysis by Swinney[19] has indicated five basic patterns of organization of state health department statistical activities: (1) no central statistical organization, (2) a division of vital statistics with some central statistical services, (3) a division of vital statistics with an independent central tabulating unit, (4) a central statistical division, with an independent division of vital records, (5) a central statistical division covering all registration and statistical activities.

In the 18 states in the first category the collection, preservation, and tabulation of the routine vital records was a function of a separate line division or bureau of vital statistics. Beyond this each major subdivision of the health department was individually responsible for all of its own record keeping, reporting, and statistical functions. Several unusual situations were found in this group. In Nevada the vital statistical and the personnel functions were merged. In South Dakota vital statistics and health education were in one division, whereas in Massachusetts vital statistics was the responsibility of the secretary of state, although a cooperative relationship with the State Health Department was maintained.

In the second category were 14 state health departments in which certain limited statistical services to other divisions were rendered by the line division or bureau of vital statistics. In most instances this had resulted from attempts at economy and efficiency by pooling all mechanical tabulating equipment and specialized statistical personnel. The usual pattern was for the functional divisions to collect and edit data and to plan tabulations. The vital statistics division then punched cards and tabulated the data, following which the completed tables were returned to the program divisions for analysis and release.

The 6 state health departments in the third category had what amounted to an adaptation of the foregoing in that they maintained a division of vital statistics and a central tabulating unit, which, however, were not united. The typical pattern here was a line division of vital statistics and a central tabulating unit as a staff agency in the division of administration.

Four state health departments had established independent units for statistical services in addition to line divisions responsible for vital records. Again as in the case of the third category, the central statistical service was organized as a staff agency responsible to the commissioner of health.

The difference, however, lay in the purpose of the central statistical unit. In this instance it had no routine administrative or operating responsibilities. Rather it existed to provide staff services and technical assistance to all parts of the department and to local health departments in the state. It served essentially for the purpose of "thinking the program through" and for planning, analysis, and interpretation. Needless to say, this necessitates highly qualified leadership and a well-trained staff.

The remaining 6 states, which formed the fifth category, had relatively recently centralized all statistical services in one unit. The pattern that was apparently emerging was to form subdivisions or sections dealing with vital records, tabulation, analysis and reports, and consultation service.

In connection with the analysis summarized above, Swinney found administrators divided into two groups with regard to centralization of statistical services. One group felt strongly that except for routine activities, such as vital records and tabulating, all statistical functions should be left in the various functional divisions. The primary reason given was the fear that centralization of statistical records and activities would detract from their adequacy and usefulness. The majority, however, felt that some form of centralized statistical unit was needed in large public health organizations to ensure efficiency, correlation of data and activities, and more profitable use of statistical personnel.

It is probably desirable that so much variation exists. Among other things variation indicates ingenuity and experimentation, two characteristics that continue to be greatly needed in this as well as many other fields of public health.

REFERENCES

1. Mattison, B. F.: The administrative value of statistics to a local health officer, Public Health Rep. **67:**747, Aug. 1952.
2. Kraus, A. S.: Efficient utilization of statistical activities in public health, Amer. J. Public Health **53:**1075, July 1963.
3. Aune, H. V.: The importance of vital records

in today's society, Public Health Rep. **74:**1029, Nov. 1959.

4. Shapiro, S., and Schachter, J.: Birth registration completeness, United States, 1950, Public Health Rep. **67:**513, June 1952.

5. Bailey, A. E.: Some recent trends in vital statistics registration practices, Amer. J. Public Health **38:**253, Feb. 1948.

6. International classification of diseases, injuries, and causes of death, Geneva, 1955, World Health Organization.

7. Mountin, J. W., and Flook, E.: Central states services affecting all branches of public health work, Public Health Rep. **58:**262, Feb. 12, 1943.

8. Ciocco, A., West, M. D., and Altenderfer, M. E.: State variation in the collection of reportable disease statistics, Amer. J. Public Health **36:**384, Apr. 1946.

9. West, M. D.: Morbidity reporting in local areas, Public Health Rep. **63:**329, March 12, 1948; and **63:**1187, Sept. 10, 1948.

10. Morbidity surveys—a symposium, Amer. J. Public Health **39:**737, June 1949.

11. Linder, F. E.: The national health survey, Science **127:**1275, May 30, 1958.

12. Langmuir, A. D.: The contribution of the survey method to epidemiology, Amer. J. Public Health **39:**747, June 1949.

13. Vital Statistics of the United States, Washington (issued annually), U. S. Government Printing Office.

14. Morbidity and Mortality Weekly Report, Washington (issued weekly), U. S. Government Printing Office.

15. Epidemiological and Vital Statistics Report, Geneva (issued monthly), World Health Organization.

16. Annual Epidemiological and Vital Statistics, Geneva (issued annually), World Health Organization.

17. Dunn, H. L.: Health and social statistics for the city, Amer. J. Public Health **37:**740, June, 1947.

18. de Shelley-Hernandez, R.: Statistics applied to biological science, Caracas, Venezuela, 1939, El Comercio, Ministerio de Hacienda.

19. Swinney, D. D.: Current organizational patterns of statistical activities in state health departments, Public Health Rep. **64:**621, May 20, 1949.

Chapter 31

Laboratory services

DEVELOPMENT OF PUBLIC HEALTH LABORATORIES

Early recognition was given to the important role played by laboratory procedures in the public health program. This may be attributed to the need for scientific guidance in an era rife with epidemic disease. It is not surprising, therefore, that most of the older public health laboratories owed their inception to some catastrophe such as an epidemic and that, generally speaking, they were developed in congested cities and towns before they became common on the state level. For example, the first municipal laboratory in the United States began operation in 1892 when New York City suffered a severe outbreak of cholera. At about the same time the first state laboratory was established in Michigan, followed by Rhode Island in 1894. Other state laboratories, however, were slow in their formation. This relatively early resort to laboratory procedure by health departments was perhaps more fortunate than is ordinarily realized. In a sense it established a philosophy or point of view and encouraged a constantly inquiring attitude. Without it many of our programs up to recent times would have been based upon sheer guesswork. The benefits that accrued from this relationship between laboratory and program were stated by William H. Welch[1] in the following terms:

The development of laboratories connected with boards of health is one which is peculiarly American. The appreciation of the need of such laboratories, of what can be accomplished by them and of the benefits which the general public derive from them, has been greater in this country than elsewhere. We have led in this particular direction. . . . The foundation of such laboratories has had

a very important stimulating influence upon boards of health, both local and state. It has introduced a scientific spirit into the work; it has brought into connection with executive officers the younger men who are full of enthusiasm with reference to studies along these lines, and I think that we may say that the general tone of boards of health has been elevated and stimulated by the foundation of laboratories of this character.

FUNCTIONS OF PUBLIC HEALTH LABORATORIES

Schaeffer[2] points to an unfortunate and contradictory phenomenon that has been occurring in laboratory science: "During an era of advancement in the biological and chemical sciences, research laboratories have flourished beyond expectation, but the service laboratories have not kept pace. This has occurred though physicians and health officers require more and greater varieties of services from clinical and public health laboratories." He explains that antibiotics have practically eliminated many infections, thereby leading to a false sense of security and largely eliminating the diagnostic microbiologic laboratory. In this respect he observes that "medical microbiology is almost a lost art and few medical bacteriologists are being trained to replace the rapidly dwindling handful of old ones." This is to be regretted and feared in view of the shrinking world, increased travel, and the concomitant risk of reintroduction of various communicable diseases.

On the other hand, although it is true that public health laboratories until recently have been primarily concerned with problems of sanitation and epidemiology, the scope of their potential role has been greatly broadened by the very changes that

568

have been occurring in society and public health in general. This is implied by the *American Journal of Public Health* in an editorial consideration of "Research and the Public Health"[3]:

As the problems of communicable disease have declined in urgency and scope in the United States, the community health program has been broadened to include, wherever feasible, other elements and situations that may adversely affect physical, social, and psychological well-being. The widening horizons of public health have in recent years come to focus on control of new aspects of the physical environment, chronic disease, and medical care. With our changing and expanding industrial technology have come environmental alterations of increasing complexity. The once dominant problems of bacterially contaminated air, water, and food have now been replaced in considerable degree by chemical pollution. The other major problem area concerns chronic disease and medical care or, more broadly, the area of personal health services.

Within the health department, the laboratory continues to serve as a guide and tool for each of the other activities. It furnishes the clue to the types and extensiveness of communicable and increasingly of noncommunicable disease problems. It not only indicates the effectiveness of the sanitation program but even provides the basis of design of engineering structures in that field. It is of great importance in certain phases of the maternal and infant health programs. In the final analysis it might be said with good reason that by itself laboratory service is of little value and that of necessity it must be used as an adjunct or in relation to other programs and activities. Beyond the component parts of the health department, although individual medical management is primarily the concern of the private practitioner, the modern public health laboratory finds it of utmost importance to assist him by ensuring, inasmuch as possible, the availability of essential aids to diagnosis, prevention, and treatment.

At the present time, therefore, the activities of at least the larger laboratories appear to fall into the following six categories:

1. Provision of facilities for physicians, hospitals, and health workers for the diagnosis, prevention, and management of disease

2. Establishment and maintenance of standards through chemical and bacteriologic examination of food, milk, water, streams, air, pharmaceuticals, narcotics, liquors, and other substances

3. Supervision, especially by state laboratories, of the practices, procedures, personnel, and products of local and private laboratories

4. Manufacture and/or distribution of sera, toxins, antitoxins, vaccines, and other biologic materials for diagnosis, prevention, and therapy; some state laboratories also determine standards of quality and potency of such substances

5. Training of technicians

6. Research

The following discussion is limited essentially to the larger laboratories located in major cities and particularly of state health departments, which, because of the populations they serve, are in a position or find it necessary to engage in a wide variety of activities. In a sense the laboratories of smaller communities that have limited facilities and resources may be considered subsidiaries or local outposts of the more extensive laboratories of larger governmental units.

All states assume responsibility for providing laboratory services at least for the diagnosis and control of communicable diseases. Ordinarily the spectrum of diseases for which such services are available is broad. Because of the number of specimens and because of state legislation pertaining to it, serologic tests for syphilis account for a significant proportion of the examinations performed by state public health laboratories. An additional reason is the inability of most laboratories in smaller jurisdictions to perform the tests and their tendency to transfer the responsibility to the larger state unit.

Because of the magnitude of the work and the customary responsibility of the state for supervision, most state health department laboratories carry on routine bacteriologic and chemical analyses of public supplies of drinking water. Private water supplies are usually tested upon special request by private citizens as well as physicians and public health workers. Frequently a fee is charged for this service. A charge for testing private water supplies is more common than for any other type of public health laboratory service; in fact, it is rare for any other charges to be made. In several instances state universities also make analyses of drinking water, either independently or cooperatively with the health department.

Interestingly facilities and procedures for the testing of food, milk, and drugs are much more varied than those relating to disease diagnosis and water examination. This is indicative of the differences of opinion, hence the complex patterns which have developed throughout the United States with regard to responsibility for surveillance over food, milk, and drugs. Although the state health department laboratories are most commonly charged with this responsibility, in 24 states, two or more agencies are involved. Most frequently the other agency is the department of agriculture, and in three instances it has exclusive jurisdiction over all aspects of milk and food laboratory control. In addition, in about a dozen instances independent state laboratories or laboratory departments, state chemists, agricultural experiment stations, livestock sanitary boards, state university laboratories, or boards of pharmacy analyze milk, foods, and drugs from standpoints of significance to public health.

Altogether 30 states have established facilities for the laboratory study and control of industrial dusts, gases, fumes, and other toxic substances to which workers may be exposed. In 25 of these the work is done by the public health laboratory; in 3 states the department of labor performs this function alone; and in the other 2 the departments of health and labor share responsibility.

At the present time one of the major functions of state health department laboratories is the distribution of biologics, pharmaceutics, and other materials for diagnosis, prevention, and therapy to local health departments and through them to hospitals and private physicians. About one half of the state laboratories manufacture at least a few of the materials they distribute. The most common are typhoid fever vaccine and silver nitrate solution for the prevention of ophthalmia neonatorum. Several states prepare rabies vaccine, diphtheria toxoid, and toxin for Schick tests. Other products occasionally manufactured in state laboratories include smallpox vaccine, diphtheria antitoxin, scarlet fever antitoxin, tuberculin, pneumonia serum, antimeningitis serum, and convalescent sera for measles, scarlet fever, and several other diseases. A few manufacture multiple antigens, particularly diphtheria-tetanus-pertussis combined antigens. In the past, several Southern states have distributed antimalarial and anthelmintic drugs.

Technical procedures, methods of transporting specimens, and reports of findings have been quite well standardized. Much of the credit for this is due the American Public Health Association, and particularly its laboratory section. This section is composed of a number of committees among which are those relating to diagnostic procedures and reagents, examination of water and sewage, examination of dairy products, analysis of frozen desserts, examination of shellfish, biology of laboratory animals, and biologic products. Each committee studies procedures and recommends those most practical for use by public health laboratories.

In the field of chronic diseases progressive public health laboratories are adding significantly to their technical armamentarium and providing an ever lengthening list of test procedures. The Clinitron, AutoAnalyzers, and similar equipment have made possible rapid, inexpensive, and broad-ranging test results. These devices have contributed greatly to the feasibility of mass screening and diagnostic programs against many chronic noncommunicable illnesses. With reference to the scope of procedures, many public health laboratories have long since performed blood grouping, blood sugars, and many now do blood cholesterols. Some already do certain other tests related to heart disease.[4] The Papanicolaou test is now commonly performed. Other laboratory procedures increasingly found include gastric acid in relation to asymptomatic cancer of the stomach, several tests for rheumatoid arthritis, and fluorescent antibody procedures as applied to rheumatic fever.[5] A few laboratories are already exploring the use of a variety of tests related to schizophrenia.[6] The public health laboratory has even become involved in genetics by virtue of tests of infants for phenylketonuria.[7] Similar biochemical tests for other genetic illnesses such as galactosemia are very apt to be added to the abilities of the public health laboratory.[8] The potential role of the laboratory in environmental health has already gone far beyond the simple tests of water, milk, and food. The greatly increased hazards of air pollution and ionizing radiation have presented the public health laboratory with great new challenges and opportunities.[9,10] Consideration has been given by Congress to the importance of this forward movement through the Community Health Services and Facilities Act of 1961. This act authorizes grants to improve and expand state laboratories and to provide training and education in the laboratory sciences.

The development of standard methods and the great increase in various legally required serologic tests have served to place responsibility upon state health department laboratories for the supervision and control of techniques used by local public and private laboratories. The origin of this role dates back about a half century when the Sanitary Code of the City of New York made the health department responsible for the supervision of clinical laboratories. Soon afterward, in 1925, the Code was amended again to establish qualifications of laboratory directors, to provide for examination of technical personnel, and to allow for inspection of laboratory premises. The laboratory of the health department was given the responsibility for enforcement.[2] The supervisory function of the public health laboratory is carried out by means of inspections, analyses in the state laboratory of duplicate test specimens from the local laboratory, licensing of local laboratories, and setting qualifications for and approval of locally employed laboratory personnel. One third of the states, for example, specifically require by law that laboratories performing serologic tests for syphilis be approved and periodically checked by the state laboratory. Nine states extend this supervision to include all types of diagnostic tests of public health significance. Increasingly, even in states with no such provisions for regulation, approval by state laboratories is being voluntarily sought by private laboratories as a mark of recognition. Unfortunately, however, in too many states there is neither licensing nor listing of the local private laboratories. In fact, a person totally untrained in laboratory science can often operate a clinical laboratory. As a result, large numbers of clinical laboratories operate without adequate or with only token supervision.[2] It is to be hoped that programs such as those made possible by the 1965 amendments to the Social Security legislation may by indirection influence this situation for the better.

No public health agency can remain progressive and effective without constantly seeking ways of improving its work, services, and methods. Although research is needed and possible in all phases of public health, one place where particularly fruitful investigations may be carried out is in the laboratory. An opportunity exists here both for pure laboratory research and for investigations carried on in conjunction with other functional divisions of the health department or other community or even national agencies. Thus the majority of large laboratories engage in special research projects in addition to their routine activities. Usually such investigations are engaged in either because of the development or discovery of a particular new problem or because of the personal interest of the laboratory worker or director. Occasionally special local funds are appropriated for particular research projects and special personnel are assigned or employed full time to carry them out. Increasingly, however, federal and private research funds are being placed at the disposal of the large, well-equipped and well-staffed public health laboratories. Frequently investigations are designed to improve currently used techniques or to compare them with new procedures. Much also has been done by public health laboratories in the development, testing, and production of new products and techniques. In addition, an increasing amount of pure research is being done. Of particular note are investigations concerned with diagnostic tests for cancer, diabetes, and fluorescent antibody techniques as well as with various aspects of influenza, rabies, pneumonia, diphtheria, pertussis, brucellosis, poliomyelitis, staphylococcic and streptococcic infections, and histoplasmosis.

LABORATORY ORGANIZATION

Despite the fact that the public health laboratory is essentially an auxiliary agency to augment the programs of the other units in the public health organization, one seldom finds it located organizationally in the manner theoretically recommended for auxiliary agencies. The practical reasons for this are the technical nature of the laboratory's activities and its frequently large size. With reference to size, in a number of states, notably Michigan, New York, California, and Massachusetts, the laboratory itself is of about the same magnitude in budget, physical size, and number of employees as the rest of the health department. The pattern, therefore, has been for the laboratories of state and large city health departments to be set up as major functional line units in the organization. Among the states only a few exceptions are found to this rule. In two states more than one bureau has laboratory functions; in one state the laboratory is in the bureau of local health services. In another it is an entirely independent agency.

The general lack of attention to the development of local laboratory facilities, because of their highly technical nature and cost, has tended to make them more or less centralized. Yet, having centralized all but the simplest procedures in the state health department laboratory, there is now a tendency toward decentralization. This usually takes the form of branch or regional counterparts of the state laboratory rather than returning to dependence upon small local laboratories.

More than half of the state health departments maintain branch laboratories at strategic points throughout their area. Usually such branch laboratories serve as localized points for the distribution of biologics and specimen equipment received from the central state laboratory and for the collection of specimens to be transmitted to the central laboratory. In addition, certain analyses that are within the competency of the local laboratory are performed there, whereas others are performed in the central laboratory for reasons of competency or efficiency.

A number of states make additional use of their supervisory authority by designating certain local public health and even private laboratories as branches or local agents. This procedure has much merit in that it encourages those laboratories to maintain their standards and stimulates others to improve theirs. A few states emphasize the development and use of local public health laboratories by subsidizing laboratories in local health departments. The subsidy may take the form of funds, personnel, or equipment.

In a few places, notably some rural counties of Maryland, the use of a joint hospital-health department laboratory has been found to be advantageous, since the additional financial resources allow the utilization of better trained personnel. Some small cities with more than one hospital have found it effective to have a single director administer the health department laboratory and the several hospital laboratories. This arrangement makes possible a well-integrated laboratory service and enables the community to obtain a director of higher caliber.

A similar problem that has occasionally arisen is concerned with the extent to which laboratory services should be centralized or decentralized within the structure of the health department itself. In the past it was not rare to find several divisions within a health department to have developed their own separate specialized laboratory service. Thus the division of communicable disease control might operate its own small laboratory in addition to the main laboratory, as might perhaps the venereal disease division, the sanitary engineering division, the food and milk division, and so on. The organization chart of State B (Fig. 10-4) provides an illustration. There are many objections to this. It involves the problem of vertical in contrast to horizontal organization and administration. The inefficiency, resulting from duplication of materials, equipment, and personnel, is obvious. It is difficult enough to find competent laboratory directors without multiplying the problem and usually settling for persons with less adequate qualifications and ability than are needed. Often the directors of the various units involved, such as engineering, have attempted personally to supervise the work of their laboratories. However, the proper direction of a laboratory is a specialized full-time responsibility and an engineer or epidemiologist rarely makes a good laboratory director. Furthermore, a multiplicity of smaller unit laboratories tends to divide the total work of the organization into tight little compartments, no one of which is aware of the others or how they might act to mutual benefit.

Three different arrangements therefore are possible: The first and by far the most desirable is the organization of a single central division or bureau of laboratory services, operating as a major unit of the health department and providing all laboratory services to all programs of the department. The second and least desirable is the operation of a series of smaller, specialized laboratories within each of a number of the functional units of the department. The third approach, which is a compromise and is sometimes made necessary out of deference to convenience, tradition, or personality, is maintenance of certain small departmental facilities for the performance of certain relatively simple procedures, in addition to a large central laboratory.

In Chapter 10, which dealt with the organizational aspects of public health, decentralization of programs and services, especially in larger cities, was discussed. Where programs are decentralized by means of health districts with district health centers, it is frequently useful to provide a small amount of space and personnel for the immediate on-the-spot performance of certain simple but important laboratory tests. The decision depends, of course, upon the nature of the programs being carried out in the district. Especially as public health agencies become more involved in programs of chronic noncommunicable disease and adult health maintenance, the provision of basic laboratory facilities in health centers will become more practical and necessary.

During recent years a number of states have experimented with the use of mobile laboratories as a substitute for or in addition to branch laboratories. Some have expressed doubt as to the usefulness of these laboratories and a few have discontinued them. It is possible that dissatisfaction might be attributed to failure to appreciate their essential purpose and therefore to use them improperly or inefficiently. Their use involves certain considerations. They should always be considered an adjunct to, rather than a substitute for, the central and branch laboratories. In this respect they should be under the technical and preferably under the administrative supervision of the central laboratory. Their effective function requires good working relationships between the staffs of the mobile laboratory, of the central laboratory, and of the local health department or local governmental officials. It is desirable that they be kept flexible in nature rather than geared for only one particular function or activity. In this way the mobile laboratory can be made to serve a multitude of purposes. In an age of good roads and rapid transit it would seem as if the mobile laboratory might occupy a significant place in the overall public health program, particularly in certain areas and for certain purposes. This is most apt to be true of emergencies, field epidemiologic investigations, stream pollution studies and control, resort sanitation, industrial hygiene activities, and some aspects of food and milk control.

The distribution of biologic products and the collection and transmission of biologic specimens require careful planning and timing on the part of the health department laboratory. Arrangements must be made for temporary storage and for prompt pick-up. Delivery and pick-up services for materials going to and from the state laboratory must be coordinated with the time schedules of public carriers such as railroad, air, and bus lines. Containers for specimens and for their safe shipment must be designed and distributed. Furthermore, provision must be made for 24-hour availability of certain products, particularly antitoxins and antisera, for use in cases of emergency. In small communities reliance is usually placed upon the cooperation and concern of the local health officer or pharmacist.

In large cities it has been possible for health departments to make very satisfactory arrangements for the provision of collection and distribution stations throughout their areas. Some are located in fire or police stations and others are in pharmacies where refrigerators are placed at the disposal of the health department. All large city health departments provide for their own messenger service for the collection of specimens and for the daily replenishment of supplies at the distribution stations. It is worthwhile to include report forms in or with the supplies made available, and many communities require that identifying data concerning cases be given at the time biologic materials are obtained from distribution stations.

REFERENCES

1. Welch, W. H.: Relations of laboratories to public health. (Lecture.)
2. Schaeffer, M.: Health department's role in improving operations of clinical laboratories, Public Health Rep. 81:71, Jan. 1966.
3. Editorial: Research and the public health, Amer. J. Public Health 57:1259, Aug. 1967.
4. Berliner, R. W., and Stewart, W. H.: The public health laboratory in the community control of heart diseases, Amer. J. Public Health 47:719, June 1957.
5. Chapman, A. L.: The chronic disease laboratory in public health, Public Health Rep. 73:1070, Dec. 1958.
6. Bachbinder, L., and Ferguson, A.: Does the public health laboratory have a role in mental health? Amer. J. Public Health 48:473, Apr. 1958.
7. Guthrie, R., and Susi, A.: A simple phenylalanine method for detecting phenylketonuria in large populations of newborn infants, Pediatrics 32:338, Sept. 1963.
8. Help from the biochemist, World Health, Aug.-Sept. 1966.
9. Hardy, A. V.: The public health laboratory—looking to the future, Amer. J. Public Health 50:927, July 1960.
10. Gilcreas, F. W., and Morgan, G. B.: The role of the public health laboratory in radiological science, Amer. J. Public Health 50:619, May 1960.

Chapter 32

Health education*

INTRODUCTION

That remarkable universal man of American history, Thomas Jefferson, once observed, "Health is no more than learning." In considering the important subject of health education the following statement is of interest:

The time has gone by when people can be dragooned into cleanliness, or be made virtuous by police regulations, and hence it is that the most thoughtful among practical reformers of the present day base their hopes of sanitary progress on the education of the masses as the real groundwork of national health. The people must be taught that good conduct, personal cleanliness, and the avoidance of all excesses, are the first principles of health, hand-in-hand in the rearing and guidance of youth. . . . They must be interested systematically in the general results of sanitary progress, and become more intimately acquainted with the social and material causes by which it is impeded.[2]

This quotation from the first report of the Maryland State Board of Health, dated 1875, emphasized that the public's health is dependent upon the public's convictions about health.

Health education in some form has always been an important activity of public health personnel. It was not until the second quarter of the century, however, that it became formally recognized as a specialty and as a major function in public health. The transition has been gradual. In the earlier eras of public health that focused upon the sanitation of the environment and the control of communicable disease, public health activity was interpreted to consist of doing things *to* and *for*

people, with reliance upon legal force whenever necessary. With the development of the newer interpretation of public health as the summation of personal health, there developed an appreciation of the need to do things *with* people and to get people to accept an increasing responsibility for their own health. This change in point of view was summarized by Governor Franklin Roosevelt in the foreword to "The Report on Public Health in New York State by the State Health Commission of 1931." He compared the report with that of 1913 as depicting ". . . the transition of the public health movement from the single problem of attaining mass health to the double task of maintaining mass health and controlling preventable disease in the individual.

"This is a more difficult task than that of establishing wholesale preventive measures in which the people themselves are not required to take an initiative. It involves the fullest use of public health education, so that citizens may understand and cooperative with activities necessary for their own welfare. Important as are the laws which the Commission has recommended, of far greater importance is intelligent action on the part of the individual and of the community."

DEVELOPMENT OF HEALTH EDUCATION

Chapter 12 includes a discussion of the development and role of the voluntary health movement in the United States. It was indicated that one of their earliest and continuing activities has been an attempt to improve the knowledge about,

---

*For a useful bibliographic guide, see Roberts, Grossman, and Griffiths: Amer. J. Public Health.[1]

hence action against, their respective disease interests on the part of the general public. Because of these early activities, priority in the field of health education may rightfully be assigned to the voluntary health agencies and especially to the antituberculosis societies. These set the pattern that was followed for about a third of a century—conscious involvement of large numbers of citizens as small contributors and/or as neighborhood volunteer workers, and the development of "impact" visual aids that depicted graphically and dramatically the medical and social consequences of the particular disease in question. Exhibits, leaflets, pamphlets, newspaper articles, health talks, lantern slides, children's parades, plays in schools, and many other imaginative techniques were used. As time passed, motion pictures, popular magazines, radio, and television were added.

In 1914 the New York City Health Department established the first bureau of health education as an official agency, followed promptly in the same year by a similar unit in the New York State Health Department. Over the years these two agencies have employed significant numbers of workers in various aspects of the field and have done outstanding work, especially in the use of mass media for popular and professional health education. Soon after the New York units were established, the Detroit Department of Health formed a separate organizational division of health education that pioneered in the development of neighborhood health groups, clubs, and guilds which intimately and effectively involved the targets of the health educational efforts, especially the socioeconomically disadvantaged, consisting for the most part of immigrants from Central Europe and both white and Negro transmigrants from the southern United States. Progress was by no means rapid; by 1929 health publications were being issued by only 52 city and 35 state health departments, and only a few had full-time directors of health education.

In the meantime, however, the field had received its specialty name, "health educa-

tion," at a conference called in 1919 by the Child Health Organization of America, which also offered the first fellowship in health education the following year. It is interesting to note that this organization was formed by a pediatrician, L. Emmett Holt, and a nurse, Sally Lucas Jean, both of whom were convinced that emphasis upon child health promotion through education and nutrition would accomplish much more than dogged, never-ending diagnosis and treatment of existing ills.[3] By 1922 there were sufficient numbers of people working in the field to merit the establishment of a separate specialty section in the American Public Health Association. However, retrogression set in and at the time that the United States became involved in World War II, a mere 13 state and local health departments reported employment of health educators (44 persons in all). Wartime needs spurred action, and special curricula were established in several of the accredited schools of public health. The rapidity of response was indicated by the fact that by 1947 over 300 persons, all of whom had completed graduate courses in recognized Schools of Public Health, were employed as health educators in official and voluntary health agencies. Concurrent was an important change in attitude on the part of health officers and other more traditional health workers from one of skepticism and suspicion to welcome and professional acceptance. This trend continued, and in 1951 the Society of Public Health Educators was formed. Also of historic significance was the formation in the same year of the International Union for Health Education of the Public.

As time passed, the philosophy, objectives, and methods of health education underwent significant change. This has been summarized by Rosen[4] as follows:

It has been recognized that it is not enough simply to present information; what counts is whether and how this knowledge is applied. Furthermore, it has been realized that the community is an organized structure, and that in health education, as in other health work, a coordinated program is needed that will touch each segment of the community in accordance with its nature and its needs. Finally, it is accepted in principle that when the members of a community have a chance to learn about their health problems and how they might deal with them, they will do so, but this was obscured during the early decades of the century by an excessive emphasis on tools and techniques.

NEEDS IN HEALTH EDUCATION

It is paradoxical that, despite extensive advances in literacy and education as well as vastly improved methods of communication, there still exists a great gap between existing medical and health protective knowledge and the public's acceptance and use of it. Professional journals are replete with reports of surveys of school children, college students, and the adult public that present discouraging and embarrassing evidence of failure in this field. Many parents still do not obtain immunization for their children, and many drivers still invite injury and death by drinking and driving and by not using seat belts. The use of cigarettes and patent medicines is still widespread. One of the handicaps of public health work, of course, is the usual absence of pain and urgency (except when an epidemic occurs). Indeed, this is becoming even more true as we progress from attacks upon communicable diseases to an attempted control of chronic illnesses. There is little difficulty in motivating to prompt action an individual with a high fever from typhoid or a severe abdominal pain from acute appendicitis. To bring about a change in dietary or behavioral habits or to secure health maintenance examinations against possible future difficulty is quite something else. Results are not so dramatic or rapid; cause and effect are not so readily apparent.

The clearly evident inadequacy and ineffectiveness of health education up to the present obviously calls for considerable evaluation and experimentation. Steps in this direction are already underway by the Society of Public Health Educators and the Public Health Education Section and the School Health Section of the American Public Health Association. The American School Health Association is similarly concerned, and it is hoped that this will become true of the National Education Association. Skillfully developed and properly used, health education can become a powerful force in social improvement and change. Its ultimate goal, of course, should be to encourage and assist the public in taking individual and group actions to protect and improve its own health.

A number of reasons have been put forward to explain the inferior status of health education at the present time[5]:

1. It is easier to sell symptomatic relief of illness or the promise of a cure than it is to sell health and prevention of disease.
2. Education is a catchall—a ready solution and means of disposition but one that is all too seldom put into action. Whenever there is a problem in a community, someone is sure to say, "The answer is education." And usually, that is where the problem rests.
3. Health education does not have high prestige. In the schools it is treated as a subordinate subject or as an additional chore to be passed out to a teacher whose main interest is not too remotely related. It is frequently made the responsibility of an athletic coach or physical training teacher.
4. In general, the people charged with health education programs lack special training and are not qualified.
5. Departments of education and health do not work together in programming, planning curricula, and raising standards of teaching health in the schools.
6. There is a lack of overall organization in the field of health education with a unified program and a single-minded objective. An effective and dynamic program of health education must include: intercommunication of ideas, selection of priorities, formulation of program, and assignment of responsibility. As matters stand now, there is a great deal of shifting of responsibility from school to home to church to community organization.

Beyond this it is self-evident that health education has been regarded too much in the past as private preserve by the professionals in public health, medicine, and education; to be perfectly honest, they have tended to be stuffy, overly didactic, and lacking in understanding of what really worries the average and less educated components of the population. This was forcefully brought out by an official of one of the most successful public relations and advertising companies in America in an address to a public health conference which he entitled "Public Health is no

Private Preserve (or things I never knew 'till now, no thanks to you)." This unusually well-educated man stated, "I was asked by your chairman to talk about selling public health. I, like most people, know very little about public health. I have no ready answers for your problems. I'm not even sure I understand the problems themselves. But I do know this: You are not communicating—you are not getting through to people. . . . I am amazed at the amount of effort, time, and money needed to safeguard my health and that of my family . . . yet the average citizen has no awareness of your efforts and actually impedes your work through ignorance."[6] The same concerns have also been voiced from within public health itself. Lifson[7] warns, "Health education is one of the subjects which sometimes has come under attack as a 'frill.' " Hoff[8] emphasizes the preconceived and rigid attitudes and interpretations of public health workers as a major obstacle.

Three conclusions appear obvious: (1) personal and community health education are fundamental to any public health advancement; (2) significant improvements are necessary in the field of personal and community health education; and (3) the major fault and challenge rests with the schools, health agencies, and the health professions, and far better joint planning and coordination of their efforts are necessary before the current sorry record is improved.

SCOPE OF HEALTH EDUCATION

The content and methodology of health education is peculiarly difficult to define. Many have tried, but it can be fairly said that all attempts seem to have something lacking or unstated. One problem is the variety of interpretations of intent and purpose of the field. Necessarily related to this are the different ways in which health educators are used by health officers and others to whom health educators report and upon whom they must depend for guidance and support. Still another problem is the variety of knowledge and techniques a competent health educator must

have in his armamentarium—pedagogy, public health, public relations, journalism, social science, and visual aids, to mention only some.

One of the best-known and still most applicable definitions of health education is one of the earliest. In 1926 Wood[9] described health education as the "sum of experiences which favorably influence habits, attitudes, and knowledge relating to individual, community, and racial health." The term "health education" usually gives consideration to at least five phases or types of activities: analysis, sensitization, publicity, education, and motivation. They are in no sense mutually exclusive, but tend to be sequential, overlap generously, and be dependent upon each other. The first, *analysis,* is of course fundamental. It involves a study of the problems of an area or a group, the factors that generated the problems and tend to maintain them, and the characteristics of the individuals or groups that may contribute to or hinder the application of sound knowledge or techniques toward the solution of the problems. The next phase is *sensitization.* Here the intent or expected result is not an addition to health knowledge per se or an evident change in the health habits of a person or a community; rather it is a process by which the individual and the community are made aware of the existence of certain things: a health department, a disease, a service. Sensitizing procedures such as slogans, spot announcements on radio or television, billboards, and the like are not expected to give the public more knowledge about a subject or to make them do something they otherwise might not do. The best examples are found in commercial advertising where a manufacturer merely attempts to make potential customers aware of the existence of his product in competition with those of other manufacturers. He may accomplish this by bombarding the public's eyes and ears, and, in some recent instances even the olfactory sense, with simple reminders of his product. The techniques used are manifold, and include everything from repetitive spot radio announcements urging one to eat "Oaties," to sky writing, huge billboards, and even the perfuming of newspaper advertisements. In doing this the manufacturer and his advertising agent do not expect the public to rush to the nearest store to purchase his product. What he does hope for is that when those who comprise the public are in a situation that requires them to make an immediate decision, "Shall I buy or not?" or "Shall I buy this brand or that?" they will choose the product the name of which is now familiar as a result of an almost subconscious sensitizing process. Therefore, when a health department by any of the audiovisual methods asks, "Is your baby protected against diphtheria?" or states, "Diphtheria kills children," it is merely sensitizing the listeners or readers so that they will be receptive to subsequent more detailed information.

The third phase of health education is *publicity*. This is closely related to the foregoing and, like it, is of considerable importance in the public relations program of the organization. In one sense, publicity might be considered an elaboration of sensitizing procedures, presenting more details about the items mentioned in the simple concise statements or exhortations. Examples of activities that might be included in this category are press releases that relate to the program of the health department, announcements of clinics available for various purposes, and statements about the seriousness of certain conditions in the community.

The fourth phase of health education is *education* in the more correct sense. In the final analysis this is really accomplished only in a rather intimate manner and involves personal contact between the one who imparts the information and those who receive it. It must be realized that education in health or in anything else is never something given by one person to another. The mere act of presenting information and knowledge accomplishes nothing. To use an extreme example, a gibbon might be exposed to the constant expostulations of the world's greatest philosophers, but it is doubtful that he would learn anything,

simply because of inability to absorb and interpret the sounds he hears. For a large segment of the human race the word inability may well be changed to unwillingness. In other words learning takes place only through the efforts of the learner. In order to impart information to increase the knowledge of others or to change concepts, personal discussions carried out in terms familiar to the listener and related to his personality and circumstances are required. Derryberry[10] has described a demonstration of the truth of this in the experience of the United States Government in selling war bonds: "The most extensive use possible was made of all known information media, including news articles, billboards, radio, exhibits, pamphlets, motion pictures, etc., in an effort to induce people to buy bonds, not only for financing the war but also for curbing inflation. When final tabulation was made, it was found that over 80% of individual purchases were made on personal solicitation, which shows the need for intimate and personal contact in order to induce overt action in a large proportion of the population."

A similar experience was observed in Detroit some years ago in connection with a program to control tuberculosis. Unusual publicity facilities were placed at the disposal of the health department. For weeks, generous front-page space and occasionally even headlines were made freely available for the purpose. News stories were written by one of the country's outstanding popular writers. Free radio time was provided for the presentation of excellent dramas, professionally prepared, produced, and enacted. The city was exposed to a profusion of posters, streetcar advertisements, pamphlets, and similar material. A significant special appropriation made possible the employment of a large number of additional public health nurses to engage primarily in home visits for the promotion of examinations for tuberculosis. After all this had gone on for a while, a study was conducted of those who responded to determine which approach prompted them to go to their physician or to a clinic for an examination. Despite the almost ideal publicity methods, it was found that the visits of the public health nurses and the backfence discussions between neighbors accounted for most of the positive responses.

The fifth or final phase of health education is concerned with *motivation*. The mere transmission of information or knowledge, even if it is accepted, is not enough, since in itself it does not necessarily imply action or a change in habit or conduct. Among those who die each year from preventable diseases are many who have been exposed to much publicity relating to them and have even acquired considerable knowledge about them. Only a fraction of the parents of children who needlessly acquire and even die from communicable disease are either ignorant of the availability of protective measures or opposed to them. In other words the acquisition of knowledge in itself is not an accomplishment; it is the extent to which that knowledge is translated into action that makes the difference.

Various aspects of this subject are discussed in Chapter 4, entitled "Social Science and Public Health." It is well recognized that, in order to motivate people to use health knowledge, it must be presented to them in a manner comprehensible and acceptable to them and which takes into consideration their basic emotional needs and wants, their cultural attitudes, beliefs, and prejudices, their fears, ambitions, jealousies, determinations, pride, malice or any combination of these.[11] Rosenstock[12] has summarized the problem well: "It is known that human behavior is determined more by one's belief about reality than by reality itself, and that people vary markedly in their interpretations of reality." As a consequence it has been pointed out that effective health education can be achieved only by linking what is taught to the endogenous motivation of the individual or group addressed. Whitehorn,[13] in seeking a working concept of human nature, has listed a basic set of motivational emotional needs and satisfactions that may be useful: (1) the desire for affection, (2) the desire for emotional security and trust, and (3) the desire for personal significance. He feels that since these sources of motivation are endogenous

or arise from within, educational efforts based upon them are more apt to strike a responsive chord and bring forth understanding and action.

In an interesting study of commercial advertising as a health education technique, inquiry was made with regard to the use of patent medicines. Of those interviewed, 60% said they used products of this nature before calling a physician. Although the majority recognized that the claims for the products were not substantiated, the investigation indicated that the patent medicines resorted to most frequently were those for which the advertising played upon emotions (especially fear), vanity, and desire for personal gain and which promised or implied unequivocal cure and relief. It is because of the foregoing considerations that the health educator is often referred to as a "catalyst," one of whose chief functions is the provision of learning situations, preferably based upon an understanding and adroit use of community organization.

PERSONNEL IN HEALTH EDUCATION

Everyone involved in or concerned with health in any way is a health educator. A long list of such persons could be produced. The most important, however, are all of the members of the health department staff, private practitioners of medicine, dentistry, and nursing, teachers, the personnel of many voluntary and community organizations, and, last but not least, parents. These are the people who in effect are on the "firing line" of health education. It is they who in their daily person-to-person contacts are responsible for the actual transmission of knowledge relating to health. In addition, as has been indicated in the section on the development of health education, in recent years there has developed a specialized worker, the health educator, who is trained to act as a combined stimulator, catalyst, correlator, coordinator, implementor, extender, and resource person for all of the potential abilities and activities of the entire staff of the health agency.[14] Beginning in 1943, training programs were set up in several of the schools of public health to provide training for this new type of personnel. Graduates of these curricula have been found increasingly useful by official and voluntary health agencies on all levels and in school health programs. Both the present actual and the potential demand for this new professional group is great, and it would appear that within a remarkably short period of time they have carved a definite niche for themselves in the health programs of the communities and states of the nation.

FUNCTIONS IN HEALTH EDUCATION

As in all other phases of the public health program, the functions in health education vary in the different levels of government. In its *Report on Educational Qualifications and Functions of Health Educators*[15] the Committee on Professional Education of the American Public Health Association listed the functions of the health educator on the community level in the following categories:

A. Program planning and evaluation
1. Study, survey, and research in assessing health education needs and possibilities
2. Analysis of present knowledge, interests, beliefs, and practices of the people in terms of aids or barriers to the educational process
B. Organization and promotion of health education activities
1. Development of groups for health action
2. Assistance in establishing and maintaining close cooperative working relationships between those agencies and groups of citizens which contribute to the health education of the public; in this the public health educator often serves as a liaison person among public, civic, professional, official, and voluntary organizations
3. Assistance in planning preservice education for public health, school, or other personnel
4. Stimulation, organization, or guidance of in-service education for employed personnel in health de-

partments, schools, or other agencies
5. Provision of technical assistance and service as a resource person in the development and guidance of health education programs in schools, parent-teacher associations, clubs, adult education services, extension services, study groups, and libraries
6. Assistance in interpreting the value of health activities to the community in the development of community interest and support
7. Leadership in the use of various educational teaching or group work procedures as applied to public health activities
C. Extension of health education through communication
1. Development, preparation, and use of mass media of communication
2. Establishment of health library facilities
3. Organization of a speaker's bureau, conferences, and meetings
4. Organization and operation of an information service

Functions in health education on the state level, by virtue of removal from the immediate scene of action, are similar in purpose and design to those of many other activities of a state health department. Derryberry[10] has suggested the following functions and activities in which a division of health education in a state health department might engage, depending upon the size of the state, its resources, the extent of its coverage with local health units, and the presence or absence of trained health educators in local areas:

1. Planning, developing, and administering a statewide program in public health education
2. Encouraging and promoting the development of programs in local health departments, utilizing trained personnel who are capable of working in all phases of the public health program and are also sufficiently competent in education to work with the schools

3. Recruiting personnel and arranging for their training and assignment
4. Assisting the medical, nursing, and sanitation personnel in their educational work by providing them with an educational mechanism and advice on effective techniques of education in various local situations
5. Consulting with local health departments and local health educators on all matters pertaining to health education
6. Maintaining relations with the press and the public, preparing articles and approving special stories and speeches by department personnel
7. Preparing or securing public health education material and distributing it through useful channels
8. Correlating the educational endeavors of the divisions or bureaus in the state health department
9. Coordinating the activities of all agencies in the state interested in health education
10. Developing and maintaining a continuing in-service program of training for public health personnel
11. Evaluating continually the materials and methods being used both in the state and in the local departments

Health education on the federal level has been a particular interest of the Public Health Service. Necessarily its attention is focused upon the national approach to problems and situations, and the encouragement of the state and, through them, local health agencies in activities in this field. Coffey[16] has presented the following particular responsibilities of the Public Health Service in health education:

1. To focus attention on health problems of national scope as they arise
2. To give consultation service and assistance in program planning and execution and in the preparation of materials when such assistance is requested
3. To stimulate the training of personnel and hold high the standards for their training and accomplishment
4. To serve as a clearing house for new ideas, methods, and materials
5. To summarize new developments in science and show its applicability to the subject matter of health education
6. To prepare high quality materials that have national application
7. To conduct an information service for the many inquiries received
8. To conduct research on methods and materials of health education and evaluate programs with the purpose of making all our efforts more effective

It is not the purpose of this book to discuss the many and various techniques in health education. Attention is called, however, to Chapter 16, which deals with public relations, much of which has a direct bearing on the subject of the moment. A few additional words are indicated to emphasize several general considerations. The term "community organization" is one of the most commonly encountered at the present time, especially in connection with health education programs. Its exact meaning often appears elusive to many. Perhaps the simplest manner of restating it would be to say, "Find out everything you can about your community, its inhabitants, interests, prejudices, facilities, subdivisions, and the like, and proceed to work through them." The first prerequisite to a sound health education program, and therefore a sound public health program, is a thoroughgoing community survey, diagnosis, or analysis. Every organized group and every influential person or agency must be noted with their particular interests and potentialities. They must be approached insofar as they represent segments of the population. The method of approach must be carefully considered.

One of the easiest mistakes that may be made is to speak a language foreign to that of one's listeners. Too many long, technical, and complicated words and phrases may be used. Public health workers have been taken severely to task in this respect.[17] One editorial statement is especially worthy of repetition and should be heeded by everyone who works in this field: "The use of jargon becomes a bad habit with public health workers. They come to depend upon it to confuse and mystify the public and to help create a favorable impression of their work. . . . But perhaps the main reason that public health workers use jargon is that it makes them feel important. It impresses the public and it adds to their own feeling of well-being to hear the long and musical words rolling from their lips. After all, it takes a pretty smart fellow to be able just to make the sounds, to say nothing of knowing what they mean and less of knowing how to translate them into appropriate and effective action."[18]

SCHOOL AND HEALTH DEPARTMENT RELATIONS

The school represents a most important learning situation for a large and significant group of the population. What is learned by a child tends to have a deep and lasting influence on his happiness, opinions, and behavior throughout his life. The child is reached and influenced primarily through two channels, his parents and his teachers. Unfortunately the influence of some parents, chiefly because of limitations in their childhood, is not always of the best. As a result the importance of the teacher in the development of desirable health knowledge and practices is doubly magnified and serves to emphasize the importance of teacher training in health and the maintenance of the personal well-being of those in this important relationship to children.

A certain amount of friction between public health agencies and departments of education seems to have resulted from their mutual interest in the development of health knowledge and instruction of children. It is strongly felt that no real cause for conflict exists. In some areas both the health department and the school department reach for the school health education program with airs of equal proprietorship. The fact is that it belongs to both of them, or more correctly, that both belong to it. Each organization has its place and its function. The personnel of health departments must always remember that

teaching is a professional specialty in itself and that in the final analysis it is the classroom teacher who does the teaching of the children. On the other hand, school personnel should bear in mind that the school health program and its educational component are merely parts of the larger total community health program. This does not necessarily imply a right for the official health department to usurp the activities of the schools in this field any more than this overall responsibility and concern entitles the health department to take over the private practice of medicine or the management of food industries. The need is obvious. What is indicated is the coordination, in friendly, professional, and cooperative terms, of the contributions and abilities of those interested in health education, whether employed in a health agency, a school system, or elsewhere. The important fact to consider at this point in time is that the job that needs to be done is very great, that neither group alone can accomplish it, and that neither group has been very successful so far. The conclusion is clear—greater resources, much better joint planning, and truly coordinated action.

Many communities employ a person referred to as a school health coordinator. Usually this person is on the staff of the school system, occasionally on the staff of health departments and sometimes employed jointly. There is an increasing tendency to require that they obtain training in a school of public health. Such professional persons in company with the health educator of the health department may accomplish wonders in the improvement of the program. Similar trends are observable on the state and federal levels, where joint planning committees and interagency consultations are frequent.

ORGANIZATION OF ACTIVITIES FOR HEALTH EDUCATION

Within public health departments the organization of activities for health education poses problems quite similar to those arising in relation to public health statistics. Although each functional unit of the agency should be engaged in health education to some degree, there are certain over-all aspects of the field that must be dealt with in a more central manner. The questions arise, therefore, whether the work should be completely centralized in one health education unit and whether such a unit should be a line or a staff agency. Every possible variation may be observed both in state and local health departments. Centralized health education units are organized sometimes as a separate line unit and sometimes as a staff agency in close proximity to the health officer. Not infrequently, on the other hand, all activities for health education are completely decentralized and dispersed throughout the various parts of the organization. Beyond these are numerous illogical arrangements, usually arising from expediency, wherein health education is placed in a division of vital statistics, of maternal and child health, or of communicable disease control. This has little to recommend it since it usually results in provincialization of the service.

Certain general conclusions may be drawn. It would seem manifestly impossible to centralize completely the activities for health education. Even if this could be accomplished, the rest of the health department would lose the major part of its effectiveness. Therefore, the functional units, augmented and supported by a central unit of health education staffed by specialists in that field, should be encouraged to engage freely in these activities. These persons, among other ways, should function as consultants and advisors to the line divisions of the agency. It would probably be best, in most circumstances, for the central health education unit to be a staff unit closely associated with the administrator, with whom overall community planning and programming may be effected.

REFERENCES

1. Roberts, B. J., Grossman, J., and Griffith, W.: The public health educator's bookshelf, Amer. J. Public Health 53:531, Apr. 1963.

2. Report of the Maryland State Board of Health, 1875 (courtesy Clemens W. Gaines, Executive Officer, 1965).

3. Rosen, G.: A history of public health, New York, 1958, MD Publications.

4. Rosen, G.: Evolving trends in health education, Canad. J. Public Health 52:499, Dec. 1961.

5. Health education: its present status, Report by the Committee on Public Health, New York Acad. of Medicine, Bull. N. Y. Acad. Med. 41: 1172, Nov. 1965.

6 Anderson, R. E.: Public health is no private preserve (or things I never knew 'till now, no thanks to you), Michigan's Health, May-June, 1965.

7. Lifson, S. S.: What's wrong with health education in the schools? Nat. Tuberc. Ass. Bull., Dec. 1965, p. 12.

8. Hoff, W.: Why health programs are not reaching the unresponsive in our communities, Public Health Rep. 81:654, July 1966.

9. Wood, T. D. In Fourth yearbook of the Department of Superintendent of the National Educational Association, Washington, 1926, National Education Association.

10. Derryberry, M.: The role of health education in a public health program, Public Health Rep. 62:1633, Nov. 1947.

11. Bauer, W. W.: What is health education? Amer. J. Public Health 37:641, June 1947.

12. Rosenstock, I. M., Derryberry, M., and Carriger B. K.: Why people fail to seek poliomyelitis vaccination, Public Health Rep. 74:98, Feb. 1959.

13. Whitehorn, J. C.: Motivating pattern of the normal individual. In Psychological dynamics of health education, New York, 1951, Columbia University Press.

14. Education for healthier living, currents in public health, Ross Laboratories Vol. 2, No. 7, July-Aug. 1962.

15. Committee on Professional Education: Educational qualifications and functions of health educators, Amer. J. Public Health 47:114, Jan. 1957.

16. Coffey, E. R.: Planning for health education in war and post-war periods—the national program, Public Health Rep. 59:904, July 1944.

17. Bross, I.: Prisoners of jargon, Amer. J. Public Health 54:918, June 1964.

18. Editorial: By his tongue shall ye know him, Amer. J. Public Health 38:264, Feb. 1948.

Chapter 33

Public health nursing

HISTORICAL DEVELOPMENT

Among the various professional persons engaged in public health work, one group, that of public health nurses, merits particular mention. Aside from the fact that a very large proportion of public health funds and positions is devoted to them, nurses are of special significance in that, considered as a group, they probably have closer personal contact with greater numbers of the public than does the rest of the professional staff of the health department. To many citizens the public health nurse represents the health department. It is she who reduces the work of the organization to its lowest common denominator—direct service to the individual in his home. As a matter of fact, many health departments owe their start to communities' having become sold on the value of the services rendered by one or two visiting nurses. One review[1] of the subject has stated it in this way:

> It is precisely in the field of the application of knowledge that the public health nurse has found her great opportunity and her greatest usefulness. In the nationwide campaigns for the early detection of cancer and mental disorders, for the elimination of venereal disease, for the training of new mothers and the teaching of the principles of hygiene to young and old; in short, in all measures for the prevention of disease and the raising of health standards, no agency is more valuable than the public health nurse.

William H. Welch stated the case more strongly by claiming that America's two greatest contributions to public health are the Panama Canal and the public health nurse.

The public health nursing movement owes its inception to William Rathbone of Liverpool, who in 1859 was impressed by the care and comfort given by a nurse to his fatally ill wife. Already a philanthropist, he promoted the establishment of a visiting nurse service for the sick poor of his city. It is somewhat surprising to find that, despite the enormous existing demand for therapeutic nursing of the sick, the first nurse, Mrs. Mary Robinson, was directed not only to give direct care to her patients but to instruct them and their families in the care of the sick, the maintenance of clean, tidy homes, and other matters that contribute to healthful living. As the previously mentioned review[1] stated:

> . . . This went far beyond mere nursing, and the work of the visiting nurse was thus bound up with and made part of a general health movement—the nurse herself becoming perforce a social worker as well as a nurse. And the highly constructive educational work all this involved put new life and vitality into the age-old charity of visiting the sick poor, gave it enormously increased importance, and brought about its later amazing development.

In order that qualified nurses would be available for the work, Rathbone enlisted the assistance of Florence Nightingale and established a training school in affiliation with the Royal Infirmary of Liverpool. Interestingly, Miss Nightingale from the beginning referred to the graduates who engaged in home visiting as "health nurses."

In 1877 in the United States, as in England, the first visiting nurses were employed by a voluntary agency, the Women's Branch of the New York City Mission. The idea soon spread to other communities. Meanwhile official health organization were being established, and it was only natural that eventually they recognized the unique contribution that nurses could make to their programs. At first, resort was made to the visiting nurses of the voluntary agencies. Thus the nurses of the New York City Mission carried out the orders of the school medical inspectors, visited the pupils' homes, instructed the mothers in general hygiene and infant care, and took sick children to the dispensary.[2]

The first visiting nursing associations per se were established in Buffalo in 1885 and in Boston and Philadelphia in 1886. Originally those of Buffalo and Philadelphia were named District Nursing Societies and that of Boston was referred to as the Boston Instructive District Nursing Association. Eventually all their names were changed to Visiting Nurse Associations. They depended upon lay contributions for their support, and small service charges where indicated. At the beginning, not only were they administratively under the direction of lay boards but the actual work of the nurses themselves was supervised by lay persons. Within a short time, however, the Philadelphia organization led the way by providing for a supervising nurse. It is interesting that each of these three early voluntary field nursing organizations is still active and influential in its respective community, and in Buffalo, until recently, the organization provided practically all of the public health nursing services for the official health department. The Philadelphia Visiting Nurse Society, as will be described subsequently, joined with the public health nursing staff of the health department in 1959.

With the expanding concept of public health, it was inevitable that nurses be employed directly by official health departments. The first city to do so was Los Angeles in 1898. The initial purpose was to provide visiting nursing care to the sick poor rather than to engage in educational or health promotional activities. The first official public health nurse, although paid with tax funds and responsible to the health officer, was assigned to the Los Angeles Settlement Association. As more nurses were added, however, there was es-

tablished in 1913 a bureau of municipal nursing in the health department. The first state to legally approve the employment of public health nurses by local boards of health was Alabama in 1907.

In earlier days of public health work it was easier to focus public attention upon special individual problems and to obtain public and private funds for their solution than it was to gain support for a broad general program. As a result most public health nursing programs were originally organized on a specialized basis; nurses were employed specifically as tuberculosis nurses, school nurses, maternal and child health nurses, communicable disease nurses, and, later, industrial nurses. This trend was given further strength by the activities of the National Tuberculosis Association, by the passage of the Sheppard-Towner Act, and by the growing interest of school officials in the health of the schoolchild. On the other hand, the demonstration of the value of county health units sponsored by the Public Health Service and the Rockefeller Foundation and of the Town and Country Nursing Service sponsored in many parts of the nation by the American National Red Cross indicated distinct advantages to the generalization of visiting nursing activities.

Over a number of years therefore one of the outstanding controversies in public health nursing administration centered around the question of specialization versus generalization of nursing services. It was argued, on the one hand, particularly by clinicians, that a nurse specially trained for tuberculosis work, for example, was equipped to render much more adequate care and service to the tuberculous patient than was a generalized nurse. Similarly, school administrators, wishing complete administrative control over the nurses working with school children, usually argued strongly for specialized school nurses. On the other hand, those favoring the generalization of nursing services had several strong arguments to put forth. One was that it was people and families who were served rather than diseases or physical situations. Furthermore it was pointed out that seldom does only one problem exist in a family, and that a specialized nurse was apt to close her eyes to all but one. A very practical objection to specialized nursing was the frequency with which a family with several health problems would be overwhelmed by the successive visits of a series of specialized nurses where a single, well-trained generalized public health nurse could cope with all situations that might arise. Eventually a concensus developed in favor of generalized public health nursing programs with but a few exceptions, e.g., industrial nursing and full-time specialized clinic activities.

THE SUPPLY OF NURSES

Nursing represents one of the greatest professional shortage areas in the health field. There are nearly 850,000 registered professional nurses in the United States. One problem is, however, that only about 530,000 are in active nursing practice and about one fourth of these are working only part time.[3] By mid-1966 the shortage of nurses in the nation was placed at 125,-000.[4] But there is still another part of the problem. Not only is the population growing but so is its expectancy for health services, including nursing. Furthermore, with the widespread coverage by health service insurance plans, Medicare, and similar programs, new sources of funds for such services have become available. By virtue of intensified recruitment, the provision of training stipends, and other devices, the number of nursing graduates significantly increased from about 34,000 in 1966 to 52,000 in 1967. In 1962 the Surgeon General's Consultant Group on Nursing actually called for 80,000 new admissions to nursing schools by 1966. However, projections into the next half decade indicate that no further increase is probable.[5] The situation is compounded by almost 1,000 vacancies on the faculties of nursing schools.

While the nursing shortage affects hospitals the most severely, other health service fields, including public health nursing, also suffer. Among the standards that have been developed throughout the years have been some dealing with the number of nurses needed in order to fulfill satisfactorily the needs of the average community. At the present time it is recommended that there be at least 1 public health nurse for each 5,000 people, and that, if bedside nursing services are included, the population base should be reduced to 2,500. Taken as a whole, the nation is still far below these minimal standards despite the great increase in the number of public health nurses. The figures available indicate a growth in the number of nurses employed in all types of public health work, except industry, from 130 in 1901 to 35,209 full-time and 2,214 part-time in 1964. Until the early 1920's the majority of field nurses were employed by voluntary agencies. Since that time the distribution has changed considerably, and the latest increase in total employment is due in large part to a gain in the number of nurses employed by local boards of education, where over the years the rise has been both constant and substantial. In contrast a steady and continuing decline is seen in the number of nurses employed both by health departments and visiting nursing societies in relation to population. Table 33-1 presents the numbers of public health nurses employed in 1964 in different types of agencies exclusive of industry.[6]

Indicative of the shortage that exists throughout the entire field of public health nursing is a comparison of those employed in local official agencies in 1964 with the minimum suggested in Emerson's report, *Local Health Units for the Nation*.[7] Table 33-1 shows that in 1964 there were 14,738 public health nurses employed full time in local health departments. This is little more than one half the number (26,390) recommended by Emerson in his report. It should be noted, furthermore, that this is despite the fact that at the time of Emerson's recommendations there were only 48 states with a population of 131,669,300, as compared to the present 50 states with about 200 million inhabitants. At the present time the national average is 1 nurse for every 12,-800 people. Very few states, most of them

Table 33-1. Nurses employed for public health work, by agencies, United States, Puerto Rico, the Virgin Islands, and Guam, January 1, 1964*

			Nurses					
			Full time			Part time		
				Supplemental			Supplemental	
Type of agency	Agencies	Total	P.H.N. duties	R.N.	L.P.N.	P.H.N. duties	R.N.	L.P.N.
Total	9,094	38,691	35,209	402	540	2,214	297	29
National agency	7	553	553					
State agency	94	1,082	1,024	25		20	12	1
Health department	54	872	831	25		10	6	
Other official	27	180	171			4	4	1
Nonofficial	13	30	22			6	2	
Local agency	8,993	37,056	33,632	377	540	2,194	285	28
Official	2,712	16,208	14,738	263	218	750	231	8
Visiting nurse association	682	4,580	3,826	46	225	448	21	14
Hospital based program	4	32	30			2		
Other nonofficial	132	361	303	4	11	40		3
Combination service	51	1,647	1,478	51	70	34	12	2
Board of education	5,412	14,228	13,257	13	16	920	21	1

*From Nurses in public health, Washington, Jan. 1964, Public Health Service Pub. No. 785 (revised).

in New England and along the Northeastern Seaboard, plus 1 or 2 western states, have a sufficient number of nurses to meet the standards of the American Public Health Association. It should be noted further that only about a third of those staff nurses working in public health nursing have received 1 year or more of academic training in public health nursing, although at supervisory level and above, a majority have had 1 or more academic years of public health training. To further illustrate the nursing personnel shortage, 1 out of every 20 budgeted positions for public health nurses in state and local health departments is currently vacant. Actually this figure is low since several states and large cities did not report and their nursing vacancies therefore were not included in the count. It is estimated that about 20,000 additional public health nurses are needed in the United States in order to meet minimum desirable standards. It is also estimated that by 1970 a total of 50,000 public health nurses will be needed. This is based upon the combination of 1 nurse per 5,000 population for local areas, the current ratio of administrative and supervisory person-

nel, the current number of nurses in state agencies, and an additional 1,500 nurses to assist in programs for the home care of the sick.[3]

Meanwhile some very significant steps have been taken during recent years to extend the effectiveness of public health nursing staffs by the training and use of a variety of auxiliary personnel.[8] Thus the increase in the number of practical nurses employed has been extraordinary—from 137,000 in 1950 to 250,000 in 1964. In the same interval, the number of approved training programs has tripled to about 900, with current graduates numbering about 35,000 each year. A similar increase has occurred in the on-the-job training and employment of other types of individuals who take some of the burden off fully qualified nurses. Thus between one half and three quarters of a million nursing aids, orderlies, and attendants will be employed in the nation's hospitals by 1970. In the community and in the home the public health nurse is receiving similar assistance; between 1950 and 1963 the number of home health aids and homemakers multiplied phenomenally, from

500 to 3,900. "In view of the health insurance provisions of Social Security [Medicare], it is expected that this category of supportive and personal care services into the home of the individual will expand even more in the decades ahead and their services will become increasingly integrated into the personal health care team."[5] Estimates of the number of individuals employed in the several categories mentioned at the beginning of 1966 are as follows[9]:

Professional nurses	621,000
Practical nurses	282,000
Aides, orderlies, attendants	500,000
Home health aids, homemakers	6,000

In addition, much of the burden of epidemiologic case finding and follow-up is being taken off the shoulders of the public health nurse by disease control investigators.

FIELD NURSING AGENCIES

In the evolution of community health programs, the contribution of nurses has been increasingly recognized on all levels.

National level

Generally speaking, field nurses today may be placed into two general categories —those employed by official health agencies primarily to carry out preventive and promotive health functions, and those engaged almost always by voluntary agencies primarily to render home nursing care to the sick. Despite some differences of opinion regarding terminology, it is convenient for our purposes to refer to the first group as public health nurses and to the second group as visiting nurses. It should be pointed out, however, that neither of these terms can be interpreted strictly. The functional differences between the two groups are becoming increasingly obscured. Both visiting nurses and public health nurses visit homes and perform what are considered public health functions. Furthermore there are many indications of a trend toward the inclusion of bedside nursing care of the sick in the functions of the publicly or officially employed field nurse. In other words the distinction between the two groups of nurses, if indeed a real distinc-

tion exists, depends merely upon the manner of their employment and compensation—in one case by government, in the other by a private yet publicly supported agency.

Two agencies of the federal government, i.e., the Public Health Service and the Children's Bureau, conduct activities in public health nursing. They operate essentially by providing grants-in-aid and consultation service to the states and through them to local health departments and by participating in the development of proper standards and qualifications. For a period of years the Office of Indian Affairs provided direct nursing service to its wards by means of public health field nurses stationed on the various reservations. In 1953 this activity was transferred to the Public Health Service. In general the work is the same as that performed by public health nurses employed in local health departments. Three nonofficial agencies that are active on the national level are the National League for Nursing, the American Nurses' Association, and the Town and Country Nursing Service of the American National Red Cross.

State level

By 1937 all of the states employed public health nurses in their state health organizations. The manner of their placement in the organization varies. The majority of state health departments have separate bureaus or divisions of public health nursing, while a few place it under maternal and child health, preventive medicine, or local health administration. Individual nurses may be assigned to functional units of the department by the nursing unit and in a few instances are employed directly by the specialized service. The functions and responsibilities of nurses in state health departments depend upon the legislative basis of the department. In the majority of instances they act as advisors to local health departments, boards of education, voluntary health agencies, and to other state agencies. In a few state health departments that have been given broader responsibilities and powers the nurses may actually supervise and administer certain direct services, local as well as state, and may have some inspectional powers such as are related to midwives, nurseries, baby boarding homes, nursing or convalescent homes, and hospitals. The latter function is becoming more important in relation to the Medicare portion of the 1965 Amendments to the Social Security legislation. Other important activities of state health department nurses include demonstrations of particular services or of total public health nursing programs and the conducting of in-service training courses.

All state health departments are active in the promotion of home public health nursing services for prenatal and postnatal patients, infants, and preschool children. In order to do so they function either through the direct assignment of state nurses to local areas, through emergency loan of state nurses to specially selected local communities, or through subsidy of local nursing programs. In recent years a number of state health departments, often in conjunction with philanthropic foundations, have experimented with the provision of nursing service for home deliveries.

Local level

On the local level nurses are employed by a number of different agencies. Outstanding, of course, is the official local health department, the nurses of which render direct personal service to individuals and families. In addition, many local boards of education employ special school nurses. Of a quasi-official nature is the nursing program of the American National Red Cross, which began in Ohio in 1912 and has since spread to many parts of the country, particularly in rural areas. From the beginning its policy has been to promote and assist in the establishment of local public health nursing programs and of full-time local health departments to which it eventually turns over its work. The American National Red Cross also played an important role in the promotion of public health nursing units in state health departments.

The majority of public health nurses employed in a nonofficial capacity are found in the many local visiting or voluntary nursing associations. These organizations are primarily concerned with bedside care of the sick. It should not be assumed, however, that their function is limited to this since the typical home visit includes much public health education and promotion as well as bedside nursing services. An important consideration in this respect is the fact that increasingly nurses of visiting nursing associations and of official health departments receive similar training and frequently interchange positions.

Two other groups that until recently provided visiting nursing services should be mentioned. Some of the larger insurance companies, particularly Metropolitan Life and John Hancock, for many years offered home nursing service to persons holding certain types of policies. The manner in which this was done varied, depending upon the size of communities, the number of policyholders, and the existence of other qualified nursing agencies in the community. In some areas nurses were employed directly by the insurance companies, while in others the service was purchased on a cost per visit or on a contract basis from local private nursing agencies. Another source of nursing service that has played an important role in some parts of the country is the large private industrial medical and health programs, many of which employ not only industrial clinic nurses but also nurses whose function it is to attend sick employees and sometimes members of their families in their homes. With the broadening scope of industrial hygiene and the interests of labor unions in health services, such programs often include health protection and promotion activities provided by industrial clinic and home visiting nurses.

Before leaving the subject of public health nursing agencies, reference should be made to the National Organization for Public Health Nursing. While it did not render direct service to the public, it played a dominant role in the advancement of this field. The NOPHN was organized in 1912 as the national professional society for those engaged or interested in this work and became recognized as the spokesman for the profession. No other single agency contributed so much to the improvement of educational and service standards and to the promotion of the public acceptance of and respect for the work of the public health nurse. By 1952, however, several other agencies had become concerned about the growing number of nursing agencies and the need for coordination. As a result, in that year the NOPHN joined the National League of Nursing Education and the Association of Collegiate Schools of Nursing to form the National League for Nursing. At the same time the bylaws of the American Nurses' Association were changed to provide for cooperation with the new National League for Nursing. Meanwhile the National Association of Colored Graduate Nurses also went out of existence and its functions were integrated into the other organizations. As a result there are now only three national nursing organizations: the American Nurses' Association, the National League for Nursing, and the American Association of Industrial Nurses.[10]

FUNCTIONS AND RESPONSIBILITIES

The following statement is accepted as the definition of public health nursing.

Public health nursing is a field of specialization within both professional nursing and the broad area of organized public health practice. It utilizes the philosophy, content, and methods of public health and the knowledges and skills of professional nursing. It is responsible for the provision of nursing service on a family centered basis for individuals and groups, at home, at work, at school, and in public health centers. Public health nursing interweaves its services with those of other health and allied workers and participates in the planning and implementation of community health programs.*

The statement of functions and qualifications for public health nurses, first prepared in 1931 by the Subcommittee on Functions of the National Organization for Public Health Nursing, has undergone several revisions. The most recent statements of functions and qualifications were prepared by a committee of the Public Health Nurses Section of the American Nurses' Association in 1964.[11] They represent the combined thinking of practitioners of public health nursing from every state and territory of the United States. These statements

*Statement presented and adopted at the National League for Nursing Biennial Convention, May 1959.

are grouped by classification and include functions, standards, and qualifications for public health nurses in staff positions; administrative, supervisory, and consultative positions are listed separately.

The following are the functions of public health nurses in staff positions employed by departments of health, boards of education, and voluntary agencies:

ASSESSING
Function I
Identifies present and potential needs and resources related to the health of individuals, families, and the community
- A. Uncovers health needs and problems through observation, interviews, analysis of records, and use of vital data
- B. Observes, explores, and evaluates the patient's physical and emotional condition, reaction to drugs or treatments
- C. Considers age, sex, culture, economic status, or geographic location that may influence the incidence or prevalence of health problems
- D. Recognizes attitudes that influence individual and community health
- E. Estimates the ability and readiness of individuals and families to recognize and meet their own health needs
- F. Identifies the availability and utilization of community resources
- G. Evaluates the urgency and complexity of the need in determining priority of action

Function II
Shares in identifying present and potential needs and resources related to the agency's program and the nurse's job responsibilities
- A. Appraises community health and social needs and resources for interpretation to administrative and planning groups
- B. Appraises the adequacy of public health nursing services in her district in relation to the community needs and the agency program
- C. Determines through her contacts with patients, families, members of related disciplines, and others, the extent of their knowledge of the agency's program
- D. Estimates the effectiveness of intra- and extra-agency communications
- E. Participates in the exploration and identification of her own needs in relation to the job

PLANNING
Function I
Plans for comprehensive nursing service to individuals and families in their homes
- A. Interprets nursing and other services of the agency to patients and families as a part of planning
- B. Plans with the individual, family, physician, and other concerned members of the health team for care which is appropriate

C. Plans with other individuals and agencies for continuity of patient care

Function II
Participates in planning for public health nursing service in special settings such as schools, places of employment, nursing homes and similar institutions, hospitals, clinics, and health conferences
A. Helps develop and arrange for public health nursing services in special settings
B. Develops plans for group teaching to meet the special needs of various groups

Function III
Contributes to planning for the development and operation of the public health agency
A. Contributes to the development of philosophy, purposes, policies, and procedures of the public health nursing services in the agency
B. Participates in planning nursing aspects of new and ongoing programs
C. Contributes to the preparation and revision of the nursing budget
D. Participates in planning the administrative procedures of the nursing office
E. Participates in planning continuing education programs for agency personnel

Function IV
Participates in planning with other agencies for community health programs
A. Advises or participates in community group planning related to nursing and health
B. Plans with professional organizations and civic groups for the improvement and advancement of the practice of nursing and public health

IMPLEMENTING
Function I
Helps provide comprehensive nursing service to individuals and families in their homes
A. Gives skilled care to patients requiring part-time professional nursing service and teaches and supervises the family and other members of the nursing team
B. Interprets extent and limitations of available nursing service
C. Gives preventive and therapeutic treatment under medical or dental direction, and teaches positive health measures
D. Utilizes her understanding of behavior patterns in giving nursing service
E. Initiates nursing measures to prevent complications and to minimize disabilities
F. Helps the individual and family to develop attitudes that permit them to make optimum use of available resources and health facilities
G. Helps the family accept and assume its responsibility for providing and arranging care, and guides it toward self-help
H. Helps the patient and family understand implications of the diagnosis and recommended

treatment consistent with their readiness and with the knowlege of the physician
I. Helps individuals and families to utilize their capabilities and make the best possible adjustment to their limitations
J. Helps individuals and families understand patterns of growth and development, and encourages attitudes and actions that will promote optimum health for each individual
K. Aids in effecting changes in the environment or in the organization of activities for the elimination or modification of health hazards
L. Communicates with other professional workers regarding the individual and family, and refers pertinent information to the appropriate agency
M. Participates in conferences with other disciplines to coordinate services and plan joint action
N. Assists the physician and dentist with examinations and treatments when nursing skills are required
O. Obtains laboratory specimens, performs diagnostic tests when indicated, and interprets the significance of the results to individuals and families when authorized
P. Participates in recruiting, training, and supervising volunteer workers
Q. Maintains necessary records and reports

Function II
Provides public health nursing service in special settings
A. Gives direct or consultative nursing services in such settings as schools, clinics, hospitals, or places of employment
B. Provides nursing service, on a demonstration or temporary basis, to convalescent and nursing homes and similar institutions
C. Carries out inspections of institutions when delegated by the licensing authority for the purpose of making nursing recommendations
D. Participates in the teaching of selected individuals and groups

Function III
Participates in the development and operation of the public health agency
A. Keeps the agency informed about changes in the community and in nursing practice which may have an effect on the program
B. Assists with orientation and guidance of new staff members, volunteers, citizen committees, and boards
C. Participates in the public information and promotion activities of the agency

Function IV
Participates in community health programs
A. Teaches basic principles of healthful living in relation to changing needs of individuals in all age groups
B. Provides for or encourages others in the community to provide for group instruction related to health

C. Represents the agency in her professional organizations and community groups when so designated

D. Interprets to the community the need for and meaning of health laws and regulations, and reports violations to the appropriate authority

E. Participates in community health surveys and epidemiologic studies, and other organized health programs

F. Interprets health and welfare needs to appropriate community groups

EVALUATING

Function I
Appraises performance
A. Evaluates the effectiveness of her nursing service to individuals and families
B. Evaluates the effectiveness of her service in health programs in special settings
C. Contributes to the evaluation of workers for whom she shares supervisory responsibility
D. Uses available help to study and evaluate her own job performance and plan for continuing professional growth

STUDYING AND RESEARCHING

Function I
Engages in surveys, studies, and research
A. Identifies problem areas related to her functions in assessing, planning, implementing, and evaluating
B. Participates in defining problems for study
C. Participates in the conduct of surveys, studies, and research related to her clinical and functional responsibilities

Function II
Applies pertinent research findings

QUALIFICATIONS OF PUBLIC HEALTH NURSES

The recommended qualifications for public health nurses in staff positions include:

A. **Licensure**
Holds a license to practice professional nursing in the state in which employed.

B. **Education**
Completion of a baccalaureate degree program approved by the National League for Nursing for public health nursing preparation or post-baccalaureate study which includes content approved by the National League for Nursing for public health nursing preparation. (It is essential that there be continued self-improvement through supervision, sharing in evaluation, utilization of educational opportunities such as staff education, workshops, institutes, self-directed reading, continuation of formal educa-

tion, and active participation in professional and related organizations.)

C. **Characteristics**
Abilities that contribute to the practice of public health nursing develop with experience and maturity. However, even at a beginner's level, each of the following qualities is required to some degree:
Willingness and ability to
1. Act with integrity
2. Understand and accept people with individual and cultural differences
3. Understand individual behavior
4. See and evaluate self in relation to others
5. Accept the public health nurse's role and interpret this role to others
6. Work with others toward a common goal
7. Adapt to the realities of a situation while adhering to fundamental principles
8. Gain satisfaction from helping others to help themselves
9. Use help from available sources
10. Maintain receptive and cooperative attitude toward change
11. Communicate effectively
12. Accept responsibility in professional and community activities
13. Observe desirable health practices

Qualifications for nurses in supervisory, administrative, and consultative positions require a master's degree with a major in administration, supervision, consultation, or in a special field, or a master's degree in public health from a school approved by the American Public Health Association.

ADMINISTRATIVE RELATIONSHIPS

An important administrative consideration influencing the value and efficiency of public health nursing programs is the nature of the relationships that exist among the various nursing and social agencies in the community, the public, and the members of other healing professions. The demand for public health nursing services is so great that if all available personnel in an area were employed in a single ideally efficient agency it would still be inadequate. This being true, it is important and necessary that agencies engaged in this work cooperate fully in order to correlate and coordinate their respective programs as much as possible for the maximum efficiency.

Relationships within the health department

The professional relationships of public health nurses take place in two areas: (1) within the health department itself, and (2) in contacts with other agencies and individuals in the community. Within the health department the relationship between the public health nursing staff and the administrative health officer is of paramount importance. All too often adequate and satisfactory relationships and understanding between the nursing staff and the health officer are falsely assumed to exist. It is not unknown for health officers merely to support the nursing program quantitatively according to standards such as 1 nurse per 5,000 population, but, once obtaining nursing personnel, to neglect to participate in the planning and administration of the public health nursing program and activities. Apparently some health officers, feeling that they know nothing about nursing problems, follow the path of least resistance by allowing the nursing division to proceed almost as if it were an independent agency. Inevitably this policy leads to difficulty both within and outside of the department. The health officer by virtue of his position is ultimately responsible for all phases of the health program of the department and, to a considerable extent, of the community as a whole. With respect to the nursing aspects of the program the health officer should carefully select a well-qualified director or supervisor, provide her with adequate administrative support, and see that general policies and interagency relationships are cleared at the top of the organization by him rather than perhaps haphazardly and inadequately lower down by his staff nurses and the staff workers of other agencies. He should maintain constant interest in the nursing program and endeavor to learn enough about it to assist the nurses to see how their activities really fit into the total community health picture. It is significant that within the past few years several of the schools of public health have established courses in public health nursing supervision and administration specifically for medical health officers.

Ross[12] has stated, "No division of nursing can rise above the level of performance set by its health officer and that no division of nursing will get far without his active and understanding support. The quality of the public health nursing program in official agencies country-wide is, in the last analysis, in the hands of health officers; if it is to become grade A only they can decide." In contrast with the foregoing are the occasional situations in which members of a nursing staff circumvent their nursing supervisor or director and approach the health officer with their problems and complaints. This practice should never be condoned for obvious administrative reasons. If permitted to come about and continue, it can result only in disastrous damage to the morale of the organization. Again it is up to the health officer and his nursing director to see that organizational channels are understood and followed by the staff nurses.

The public health nurse and the staff working in environmental health may on the surface seem unrelated. However, they are part of the same organization and should work in a helpful as well as cordial relationship. In the course of her daily field visits the alert public health nurse is certain to become aware of many insanitary situations. Often they have a direct or indirect bearing upon her own professional interests and activities. A policy of prompt and effective intra-agency referral should be developed to handle such situations. The same applies conversely to the engineer and sanitarian.

Relationships with other nursing agencies

One of the most important extra-agency relationships of public health nurses is with the staffs of other agencies that render nursing services in the community. In view of the necessity of maintaining desirable interagency relationships and of the considerable scarcity of nursing personnel at the present time, it is important that public health nursing functions be carefully analyzed in order to make the most efficient use of the time of those employed. One writer[13] has stated: "The discriminating review of our nursing functions which was forced upon us as a war expediency helped us to set up standards of priority in our home visiting programs which should continue to be of assistance to us in our present and future planning. However, this review also exposed the fact that the qualities of ready adaptability which have made public health nurses such a valuable adjunct to public health staffs have also resulted in wasteful use of our nurses' professional skills. We found that many of the time-consuming duties our nurses had carried did not require highly technical skill. However, they absorbed so much of the time of our well-prepared nurses that the teaching and other skills they had acquired were not utilized to the best advantage."

Among the sound recommendations that have recently been made and increasingly followed are those for the elimination of public health nurses in strictly clinical activities, the supervised use of nurses without public health training, practical nurses, nurse aids, community service assistants, neighborhood health workers, and lay volunteers for certain activities; and the elimination insofar as possible of strictly clerical activities of public health nurses by the employment of an adequate office staff and the constant scrutiny of record requirements. By such means the strictly public health nursing activities of many agencies may be increased considerably.

Consolidation of nursing services

There is little if any justification for more than two field nursing groups in any given community: (1) the public health nurses working as employees of the official health department and (2) the staff of the nonofficial visiting nursing association. Beyond this the trend has been to explore ways of effectively and equitably merging even these two groups. Regardless of the number involved, the correlation and coordination of the work of all agencies providing nursing services in a community

are obviously necessary and desirable in order best to serve the needs and interests of the public. Since there is no one answer to how this may be accomplished, each community must work out a solution best suited to its particular needs and backgrounds. The number and variety of possible arrangements in a given community may be somewhat as follows. If there are several voluntary or nonofficial agencies such as a visiting nursing association, cancer societies, tuberculosis societies, and industrial health organizations that render nursing services in the community, they may (1) remain completely independent of each other in an inefficient uncoordinated manner, (2) retain their individual identities but coordinate their programs by means of a central nursing advisory committee in which each agency participates, or (3) combine their programs to form a single community public health nursing agency. The voluntary agencies singly or united may limit their activities to bedside care, leaving most or all educational, promotional, and legal control measures to the nurses of the official health department. On the other hand, the health department may delegate some or even all of its public health nursing responsibilities to the voluntary nursing agency. In the few communities where this procedure is followed, it is usually attributable to two influences, i.e., the existence of a long-established, well-supported, and accepted visiting nursing association, and a weak official health department or one of relatively recent origin and tenuous support.

The completely satisfactory consolidation of community nursing services is as yet relatively rare, usually strongly resisted, and in some situations premature. One of the most successful solutions developed up to the present time is that effected in Seattle, Wash. The official and voluntary nursing agencies agreed upon a cooperative, completely generalized public health nursing program that includes all preventive, promotive, educational, and bedside services but retains the board of directors of the voluntary nursing agency as an advisory committee that controls its own contribution to the total cost of the program by means of an annual contract with the official health department. Where carefully prepared for and put into effect, this plan has worked well and has brought about an increased efficiency and economy, and both groups of nurses have found more professional job-appeal and stimulation from it.

In 1959, Philadelphia proceeded to merge its several field nursing services in still a different manner that appears to be quite successful and acceptable to all concerned.[14] There were three groups involved: (1) the nursing staff of the department of public health, (2) the nursing staff of the long-established and highly reputed Visiting Nurse Society of Philadelphia, and (3) the nursing staff of a smaller voluntary nursing agency restricted to one section of the city. After careful study and planning by representatives of all three agencies plus a number of additional unaffiliated citizens and consultants, it was decided that no one agency should absorb the others. Instead a completely new and distinct agency was established— the Community Nursing Services of Philadelphia. Each of the three existing agencies formally agreed to place at the disposal of the new organization all of its personnel and noncapital material resources. Each contributed a proportionate share of funds to employ an outstanding public health nursing administrator, her secretary, and part-time financial and legal assistance. These are literally the only direct employees of the new organization.

It was agreed that the sum of the nature and level of services of the respective cooperating agencies at the time of the merger would serve as the base line of activities, any addition to or subtraction from which would require concurrence by the Board of Directors of the new Community Nursing Services organization. This consists of individuals equally designated by the city government and the directors of the Visiting Nurse Society (which still continues its separate existence in order to own property, to accept gifts and contributions, and to receive monetary support from the United Fund). The Commissioner of

Health is an ex officio member of the Community Nursing Services' board of directors and the director of the department's Community Health Services routinely meets with the Board as a consultant and advisor.

As a first step a group of particularly well-suited and experienced nurses from all three agencies worked together in one district of the city for 1 year in order to find potential operational trouble spots, develop new policies, records, and the like. Meanwhile an extensive indoctrination and retraining program was begun on a phased basis with the remainder of the personnel. As each new group was ready to begin a merged operation in some additional district of the city, some of those who had already been working in the trial area were transferred to help get them started. The top administrative and consultative staff is housed in the Community Health Services headquarters building, and in all cases the Community Nursing Services' field nursing staffs are housed in district health centers with the respective multidisciplinary staff of the general health program.

Meanwhile a Medical Advisory Committee was established and began to function in connection with the many technical problems that continually arise in a nursing program. In addition, in order to maintain a balanced and up-to-date activity a program committee was established to review any suggested program changes of major import, to study community needs, and to make recommendations to the board of directors regarding any indicated policy and program changes. By agreement the director of Community Health Services is an ex officio member of the medical advisory committee and is chairman of the program committee. This assures a constant channel to and from the general health program of the community. To date, the organization and its program have been functioning well and smoothly, and there is reason to feel that the community is obtaining more and better service per nurse and per dollar expended. Probably the greatest virtue of this approach is that no one organization can feel that it was absorbed or swallowed by any other organization or group. To the contrary, the very structure connotes and requires cooperative action.

With reference to the joining or merger of nursing services, in 1946 The Association of State and Territorial Health Officers adopted as a general guide a resolution that included the following recommendations:

The community should adopt one of three patterns of organization that will provide the type of coordinated public health service most feasible under local conditions and that will best fit into the general plan advocated by the state department of health in each state. The organization patterns are:
  A. All public health nursing service, including care of the sick at home, administered and supported by the health department. This is the most satisfactory pattern for rural communities.
  B. Preventive services carried by the health department, with one voluntary agency working in close coordination with the health department, carrying responsibility for bedside nursing and some special fields. At present this type of organization is the most usual one in large cities.
  C. A combination service jointly administered and jointly financed by official and voluntary agencies with all field service rendered by a single group of public health nurses. Such a combination of services is especially desirable in smaller cities because it provides more and better service for each dollar expended.

Medical relationships

The nurse in public health work has traditionally served on the right hand of the physician. Therefore the relationship of the public health nurse with physicians practicing in her community has become of great importance. In most of her daily work the public health nurse repeatedly comes in contact with people who either are or should be under the care of a physician. She must always realize that private physicians as a group constitute the most powerful and most important weapon against ill health. Accordingly, the public health nurse, working in the field with families and individuals, must assume as one of her primary functions the interpretation of medical service in the community. She must act as a sort of implementor, seeking out those who need the care of physicians, helping them to obtain it, and assisting them in putting the advice of their physician into effect.

It is advantageous to a health department and particularly to its nursing staff that there be a medical advisory committee with which to discuss, clear, and implement matters of medical policy. The members of the committee should be appointed by the local medical society. Frequently the public health committee of the medical society serves the purpose adequately. A committee of this nature is particularly helpful in planning new projects or programs in which the public health nursing staff may be engaged. Another valuable service of the medical advisory committee is the formulation of written policies for the nurses of the health department. It is obviously of mutual benefit for the director of nurses as well as the health officer to meet with the medical advisory committee.

On entering a home, the public health nurse should whenever possible relate her visit to the wishes of the family physician. In order to do this successfully the astute public health nurse should acquaint herself with the wishes and policies of each physician in her area and constantly keep him apprised concerning the status of his patients. This she may do by means of personal interviews, telephone conversations, or written reports. Some agencies have a policy that the first contact with a physician must be through an interview or at least by phone. These policies are basic to good relationships and are appreciated by medical practitioners.

It is important that public health nurses observe professional ethics the same as they do in the hospital situation. In the typical community everyone who receives nursing care, particularly of a bedside nature, should be under medical supervision. Permission and instructions should be obtained from the attending physician beforehand in order to make the nursing services of greatest value, to maintain desirable patient-physician relationships, and to develop a feeling of professional partnership between the public health nurse and the private physician. Diagnoses and treatments must never be criticized or contradicted. If the nurse feels that she possesses information that might alter the medical management of the case, she should discuss it in a cordial, respectful manner with the medical attendant, but never with the patient or his family.

The selection of a physician should be the prerogative of the patient to be served. Frequently the nurse, and for that matter other health department employees, is asked to name an acceptable medical attendant. If possible no single physician should ever be suggested. The person making the request should be given the names and addresses of several capable and creditable practitioners, preferably from a list agreed upon by the local medical society. The complaint is sometimes heard that public health nurses take patients away from private physicians by referring them to health department and other free clinics. Unfortunately this claim occasionally may have been justified. The amount of the services for which private physicians are uncompensated is fairly common knowledge. Many prefer to maintain contact with their patients through poor times as well as good. This being true, in the interests of good professional relationship it is important that no such referral ever be made except after the signed release of the patient by his physician.

Community nursing council

Somewhat similar in nature and purpose to the medical advisory committee that has been previously recommended is a community nursing council. This advisory group should assist in studying, planning, improving, and coordinating all of the nursing activities in the community. Its membership is usually fairly large, including representatives from all official and nonofficial agencies that render nursing services, from organized professional groups such as medicine, dentistry, nursing, and social work, and from the public at large.

At the present time a great many communities have a council of social agencies, often in close affiliation with a community chest or fund. The council plays a most important role in the development of joint analyses, planning, and implementation by all of the many social agencies that exist in the typical community. It usually functions by means of a number of standing and ad hoc committees with representatives of various interested and pertinent agencies. The health committee, which is almost universally one of the standing committees, often has a subcommittee on public health nursing. Occasionally this subcommittee serves effectively in the absence of a community nursing council.

PUBLIC HEALTH NURSING AND SOCIAL WORK

The association of the official health nursing program with the other social agencies in the community brings out the fact that in a certain sense the public health nurse is essentially a specialized type of social worker. Her approach to individual and family problems, however, must of necessity be from a somewhat different basic point of view from that of the usual professional social case worker. Nevertheless, because of the complex nature of all social problems, of which illness and its prevention are one, mutual understanding and cooperation between the two groups is of great importance. The public health nurse should first be familiar with each of the social agencies in her community and second should know what each does, where its interests and contributions cut across, supplement, or complement those of the public health nursing program. She should have available for ready reference a directory or file indicating the interests, resources, location, and leadership of each one.

Usually the social welfare programs consist of six basic community services: child welfare services, family services, medical social services, psychiatric social work, public assistance, and recreation. Occasionally most or all of these are found in a single agency. However, the usual pattern is for a number of official and nonofficial agencies to be involved. Some of the types of programs in which they are variously concerned with administering are those dealing with aid to dependent children, the care of neglected and delinquent children, child guidance, mental hygiene clinics, old-age assistance, unemployment insurance, aid to the blind, vocational rehabilitation, and retirement.

One of the important practical reasons for familiarity with the social agencies of a community is for purposes of referral. A case of tuberculosis, for example, may appear to be primarily the concern of the health department through its public health nurse. However, problems of hospitalization and its costs, family support in the absence of the breadwinner, the placement of dependent children, and rehabilitation, to mention but a few, will usually arise. The public health nurse cannot solve all of these singlehandedly. She must therefore refer certain aspects of the total family problem, which has been crystalized by the appearance of tuberculosis, to other appropriate community resources.

Of great value to the nurse in such instances is the existence of a social service exchange. This is a clearing house wherein are registered identifying data regarding cases on the registers of the various community agencies. Its purpose is to enable all community agencies to serve the needs of the distressed individual or family more satisfactorily. The following types of patients or families should usually be registered by public health nurses: (1) those with pressing or complex social problems, (2) those to be referred to social agencies or other health agencies, (3) those having long-time health problems such as tuberculosis, (4) those receiving free services for which a charge is usually made, and (5) readmissions that were previously registered with the exchange. These patients or families are cleared again as a means of obtaining new data about them.

ADMINISTRATIVE AIDS IN PUBLIC HEALTH NURSING

As in other professional areas, public health nursing has found it practical to apply certain well-proved administrative aids.

Supervision

Unquestionably the most valuable administrative aid is the supervision provided at each level within a public health nursing agency. Supervision is necessary for the properly balanced development of the nursing service to public health programs and for the maintenance of its standards. Total responsibility for such supervision rests upon the nurse administrator and, depending upon the size of the agency, assistants and one or more supervisors. At the staff level supervision ensures the quality and quantity of the service through both administrative and educational processes. With a ratio of one supervisor to every six to eight staff nurses, it should be possible for the supervisor to offer sufficient guidance and counsel to the field or staff nurses in order to maintain the standard of the service offered and individually develop each staff nurse to the maximum of her ability to serve the patient and his family. The nursing supervisor is in fact also a liaison person who serves as a two-way link between the staff nurses and the administrative officers of the agency. The supervisor interprets policies and methods of application and may also transmit the impressions of the staff, together with suggestions for additions or changes in policies, to the administration centers of the agency. In this way it is possible for the field staff to play an important role in the formation or modification of policies and program.

Standard procedures

In any situation where a number of persons perform similar work toward a common purpose, it is desirable that they each follow the same procedures with regard to certain aspects of their work. In order to avoid misunderstanding and confusion, it is helpful, even in the smaller agencies, to have available a manual that sets forth clearly the policies of the agency and details of technical procedure. This should include statements of the exact responsibilities and authority of the personnel, standing orders used by the agency, and descriptions of techniques that are considered safe, effective, and ethically acceptable. While each agency will find it necessary to develop its own manual, attention is directed to the *Manual of Public Health Nursing*, which has been prepared and is periodically revised by the National League for Nursing (formerly the NOPHN). Many state health departments have also prepared excellent nursing manuals for use by local health departments. There also should be a record manual in which the purpose and proper use of each record used by the public health nursing staff is explained and illustrated. It must be remembered that as valuable as these administrative manuals are they quickly become useless unless continually kept up to date.

Clerical staff

Although much of the recording, particularly that relating to details of field visits, must of necessity be done by the nurses themselves, there is much clerical work that is most efficiently carried on by an office clerical staff. Despite this, it is by no means uncommon to find the professional nurses of many organizations devoting large proportions of their worktime to details of recordkeeping and analysis in the office. This is particularly unfortunate in the face of significant shortage in nursing personnel. The false reasoning appears to be prevalent that, as long as nurses must be employed in the public health nursing program, they might as well do all or most of the clerical work involved. It should always be realized that the records are also a necessary part of the program and that proper personnel for their handling is wholly justified. Furthermore, it is well to remember that the use of the relatively expensive time of a professionally trained public health nurse for office work, which may more efficiently and effectively be turned over to lesser trained employees in lower salary scales, is poor administration.

REFERENCES

1. Department of Philanthropic Information, Central Hanover Bank and Trust Co.: The public health nurse, New York, 1938, reprinted by the National Organization for Public Health Nursing.
2. Waters, Y.: Visiting nursing in the United States, New York, 1909, Charities Publication Committee.
3. Facts about nursing, New York, 1966, American Nurses' Association.
4. Stewart, W. H.: The challenge to nursing, Public Health Rep. **82:**92, Feb. 1967.
5. National Commission on Community Health Services: Health manpower, Washington, 1967, Public Affairs Press.
6. Nurses in public health, Washington, 1964, Public Health Service Pub. No. 785 (revised).
7. Emerson, H.: Local health units for the nation, New York, 1945, Commonwealth Fund.
8. Freeman, R., and Holmes, E.: Administration of public health services, Philadelphia, 1960, W. B. Saunders Co.
9. Health resources statistics, Washington, 1965, Public Health Service Pub. No. 1509.
10. New structure of nursing organizations, Public Health Rep. **67:**1258, Dec. 1952.
11. Functions and qualifications in the practice of public health nursing, New York, 1964, Public Health Nurses Section, American Nurses' Association.
12. Ross, G.: Is the health officer fulfilling his responsibility in relation to the nursing program? Amer. J. Public Health **29:**305, Apr. 1939.
13. Johnson, M. L.: Public health nursing administration in the changing order, Public Health Nurs. **39:**333, July 1947.
14. Wilson, D., Andrews, M., and Hall, M.: Community nursing services of Philadelphia, Nurs. Outlook **9:**612, Oct. 1961.

Chapter 34

Social services

INTRODUCTION

In the chapter on social pathology emphasis was given to the complex nature of the problems of people. All public health problems were shown to have components that involve economics, education, cultural attitudes, and many other factors. In the normal conduct of their activities public health workers must involve themselves to some degree in the solution of these other aspects of the problems with which they deal. Public health nurses have been particularly active and successful in this regard. However, it must be realized that the recognition and adequate handling of such problems and the dealing with certain types of individuals and agencies often require special training and skills with which the traditional professional public health worker has been only partially provided. It is only relatively recently that official public health agencies have realized the potential value and contribution of the social worker to the public health program.

Public health workers and social workers should understand and relate to each other with relative ease and to mutual advantage since both are concerned with the multifaceted problems of individuals and families. To be successful, both professions must be family and society oriented rather than merely individual oriented. Social case work, public health nursing, and in fact public health activities in general attempt to aid the individual or group to understand its problems, to rationalize, and to explain. As health workers become more involved in the implementation of recent health legislation, especially the Regional Medical Programs: Heart, Cancer, and Stroke Amendments of 1965 (P.L. 89-239); the Medicare, Medicaid, and Comprehensive Child Health Amendments of 1965 of the Social Security Law (P.L. 89-97); and the Comprehensive Health Planning and Public Health Service Amendments of 1966 (P.L. 87-749), a much broader viewpoint than has been followed in the past will be even more necessary.

Barnett[1] has stated the case clearly in a background paper prepared for the Third National Conference on Public Health Training:

If health is perceived to include more than medical or biologic entities, and is a by-product of social systems, then social work is intimately related to public health. Family planning, alcoholism, suicide and drug addiction are public health and social problems. The major social problems of today—juvenile delinquency, racial discrimination and violence, poverty, crime, child neglect, marital incompatibility and divorce, deterioration of the inner city and expanding suburbia relate to health and to welfare. These are social and health problems. These situations are crucial. In planning it is recognized that health and social problems are interrelated and have interwoven etiologies. Thus far, social problem intervention has been carried out through one social system and health problem intervention through another. There has not been consensus on social-health issues, problems, and decisions either by the people in need, the professional service groups, or the decision makers. Medicine, education, and social work are concerned with the individual, the family, and the community. They all have a concern for prevention, early casefinding and early mobilization of high quality care provided through a network of specialized services. The hitherto sharp lines of demarcation between institutional care and home care, physical disability and mental disability, health and welfare needs, are blurring. There is a general movement toward a more holistic interpretation and operational definition of the principles of primary, secondary, and tertiary prevention.

DEVELOPMENT OF THE FIELD

Social work in relation to health and medical programs had its beginnings early in the twentieth century when Dr. Richard Cabot and Ida Cannon introduced the concept at the Massachusetts General Hospital. They based their action on the philosophy that the patient's understanding and cooperation were needed to overcome illness, over and above anything the physician and the hospital might do. Furthermore, they recognized that there were many other factors involved in recovery, among them the family economy, the living conditions in the home and neighborhood, social relationships, and the like. They recognized also that there were usually available in the community numerous resources that might be tapped for the best ultimate solution of all aspects of the case, provided the physician had time to seek them out or if he had someone to do it for him and the patient. The success and spread of these ideas in medical and hospital practice are well known. Social work and its involvement in health and medical programs has progressed considerably as a profession since it was presented to hospitals as an economy measure to preclude giving free care to people who might be able to pay. From this it passed to a concern for assisting individuals with the social and economic problems that contributed to or arose out of their medical problems.[2] Today, as indicated by Silver and Stiber,[3] the emphasis is more on prevention, and the social worker's role in the health team is "to seek out potential sources of disaster that lie within the personality of individuals or family relationships, and attempt to modify the situation favorably." As they suggest, it may involve working with a child in a family rather than directly with his disturbed mother or with a husband rather than his sick wife. In other words the emphasis now is often on strengthening the supporting factors as much as on helping to treat the individual who is ill. Under such circumstances, however, the social worker is confronted with a difficult decision as to the most effective balance between the nature and extent of services to give to persons who already have

problems and need immediate help as against those who are in situations or groups that make them vulnerable to potentially harmful societal stresses.[4] In the latter role the emphasis must be on analysis, anticipation, and neutralization or at least diversion of the undesirable social forces.

PRESENT STATUS

At this time there are 70 schools of social work in the United States and Canada accredited by the Council on Social Work Education, with several additional schools seeking accreditation. The number of graduates increased from 1,772 in 1955 to 3,967 in 1966, and at the close of 1966 there were 10,365 students enrolled.[5] An estimated 5,800 social workers are engaged at general and allied special hospitals, and about 7,500 work in mental institutions.[6] Following the adoption of their services by hospitals, numerous voluntary health agencies began to employ social workers, and more recently, because of the increasing emphasis upon the social and community aspects of health as well as the trend to integrate preventive and promotive health activities with therapeutic medical care and rehabilitation, increasing numbers of official health agencies have been adding social workers to their staffs.

Despite this, the valuable adjunct of social work is still utilized only to a fraction of its potential by health agencies. Currently only one quarter of all hospitals in the United States have social services available in the hospital to the patients who need them.[7] By 1950 there were only slightly more than 400 positions for qualified social workers in health agencies in the United States, exclusive of positions in hospitals, clinics, and other medical care institutions. Most positions were on the staffs of official state and local health departments and of agencies concerned with crippled children or vocational rehabilitation services. Others were on the staffs of voluntary health agencies on national, state, and local levels. During the following decade from 1950 to 1960, there occurred only a 3% increase in employment of medical and psychiatric social workers by governmental noninstitutional health agencies and only a 1% increase by voluntary health agencies. A study[8] of 131 state and local health departments in 1961 showed a social work vacancy rate of 15.8% in contrast with an overall vacancy rate of 7.7%. Social work had the highest percentage of vacancies of any category in the health field. Ironically, despite the overall shortage of qualified personnel in this field, another study revealed that of all social workers with 2 years of training and a master's degree, 47% reported field instruction in either medical or psychiatric social work.[9] Between 1960 and 1965 the number who sought field instruction in a health setting increased by 9.3%. At present, health programs rank fourth in the 10 possible fields of social work practice among students and graduates.[5] It appears therefore that far more of the inadequate number of social workers wish to work in the health field than can find satisfactory employment in it. The social and legislative advances of the past few years are almost certain, however, to bring about a marked acceleration in the employment of social workers in the health field. This will be necessary in view of the increased emphasis upon comprehensiveness and continuity of care on a family and neighborhood basis, mental health programs, the health needs of the socioeconomically disadvantaged, aged dependents, and addictive diseases. It is difficult if indeed possible to estimate the number of social workers ultimately needed in health programs in view of the extremely labile and transitional nature of the current situation.[7] This very difficulty lends weight to Wittman's[10] comment, "There is an urgent need to capitalize on the current upsurge of interest in expansion of health services. . . . There will be high value in the achievement of more precise definitions of practice in public health social work and medical social work. An immediate task for public health social work is the exploration of the potential contributions of group work training and preparation in community organization in the health services. There should be more experimentation with com-

binations of practice methods which would seem to lend themselves in a better way to improved and extended health services."

ROLE OF THE SOCIAL WORKER IN PUBLIC HEALTH

The range of the social worker's activities in a health agency is necessarily determined by the size, scope, and changing purposes and priorities of the agency, the vision and understanding of its administration, and the availability of social work personnel. One basic question must be answered with respect to their function in a health department: What is the extent of direct service through personal contact with individuals in need of assistance, in contrast with working essentially through other members of the staff, especially the public health nursing staff? An ancillary factor here is the extent to which other members of the staff have been prepared to understand and accept the potential professional contribution of the social worker. In most instances in which social workers have been brought into programs of local health departments, many individual and family contacts were initially anticipated and emphasized. Repeatedly, however, it has been found that the most efficient and fruitful use of the limited number of social workers and of their time is as staff consultants, fellow program planners, and as liaisons with the many other pertinent community agencies.[11-14]

The increased need for and employment of social workers in public health programs led to the establishment in the Committee on Professional Education of the American Public Health Association of a subcommittee on Educational Qualifications of Social Workers in Public Health Programs. This subcommittee, in collaboration with the American Association of Medical Social Workers, not only developed a series of sound qualifications for the different levels of social work in health agencies but also produced the following excellent statement of social work functions in health and medical programs[15]:

1. **Social work consultation services.** Consultation is a major responsibility of social workers

in public health. It is often available on any aspect of the health department's program. More commonly it is related to the social problems of an individual or family, to problems met by other agencies, to social needs within the community, to coordination of the services of the health department with other community services, to agency administration, and to program and policy development within the department. Depending on the situation, the social worker may provide consultation service alone or as a member of an interprofessional team, as in evaluation of particular aspects of a community or institutional program.

2. **Program planning, implementation, and policy formulation.** Social workers in public health usually have responsibility for participating in program planning and policy development in the agency. On the basis of their professional equipment and the cumulative evidence from day-to-day activity, they are generally in a position to know how policies affect individuals or groups, or what standards and programs need to be strengthened, modified, or developed.

Social workers participate, with other personnel, in the development of joint projects; in the stimulation of activity on problems which fall within the jurisdiction of the health agency; and in the determination of program priorities. As a member of an interprofessional staff, social workers have the added responsibility of conferring with and advising health officers and program chiefs and supervisors in other professional areas on appropriate matters, or help in determining the most satisfactory solutions to social problems.

In most health agencies, administrative and supervisory responsibilities for the social work services are assigned to one person, who is often designated chief social worker, director of social work, or chief social work program consultant.

In some instances, primarily in mental health agencies, social workers carry out the major administrative responsibility for development of the total program of the agency.

3. **Social work services to individuals and families, social case work.** Social case work in public health involves social study and evaluation leading to services for individuals or families who are having difficulty in social functioning, primarily as it affects their health and their ability to use health services. The problems may be those "which impinge upon the family unit or individual from the social or physical environment" or those "which the individual brings into being, in whole or in part, by modes of behavior and interaction between himself and other persons and situations." Individuals or families needing social case work may be brought to the attention of

the social case worker by the members of the health team, by other agencies, by the individual or family, or they may belong to a group already identified, needing social case work on the basis of diagnosis or the type of situation. Persons within selected categories may be routinely referred for the purpose of identifying social factors which affect the individual's health problems or his use of needed health and medical services. The social worker initiates case work services in instances where resolution of social and emotional problems helps to prevent problems or facilitates care. Collaboration with other professional staff is an essential part of the case work process.

Social case work service may be provided temporarily for the purposes of demonstration, in order to develop methods of effective referrals to appropriate agencies, or to facilitate more comprehensive study and treatment by the health agency.

Opportunity for direct case work services is most often provided in local agencies, less frequently in state programs, and least often in programs at the national level.

4. **Social work services to groups.** Increased use of the group process in resolving social problems is a definite trend in social work in public health. The social worker in public health may act as leader of groups of patients or family members, or as a consultant or resource person to groups or to their leaders. This group process may be used by social workers with patients in a single diagnostic category, with relatives of patients who have the same health problem, or with other groups where there is a health need.

Social group workers, especially trained in social group work methods, have been used more frequently in hospitals and mental health programs than in other public health programs, although the opportunities in all are apparent.

5. **Social work services to the community.** All members of the public health team contribute to the provision of community services. In public health, the social worker places a major emphasis on this activity, in which he applies his social work knowledge of individuals, groups, and communities and of community process, his understanding of social welfare as a social institution, and his knowledge of social work organization to the task of community planning.

The social worker in public health is in a strategic position to identify, evaluate, and document social problem, relating to health needs, to discover ways of preventing them, and to plan new services or to strengthen those already in existence. He serves also as an interpreter of social resources to other team members and of health services to social agencies. He thus assists in improving collaboration and in coordination of programs for health and social welfare, and in modifying or developing services to meet new needs.

Social workers especially trained in the social work method of community organization have been used more often in voluntary health programs than in public health departments.

6. **Research, studies, and surveys.** Research is carried on by social workers, both independently and in collaboration with other professions in public health, mental health, and medical care programs.

7. **Educational responsibilities.** The social worker is responsible for the supervision of social work students assigned to the agency for field instruction. He also participates in the preparation of students from other professions with respect to promoting an understanding of the social and health needs of individuals, groups, and communities, and ways of preventing and meeting these needs. He contributes to and benefits from the educational program of the health agency by participation in programs of staff education within the agency and in the community.

As a conclusion, attention should be drawn to a timely statement by Wittman.[10] "The social work profession is only one of several concerned with means for the prevention and treatment of disease and disability in this country. It should make every effort to take its place beside the others in a concerted attack on problems of ill health."

REFERENCES

1. Barnett, E. M.: Social work training needs. Background paper prepared for Third National Conference on Public Health Training, Washington, Aug. 1967.
2. Goldstine, D., editor: Readings in the theory and practice of medical social work, Chicago, 1954, University of Chicago Press.
3. Silver, G., and Stiber, C.: The social worker and the physician, J. Med. Educ. **32**:324, May, 1957.
4. Rice, E. P.: Concepts of prevention as applied to the practice of social work, Amer. J. Public Health **52**:266, Feb. 1962.
5. Annual statistics on social work education, 1966-67, New York, Council on Social Work Education.
6. Selected characteristics of social workers, mental health manpower, Current Statistical and Activities Report, No. 6, Public Health Service, May 1965.
7. Closing the gap in social work manpower. Task Force Report on Social Work Education and Manpower, Washington, 1965, Department of Health, Education, and Welfare.
8. Hill, E. L., and Kramer, L. M.: Training for service and leadership in the health professions, Department of Health, Education, and Welfare Indicators, Aug. 1964.
9. Salaries and working conditions of social welfare manpower in 1960, New York, 1961, National Social Welfare Assembly, Inc.
10. Wittman, M.: Social work manpower in the health services, Amer. J. Public Health **55**:393, Mar. 1965.
11. Spielholz, J. B., and Brakel, I. V.: The medical social worker in a county health department, Amer. J. Public Health **37**:733, June 1947.
12. French, W. J., and Wiser, G.: The use of the medical social service by a county health department, Amer. J. Public Health **38**:1555, Nov. 1948.
13. Grant, M.: Social service in a health department, Amer. J. Public Health **43**:1545, Dec. 1953.
14. Haselgrove, M.: The social worker in public health, Quart. Bull. Dept. Pub. Health of South Australia **97**:35, Jan. 1956.
15. Educational qualifications of social workers in public health programs, Amer. J. Public Health, **52**:317, Feb. 1962.

Chapter 35

Nutrition services

FOOD AND THE HEALTH OF NATIONS

In a dissertation written in 1851 on the subject "Food and the Development of Man,"[1] Otto Ule stated as follows:

Of all the influences which determine the life of the individual, and on which his weal and woe depend, undoubtedly the nature of his food is one of the weightiest. Every one has for himself experienced how not only the strength of his muscles, but also the course of his thought and his whole mental tone, is affected by the nature of his food. . . . The foods we use must contain the indispensable elements of nutrition in due proportion; our food must be mixed, varied, and alternating. And what is here said with regard to individuals, holds good also for nations. The foodstuffs of an energetic population are up to the standard only when they are multifariously blended, and when there is a due proportion of substances belonging to the three groups mentioned above.* Now, this relation between the nutrition and the physical and the mental development of people must be apparent in the history of their civilization. Where the food is insufficient, fluctuating between want and excess, uniform and undiversified, the capacity of the people for work must be inferior; their bodily strength and their mental culture must be of a low grade.

The importance of nutrition on a national scale was probably fully realized for the first time in this country as a result of the White House Conference on Child Health called in 1930 by President Hoover. Although not at first anticipated, nutrition loomed as a factor of predominant concern, not only because of its specific importance but especially because of its relationship to so many other circumstances related to the well-being of children. Shortly thereafter, the League of Nations began what was called a world food movement in an attempt to remedy the dire nutritional difficulties of so much of the world population which resulted from the economic depression. It emphasized the importance of adequate diets to health and suggested that agriculture by supplying the necessary foods to the world could overcome the depression not only for itself but for the many industries related to it. Under the League's auspices many studies of the relation of nutrition to the health of various groups were carried out. Two specific results were the formulation of the first table of optimum dietary standards and the organization of national nutrition committees in about 20 countries. Boudreau[2] states, "It was the belief of many that had this movement been started early enough the train of events leading to the Second World War might have been halted." Few things cause discontent as much as hunger, especially in the midst of plenty.

Most of the fruits of war are bitter. Let us consider some of its better fruits. Much has been heard during recent years of the use of food as a weapon. The idea is not new. Captains of war recognized early the relationship between food and conquest. All would-be conquerors, from Caesar to Napoleon and Hitler, had as one of their fundamental military precepts that an army travels on its stomach and saw to it that their soldiers received the best food available. The use of siege as a means of subjugation is so old as to be obscure in its origin. The cutting off of the supply of food was, of course, its chief purpose. The technique is continued in modern times in the form of embargoes, blockades, and mine fields. Once conquest was effected, the im-

---

*The three groups the author mentioned are blood-formers or albuminates, heat-producers or respiratory foods rich in carbon, and the nutritive salts.

portance of food did not diminish; if any-thing, it increased. The Roman soldier has been described as entering conquered lands carrying sacks of flour on the point of his lance. To keep the conquered peoples con-tented, their Roman rulers gave them bread and circuses. In this connection it is inter-esting to note the position of bakers in the Roman state. During the Roman Empire bakers were considered as persons impor-tant to the welfare of the nation and were made civil servants, licensed and paid by a department of food supply. It might be asked why a state such as Rome, which was anything but socialistic, followed such a nu-tritional policy. Undoubtedly it was because in the period of the Roman Imperium bread had become a political factor of enor-mous importance. A sufficient supply of bread meant social peace; lack of it implied hunger and bloody revolution.

During World War II food was used as a weapon as usual but this time as a defen-sive weapon as well as for offense. The story of the stupendous efforts of the Allied Na-tions to produce not only more food than ever but also food of a better quality in the face of many difficulties is too well known to justify retelling. Not so well real-ized, however, is the effect of this effort on the general health and well-being of the countries involved. Taken as a whole, it is entirely justifiable to state that not only did the millions of young men and women who were in uniform get better meals than they otherwise would have obtained, but also the civilians benefited enormously from an educational standpoint and from the substitution of nutritionally more desirable foods for those which were scarce and less beneficial. The effects of this are sure to be far-reaching and, it is hoped, long-last-ing.[3,4]

Dr. Frank G. Boudreau, Executive Direc-tor of the Milbank Memorial Fund and his co-chairman on the Food and Nutrition Board of the National Research Council, Dr. Russell M. Wilder,[5] have given some in-dications of these effects:

It is perhaps too early to appraise the contribu-tion of workers in nutrition to the winning of this war, but some credit undoutedly is due them for the fact that the country has come out of the war with unusually good health reports. Infant mortality has continued its decline despite the war, and in contrast to the usual experience in war. Deaths from tuberculosis have not increased as they always did before in war; indeed a new all-time low record has been obtained. The figures for maternal mor-tality are better than they were before the war, and the same is true for virtually all death rates which reflect in any way the influence of diet on the pub-lic health. We might be less assured of the contribu-tion of nutrition to these better records were it not that in Great Britain the fall in these rates has been even more pronounced, and over there all environ-mental factors except nutrition were worsened by the war.

The situation in Great Britain was sum-marized by Dr. H. E. Magee,[6] Consultant in Nutrition to the British Ministry of Health, in a paper published in the *British Medical Journal* in March 1946:

The war-time food policy was the first large-scale application of the science of nutrition to the population of the United Kingdom . . . . A diet more than ever before in conformity with physi-ological requirements became available to everyone, irrespective of income.

The other environmental factors which might in-fluence the public health had, on the whole, deteri-orated under the stress of war. The public health far from deteriorating, was maintained and even in many respects improved. The rates of infantile, neo-natal mortality, and the still-birth rate reached the lowest levels ever. The incidence of anemia declined, the growth-rate and the condition of the teeth of school children were improved, and the general state of nutrition of the population as a whole was up to or above prewar standards. We are therefore entitled to conclude that the new knowledge of nu-trition can be applied to communities with the ex-pectation that concrete benefit to their state of well-being will result.

This was supported by Sir William Jame-son,[7] Chief Medical Officer to the Ministry of Health of England and Wales, who said, "This can't be just an accident. All that's been done to safeguard mothers and chil-dren must have had some effect—such things as the national milk scheme, vitamin sup-plements for mothers and children, the great extension of schemes for school meals and milk in schools. There are doubtless other factors—full employment and higher purchasing power in many families, espe-cially in the old depressed areas; as well as the careful planning from a nutritional point of view of the restricted amount of

food available for the nation." His conclusion was that "nutrition is the very essence and basis of national health."

NUTRITION IN THE WORLD COMMUNITY

A measure of the importance of food to
people other than its value in times of
strife is the proportion of the productive resources that is devoted to providing it. The
figure is always considerable, varying from
about 37% of the total productive resources
of the United States to about 90% in
China. It depends on many factors such as
wealth, social constitution, the nature of the
soil, the national economy, industrialization, scientific development, and transportation. Of great importance are habits, customs, and education. "Food does more than
satisfy hunger and provide pleasure, it also
helps man to reach his genetic potential.
The health and well-being of the people
of the world now and in the future depend
upon how efficiently man develops, protects,
and uses his food supply. Unfortunately
the gap between the world's population
and its food supply is widening; therefore
every person now alive has a responsibility
to make good use of today's food supply to prevent further widening of this
gap."[8]

It is difficult to determine the exact number of people in the world who are underfed, but the fragmentary evidence available
indicates that more than 1 billion people
are not receiving enough food to carry out
useful, productive lives.[9] The most vulnerable group to suffer from malnutrition consists of young children under the age of
4 years. Their malnourished state, complicated by disease, may lead to death. "It
is estimated that 350 million children or
70% of the world population under six are
stunted by protein-calorie malnutrition."[10]
Relatively minor infectious diseases like
measles, whooping cough, or chickenpox
often become fatal. The protein-calorie deficiency is known by different names around
the world where diets are habitually poor;
in South America it is *culebrilla,* in Africa
kwashiorkor. The United Nations, recognizing protein-calorie malnutrition as a
major world public health problem, has
charged three agencies—FAO, WHO, and
UNICEF—to aid in solving the dilemma.

With the great advances in the science of
nutrition it may seem a strange paradox
that so much malnutrition still exists, but
it must be realized that there is always a
great lag between research and interpretation to the masses. In the field of nutrition
there is not only a lag in interpretation but
also in human resistance. Food has been
said to represent the crossroads of emotion,
religion, tradition, and habit—and food
habits usually are changed very slowly. In
addition to ignorance, prejudice, and poverty, however, agricultural practices and
economic policies also play their part in the
total picture of malnutrition. World leaders
are beginning to realize that people are ra-
tioned by economic status and agricultural
practices as well as by an understanding of
their needs. Food intakes often reflect external circumstances rather than the fundamental needs, and some of these external
circumstances are man made and can be
man controlled.

Significant steps have been taken to avoid
a repetition of the failure to control some
of these man-made external circumstances
following World War I. At the United Nations Conference on Food and Agriculture,
held in Hot Springs, Va., May 18 to June
3, 1943, 44 nations agreed to work together
to secure a lasting peace through freedom
from want. In the records of this conference[11] the bearing of nutrition on human
health was well stated in four short sentences:

1. The kind of diet which man requires for
   health has been established.
2. Investigations in many parts of the world
   have shown that the diets consumed by the
   greater part of mankind are nutritionally unsatisfactory.
3. Diets which do not conform with the principles of satisfactory nutrition lead to impaired physical development, ill health and
   untimely death.
4. Through diet a new level of health can be
   attained, enabling mankind to develop inherited capacities to the fullest extent.*

---

*Consumption levels and requirements, United Na-
tions Conference on Food and Agriculture, Final
Act and Section Reports, Appendix 1, Report of Section 1.

In planning the United Nations organization one of the earliest considerations was the establishment of the Food and Agriculture Organization as one of the specialized agencies of the United Nations. The meeting of the Preparatory Commission held in Washington from October 28, 1946 to January 24, 1947 was attended by representatives of 17 nations: Australia, Belgium, Brazil, Canada, China, Cuba, Czechoslovakia, Denmark, Egypt, France, India, Netherlands, Philippine Republic, Poland, United Kingdom, and the United States of America, with Thailand present in discussions concerning rice. Russia and Argentina were invited to send representatives; the latter sent observers. Other international organizations represented included the International Bank for Reconstruction and Development, the International Labor Office, the International Monetary Fund, the United Nations Economic and Social Council, and the World Health Organization.

The Food and Agriculture Organization recognized the following challenges:

1. How to expand the total food production of the world
2. How to increase buying power so people who are now poor and underfed can buy the additional foods they need to maintain health
3. How to improve distribution between nations, so farm prices will be stable, and so starvation and surpluses will not exist side by side

The organization felt that responsibility rested with national governments and that the functions of the international organizations might consist of research, supplying information and consultation, encouraging cooperation, and assistance in making farming more efficient with the result that many farm workers in the less developed nations might transfer to small industries. It also hopes to play a part in the stabilization of agricultural prices as a step toward reaching a balance between production and consumption. A conference such as this would not have been held even 25 years earlier because the relation of nutrition to the health, peace, and happiness of the world had only recently been recognized. Of the member governments, 104 are now members of the Food and Agriculture Organization, and representatives of these governments meet annually to review the world situation in food and agriculture, forestry and fishery, to discuss common problems, and to agree on common action. Representatives of 18 governments comprise a smaller council and act between the annual sessions on the decisions made by the Conference.

What can be expected for the future of these international efforts? The possibilities were well expressed by Sir John Boyd Orr,[12] once Director General of the FAO:

> I feel confident that both the highly industrialized countries and the underdeveloped countries will realize that cooperation in making this new machinery work is in their own interests . . . and that they will cooperate wholeheartedly. . . . In that case, we can look ahead to a happier future in which there will be food for the people, prosperity for agriculture, and an expansion of world trade, all of which are absolutely essential for a permanent peace.

In 1962 the Food and Agriculture Organization (FAO) and the United Nations created a 3-year World Food Program. It had two advantages: (1) its multilateral sponsorship precluded any accusation of political or economic intent, and (2) nations other than the United States could contribute surplus supplies and personnel to it. The World Food Program has been extended for another 3 years.[11] The Food for Peace Programs have three general goals: (1) to obtain higher protein foods for distribution, (2) enrichment and fortification of available foods, (3) formulated food development. "A formulated food is a single food which can serve either as a beverage or a gruel, or perhaps even in bread—a food which includes all nutrients a child requires."

The United States in an effort to support the United Nations FAO program passed P.L. 480. The following summarizes some of the main points of this law,[13] which was effective between 1954 and 1962:

TITLE I: Millions of tons of food have been shipped to foreign ports, paid for in local currencies and then the currencies made available to the recipient nation as aid to local developmental projects.

TITLE II: Some 60 countries received food grants

until 1962 valued at about $800 million. These were government-to-government grants. Foods were made available through the Food and Agriculture Organization of the U.N.

TITLE III: Foods were made available to needy countries through the intermediary of UNICEF and non-profit voluntary relief agencies such as CARE and religious groups. Most foods under this title have been used for child feeding.

TITLE IV: Includes a barter program under which, by 1962, about $1.5 billion of supplies had been exported.

TITLE V: Provides foods on long-term dollar credit.

Many world powers and philanthropic organizations have contributed to easing the critical food shortage in the underdeveloped countries in a variety of ways, by supplying fertilizer, technical aid, and surplus foods.

THE DETERMINANTS OF DIET

With all the cooperation among agencies, countries, and individual scientists, many practical problems remain to be solved by education, by agricultural and industrial production, by better food sanitation procedures, and by proper food storage.[14] One of the most difficult problems relates to the eating customs and habits to which a people are accustomed. Reeducation in this regard usually is very difficult. Even to list the factors which decide the nature of the diet of an individual or of a community or nation is a formidable task. They may however be placed within a relatively few categories. Adapting from Margaret Mead,[15] they might be said to depend on six types of influences: (1) physiologic needs, (2) social organization, (3) advances in food technology, (4) economic resources and cost, (5) attributes of food, and (6) psychologic attitudes. Merrill[16] has compressed these in indicating that we must remain cognizant of the factors that influence food intakes. He grouped them into four headings: geographic factors, biotic factors, economic factors, and cultural factors.

"Men eat," he says, "not only what the soil and the climate allow them to eat, not only what the saleability and desirability of the products they grow allow them to purchase from their neighbors, but essentially they eat what they saw their parents and grandparents eat before them."

Physiologic needs are affected by at least two types of desires: the wish to avoid the discomfort of hunger and the desire for health and vigor. For most people the former is probably the factor of predominant concern. The extent to which the feeling of hunger is produced varies to a considerable degree with the energy expenditure, which is influenced by hundreds of such diverse factors as the extent of industrial and agricultural mechanization, indoor and outdoor temperatures, recreation, and methods of earning a living.

With regard to the physical attributes of foods and psychologic attitudes toward them it is obvious that different foods have different characteristics which may tend to make them pleasant or unpleasant, desirable or undesirable, practical or impractical to the individual. Among these are flavor, odor, texture, color, form, temperature, nutritive value, cleanliness, and perishability. It would be a rare person indeed who could honestly deny having some food habits based on such factors. This, of course, is closely interrelated to the question of psychologic attitudes toward food. Some foods are shunned for fear that they might be fattening, poor mixers, or what not. Some foods are identified with low social or economic status (example: corned beef and cabbage); others are identified with affluence (example: lobster). Certain foods are symbols of hospitality, for example, wines, and in some circles, ice cream. Of common knowledge is the relationship between certain foods and religion. It is not without significance that every known religion has rules relating to some foods.

Because of some and in spite of other factors influencing dietary habits and customs, some rather remarkable changes have taken place in the types and amounts of foods consumed by the American public during the past half century and particulary during the war years. The most outstanding changes have been steady increases in the consumption of dairy products, citrus fruits and juices, and leafy, green and yellow vegetables. Steady downward trends occurred in the consumption of potatoes, grain products, and some fruits.

Such changes in food consumption have

naturally had an effect on the intake of the various specific nutrients. Surprisingly enough the number of calories has remained more or less constant, except for a short drop during and after World War I and during 1935, a year of both economic depression and drought. While the use of potatoes and cereals has declined, the increase in use of fats, oils, and sugar has made up the otherwise lost calories. Per capita intake of protein decreased steadily from 1909 to 1933. It increased sharply in 1934 because the drought in that year necessitated slaughtering of many animals for lack of pasture and feed. As a result the amount of protein available in 1935 was the lowest for the entire period 1909 to 1945. Since then the figure has increased until now it is equal to the 1909 figure. The recent increase, however, is due in part to increased consumption of milk and eggs as well as the return to normal of the use of meat, poultry, and fish.

The greatly increased use of dairy products has resulted in marked increases in calcium and riboflavin. The bread and flour enrichment program also contributed to the riboflavin increase as it did to the increase in thiamine, niacin, and iron. The latter decreased with the decrease in consumption of meats and grain products. Some return was occurring, however, with increases in meat consumption when the enrichment program went into effect, causing an increase of 15%. With the greatly increased use of leafy, green and yellow vegetables, a marked increase in the amount of vitamin A available has taken place. A similar change in the amount of ascorbic acid has resulted from the increased consumption of tomatoes and citrus fruits.

Taken as a whole, although the situation preceding World War II tended to be somewhat unfavorable, the changes in the food habits of the American public in the more recent past seem definitely encouraging with significant increases in most of the essential nutrients, coupled with a continuing awareness of "excess baggage," partly based on increased appreciation of the relationship between obesity and cardiac ailments.

PUBLIC HEALTH NUTRITION IN THE UNITED STATES

Recent changes in our social organization have had far-reaching effects on our national food habits. It is conceivable that the process of Americanization involving the intermarriage of many nationalities results in considerable interchange of dietary customs, ideas, and habits. Increased travel enables individuals to experience many new types of foods and cooking. Of course, the one social change which has had the most far-reaching effect has been the shift of our civilization from an agrarian way of life to an industrialized, urban existence. This has resulted in a considerable shift away not only from the production of food at home but also from eating at home with the development of school lunches, the workingman's lunch box, restaurants, cafés, drugstore lunch counters, and drive-ins. Eating at home often tends to promote a habitual and limited choice of food whereas eating in groups outside causes a trend toward greater variety, interest, and choice. However, it must be remembered that steam tables often provide food of impaired vitamin content.

Many of the food problems caused by our urbanization have eventually been met to an amazing degree by developments in the field of food technology which have played a dominant role in recent changes in our food habits. Rolling daily on our railroads are thousands of refrigerator cars, possibly one of our civilization's most significant inventions. More recently the building of good highways has made possible the use of fleets of food trucks and milk tank cars. Canning, dehydration, and quick freezing have produced great changes in our dietary lives. Now, only the smallest communities lack frozen food lockers and supermarkets. These and many other developments have made commonplace types of foods that only a short time ago were seasonable, rare, expensive, or exotic. Today's citizen of Middletown may have milk from Illinois, cereal from the Dakotas, oranges from Florida, avocados from California, pineapples from Hawaii, celery from Michigan, eggs from New Jersey.

Of course, the mere desire for food and

its availability do not necessarily ensure procurement. After all, food is a commodity and can be had only for a price. It is logical therefore that those who are economically handicapped cannot afford any but the simplest and cheapest food habits. Furthermore, they cannot afford the auxiliary factors influencing dietary development such as education, travel, and the like. As a result, large numbers of our low-income population suffer from marginal or frank deficiency diseases, often in the face of food surplus. For the rural family in these circumstances much good has been done by the Agricultural Extension Services in promoting vegetable gardens in addition to cash crops, home canning, and other methods of food preservation, the construction of food cellars, and instruction in soil care and crop planning.

For urban populations with low incomes the problem has been more difficult. The school lunch program represented in its inception an attempt to supplement the diets of children of this group of the population but later spread to become a means of providing a noon lunch for all children who could not conveniently return home at midday. Since 1946 the school lunch program has grown and now serves 19 million children. "Attesting to the value and potential of school feeding, the 89th Congress passed the Child Nutrition Act of 1966, authorizing a School Breakfast Program together with a Special Milk Program."[17] The Department of Agriculture anticipates that by 1975 the school lunch program will be serving from 42 to 46 million children.[18]

Although the school lunch program is generally considered to be a joint affair between federal, state, and local authorities, it is of greatest importance that the principal, teachers, parents, and school lunch managers be interested in and understand the program. On a federal level information regarding the establishment and management of the program and the use of surplus foods is available through the United States Department of Agriculture. On a state level inquiry can be made through the state health department and through the state department of education. On the local level health departments and school authorities can obtain all necessary information for the technical information necessary to the establishment and management of a school lunch program. However, the technique of serving food is not enough; the art of incorporating nutrition education into the entire curriculum so that the feeding experience is really a laboratory demonstration is essential if the aim of developing good food habits in children not only for the school year but for life is to be reached. Todhunter[19] has aptly described some goals that must be attained if the school lunch is to contribute to the nutritional well-being of the child:

1. Educators and school administrators must understand the importance of nutrition for school children and recognize the value of the school lunch in nutrition education.
2. The school lunch must be a part of the total school program. Teachers need to have training which will provide sufficient background in nutrition to be able to give children adequate guidance in food selection and the development of desirable food habits.
3. The school lunch program must be managed by trained lunch managers, assisted by employees who have been given adequate training for their specific jobs.
4. The school lunch must be eaten by "trained" children—that is, children who are learning about foods in relation to nutrition and health and who recognize the school lunchroom as a laboratory for educational experiences.
5. The school lunch program must run on a non-profit basis, financed in the same way that other school services are financed. The sale of nonessential foods and beverages at lunch times or at any other period of the school day should not be permitted.
6. There must be further research and study of the nutritional needs of children, of ways of developing new food habits, and of how to teach nutrition to boys and girls so that they will put into practice what they are taught.
7. Nutritionists, dietitians, public health workers, and health educators must be alert to the significance of the school lunch as a contribution to the nutritional well-being of the child and must direct their efforts to the fulfillment of such a program as has been described.

Nutrition education can and should be a part of the total school curriculum. History, for example, cannot be adequately taught without some emphasis of the part that food or the lack of it has played in the major developments and tragedies of the world. Many factors such as religion, emotions, agricultural practice, and income must all be considered in the study of racial and individual food habits. Food habits are slowly developed. Once formed, they are even more slowly changed. Nutrition education and the true appreciation of the part that food plays in the attainment of total health are slowly acquired. Consequently, nutrition education and application cannot be limited to one class, one semester, or 1 year at one of the age levels if its true value is to be translated into healthier, happier children and adults.

The extensive urbanization of the United States and the diminished ability of the small farmer to make a profitable living has had an adverse affect on many families as pointed out by Alvin L. Schorr[20] in his book, *Poor Kids:*

> In 1963, of the 69 million children in the United States who lived in families, 15.6 million were poor.
> Depending upon one's definition of poverty, the number of poor children can be enlarged or diminished. It may be well, therefore, to be explicit about what this figure means. The portion of income that a family uses for food may be regarded as a rough indicator of its prosperity. That is, as total income goes up, a smaller and smaller percentage is devoted to food. The poorest families spend a third or more of their income on food; other families generally spend a smaller proportion. The point at which total income is less than three times the cost of the basic nutritional requirements of a family (of specific size and ages) may be viewed as the brink of poverty. Basic requirements are determined here—some will think too stringently by the economy food plan developed by the Department of Agriculture. The economy food plan is for "temporary or emergency use when funds are low." In the long run it cannot provide an adequate diet. It is by this standard that almost one fourth of the children in the United States are counted as poor.

During the depression of the early 1930's the federal government, in order to combat a general inability to obtain food, established the Federal Surplus Relief Corporation, later reorganized as the Federal Surplus Commodities Corporation, which, working with other agencies, provided food for school lunches and other programs. In

1939 an unprecedented program was started by the Department of Agriculture for supplying low-income families and those on relief with foods at public expense. One of the interesting points on this program was that the foods, which consisted of surpluses, were distributed not by a government agency but by grocers. Known as the Food Stamp Plan, a form of scrip was printed and distributed to low-income and relief families who could use it at markets of their choice and within certain limits for the foods of their choice. The grocer could subsequently turn in his accumulated stamps to the federal agency for reimbursement. The Federal Surplus Commodities Corporation actually served as a food-purchasing agent, bidding for surplus foods and then arranging for distribution and packaging. Throughout, however, supplies flowed through the regular channels of trade. The plan as a whole was quite successful in that it satisfied private enterprise and at the same time allowed the recipient of the food to enjoy more nearly the status of the independent purchaser. The magnitude of the program is evident from the total sum of $235 million made available by Congress for the removal of agricultural surpluses in 1940 and 1941. Considerable conscious and subconscious nutritional and dietary education resulted from the plan, and it had a definite and considerable effect on the eating habits of a large fraction of the nation's population.

Along the same line, more recently in 1961, Congress enacted a 3-year pilot program to improve the nutritional status of low-income families by the provision of food stamps. Eight economically depressed areas were selected for study. After 3 years the low-income families who had participated in the pilot project showed better diets than the families who had not participated. As a result, the program was expanded in 1964 to cover 43 areas in 22 states. "Findings showed food stamp families made significant increases in the value of food purchased with more than 80 percent of this increase accounted for by animal products—meat, poultry, fish, milk and eggs—and by fresh fruits and vegetables."[21]

RELATION OF NUTRITION TO SELECTED HEALTH PROBLEMS

In perhaps no phase of the public health program is nutrition more important than in the maternal and infant health activities. Although the relationship of the nutrition of the expectant mother to the nutrition and health of her fetus seems self-evident, it is only recently that sound, scientific proof has been forthcoming. Prominent among the workers whose studies have stimulated great interest in this field are Ebbs, Tisdall, and Scott[22] at the University of Toronto; Burke, Stuart, and their co-workers[23] at Harvard; and Warkany[24] at the University of Cincinnati. Studies have now been reported from many countries and from many laboratories within this country, the results of which all point in one direction: Mothers who are well nourished protect their health and the health of their babies; mothers who are not well nourished jeopardize their own physical well-being and give birth to infants not adequately equipped to withstand the trauma of extra-uterine life. In addition, a greater proportion of the miscarriages and stillbirths have been reported in the poorly nourished mothers. Reports further indicate that, although both the fetus and the mother may be affected by the mother's poor nutritional status, the fetus tends to suffer the most. It is also recognized that only to a limited extent is the fetus a parasite, and that extent is limited apparently by the mother's nutritional state. If the findings reported in several studies applied to all women in this country, as they well may, better nutrition of all pregnant American women would result in over 1 million American babies each year starting their lives at a higher level of health.

Many questions remain to be answered. For example, does inadequate nutrition on the part of the mother play a role in the development of congenital anomalies? Can a woman poorly nourished all of her life compensate for long-term poor nutrition by consuming adequate food during the period of pregnancy? What are the added risks for the woman who at conception is malnourished? In spite of the fact that research groups have not yet been able to unravel all of the confusion out of this important aspect of preventive medicine, we have adequate knowledge of the relation of nutrition to the health of both the mother and the baby to use all resources at hand to encourage the best state of nutrition possible in all pregnant women. Furthermore, we realize that good nutrition throughout the entire prior life-span is essential if optimal nutrition is desired in the offspring. Nutritional status, good or bad, cannot be turned on and off like a faucet. Adequate nutrition during pregnancy requires adequate nutrition before pregnancy.

How then should the pregnant woman's diet be managed? The circumstances of the problem place the responsibility squarely in the hands of the practicing physician to whom she goes for care. Her diet should be neither ignored nor considered merely in terms of a table of standards. Each woman is an individual and should be treated as such, and the physician is neglecting a duty to his patient if he fails to study her dietary problems as carefully as he checks her blood pressure. Public health nurses and nutritionists can assist the physician by further interpreting the nutritional needs of pregnancy and lactation to women individually or in mothers' classes.[25]

Once the woman has delivered herself of her infant, it has certain nutritional requirements and dietary problems peculiar to its early age. Many factors are involved including its lack of teeth, limited digestive powers, enormous needs for growth, and its need to acquire a taste for foods of a variety of flavors and textures. The mother also has nutritional needs peculiar to her own recovery from the physiologic strain of pregnancy and to the production of adequate breast milk for the feeding of her infant. The advantages of breast feeding are many and will not be recounted here, except to make passing reference to one that is related to mental health. Suffice it to say that food habits, good or bad, are established very early; the security, comfort, and ideal food that breast feeding affords start the infant out with mealtime being a psychologically as well as physiologically satisfying experience.

Federal agencies are cognizant of the problems of the medical and nutritional needs of the prenatal population and in 1965 under the guidance of the Children's Bureau made funds available to local and state groups for comprehensive maternity and infant care projects.[26] These MIC projects throughout the country should be able to provide services to the 20- to 29-year-old group of women who by 1973 will number 16.9 million.[27]

The school health program is perhaps the activity to which nutrition is next most closely allied. Its relationship here is threefold: (1) the assurance of a satisfactory midday meal while the child is away from home, (2) the imparting of sound nutritional information, and (3) growing out of proper integration of the first two, the development of desirable nutritional habits.

Major obstacles to the inclusion of more nutrition education in school curriculums would appear to be the lack of understanding of educational concepts on the part of the nutrition specialists and the lack of workable information about nutrition on the part of the teachers. In the past teachers' colleges have not provided their students with an adequate background in health, and nutrition has been particularly neglected. Consequently, graduate in-service nutrition education is now being given in many states. The training is offered by one or several agencies or institutions employing personnel who are experienced in both the field of education and the field of nutrition. Among the groups assisting with such training programs are county, city, and state health departments; colleges and universities, particularly those engaged in training home economics teachers; the American National Red Cross; and government agencies such as the Agricultural Extension Service.

Graded programs in nutrition are now receiving increased attention, and both commercial and academic groups as well as the official and nonofficial agencies are making available helpful guides planned on graded levels. The use of tools appropriate to the age and interest of all grade levels is an absolute necessity in this as in all health fields. In the primary grades the emphasis is best placed on food, i.e., how it grows, how it tastes, etc. In the upper elementary grades, simplified technical information is developed, such as the need of particular foods for growth. In the high schools the scientific approach will hold the student's interest provided that his earlier nutrition education has given him the information necessary for this more mature approach.

Nutrition education that can accompany a well-managed school lunch program holds great potentialities, but these potentialities are far from realization in many school feeding programs. Schools that feed but do not teach are falling short of one of the aims of providing a lunch at school. Through the school lunch children have an opportunity to become acquainted with foods not familiar to them and simultaneously to learn good patterns of eating by practicing them throughout their school years at the noon meal, at least. The school lunch program should be a part of the broad health program for all children in a school.

Children with special health problems, i.e., physical, mental, or economic handicaps, also need the services of a nutritionist. The feeding of premature infants is the responsibility of the physician, but a nutritionist can aid him. The child in the preschool age group needs an adequate diet to develop his full potential. As President Lyndon Johnson[28] pointed out in 1967, the program Head Start "has dramatically exposed the nutritional needs of poverty's children. More than 1.5 million preschoolers are not getting the nourishing food vital to strong and healthy bodies." The President also proposed child and parent centers that would meet a wide spectrum of the following needs: (1) health and welfare services, (2) nutritious meals for needy preschoolers, (3) counseling for parents in prenatal and infant care and instruction in household management, accident prevention, and nutrition, (4) day care for children under 3 years old, and (5) a training base for specialists in child development.

Mentally handicapped children are increasing in number and require special help in meeting their dietary needs. "Nutritional factors may be directly involved in retardation in conditions due to inborn errors of metabolism, such as phenylketonuria and galactosemia. Mental retardation may result if these conditions are not detected early and accompanying medical and specific dietary treatment provided."[29] The 1963 Maternal and Child Health and Mental Retardation Planning Amendments increased the crippled children's services "so that care may be provided to children handicapped by any form of disability or long-term illness."[30]

Welfare departments and juvenile courts, migrant workers programs, child care facilities, all can use consultant services of the nutritionist or dietician. The nutritionist must be perceptive to programs that can incorporate her services and must be flexible enough to meet the variety of needs in children and youth programs to which she can offer valuable consultative service.

One of the greatest concerns with regard to an aging and an aged population is nutrition. In many respects the former group is of more importance than the latter because there are many more people growing old than there are those already infirm by virtue of age. Far more can be accomplished for those who are aging than for those already advanced in years. Furthermore, the circumstances of middle life determine in large part whether the subsequent advanced years will be healthy or infirm. If life is worth prolonging, it is worth nurturing in a healthy condition rather than in a state of chronic illness and dependency. Man's most productive years should be during the fifth and sixth decades, yet it is here that incapacitating chronic illness strikes so often. Arteriosclerosis, hypertension, arthritis, diabetes mellitus, degenerative conditions of the kidneys and liver, cancer, and various other disorders increasingly are becoming dominant challenges to the public health and medical professions. These are all conditions of as yet somewhat uncertain etiology. However, it is known that the way of life has much to do with the de-

velopment of all of them and considerable research indicates a frequent direct or indirect relationship with nutrition.

Certain facts about the older population should be borne in mind. In general, they tend toward a more sedentary type of existence involving less physical activity. A larger percentage of their time is spent indoors where the temperature is warm. The period of tissue and organ development is largely past, and certain changes in food habits have been enforced by virtue of impaired dental function, elimination difficulties, and various physiologic changes. One of the most common results is the acquisition of excess weight. One thing that is certain is the effect of overweight and obesity on life expectancy. From middle age onward there is almost a direct line relationship—the age-specific death rates are increased roughly 10% for each 10 pounds of excess weight. Thus an excess of 25 pounds will lessen life expectancy by 25%. The exact reasons for this are not entirely clear because the premature deaths are not all just due to cardiac failure from carrying an overload. For example, the incidence of diabetes mellitus is two and one half times as great and of cardiovascular and renal disease one and one half times as great in the obese as in those of average weight.[31,32] Sebrell[33] has pointed out the following:

. . . As we pass through the middle years, the percentage of body fat usually rises, though the overall weight may remain the same. Thus, among groups of standard weight, fat may comprise only 10 per cent of the body weight in younger men, as compared with 21 per cent in older ones. The prevalence of obesity increases to about age 40 for men and 50 for women, and declines after age 60. This decline is due not only to loss of fat, but also to the loss of fat people.

The fact that obesity is correlated with aging and chronic disease does not in itself imply a causal relation. Unknown etiological factors may be common to these conditions. In various studies, however, caloric restriction has prevented cancer in mice, prolonged greatly the life of rats, and reduced the signs of diabetes in humans. Moreover, striking decreases in the incidence and severity of diabetes and hypertension accompanied undernutrition and loss of weight in certain European countries during both World Wars.

In the final analysis, all obesity results from overeating in relation to one's physiologic and environmental needs. The second of these factors has tended to be overlooked, indicating the importance of obtaining assistance from workers in several other fields in the development and conduct of obesity control programs. Sometimes, for example, excessive eating is an expression of disturbed emotional balance, as Waife[34] puts it, a substitute for some lack in the pattern of living, as the vicarious satisfaction for emotional starvation. The possible psychologic roots of excessive eating are many. "Paucity of companionship, love, and affection, dearth of opportunities for expression of personality, meager sources of pleasure, and sensuous gratification are some of the factors. Fear of economic insecurity, frustration from undesired social position, shame for inadequate capabilities, and shyness are often compensated by overeating." The discovery and solution of these causative problems may be more successful if the services of psychiatrists, psychologists, and social anthropologists are incorporated in certain phases of the public health nutritional activities.

With one out of every three Americans who are 20% overweight,[35] a variety of formula foods, fad diets, and medications have become a psychologic crutch. Apparently the overweight person would rather not revert to a proper and adequate diet. Diet was originally a Greek word meaning "way of life," and control of weight is a lifelong series of habits that must be cultivated.

In contrast with obesity in the middle and advanced years is the problem of underweight and excessive leanness due to caloric restriction. The reasons for this may be impaired dental function, allergic difficulties, disinterest in eating because of living alone or, as in many instances of overeating, for emotional reasons such as anorexia nervosa. When this occurs there is not only lessened resistance to tuberculosis and to various acute infections, but there may also result serious disability from ocular, vasomotor, endocrine, and skeletal changes. In addition, there is the risk of mild to full-blown avitaminoses, particularly pellagra, beriberi, and scurvy. These in turn may aggravate further the underlying causes by bringing about additional oral or psychic conditions.[36]

Although all concerned agree that much is still to be learned about the relationships between nutrition, chronic diseases, and the aging process, there is ample justification, if not urgency, for public health agencies to use in their planning and to disseminate among the public the very considerable knowledge that is available and also to stimulate motivational research. In addition, there is a need, as Keys[37] suggests, to protect the public from nutritional nostrums: "Part of the problem of providing nutritional help for older persons consists in countering the claims of the food faddists, the purveyors of special nostrums offered for nutritional purposes, and the writers who find a ready sale for books and articles promising miracles from peculiar diets. The older person who observes deteriorative changes in himself is especially vulnerable; the greater the loss of the sense of well-being, the stronger is the urge to believe any promise of help."

Interest of Congress in the nutritional aspects of aging is reflected in the Medicare amendments to the Social Security Act. Written into the Conditions of Participation for Extended Care Facilities are requirements for the dietary supervision and adequacy of meals. The Home Health Care section has given the professional worker an obvious responsibility for all of the acute and chronic nutritional implications of the aged.

In the field of oral hygiene and public health dentistry good nutrition practices play a primary role. Conversely, there is much that the dental worker can do to promote healthier food habits.[38] It begins with the diet of the expectant mother and continues with the nature of the feedings and the subsequent more substantial diet of the infant. Also the relationship between dietary inadequacies and the development of pathologic conditions of the gingivae may be mentioned. As Massler[39] emphasizes, "The physical character of the food is not a nutritional factor but it is an important dietary consideration. The natural cleansing action of the food is an important adjunct to good oral hygiene. The detergent action of the food must supplement the toothbrush in preventing the accumulation of food debris, with subsequent caries and local gingivitis. Since relatively few individuals use the toothbrush correctly or effectively, the physical character of the food is an important consideration in planning a well-balanced diet."

A further consideration of considerable consequence is the effect that a diet high in carbohydrates, especially free sugars, has on the growth of lactobacilli in dental plaques with resulting carious breakdown of the enamel and other tooth substance.[40] Certainly here is a fruitful area in the realm of public health nutrition for the partial solution of a difficult problem of extensive magnitude.

THE PLACE OF NUTRITION IN THE PUBLIC HEALTH PROGRAM

Nutrition should be considered an important activity of a health department because good nutrition is a prerequisite of good health and because good health is necessary for the full realization of useful, enjoyable lives. When we speak of good health and nutrition, we should not mean just adequate health and nutrition but rather those qualities plus a reserve; in other words, health and nutrition might be thought of in three gradations: negative, borderline (or just adequate), and positive. It is for the latter that we must strive.

From what point of view should a department of public health be concerned with problems of nutrition? It should not be in terms of dispensing foods or nutritive concentrates to the undernourished and needy because that constitutes a part of public welfare. Nor should it be in terms of studying and examining individuals as such and rendering therapeutic assistance because that represents part of the private practice of medicine. Rather, as with all other problems, the health department's approach to nutrition should be all-embracing, viewing the people as a whole and not as individuals. This applies to both investigative and remedial activities.

Because of shortages of funds and especially because of insufficient numbers of adequately trained personnel, relatively few local health departments, except those in large urban centers, have special or distinct programs of public health nutrition. Many other reasons exist to indicate the desirability of operating the public health nutrition programs on the state level. Many states have state nutrition committees that may serve as nuclei around which to build the program. Some of the most intimately related agencies, such as the Agricultural Extension Programs, are organized on the state level. Many, if not most of the problems involved, are statewide rather than countywide. Finally, as will be seen, the type of program visualized would involve local contacts by the accepted local public health personnel rather than by the nutrition staff whose function would be most efficient and fruitful in an advisory and consultative capacity. Because of this, it would appear most practical to limit attention essentially to programs carried out on the state level, which after all exist in large part to assist and support the efforts of local health personnel.

The first states to employ nutritionists were Massachusetts and New York in 1917, and they have maintained continuous service ever since. At first, their activities were merely those of specialized educators working essentially with the schools. Gradually they expanded their interests to include work with tuberculosis clinics, community education, and staff education. Largely as a result of federal funds made available under the Maternity and Infancy Act (Sheppard-Towner Act), Illinois, Michigan, Mississippi, and Connecticut began nutrition services. Because of the source of federal funds, the Children's Bureau, these activities were all placed in the respective state divisions of maternal and child hygiene. In 1929 the law was repealed, and because of the economic depression, only Connecticut, Massachusetts, and New York continued the activities. In 1935 the passage of the Social Security Act enabled the Children's Bureau, and through it the states, to pick up where they left off. Soon afterward, the war, with its attendant food shortages and rationing plus the disturbing results of draft examinations, made the public and health officials more nutrition conscious than ever before in history. As a result, by 1948, 50 out of 53 state and territorial official health agencies were budgeting funds for the employment of 170 nutritionists. At first, most of the nutrition services were financed by outside funds. Thus in 1945 and 1946, 63% came from the Children's Bureau, 9% from the Public Health Service, and only 28% from the states.[41] Since then state and local health departments have increasingly assumed the responsibility for these activities.

ORGANIZATION AND FUNCTIONS OF STATE NUTRITION PROGRAM

Up to the present there has been much difference of opinion concerning the manner in which a nutrition program should fit into the structure of a state health department. In some states it has been organized as a separate division or as a staff agency directly responsible to the commissioner. In others it has been placed in divisions of medical services, public health nursing, and local health services. Most commonly it has been allocated to the bureau or division of maternal and child health. Undoubtedly this has come about as a result of the noteworthy pioneering of the United States Children's Bureau, and a suggestion for a different arrangement should not be construed as an attempt to detract from the credit due its far-sighted leadership. Rather, it is felt that public health activity in the field of nutrition is of such importance as to justify its inclusion as a more fundamental activity of wider scope rather than to risk the possibility of its benefits becoming limited to one or two groups in society, in this case children and expectant mothers.

While each state must of necessity organize its program with consideration to its peculiar problems, facilities, and organizational history, it is believed that the most logical place for the state nutrition program in most instances is in the division of local health services. As will be seen from what follows, the outstanding function of the state health department in nutrition, as in most other fields, is to provide leadership, guidance, consultation, and advice to those working on the local level where the public is ultimately found. The tested pattern is the result of accomplishing these aims by means of channeling the services of the state specialists through a division of local health services. This administrative technique has proved itself to make for economy, efficiency, and coordination from the viewpoints of both the state and local staffs.

The nutrition program should be under the direction of an individual who is immediately responsible to the director of local health services. The ideal qualifications of the director of nutrition should include a medical education with special clinical experience in nutritional diseases, a basic background in biochemistry, and training and experience in public health. The obvious difficulty in obtaining such a person can be solved to some extent by careful choice of the personnel who will carry out the detailed activities of the program under his direction. The most important qualifications are the medical and public health backgrounds, which will enable the director of nutrition to give the necessary medical guidance and to integrate the program into the other activities of the health department. The program should be so organized as to carry out a double purpose: first, because of the ever present need and the unusual present demand for education and promotion in the field of nutrition, a service program should be organized; second, since it behooves all progressive health departments to assume some responsibility for evaluation and the advancement of knowledge, especially as it relates to potential public health practice, a research program is advisable.

LOCAL NUTRITION PROGRAMS

In order to carry out any corrective and promotive program on a sound basis, it is desirable, if possible, to determine at the outset the type and extent of existing problems and to furnish a base line from which to appraise any changes that might be due to subsequent activities on the one hand or economic and biologic influences on the other. It is necessary therefore that everything possibly related to the state of nutrition of the people in the area be carefully considered and studied. The nutrition staff should accumulate and appraise data about groups of individuals or districts of the jurisdiction that might be of value in the service program. This involves (1) a study of the material and economic resources of the community, i.e., types and amounts of foods produced, exported, retained, imported, (2) a study of food production potentialities, (3) a study of food preparation customs, (4) a study of actual food consumption patterns, (5) a study of the nutritional status of the population, including an appraisal of the incidence, distribution, and types of deficiency diseases.

Depending on the amount of funds and personnel available, the latter activity may vary considerably from a mere study of reports of illness and death to the carrying out of extensive surveys on representative groups of the population.

Within recent decades the survey method of approach has been applied to the field of nutrition in an attempt to evaluate existing nutritional conditions of populations. The procedure that has been developed is a threefold approach, using clinical examinations and histories, dietary analyses and/or food inventories, and various laboratory tests which have been developed. Admittedly all of these procedures are subject to considerable variation and error due to the influence of the personal factor in clinical examinations and the listing of food intake, the difficulty of measuring food accurately, the variables introduced by various types of cooking, and the fact that many of the laboratory tests are still in the developmental stage. Nevertheless, by recognizing these drawbacks and by reasonable applications of the results, the survey method can be useful in indicating outstanding problems in any given area. These procedures are admittedly too costly for most local health departments at this time. However, in some areas they have been carried on as a cooperative enterprise of the health department and the departments of home economics,

biochemistry, and medicine of universities.

It was previously stated that a health department's service activities in nutrition should not be of the nature of dispensing public welfare. If not, then what remedial measures can be taken? They can take the form of ever increasing education by showing the people what is wrong, by teaching them why it is wrong, and finally by assisting them in their efforts to overcome the problems themselves. To accomplish this end sometimes involves the breakdown of almost traditionally faulty diet habits and the translation of scientific diet analysis and planning into readily understandable and usable layman's terms. As one writer aptly put it, the facts of good nutrition must be made part of the local folklore.

A change in the mores of a people, especially as related to such a self-preserving function as nourishment, is usually accomplished slowly and with considerable difficulty. In the process we must deal with deeply ingrained racial, regional, and familial customs and with prejudices, prides, jealousies, and even superstitions and fears. To tell individuals and communities what is wrong and what remedies are needed is not enough. The more subtle, the more fruitful, the more enduring approach is one that maneuvers community thought into the position of itself recognizing the needs and the remedies at hand. In essence, we must show communities and families how they can help themselves.

How may this be done? In most communities in the United States there already exist many agencies and individuals not only interested in but actually already engaged in the promotion of better nutrition. State and local departments of education, welfare, and health, home demonstration agents, county farm agents, the state agricultural extension services, the federal Departments of Agriculture and Labor, the American Red Cross, home economics teachers, community garden, canning, and lunchroom projects, and many more are already in the front lines of activity. Working separately, there results not only some duplication of effort but also failure to recognize the existence of some problems that are perhaps of too great a magnitude for any one agency although not for the concerted effort of the whole group. The development of intelligent cooperation and initiative among all these groups through health department leadership, then, is one function of a public health nutrition service. In other words, much of the function of the health department is that of a coordinator and catalyst for existing community resources.

Beyond this, consultative service should be offered by well-qualified nutritionists to the various persons and agencies mentioned, the end in view being to demonstrate how nutrition education can be injected into daily routine without adding appreciably to the daily burden.

These phases of the work should be under the immediate supervision of a well-trained, experienced, and personable nutritionist with a knowledge of the state and its governmental and voluntary agencies. Working under her direction should be a number of regional consulting nutritionists and possibly one or more institutional nutritionists with a special background in institutional dietetics. The state should be divided into regions roughly comparable in size, number of counties, population, inclusion of large cities, industries, etc. It is to be suggested that, at first, activities be restricted to counties with full-time public health services since their existence will facilitate public acquaintance and acceptance of the work of the nutritionist. The length of time to be spent in each local area, the frequency of visits, and the particular type of activity and approach should be worked out on the basis of cumulative experience in the locality by the regional nutritionist herself. In some places frequent visits of short duration or irregular visits of several weeks' duration may be more successful than regularly scheduled routine visits of 1 week.

At all times the nutritionist should keep in mind the actual and potential contributions that local home economists, teachers, home demonstration agents, and many others can make and should plan accordingly to promote the use of their services

whenever possible. She should remember that efforts on her part to render direct service to the public will reach only a few and that her real contribution is to promote the use of local talent and facilities for nutritional betterment by timely suggestions, correlation, and cooperation.

The rapid expansion of nutrition services in both public and private health agencies in recent years has lead the Foods and Nutrition Section of the American Public Health Association to formulate the following statement of functions of a nutrition service to be adapted to the local conditions in an area.[42]

1. To determine the nature and magnitude of nutrition needs and to establish long-range objectives and short-term program goals.
2. To work toward the integration and coordination of nutrition service with all other appropriate services within the health agency.
3. To keep own agency informed and to work with other official agencies and organizations engaged in food and nutrition programs in a coordinated approach to the improvement of the population's nutrition status.
4. To provide a nutrition education program, including inservice education. Such a program should lead to the establishment, improvement (when indicated), and maintenance of sound eating habits throughout life, and should thereby foster the promotion of nutritional health and prevention of disease.
5. To provide consultation services on nutrition problems, on developments in nutrition research, and on the administration of nutrition aspects of programs within the agency, to professional personnel—such as physicians, nurses, and dietitians—and to groups, organizations, and other agencies.
6. To emphasize nutrition services for persons most susceptible to nutritional difficulties, for example, expectant and nursing mothers, infants and children, adolescents, the aged, those with chronic illness or physical handicap, and those with limited food budgets or restricted sources of food. The persons responsible for nutrition of such groups should be given practical instructions on the planning and value of an adequate diet, how to use available foods, and how to make prescribed dietary modifications.
7. To promote programs for adequate nutrition and food service and the provisions of suitable physical facilities by offering consultation, technical assistance, and training programs to management and food service personnel in institutions of all kinds, such as hospitals, penal institutions, sanatoriums,

nursing homes, homes for the aged, industrial establishments, child care institutions and day care centers, and schools and colleges. This should make the administrative and food service personnel aware of the nutritional needs of the people they serve, and better able to meet those needs.

8. To develop, evaluate, and promote the use of nutrition education materials.
9. To participate in (or conduct) studies and investigations on the relationship of dietary factors to health and to disease.
10. To provide direct nutrition services where indicated.
11. To evaluate continually the effectiveness of the public health nutrition programs.
12. To record, report, or summarize progress and activities at regular intervals.[29]

With the rapid expansion of the services of the public health nutritionist, there is a critical need to evaluate the services they render and determine what services could be delegated to other personnel. The 6 or 7 years of training required is barely enough to fit in all the many experiences needed to face the complex nutrition problems in urban and rural society in an age of advancing technology. The University of California has developed a 5-year program that produces graduates with a master's degree, ADA internship, and some experience in public health. Japan meets its personnel needs by graduating 2-year nutrition technicians. Just as the hospital dietician has promoted the use of food service supervisors, so must the public health nutritionist look for ways of extending her services through lesser trained workers. The underdeveloped nations have selected village workers, trained them for 1 year, and returned them to their homes to teach health and nutrition to their peers. Might not this principle be used to teach women in the ghetto areas of our cities, to saturate the neighborhoods with adequate nutrition information on food buying and budgeting, and to provide enough sound nutrition information so that people would not become vulnerable to fallacious practices and beliefs?

LEGISLATION FOR ENRICHMENT OF FOODS

One other type of activity in the field of nutrition that should be mentioned con-

cerns a more centralized and forceful kind of activity. This is the possibility of a community or of a state attacking nutritional problems at their source, i.e., the place of production or distribution of a product. Perhaps the earliest example of this sort was the addition of iodine in the form of sodium or potassium iodide to public water supplies, chocolate, and, more practically, to table salt.

During periods of war animal foods become scarce because animals are expensive to feed and to produce; cereal products are consumed in greater quantities for they are the least expensive to produce in terms of acreage, man-hours, and cost. Consequently it was apparent to the Food and Nutrition Board of the National Research Council during the World War II period that cereals as a major part of the nation's diet must offer adequate nutrients.

On January 18, 1943, a government order known as War Food Order No. 1 went into effect. This order required that all white bread be enriched to meet the requirements of the order in thiamine, niacin, riboflavin, and iron. It remained in effect until October 18, 1946. By extending the practice of enrichment to low-priced bread, this program brought its benefits to low-income groups where the need was greatest. Since the War Food Order was an emergency measure and in peacetime inapplicable to interstate situations, an increasing number of states have passed legislation for the continuance of a policy of enrichment of all white flour and bread within their borders. By now, well over half of the states have adopted flour and bread enrichment legislation.

Because corn is a staple food in the southern states and substantially replaces white flour products, the Food and Nutrition Board recommends the enrichment of all corn products to the level of federal standards in areas where the consumption of corn is substantial. In some areas of the South the enrichment of corn products has met with remarkable success. For example, during a period of about 15 months the Alabama Extension Service persuaded over 450 corn mills representing about 90% of the state's milling industry to begin voluntary enrichment of corn meal. South Carolina inaugurated its program in 1943, and the program has been continuously successful. In March 1949 the South Carolina legislature strengthened the program by amending the state's degerminated corn products enrichment law, making it mandatory to enrich all types of corn meal and grits sold for human consumption. Georgia, Mississippi, and North Carolina also have corn enrichment laws. In some areas the corn enrichment program has been delayed principally because of the nature of the corn milling industry; some products are degerminated while others are not, and a large proportion of both kinds is marketed through small mills.

The repeal by some states of legislation that imposes class or restrictive taxation on margarine and the enactment of laws providing for its enrichment by the addition of 15,000 units of vitamin A per pound are further examples of centralized approach to the problem of ensuring adequate food, especially to low-income groups. A particularly important step forward was made on March 16, 1950, when the United States Congress enacted P.L. 459, which repealed the federal tax on margarine.

REFERENCES

1. Ule, O.: Food and the development of man (translated from the German by J. Fitzgerald, from Die Natur, 1851), Pop. Sci. Month. 5:591, 1874.
2. Boudreau, F. G.: Nutrition in war and peace. Milbank Mem. Fund Quart. 25:232, July 1947.
3. Boudreau, F. G.: Future implications of the nutritive value of the American wartime diet, Amer. J. Public Health 85:243, Mar. 1945.
4. King, C. G., and Salthe, O.: Developments in the science of nutrition during World War II, Amer. J. Public Health 36:879, Aug. 1946.
5. Boudreau, F. G., and Wilder, R. M.: The Food and Nutrition Board of the National Research Council: a review of its accomplishments and a forecast of its future, Fed. Proc. 5:267, June 1946.
6. Magee, H. E.: Application of nutrition to public health, some lessons from the war, Brit. Med. J. 1:475, Mar. 1946.
7. Jameson, W.: The place of nutrition in a public health program, Amer. J. Public Health 37:1371, Nov. 1947.
8. White, P. L.: Let's talk about food, Chicago, 1967, American Medical Association.
9. Reid, A. C.: Freedom from hunger, J. Amer. Med. Wom. Ass. 18(5):395, May 1963.
10. Randal, J.: Hunger: Does it cause brain damage? Think, p. 3, Nov.–Dec. 1966.
11. Consumption levels and requirements, United Nations Conference on Food and Agriculture, Final Act and Section Reports, Appendix 1, Report of Section 1.
12. Orr, J. B.: Nutrition and human welfare, Nutr. Abstr. Rev. 11:3, July 1941.
13. Van Veen: U. S. food production and world food needs, J. Amer. Dent. Ass. 48(6):473, June 1966.
14. King, C. G.: Trends in international nutrition programs, J. Amer. Dent. Ass. 48 (4):267, Apr. 1966.
15. Mead, M.: The factor of food habits, Ann. Amer. Acad. Polit. & Soc. Sci. 225:136, Jan. 1943.
16. Merrill, M. H.: Meeting the challenges of the coming decades—the role of medicine in nutrition. Talk given at the Western Hemisphere Nutrition Conference, Chicago, Nov. 1965.
17. Leverton, R.: Food and nutrition news, National Livestock and Meat Board, Vol. 38, No. 6, Mar. 1967.
18. Weckster, N. A.: V.F.M. trends, Volume Feeding Management, Sept. 1965.
19. Todhunter, E. N.: Child feeding problems and the school lunch program, J. Amer. Diet. Ass. 24:422, May 1948.
20. Schorr, A. L.: Poor kids, New York, 1966, Basic Books, Inc.
21. Currents in public health, Ross Laboratories, Vol. 5, No. 2, Feb. 1965.
22. Ebbs, J., Tisdall, F., and Scott, W.: The influence of prenatal diet on the mother and child, J. Nutr. 22:515, Nov. 1941.
23. Burke, B., Beal, V., Kirkwood, S., and Stuart, H.: Nutrition studies during pregnancy, Amer. J. Obstet. Gynec. 46:38, July 1943.
24. Warkany, J.: Manifestations of prenatal nutritional deficiency. In Harris, R. S., and Thimann, K. V., editors: Vitamins and hormones, advances in research and applications, New York, 1945, Academic Press, Inc., Vol. 3.
25. Lowenberg, M.: Coordinating maternity care: the role of nutrition, Amer. J. Public Health 41:13, Nov. 1951.
26. Hill, M., editor: Nutrition program news, U.S.D.A., May–June 1967.
27. Barr, A.: Report of the Nutrition Institute in Maternity and Child Care, Oklahoma City, Oct. 6-8, 1964.
28. Johnson, L. B.: The White House message on America's children and youth, Feb. 8, 1967.
29. Shoun, F. N.: An overview of nutrition programs for children in the United States, The nutritionist in health and welfare programs for children, Pittsburgh, 1962, University of Pittsburgh Press.
30. Egan, M. C.: Opportunities for nutritionist and dietitians in rehabilitation programs, J. Amer. Dent. Ass. 49(4):295, Oct. 1966.

31. Vilter, R. W., and Thompson, C.: Nutrition and the control of chronic disease, Public Health Rep. **66**:632, May 1951.
32. McCay, C.: Effect of restricted feeding upon aging and chronic disease in rats and dogs, Amer. J. Public Health **37**:521, May 1947.
33. Sebrell, W. H.: Potentialities in chronic disease, Public Health Rep. **68**:737, Aug. 1953.
34. Waife, S.: The pathogenesis of obesity, Amer. Pract. **2**:47, Sept. 1947.
35. The National Observer, Jan. 13, 1964.
36. Editorial: Nutrition and vital resistance, Amer. J. Public Health **37**:915, July 1947.
37. Keys, A.: Nutrition for the later years of life, Public Health Rep. **67**:484, May, 1952.
38. Davis, W.: What can the dental health worker teach regarding nutrition and diet? Amer. J. Public Health **31**:715, July 1941.
39. Massler, M.: Nutrition and the oral tissues, Amer. J. Public Health **35**:926, Sept. 1945.
40. Jay, P.: The role of sugar in the etiology of dental caries, J. Amer. Dent. Ass. **27**:393, Mar. 1940.
41. Report to Food and Nutrition Board, National Research Council, nutrition programs in state health departments, Public Health Rep. **65**:417, Mar. 1950.
42. Educational qualifications of nutritionists in health agencies, Amer. J. Public Health **52** (1):116, Jan. 1962.

Part V

The future
of
public health

The role of the prognosticator at any time and under all circumstances is fraught with difficulties and dangers. Change is known to be inevitable in a biologic complex such as that in which we humans play a dominant role. The nature and extent of the change, however, present quite different questions. It is here that one challenges credulity, stubs one's intellectual toes, and risks one's reputation. Nevertheless, prognostication is justified and serves a useful purpose. When based upon considered analysis and judgment of things past and present, it forms the best possible and in fact the only reasonable basis for determining sound planning and action for the future.

Chapter 36

The past as prologue

INTRODUCTION

During recent years public health workers in the United States have experienced increasing introspection and have raised a number of provocative questions: What is the future of our profession? Have we served our essential purpose and should we begin to phase out? Is public health at crossroads? Have our training and our programs kept up with the times, or have we become passé? Are we sufficiently dynamic or have we become static? What are the next steps in public health? Questions such as these increasingly have been the keynotes or themes of local, state, and national professional meetings and discussions. Events of the past several years have made increasingly critical the need to find adequate answers to these and related questions.

What is the background against which we should judge ourselves and determine the future course of public health? At this point it is insufficient merely to look over one's shoulder at the events of the past 5, 10, or 25 years. Rather, it is necessary to turn full-face about and view our entire past as a species in order to obtain a proper perspective.

A LOOK AT THE PAST

Our planet was formed about 3 billion years ago. Based upon the discoveries of Dr. Louis Leakey in the Olduvai Gorge of Tanzania, it was only 500,000 to 1 million years ago that the first creature that might be called man appeared. He was distinguished by his ability to grasp with an opposing thumb and by his development of the power of conceptual thought and means of transmitting the results of his thinking, information, and knowledge to others. Although he possessed these remarkable innovations, man nevertheless progressed very slowly and tortuously. For all except a very small part of his history the conditions of his existence have been decidedly primitive, and, indeed, in major parts of the world today they remain so. This primitive existence consisted of obtaining food, avoiding death from the elements, wild beasts, and other men, reproducing, and attempting to establish an understanding of and relationship with some superhuman force or being. For most of the period man obtained food merely as a predator living off the fruits of the land as they occurred naturally. This, of course, had its limitations.

Eventually, after some hundreds of thousands of years, man made and applied a number of truly fundamental discoveries, i.e., the control of fire, the domestication of animals, and the development of planned agriculture. These three great advances led to further discoveries and made possible all subsequent development of the species. However, they all took time. Thus countless generations passed before man progressed beyond the digging stick, before he smelted metal and made useful tools therefrom, and before he developed even simple methods of food preservation. Only recently and only in certain areas did man reach the point at which he could produce not only enough food for himself and his family but also a surplus with which to support the now specialized fabricators of his tools and clothing. The latter began to concentrate in convenient places, usually determined by proximity to natural means of transport or to natural strongholds. Thus the first urban centers came into being, and with them came new problems, including many of a public health nature. These urban centers with their attendant developing cultures probably first appeared about 3500 B.C. in the Tigris and Euphrates valleys of Mesopotamia and in the Nile valley of Egypt. Similar unique centers developed subsequently in Crete, in the Indus valley, along the lower Yellow River of China, in Central America, and on the coast and Andean highlands of what are now Peru and Bolivia.

The urban centers became increasingly important for a number of reasons, i.e., as trading places, as headquarters for those who governed and the military who supported them, as convenient and desirable living locations for those who in one way or another had gained control over large areas of land and all they contained, as the focal points for the religions that developed, as repositories of acquired knowledge, and eventually as centers of learning and research. Gradually some of these urban civilizations grew, reached their zeniths, then faded due to conquest, plague, or famine. Others grew, spread, and continued their influence in adapted forms in other parts of the world. Remarkable throughout most of this period, however, was the slowness of improvement and the small number of people involved.

At the time the Roman Empire reached its peak in the second century A.D., Italy had a population of only about 14 million, almost 10% of which resided in Rome. By the time of the Norman Conquest in 1066 A.D. there were only about 1 million people in the British Isles. As recent as the beginning of the eighteenth century the population of the British Isles had grown only to about 7 million persons, almost 10% of whom inhabited the city of London. From about this point on in history, however, great discoveries and events began to occur at an accelerating rate: the discovery, exploration, and colonization of new lands; the use of coal; the discovery of steam power and its application to transportation and industry; advances in medical and related sciences; the belated planting and nurturing

of the seeds of social consciousness and democratic self-government. These and other types of revolutions led to a sudden spurt in the size and distribution of the human race, in effect, to a human explosion. As previously pointed out, to appreciate the recency and magnitude of this human explosion, it should be realized that, whereas during the tremendous period before 1650 A.D. the world population grew to only 450 million, in the mere 300 years since there has been a sevenfold increase to almost 3.5 billion.

Even from this very sketchy résumé of man's background, it is clear that public health is still a very new concept, that man has been exposed to its benefits for only a tiny fraction of his total time span, and that of necessity up to the present the quite new public health profession has been addressing itself essentially to a vast accumulated backlog of problems and needs, and, incidentally, with signal success.

If our eventual goal is the ultimate possible length and quality of human life, considering all of man's past, present, and future, it may be contended that public health through time must consist of three phases, i.e., cleanup, repair, and building. It is clear that we have been devoting our attention so far to the first and to some extent the second of these, and it is hoped that the continuation of this period will be of limited duration. It is the construction phase, the positive building and maintenance of good health, that must endure through the long period of man's future as our goal. This is the goal that henceforth should occupy a major share of the attention and effort of society in general and of public health workers in particular. In other words we have merely begun, and the best is yet to come.

OUR EXPLODING ERA

Irvine[1] has observed, "The public health is necessarily a reflection of the times, our culture, our social system, and level of knowledge." To understand our proper place and role in the present and future and to understand the environment in which we must work, let us again examine the world at large. We are living in the midst of what is undoubtedly the most revolutionary period of man's history. Historically it had its origin in the remarkable period of the late eighteenth century, which saw, among other things, the French and American Revolutions and the Industrial Revolution. In a sense this period might be considered to represent the lighting of the fuse, and the present full force of its consequences to represent a series of intimately interrelated explosions, i.e., demographic, economic, social and political, cultural, and scientific and technologic. All of these revolutions or explosions bear great significance to the direction that public health must take in the future.

The demographic revolution
Because of its complexity and the number of variables involved, an adequate explanation of the current demographic revolution is not easy. Some of the many factors were discussed briefly elsewhere in this book. With specific reference to the United States, several recent phenomena of consequence may be noted. We have never experienced such an increase in marriages, such a reduction in the average age of marriage and parenthood, and such an absolute and relative increase in births as has occurred since 1940. All of these have had a positive effect upon the population. Even if the marked reversal of the average size of the family were not continued, the mere lowering of the average age of marriage and parenthood, with a shorter interval between generations, would result in a larger number of people living at any given moment.

Barring unforeseen adverse economic or other events, the number of births may be expected to continue to increase. The millions of babies born during the late 1940's and early 1950's became marriageable during the 1960's, producing an additional spurt in the number of births. Expectations are therefore for over 5 million annual births by 1970, and almost 6 million by 1975. Added to this is the effect of greater longevity due to the successful application of public health measures, improved nutrition, and similar beneficial factors. At the

turn of the century, of every 1,000 infants born alive, approximately 200 died within their first year. Now fewer than 24 succumb. Notestein[2] emphasized this by pointing out that a white female born in the United States now has a better chance of living to the age of 60 years than she had of surviving to her fifth birthday in 1900. Nor have the benefits been restricted to children. In 1900 more than 25% of children born in the United States faced the prospect of becoming orphans by the time they reached 18 years of age. This grim figure, fraught with so many social implications, has now been reduced to 7%.

The unforeseen dramatic extension of the length of life is well illustrated by the many correct predictions of the imaginative Jules Verne. In most things, time proved him to be amazingly accurate. However, in 1890, when the average length of life was 37 years, he optimistically predicted that 1,000 years later, by the year 2890, the average life-span would reach 58 years! Actually, life expectancy at birth has increased from 47.3 years in 1900 to over 70 years at the present time, with a high of almost 75 years for white females. Undoubtedly this trend will continue for some time, and it is entirely conceivable that by 1980 the average age expectancy of life at birth might be 80 years. As a result it is reasonably certain that our population will increase 10 to 12% per decade during the next two to three decades. This will bring about a total population in 1980 of about 250 million people.

One result of the foregoing is that, while in 1900 only 13 million persons, or 18% of the total population, were in the age group over 45 years of age, now the corresponding figures are about 67 million and about 33%. Furthermore, it is estimated that by 1975 almost 50% of the labor force in the United States will be over 40 years of age. Similar shifts are occurring at the other end of the scale. Thus it is estimated that within a decade, while 10% of our people will be over 65, about 50% will be under 25 years of age. In brief, then, the current population boom is characterized by marked increases at both ends of the life-span. Incidentally, these are the periods of life that ordinarily demand the greatest amount of medical and public health attention.

The economic revolution

There are many characteristics of the current economic revolution that do and will affect the nature of public health problems and programs. There is a distinct and rapid trend toward economic equality among people. In the United States, for example, this is evidenced by continued broadening of the social security coverage, the development of the concept of the guaranteed annual wage for industrial workers, the increased purchase of insurance and retirement policies, and the ever widening ownership of corporate stock. As a result of this trend the standard of living among all groups and classes of the population has been equalizing and is going up steadily and markedly. Already it has reached a level beyond the expectations of only a few years ago.

The social and political revolution

The effects of the rapidly expanding economy are closely linked with the recent striking social and political changes. It is interesting that in introducing a colloquium on "Governing Urban Society," James E. Webb,[3] Administrator of the National Aeronautics and Space Administration, predicted the following:

There is a strong possibility that this century will be noted neither for its technology nor for its science. For today there is a growing conviction among people and among nations that it may now be possible to eliminate human suffering and human misery—that it may now be possible to build a world society which offers human dignity and the opportunity for self realization to all. Despite the enormity of such an undertaking, it is significant that the question is no longer whether such a goal *should* be met; nor is the question now whether such a goal *can* be met. The questions perplexing us today are those of *how* the goal can be achieved and *how long* will be required. . . . Perhaps this alone is enough to distinguish the twentieth century far more profoundly than could achievements in science and technology.

As applied specifically to the United States at this time, one can point to the overriding concerns for an all-out drive to eliminate all remaining pockets of poverty, the provision of equal opportunity, and the guarantee of complete civil rights to everyone.

Increased labor has not been the price of the rapid improvements in the standard of living. Quite the contrary, the annual days of work required, if anything, are becoming fewer, and work itself is becoming physically easier. With the increasing use of electronics and automation and the beginning availability of atomic power, even more marked changes may be expected. These changes apply to farming as well as to industry, as evidenced by the fact that, whereas 50 years ago the United States required 13 million farmers for a population of 106 million, now only 7 million farmers are needed for a population of 200 million. It is anticipated by the Secretary of Agriculture that in the year 2000, with a population of over 300 million, only about 2 million farmers will be necessary.[4] A work week of as few as 3 or 4 days is not impossible to anticipate. The implications of more time for cultural and recreational pursuits, on the one hand, and of additional behavioral and mental health problems, on the other hand, should not be overlooked. Expanded use of automation will mean less tedium, less job fatigue, and fewer opportunities for industrial accidents and illness. It should be noted that the number of women in the labor force has increased to about 30% of the total. Significant also is the change in the types of women's occupations, from domestic, farm, and semiskilled labor to clerical, semiskilled, skilled, and professional activities. Possible consequences may be an increase in the number of women involved in industrial and vehicular accidents and in the number who have physical and mental disabilities attributable to chronic tensions.

Of great social significance is the strong trend toward urbanization and metropolitanization. In the past 50 years the urban population has increased from one half to about three quarters of the total population of the United States, with only 15% now left on farms. Even so, the 15% living on farms produce surpluses of many food products. The last two decades have seen the appearance around every city of large numbers of relatively self-sufficient suburban developments of moderate priced homes or apartment dwellings, usually centered around self-contained decentralized shopping and recreational centers. It would appear that these are destined to become the social, economic, and political units of the future and should represent important points of impact for public health education and the programs it promotes.

The combination of expressways, industrial decentralization, suburbanization, and metropolitanization has led to the appearance of two new phenomena: the town that appears almost overnight around a single decentralized industrial park, and the so-called "strip city," which results from the coalescence of a number of cities or metropolises and their merged suburbia. An excellent example is the continuous strip that extends from New York City to Washington, D. C. A number of others are in various stages of formation in other parts of the country. These phenomena bring with them many new and challenging problems in public health, sanitary engineering, and the provision of medical and hospital care. Prominent among these problems is the "central rot" of the older cities and the concentration in them of socially and economically underprivileged groups—the elderly and chronically ill, the undereducated, and the various emergent groups. In addition are the needs for urban redevelopment, problems of stream and air pollution, the development of suburban slums, and the search for a tax base for the financing of local services.

One other characteristic of the present social change is the remarkable mobility of the average American. What with work car pools, frequent changes in employment, business trips, and vacations, a viewer from the higher atmosphere would obtain an impression of Brownian movement. The extent of the movement may be realized by the fact that one fifth of the population now changes residence each year. The shallow social roots that result have far-reaching implications with regard to family stability and cohesiveness, the patient-physician relationship, and the epidemiologic factors of susceptible-immune ratios and exposure. In addition to the millions of travelers within the country, more than 1 million United States citizens travel abroad each year, and millions more cross the borders into Mexico and Canada. In the process of visiting all parts of the world, United States tourists spent approximately $1.5 billion each year. The injection of this amount of money into other national economies must have some ultimate beneficial effect upon their standards of living, including health services.

The cultural revolution

John W. Gardner,[5] Secretary of Health, Education, and Welfare, in opening The White House Conference on Health in 1965, observed, "Health frees the individual to live up to his potential." Hints of the significant cultural changes to come are many. Already there is ever increasing attention given to education, both quantitatively and qualitatively. This is as true for adults as it is for children. There is more time for leisure, social interests, family activities, and intelligent consideration of current social and political issues, including those related to personal and community health, and the needs for and possible methods of providing adequate medical and hospital care for all. The combination of rising labor costs and of more free time has brought about a considerable interest in hobbies and do-it-yourself activities; these activities are good for mental health, on the one hand, but risky in terms of increased chances for home accidents, on the other hand. With the lowered age at marriage, parents may really be young with their children, and the trend toward disintegration of family ties appears to have been stopped and reversed. These factors cannot help contributing to improved family relationships and better mental health. Furthermore, younger mothers, with better education, more leisure, and a somewhat more sophisticated outlook, will of course have an effect on the birthrate, family size, child health, maternal health, and insistence upon adequate medical and institutional care. This is part of the phenomenon to which several have called attention: the shift from the era of the dominant father to the era of the dominant mother, and especially of the dominant child.

The scientific and technologic revolution

In the crucible in which the scientific and technologic revolution is occurring, many wonders that bid well for the future may be found. The British scientist Bronowski[6] foresees three outstanding scientific changes which will dominate the next 50 years: (1) change in the source and use of energy, i.e., nuclear fission, (2) change in the control of energy, i.e., automation, and (3) results of the biologic revolution. The amazing advances in the medical and surgical fields are common popular knowledge and undoubtedly will become increasingly popular news items. One thing is clear—people want to know about anything that will make them well and keep them that way.

New techniques, instruments, drugs, and antibiotics are appearing with a dizzy rapidity that makes it literally impossible to remain adequately informed. There would appear to be no limit in this field, and the future is certain to bring forth products more remarkable than those already developed. It has been estimated that the rate of major medical developments has been about one per century before 1900, about one per decade between 1900 and 1940, and one or more per year since 1940. New pharmaceuticals are being developed, tested, and mass-produced on a calculated investigative production-line basis. This is reflected in a survey which disclosed that 90% of the prescriptions now written in the United States are for medications and prophylactic products that did not even exist 10 years ago.[7] Oral agents for immunization against several infections are now being tried with apparent good results, and the ultimate development of a universal antigen is not beyond the realm of possibility. Significant pharmaceutical cracks have been made in the walls of certain cardiovascular diseases. Within the 2 weeks prior to this writing (early 1968) there was announced the synthesis of viable, infectious, and reproducing DNA and the first successful transplant of a normal human heart from a fatal accident case to a patient with a defective heart. During the past 15 years the death rate from stroke among American males aged 45 through 64 dropped from 128 to 94 per 100,000, while the death rate from hypertension in the same group declined from 93 to 43 per 100,000. The amount of decline was even greater among females. Because of the dramatic pharmaceutical and surgical advances, numerous scientists are already sufficiently optimistic to anticipate the relegation of deaths from heart disease to a secondary role by the end of the twentieth century. Similar great advances are being made with reference to a number of metabolic diseases, especially arthritis, and certain mental illnesses. Another advance of considerable significance is the recent appearance of an effective and safe oral contraceptive based upon progestational steroids. As an additional example, it is probable that eventually a chemical or hormonal means of significantly delaying menopause will be developed. Meanwhile there are already in wide use oral hormonal substances that minimize menopausal distress. The social, moral, medical, economic, and demographic effects of such discoveries are far reaching.

An area of important technical advance is in the construction industry. New materials and methods of construction of dwellings are being tried on large scales. It may be expected that out of these efforts will come more satisfactory and more sanitary low-cost and medium-cost housing, which will help to eradicate one of the contributing causes of physical and mental ill health and juvenile and adult delinquency. At the same time it may be anticipated that increased activities in the fields of community planning and traffic engineering will result in fewer vehicular accidents.

Of all technical advances, those relating to the use of nuclear energy of course overwhelm everything else. We are all increasingly aware of and concerned about the problems it will bring as well as its blessings. On the one hand, public health workers view hopefully its application to the treatment of malignancies, to portable x-ray equipment, to food preservation, to sewage treatment, and many other things.

On the other hand, we must view with concern the problems of civil defense, disposal of radioactive industrial wastes, and the like. The potentialities of the peaceful application of nuclear energy are so great, however, as to contraindicate anything but a hopeful, optimistic viewpoint of the future.

General David Sarnoff, speaking as Chairman of the Board of R.C.A., made the challenging comment: "Our atomic age is like a knife; in the hands of a surgeon it can save a life; in the hands of an assassin it can take one. But to blame the knife is ridiculous."

COURSE OF ACTION

In the light of man's past history and of all of these momentous current events, what must be our course of action in the field of public health? Reference was made previously to the three phases—cleanup, repair, and building—that public health must consist of through time. It would seem logical that their counterparts during this present period of public health history should be (1) consolidation of past successes, (2) remediation of the backlog of disabilities, and (3) a truly vigorous, carefully planned attack upon both new problems and unsolved old problems.

Consolidation of past successes

Consolidation of past successes really consists of unfinished business. There is a tremendous amount yet to be accomplished in the areas for which we now have quite adequate tools and knowledge for rather complete success. Consider the area of health statistics. The gathering and processing of relevant data form an essential part of the approach whereby the problems that confront us are studied, understood, and attacked. Excellent and current data are available on the circumstances surrounding births and deaths in the United States. But we still fall far short of the more important goal of satisfactory morbidity data, i.e., the incidence and distribution through time and space of illness, the types of illnesses, proneness to illness, and many other analyses. There is a serious need, particularly at this time, to extend the use of

proved procedures such as sampling techniques and the full collation of available data. The recently established continuous National Health Survey will be of assistance. Beyond this, public health agencies, the medical profession, hospitals and clinics, insurance companies, business and industry, and various social agencies must soon work out a much more adequate means of standardizing and pooling their respective data concerning illness. Similarly more extensive use must be made of longitudinal studies of health and disease. In addition there are certain customary categories such as cardiovascular disease and cancer that should be broken down in order to pinpoint and expedite our future attack upon their components. What is greatly needed of course is a comprehensive community, state, and national epidemiologic intelligence and surveillance system that would constantly keep score and point up the problems as they are still developing.

There is still a vast amount of unfinished business in the control of diseases against which we already have quite effective tools. It is entirely reasonable to visualize that during the next 20 to 25 years tuberculosis, the venereal diseases, poliomyelitis, brucellosis, meningococcic meningitis, tetanus, rabies, trichinosis, and a number of other diseases might for all practical purposes be eradicated in this country and even in the world. Tuberculosis and syphilis still account for about 10,000 deaths per year in the United States. Certainly these deaths are needless in view of our expanding economy, our existing knowledge, the increased availability of hospital beds, isoniazids, PAS, and the ever broadening spectrum of antibiotics.

Eradication is admittedly a strong word; but 25 years ago how many people would have believed that by now deaths from typhoid fever, smallpox, malaria, typhus fever, diphtheria, scarlet fever, pertussis, measles, and a number of other previously important diseases would no longer occur to any practical extent in the United States? Yet, today these triumphs are realities. On the international level, a number of countries are already working with the World

Health Organization toward the goal of worldwide eradication of malaria.

There are still many other diseases which, although not yet eradicable, can be depressed to a fraction of their present level. Among these are pneumonia, influenza, dysenteries, diabetes, appendicitis, and many maternal and infant deaths. Not including the approximately 100,000 infant deaths, these conditions alone result in the loss of almost 100,000 lives each year. If the United States enjoyed the rates of the less affluent Netherlands, it would lose only 54,000 infants each year instead of the current 100,-000. Similarly, with reference to total deaths, this country would experience only 1.6 million deaths annually instead of the current 1.8 million—a saving of 200,000 lives a year. A nonfatal but very important pathologic condition that can be expected to decrease substantially is dental caries.

In the area of environmental health an enormous amount of consolidation awaits fulfillment. As pointed out elsewhere, there are still nearly 5,500 communities, each with populations of from 200 to 500, a total of from 2 to 3 million people, that have no public water systems; almost 15,000 communities, containing about 80 million people, have waterworks in need of improvement or extension. Over 9,000 towns, with about 6.5 million people, need sewerage systems; about 10,000 other communities, containing about 80 million people, have sewerage systems that need improvement or extension. In rural areas more than 33 million people still lack satisfactory excreta disposal facilities of even the simplest type.

Many of the sanitary shortcomings mentioned relate to the expanding suburban areas. There is a great need to discover and develop more adequate solutions to the environmental health problems of these areas. The political scientist will probably contribute to this as significantly as does the sanitation scientist.

Disease outbreaks traceable to food, milk, or water, while fewer each year, still occur to a significant extent. Workers in the field of environmental health still have before them the application or provision of customary sanitary services and safeguards to

the great number of new suburban communities, the extension of industrial safety and hygiene to the large number of smaller plants, and the challenge of the rapid economic and industrial development of the South and West.

A great social challenge still facing public health workers and others is the complete equalization of opportunities for health among the races. The unpleasant fact is that the age-adjusted death rate for whites in the United States is currently 7.1 per 1,000, in contrast to a rate of 10.3 per 1,000 Negroes. Similarly the infant mortality for white babies is 21.5 per 1,000 live births, in comparison with 40.3 per 1,000 live births of Negro babies. With reference to life expectancy at birth, for white males it is 67.7 years, in contrast to 61.1 years for nonwhite males. For females the comparison is 74.6 years for white females to 67.2 years for nonwhite females. Obviously these discrepancies can no longer be tolerated in an affluent civilized society. The relationship of poverty to illness, disability, and malnutrition is now accepted. With greater equalization of educational and employment opportunities, wealth, foods, and goods, and the ever rising standard of living, the differences in health potential should become much less. In order to accomplish this, however, the development of a more effective working interrelationship among agencies in related fields will be necessary as well as the development of new and more effective methods of providing comprehensive health services on a neighborhood basis.

For quite a few years investigators have discussed and promoted the concept of complete coverage of the nation with adequate local health services. Yet, many significant areas remain unserved, or are served by too few professional workers. Also it must be realized that more is involved than the mere quantitative filling-in of a geographic jigsaw puzzle. Quality of personnel and comprehensiveness of programs are involved too, with adequate backup by suitable hospital, convalescent, and rehabilitative services. In addition, there is the necessity of further practical administrative decentralization of local health services to serve more adequately the multiplying and growing neighborhood and suburban housing developments, possibly through their trading centers, and with appropriate participation by those who are to be served.

Perhaps the most important point for consolidation, and one which affects most of the others, is assurance of the availability of adequate medical and hospital services for all of our population. The development of this has been very difficult because of many complex economic problems and traditional political and professional philosophies. Actually, much progress has been made in recent years, especially by means of voluntary group medical and hospital insurance, now augmented by Titles V, XVIII, and XIX of the Social Security Amendments of 1965, the subject of detailed discussion in Chapter 25. With regard to future developments, it is hoped that the public health profession will play a significant role as a catalyzer, a coordinator, and possibly as an administrative agent for all interested parties. Whereas the basic problem at the moment is to provide a way to lighten the burden caused by catastrophic illness or injury, we must also consider it in the light of the eventual development of an all-inclusive medical, hospital, nursing, and social service with strong if not major emphasis upon positive health promotion, early diagnosis, and prevention of disease. Unfortunately all but very few so-called health insurance plans are actually nothing but episodic therapeutic medical care plans with no benefits for disease preventive or health promotive services.

In order to meet the foregoing needs certain personnel problems must be solved. We must develop more successful methods of recruitment into all of the health fields. A more aggressive and carefully planned approach to high school and college students must be pursued. But before we attempt to interest students in our field, we must define our future goals and must ourselves be sure of what we are trying to accomplish and in what we are trying to interest them. Needless to emphasize, more

reasonable salaries and benefits must be secured for public health workers. Beyond this, however, is the necessity to work out some equitable means of transfer of accumulated benefits, such as retirement and pension rights, from one location to another when public health workers change their locus of employment.

Over a relatively short interval of history we have witnessed the development of numerous splendid training centers related to the health sciences: schools of medicine, nursing, engineering, and public health. They have developed high standards and practical methods of teaching and have contributed greatly to the world's knowledge through their research. Nevertheless, it would seem imperative that their goals, curricula, and facilities be reviewed particularly carefully and continuously at this time in relation to the revolutionary changes that are occurring with such rapidity and are shaping the future. It is quite probable that a rather considerable retooling job is needed in all quarters. Certainly the time has come for health workers in all fields to have a much better background than heretofore in sociology, social pathology, behavioral science, community analysis and dynamics, and political science. Medical schools as well as schools of public health must place more stress upon subjects such as the medical and health problems that arise from exposure to fissionable material, accident prevention, mental health, chronic disease control, physical medicine and rehabilitation, and especially geriatrics and preventive and promotive medicine. The health department of tomorrow will obviously have to include geriatricians, as yesterday it included the services of pediatricians.

A final personnel problem is the inability to supply and pay for a qualified staff of sufficient size to meet the needs and demands of the citizenry. This is especially true on the local level. As a result we must be willing to explore possible satisfactory compromises that will provide more efficient service to more people. The potentialities of joint employment with other health agencies and with agencies in related fields should be explored further. We must experiment much further with the use of auxiliary personnel such as nonmedical administrators, epidemiologic field investigators, nurses' aides, and neighborhood health workers recruited from the neighborhoods in which they serve. Proper relationships and division of responsibilities must be worked out between sanitary engineers and sanitarians and between public health nurses and medical social workers. It may be useful to consider blends of public health nurses, social workers, health educators, and other personnel. Possibly we may find it worth while to develop some entirely new categories of personnel that will more adequately meet the new challenges which are on the horizon.

Remediation of the backlog of disabilities

What sometimes has been referred to as the fourth phase of medicine forms the second part of our present and future concern —the remediation of the great backlog of disabilities to the point where the certain amount of inevitable current disabilities may be handled with relative ease and economic efficiency. Two aspects of this are important for us to realize at this time, i.e., the size of the backlog and its economic significance. With regard to extent, it has been estimated that there has accumulated in the United States at the present about 2.5 million persons with orthopedic impairments, about the same number with unremedied hearing defects, and about a quarter of a million blind individuals. Furthermore, about a quarter of a million disabilities due to accidents, illness, or congenital defects are added each year.

Recent experience, particularly during World War II, has established the fact that a very large number of all types of handicapped persons are capable of making real and significant social and economic contributions if given an opportunity to readjust to the demands of working and living situations. In every community there are disabled persons in need of assistance, but how many public health agencies have really addressed themselves to this challenge? The public health agency obviously

cannot be expected to do the whole job, but it can serve as the catalyzer in the first instance for the establishment of a sound program, as a rallying point for all public and private agencies involved. Beyond that, it may provide certain specific activities in the field of physical and mental rehabilitation. It may also make known to the public and to special groups the needs, methods, and opportunities for prevention and rehabilitation of disabilities. It is impossible of course to predict, but the incidence of disabilities may not necessarily continue at its present level. Progress in control of tuberculosis, immunization against poliomyelitis, prevention of a few of the congenital malformations, potential advances in the prevention of accidents or better management of their consequences, and prevention of cardiovascular diseases and mental illness may result in a smaller annual addition to the number of disabilities.

Attack on new and unsolved old problems

There are so many new areas left for aggressive pioneering attack that it is difficult to know where to begin. All of these are problems to which various persons, groups, or agencies have addressed themselves to some extent. It must be admitted, however, that in many respects our efforts have been partial, poorly planned, and uncoordinated. Of one thing we can be sure—the abatement and if possible the control of the so-called chronic noncommunicable diseases will be one of our major concerns for quite some time into the future. With regard to these conditions, the importance of early diagnosis of predisposition or actual illness has logically been stressed. In this connection, periodic physical or so-called health examinations have been discussed and promoted for many years. Yet it must be admitted that the reception of the idea both by the public and unfortunately by many of the medical profession has been disappointingly poor. There are a number of reasons for this, each representing a challenge. There is the matter of economics. The physician is entitled to a fee for his professional service. But many people are either not sufficiently sophisticated to seek out or not economically able to afford medical attention in the absence of a frank illness or disability. A serious deterrent is general medical disinterest in the periodic physical examination. One has only to canvass a number of conscientious enlightened citizens who have sought to obtain this sort of medical service to learn of their all too common disillusionment. Too often the physician is so preoccupied and overloaded with patients who have frank ills and injuries that he essentially pats the apparently well patient on the back, tells him he appears healthy, and sends him on his way. In addition, as mentioned previously, the fact that health insurance plans still pay only for illness or injury rather than health serves as a powerful economic and psychologic deterrent. There are also the factors of misguided modesty or fear which delay many people from seeking periodic physical examinations until the development of definite signs or symptoms drives them to it. All of these deterrents represent real challenges for the medical profession, medical educators, medical economists, public health administrators, public health educators, and behavioral scientists.

Let us pass on to some of the chronic noncommunicable diseases that are now of such high incidence and consider briefly some of the prospects for the future. The total picture, although at the moment somewhat overwhelming, is not necessarily entirely dark. Recognition must be given to the remarkable advances that have been made in only very recent years in the better understanding of the physical chemistry and physiopathology of many of these diseases and to the progress in the fields of biochemistry, pharmacology, and chemical and industrial antibiotic production. Consider cardiovascular disease, the current captain of the causes of death. It accounts for 50% of the total death toll in the United States. Actually it is a complex of different conditions, i.e., congenital heart disease, rheumatic heart disease, arteriosclerotic heart disease, hypertensive heart disease, cardiac syphilis, thyroid heart disease, and various other organic and functional cardiac conditions. Some of these are

potentially eradicable, while the incidence and seriousness of others may be reduced. Eradication of heart disease due to rheumatic fever, syphilis, and thyroid dysfunction is well within the realm of possibility. Some reduction in congenital heart disease may be expected from the assurance of rubella and other viral infections in woman before marriage and pregnancy. Discovery of the significance of familial tendency, obesity, and personality also have done much to point to ways of prevention or abatement of hypertension. More recently the discovery of the dramatic effects of tranquilizers, guanethidine, mecamylamine, and other drugs on hypertension, with few adverse effects, opens a whole new vista for speculation.

Recent developments provided a possible means of prevention of atherosclerosis. There are indications that this condition may be delayed or its effects kept to a minimum by lipotropic factors such as choline and inositol, which reduce high blood cholesterol levels. It may be possible to prevent or control the disease by a diet low in cholesterol.

The practical potentials in this field are illustrated by recent analyses which indicate that during the decade that ended in 1965 death rates from heart disease declined by 5%; from hypertension, 46%; from stroke, 20%; and from rheumatic heart disease, 33%. Although coronary heart disease death rates rose 11%, they have since fallen by 2%. It is not at all unreasonable to expect the national Heart Disease, Cancer, and Stroke program to accelerate the decline in incidence of these current major killers.

In all of these and related situations there are many possible points of action for public health agencies; i.e., administrative organization, promotion, and possibly management of positive health maintenance by means of periodic health examinations; use of chest x-ray examinations for screening of certain cardiac defects and tuberculosis; generalized and individualized nutrition education, especially with regard to obesity; adequate provision of protective factors, and in some instances low cholesterol diets;

activities in the field of mental health especially as it relates to personality factors; and general health education. Two important and encouraging points should be borne in mind with regard to cardiovascular diseases: (1) the inevitable beneficial effect of the recent considerable and widespread improvement in the standard of living, including nutrition; and (2) the fact that sulfonamides, penicillin, and the host of other antibiotics have been used for only about 20 years. There is reason to expect that we have not yet even begun to reap some of the long-term delayed-action benefits of these and other factors and that their effects will show up in part in future lowered incidence of some of the cardiovascular diseases.

Cancer represents perhaps the most difficult disease problem for the present and for the future. There seems to be no question of a real increase. Some reasons for encouragement do exist, however. Detection at earlier stages of cancerous lesions not readily accessible is becoming more common through the wider use of radioactive tracers and the Papanicolaou technique of cytologic examination. The health officer might well devote attention to the physical and economic availability of these procedures to all who might benefit from them. Considerable progress is being made also in treatment with radioactive isotopes, improved deep x-ray equipment, and improved surgical techniques. The large sums of money now going into research on the causes, prevention, and treatment of cancer also give reason for a substantial degree of optimism. Meanwhile public health personnel may participate further not only through increased general public education but also by extending control over certain environmental factors, urging and arranging for periodic physical and laboratory examinations, and encouraging continued and extended good obstetric and gynecologic practice. Most specifically, all health workers have a great responsibility to work toward the reduction and elimination of cigarette smoking, which has been shown so conclusively to be involved in cancer of the lung and larynx as well

as emphysema and coronary heart disease.

About a half million people suffering from mental disorders now occupy about one half of the hospital beds in this country, and the number is increasing. There is some question, however, as to whether the increase in mental disorders is real or apparent. The public is much more aware of the problem than ever before and is now willing to discuss it in other than hushed terms. As a result many more people are seeking treatment than previously. Also more conditions are being recognized as mental aberrations. The shortages of hospital beds, psychiatrists, and psychiatric social workers and the inadequate psychiatric training among public health personnel are serious problems. On the other hand, in addition to improved fever and shock therapy, the door to a new approach has been opened by the discovery of some remarkably effective drugs such as tranquilizers. If, as previously predicted, a means of putting off menopausal changes is developed, a significant result should be a decrease in involutional melancholia and senile psychosis. Suicide is a generally ignored but major cause of death. Here is a significant field related to sociology, psychiatry, mental health, and community education that public health workers with very few exceptions have completely ignored. Local health departments, in addition to public education, should provide or arrange for around-the-clock guidance services for despondent individuals, somewhat similar to the activities of Alcoholics Anonymous. Such a program should use the collaborative help of religious, medical, and other groups in the community. Related to this is the potential contribution that public health workers might make to the solution of the problem of juvenile delinquency and other manifestations of the disease-delinquency-dependency syndrome, discussed at length in Chapter 5.

Finally, to touch briefly on a completely different area for pioneering, that of environmental health, consider the relatively meager and ineffective manner in which we individually and collectively have addressed ourselves to the public health aspects of the control of stream pollution and air pollution, the disposal of radioactive wastes, the prevention of home accidents, and improvement of inadequate housing. These are "musts" and will continue to be so into the future.

CONCLUSION

Challenges?—No end of them. Shortly before his death, the great inventor and industrialist Charles F. Kettering said, "The achievements of the past 50 years will be dwarfed by the things to come if we just keep our minds open and willingly contribute each day an honest day's work." This is well complemented by a statement by General David Sarnoff, "We may be a privileged generation who, by taming our fears, our hungers, our terrible weapons, are asked to pay the price of the transition to a golden hour."

As participants in one of the most successful and significant endeavors in history, we must each keep our minds open and contribute a share of thoughtful imagination to the solution of the fascinating challenges of the future, and in so doing remember that intelligent mankind is still very young and that the future will last a long, long time.

REFERENCES

1. Irvine, E. D.: Public health: what of the future? J. Royal Soc. Health 2:106, 1962.
2. Notestein, F. W.: As the nation grows younger, The Atlantic 200:131, Oct. 1957.
3. Webb, J. E.: Governing urban society: new scientific approaches, Philadelphia, 1967, American Academy of Political and Social Scientists.
4. Freeman, O. L.: Agriculture/2000. Address presented to the National Science Teacher's Association, Detroit, Mar. 20, 1967 (mimeographed).
5. Gardner, J. W.: A great move forward. Address presented at the White House Conference on Health, Washington, Nov. 3, 1965 (mimeographed).
6. Bronowski, J.: The shape of the future, J. Royal Soc. Health 3:127, 1962.
7. News item: Amer. Med. Ass. News, Dec. 29, 1958.

Author index

Newsholme, A., 23
Nightingale, Florence, 585
Norton, J. W. R., 431
Notestein, F. W., 629
Notkin, H., 492

O

O'Harrow, D., 519
Orr, J. B., 609
Osborne, F., 100
Osler, W., 14, 241
Otis, T. W., Jr., 333
Owen, Robert, 471

P

Palmer, C., 407, 410, 411, 412, 413
Palmer, G. T., 275
Palmerlee, F., 411
Palsgrove, J. E., 408
Pan, C., 104
Parkhurst, E., 515
Parran, T., 250
Parrish, H. M., 433
Parsons, T., 88
Pasternack, M., 414
Patterson, R. S., 26
Patty, F. A., 533
Paul, B. D., 64, 76, 248, 415
Paul, V., 61
Pelkins, A., 71
Penchansky, R., 416
Pennell, M. Y., 402
Perlman, M., 121
Petersen, E. L., 386
Peterson, P. Q., 254
Petty, William, 114
Pfiffner, J., McD., 189, 194, 211, 263, 289, 322
Phillips, J. C., 141
Piersol, G. M., 396
Pinel, Philippe, 424
Pitney, E., 413
Platt, P. S., 243-246, 248
Pogt, W., 100
Polsby, N. W., 145
Pond, C. B., 135
Pond, M. A., 83, 541
Porterfield, J. D., 424
Potter, R. G., 105
Prescot, W. H., 22
Prescott, S. C., 505
Preshaus, R., 189, 194, 211
Press, E., 540, 542
Prindle, R. A., 510
Pritzker, T., 414
Prothro, W. B., 447

R

Randal, J., 608
Randall, C. B., 199
Rathbone, William, 585
Reed, L. S., 427, 478
Reid, A. C., 608
Reston, J., 154

Rhyne, C. S., 415
Rice, E. P., 602
Rich, W. H., 355
Richardson, B. J., 20
Richardson, E. L., 250
Richardson, H. D., 87, 88
Robb, R., 188
Roberts, B. J., 575
Roberts, H., 540
Robins, E., 435
Robinson, G. C., 463
Robinson, R. L., 429
Rogers, F. B., 3, 14
Roemer, M. I., 9
Roemer, R., 415
Rogotzkie, R., 505
Rolph, C. H., 100
Roosevelt, F. D., 245
Rosen, G., 3, 4, 14, 81, 471, 575, 576
Rosen, H., 88
Rosenau, M. J., 3, 12, 251, 252
Rosenstock, I. M., 580
Roskopf, R., 515
Ross, G., 592
Ross, M., 436
Ross, R. M., 140
Ruderman, A. P., 121
Rudolfs, W., 505
Rusk, H. A., 486, 487, 491
Russ, H., 34
Russell, P., 47, 50
Ryle, J. A., 80, 81

S

Safford, B. M., 416
Salthe, O., 607
Sand, R., 462
Sanders, D. S., 216, 288, 424
Sargent, E. G., 402
Sayre, W. S., 189
Schachter, J., 547
Schaefer, M., 279, 281, 568, 571
Schleh, E. C., 199
Schlesinger, E. R., 368
Schmidt, W. M., 367
Schneider, D. M., 67
Scholz, G. C., 414
Schorr, A. L., 613
Schottstaedt, W. W., 80, 87, 88
Schulzinger, M. S., 543
Scott, J., 513
Scott, W., 614
Seagle, W., 161
Sears, P. B., 102
Sebrell, W. H., 616
Sedgwick, William T., 41
Seipp, C., 280
Sensenich, H., 486
Shafer, J. K., 352
Shakespeare, William, 12
Shattuck, Lemuel, 24, 25, 34, 79, 471

Shavely, T. R., 151, 153
Shei, P. C., 105
Shneidman, E. S., 433, 436, 437, 438
Shoun, F. N., 616
Shryock, R. H., 9, 460
Shubick, H. J., 224
Silver, G., 602
Silverman, C., 353
Simmons, L. W., 79, 85, 90, 91, 93
Simon, Sir John, 21, 22
Simpson, D. F., 254
Sinai, N., 37
Skinner, E. F., 58
Slee, V. N., 122
Smillie, W. G., 27, 28
Smith, Adam, 114
Smith, B., 144
Smith, G., 6
Smith, H. B., 413
Smith, L. M., 402
Smith, M. C., 413
Smith, S., 27, 28
Snider, C., 129, 136, 139
Somers, A. R., 478
Somers, H. M., 478
Southwood-Smith, 20, 461, 471
Sparer, P. J., 431
Spielholz, J. B., 603
St. J. Perrott, G., 426
Stead, F. M., 497
Stearn, B. J., 79
Steel, E. W., 504
Steiger, W. A., 80
Steigerwald, B. J., 513
Stewart, W. H., 570, 587
Stiber, C., 602
Stieglitz, E. J., 397
Stockle, R., 275
Stokes, E. D., 145
Stoll, N. R., 48
Stolnitz, J., 104
Stone, D. C., xi
Stotland, E., 435
Stroud, H., 418
Strow, C. W., 144, 489
Stuart, H., 614
Susi, A., 571
Swinney, D. D., 565
Sydenstricker, E., 82

T

Tauber, I. B., 103
Taylor, E. J., 487, 491
Terris, N., 4
Terry, M. C., 355
Thomas, H. A., 515
Thompson, C., 616
Thompson, D. J., 512
Thompson, M. H., 515
Tiboni, E., 540
Tisdall, F., 614
Tobey, J. A., 175, 176, 178, 179, 180, 415

Subject index